Nerve Injuries and their Repair

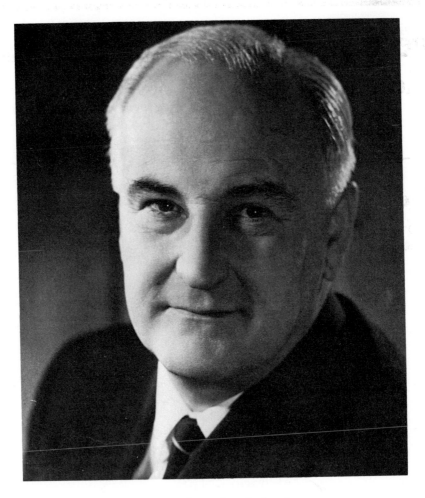

Sir Sydney Sunderland

Nerve Injuries and their Repair
A Critical Appraisal

Sir Sydney Sunderland
Kt CMG, MD, BS, DSc, Hon.LLD (Melb. & Monash),
Hon.MD (Tas. & Q'ld), Hon.FRACS, FRACP, FAA

Professor Emeritus of Experimental Neurology, University of Melbourne

CHURCHILL LIVINGSTONE
EDINBURGH LONDON MELBOURNE AND NEW YORK 1991

CHURCHILL LIVINGSTONE
Medical Division of Longman Group UK Limited

Distributed in the United States of America by Churchill
Livingstone Inc., 1560 Broadway, New York, N.Y. 10036,
and by associated companies, branches and representatives
throughout the world.

First published 1991

ISBN 0-443-04161-X

British Library Cataloguing in Publication Data
Sunderland, Sir, Sydney
  Nerve injuries and their repair.
  1. Man. Nerves. Injuries. Surgery
  I. Title
  617.483
Library of Congress Cataloging in Publication Data
Sunderland, Sydney, Sir.
    Nerve injuries and their repair: a critical appraisal/Sir
  Sydney Sunderland.
      p. cm.
    Includes index.
    0443041061X
    1. Nerves, Peripheral—Wounds and injuries.   I. Title.
    [DNLM: 1. Peripheral Nerves—injuries. 2. Peripheral
Nerves—surgery. WL 500 S958na]
RD595.S887 1991
617.4'83044—dc20
DNLM/DLC
for Library of Congress   90-2408

Printed in Great Britain by The Bath Press, Avon

Preface

The first edition of *Nerves and Nerve Injuries* was published in 1968 and a second edition in 1978. Both have been reprinted. A continuing demand for the book raises the question of whether a new, revised and rewritten edition is required. Careful reflection has convinced the author that such an edition is not warranted at this time.

The author believes that any new edition can only be justified if most of the contents have been subjected to changes, alterations and additions that are sufficiently substantial and relevant to warrant its replacement for an earlier edition.

In the case of *Nerves and Nerve Injuries*, the bulk of the contents relate to basic factual information of considerable clinical interest and significance that will not change in centuries. Instead of a third edition, what is really needed is a satellite or companion volume to the major work that addresses itself to those areas that call for amendment and for the inclusion of new and relevant information on nerve injury and nerve repair. This will explain the title of this book, *Nerve Injuries and their Repair. A Critical Appraisal*, and the motivation behind the selection of its contents.

This book is concerned solely with the subject of nerve injury and nerve repair. Non-traumatic causes of nerve dysfunction have been omitted intentionally.

Having in mind the wide-ranging nature of the book and the fact that it will be frequently used for reference purposes it is believed that some repetition is necessary and justifiable lest too many cross references destroy the continuity of an account. It is hoped that the understanding reader will appreciate this point.

Finally, the contents are based on the experiences and thoughts of one who has been involved in the laboratory investigation, study and clinical management of nerve injuries for more than 50 years. Such studies have at all times been directed to the elucidation of those principles on which the clinical management of nerve injuries should be based.

Melbourne 1991   Sir Sydney Sunderland

Acknowledgements

Though this saga of nerve injury, regeneration and repair has been a solo effort there are some to whom the author will always remain indebted for their friendship, generous help and support.

That the book is dedicated to my wife is the best I can do, inadequate though it is, to express my indebtedness to her for her monumental contribution to the completion of the book. She has typed and checked the entire manuscript several times and without her constant support and encouragement over the years the task would never have been undertaken let alone completed.

Though in my 80th year and 15 years into retirement, the Anatomy Department of the University of Melbourne, through the kind offices of Professor Ian Darien-Smith, has provided me over the years with accommodation and facilities while Professor Graeme Ryan, Dean of the Faculty of Medicine, has thoughtfully arranged for the Faculty to fund the final preparation of the manuscript for transmission to the publishers.

Churchill Livingstone has brought its customary skills and experience to the publication of the book and for this I thank them. My thanks are also due to Mrs Meldrum, Medical Librarian at the Alfred Hospital, who has been most helpful in tracking down and checking source material.

Lastly, this is an appropriate place and opportunity to acknowledge the debt I owe to colleagues in North America, Europe and elsewhere who have always given freely and generously of their time and experience during fruitful discussions and debate at international meetings and during the course of personal visits. I have indeed been fortunate in my clinical and laboratory contacts over the past 50 years. They are too numerous to name and too important to be overlooked. Clearly I owe much to the camaraderie that exists between workers in widely separated parts of the world but linked by a common cause and interest directed to achieving the best possible result from nerve repair by way of an unremitting search for the knowledge on which this depends.

Sir Sydney Sunderland

To
Nina Gwendoline

Contents

General considerations

1. Introduction

The old order changeth, yielding place to new,
And God fulfils Himself in many ways,
Lest one good custom should corrupt the world.
                    Tennyson. *Morte d'Arthur*.

One of the advantages of the first, and subsequently the second, edition of *Nerves and Nerve Injuries* is that it is the work of a single author who, at the time the book was written, could claim personal involvement both as a clinician and as a laboratory investigator capable of exploiting several scientific disciplines. Under these conditions knowledge from both clinical and experimental sources could be integrated in an orderly and meaningful way so that the central theme of nerve injury and nerve repair could be pursued on a broad and coordinated front.

Today the situation is different, for it is becoming increasingly difficult to preserve the closest possible integration of information pouring in from clinical and experimental sources. Spectacular developments in molecular biology, pharmacology, biochemistry, and electroneurophysiology, and the application of the complex technology required to support them, have outstripped the capacity of any one individual to handle the detail in every scientific discipline with any real authority or understanding. This largely explains why some of the subject matter in the Second Edition of *Nerves and Nerve Injuries* has been omitted from this companion volume, special attention now being given to those aspects of the subject in which the author has had a particular and lasting interest.

There is the further point that much of the recent published work in these various scientific disciplines has only an obscure relationship to the central theme of this text. Despite this, it has been possible to retain the essential objective of bringing all relevant aspects of the topics selected for inclusion together in an orderly and meaningful way.

The literature relating to nerve injury and nerve repair over the past 10 years remains a problem. Today we are confronted with a growing and confused mass of facts, often of an isolated and unrelated character, that clinicians and experimentalists pour daily in a continuous stream into the literature. As a result, the volume of papers, monographs, journals and books is approaching dimensions that are rapidly reaching the point of discouraging and defying readers.

While acknowledging that fact finding is the objective of any scientific enquiry, and that facts should be the ultimate court of appeal when an element of uncertainty, inconsistency or disagreement arises, we are now exposed to the real danger of becoming so preoccupied with accumulating new facts, often of an isolated and fragmentary nature, that too little time is left for their rational analysis. As a result, a synoptic and balanced appreciation of a subject becomes exceedingly difficult and general principles tend to become obscured in a mass of irrelevant detail.

What is also disturbing is that even a cursory examination of the current literature reveals an astonishing disregard for information that is already available, so that much of what is being reported continues to be either repetitious or irrelevant, or both, even though it may be supported in this technological age by an arsenal of gadgetry. Far too much time and effort are being spent 'rediscovering the wheel'.

Accordingly, the author has purposely refrained from including a comprehensive list of recent publications on the subject, redundant material being disregarded in favour of key references that con-

3

vey information that is original, has broken new ground, settled controversial issues or has introduced new and promising concepts. The intention, then, has been to retrieve from a morass of detail information of proven validity and to rescue from oblivion those facts that it is our wisdom to remember but our weakness to forget. Information does not need to be new to be important.

Finally, a persisting obstacle to improving the results of nerve repair today on a broader front is the failure by some to take advantage of information that has already been made available. The need to reduce the gap between what is known and what is practised remains a continuing challenge.

In a book of this nature there will always be the problem of deciding what to include and what to omit and such decisions must be largely a matter of personal judgement and a reflection of individual interpretation and emphasis.

Mediaeval surgeons believed that operative detail and surgical techniques could not be learnt from books but only by serving an apprenticeship under the tutelage of an experienced surgeon and by observing and assisting him in his craft. Thus, as long ago as the 15th century, Leonard of Bertapaglia wrote 'You must accompany and observe the qualified physician, seeing him work before you yourself practise, for by observing terrible accidents, you will discern the methods employed by those who treat them and thus attain the perfection of the masters.' This advice is as sound today as it was in mediaeval times and explains the omission from this text of descriptive details of operative procedures. Accordingly, the text is concerned with principles and changing attitudes and ideas regarding the management of these injuries and not with the details of changing operative techniques. At the same time the necessity for preserving and encouraging the highest standards of technical skills and achievement is obvious and is strongly endorsed.

After 50 years of unbroken endeavour in this field of activity, the preparation of this text has provided the author with an opportunity to pause and look back over the past and, by avoiding the tyranny of detail, to obtain a more general view of the subject, to contemplate its wider relations and so to crystallise his own thinking on the many

problems in nerve injury and nerve repair that continue to baffle and to confuse us. In the process of doing so it becomes possible to sift the 'chaff from the grain', to discard what is outmoded and has been disproved, to include what is genuinely new and confirmed, to separate fact from fiction and fantasy, and, finally, to offer suggestions on the direction that future research might be expected to take to correct and eliminate persisting imperfections and gaps in our knowledge. Finally, where genuine doubt and uncertainty still persist, this is recognised and included as a challenge to the imagination and a stimulus to experimental initiative directed to new and more fruitful lines of investigation.

In essence, then, this book is based on one individual's observations, experiences, and personal views and thoughts that have accumulated during half a century of personal involvement with nerve injury, nerve regeneration and nerve repair. This covers a period of unprecedented experimental and clinical activity in many countries, as the result of which much new factual information has been added to the storehouse of knowledge while many old concepts have either required amendment or been shown to be false and discarded.

Interestingly enough, the rethinking generated by all this restless activity has revealed that many contradictions disappear when the *observations* and not the *conclusions* of investigators are compared, and that, while principles might remain sacrosanct, their clinical significance and clinical application have taken on new dimensions as the point of vision has altered in a rejuvenated and greatly changed clinical setting.

Finally, this book is not a substitute or replacement for *Nerves and Nerve Injuries* which should be consulted at all times for the details that have survived unchanged, and for the established information on which categorical statements in the present work have been based.

REFERENCES

Ladenheim J C 1989 Leonard of Bertapaglia: On nerve injuries and skull fractures. Futura Publishing Company, New York

2. Terminology relating to nerves, nerve injury and nerve repair

The careless and misleading use of terms in medical reporting is a common source of confusion and misunderstanding when interpreting and comparing the observations and writings of different authors.

Often a term is used in a manner that is clearly in conflict with correct usage, the author often compounding the error by failing to specify the meaning that he is attaching to the term. While errors introduced in this way may be corrected by following the text, there are those occasions when an element of uncertainty persists. For example, *perineural* is often used when *perineurial* is intended. Perineural means about or surrounding the nerve trunk and relates to epineurial tissue. Perineurial, on the other hand, refers to the perineurium, whose structural features and physiological properties differ significantly from those of epineurial tissue.

Again, it is not unusual for a term, particularly when first introduced into the literature, to be interpreted and used in different ways by different individuals. The availability and use of several terms, all with the same meaning, also adds to the confusion.

Finally, it should be remembered that there is a considerable literature on the subject of nerve injury and nerve repair in languages other than English, each of which employs its own terminology with terms that sometimes differ in a potentially misleading way from what would be regarded as the corresponding term in English. Such differences are inevitable and should be recognised and understood if errors in interpretation are to be avoided.

Clearly, what is needed is a universally accepted standard nomenclature for terms that are in common use in peripheral nerve literature, particularly those relating to nerve injury, nerve regeneration and nerve repair. Where synonyms are available it is suggested that there are advantages in retaining one and adopting it for general use.

The sole intention of this chapter is to direct attention to the importance of this subject. Information relating to individual terms is not provided here but is included as an introductory section on terminology in those chapters in which the term is logically located and where the definitions given leave no doubt as to precisely what is meant when a certain term is used in this book.

The passage of time will, no doubt, necessitate additions to the lists which serve only as a framework to meet the needs of future developments and new information.

3. Animal experimentation and the solution of clinical problems

The proper study of mankind is man.

Pope

That animal experimentation has told us much about the biological processes involved in axon degeneration and regeneration is beyond question. Against this background of success, the conviction has now developed that animal experimentation should be the initial step in the investigation of any clinical problem from which, it is confidently expected, important clues and answers will inevitably flow.

The outstanding contributions that animal experimentation has made to progress should not, however, blind us to the fact that this approach is not without its shortcomings and limitations. Models for studying nerve injury and nerve repair, so conveniently offered by the experimental animal, seldom match those special conditions encountered in clinical practice and frequently differ from them in several significant respects. As a consequence information so obtained may have little, if any, clinical relevance and may even be misleading.

Experimental investigations have often been employed to test, inter alia, the relative merits of different methods of nerve repair using a variety of techniques and materials. In these investigations comparisons have usually been based on four sets of observations:

1. The numbers, and histological features, of regenerating axons in the nerve below the repair.
2. The distance covered by regenerating axons within a given time.
3. The application of neurophysiological techniques to detect, study, and track regenerating axons as they grow down the nerve.
4. The recovery of function based on the study of reflex responses, muscle contraction, and forepaw and hind limb movements.

There are several reasons why extrapolation to the clinical situation of animal data obtained in these ways should be treated with considerable caution.

1. To generalise, it appears from a survey of the literature that neuroscientists are primarily concerned with axon regeneration as a biological phenomenon, whereas the clinician's principal concern is the restoration of function. However, for axon regeneration to be functionally effective it is essential that regenerating axons should reach and re-establish connections with their original, or at least functionally related, end organs and this they often fail to do.

Among the many complex anatomical and pathological processes involved in axon regeneration, some have the potential to obstruct and misdirect axons during their growth. Where this occurs the restored pattern of innervation is left incomplete and imperfect in comparison with the original and function suffers accordingly.

Of special significance in this respect is whether there are neurotropic influences generated at the distal nerve stump that counteract this loss of axons by sorting out and organising axon growth in such a way as to ensure that each axon re-establishes its original, or at least a functionally related, terminal relationship. Such selectivity would simplify the surgeon's task in that neurotropic influences would ensure the restoration of functionally useful connections.

Because of its crucial importance to nerve repair, a separate chapter (p. 155) is devoted to this subject in which it will be shown that there are no such neurotropic influences operating to direct axons back to their old end organs.

All this means that the presence of regenerating axons in a mixed nerve below the repair is no guarantee that those axons are destined for functionally relevant destinations. This explains why:

a. the quality of the recovery after nerve repair is determined by the final destination of regenerating axons;
b. it is possible to have good axon regeneration but a poor functional result;
c. it is essential to draw a distinction between useful and wasteful regeneration;
d. the mere presence of regenerating axons below the repair is, in itself, an unreliable guide to the functional outcome of that regeneration. It is for this reason that, after the repair of a mixed nerve, an advancing Hoffmann–Tinel's sign, that registers the descent of sensory 'axon' tips, is of doubtful prognostic significance.

To recapitulate, while such experimental methods reflect the potential for axon growth they fail to differentiate between useful and wasteful regeneration, provide no clue as to the final destination of the regenerating axons and leave unanswered the all-important question of the recovery of function.

2. With animal experimentation, man has the advantage of dictating the terms and conditions of the experiment whereas in the clinical situation this is denied him.

In the experimental animal, trauma to the limb is minimal, the nerve is cleanly transected, and steps are taken to prevent wound infection and to ensure that the repaired section of the nerve is left occupying a satisfactory bed. These artificially created conditions are in marked contrast to the mutilating injuries commonly occurring in civilian accidents and battle casualties. In such injuries a considerable length of the nerve may have been destroyed or severely lacerated, the neighbouring tissues extensively damaged, and the wound infected. Residual scarring may also result in the formation of restrictive adhesions and an unsatisfactory bed for the nerve.

3. In man, both the repair of the nerve and the outcome of axon regeneration are subject to constraints imposed by the complex multifasciculated structure of peripheral nerves. These conditions cannot be matched in animals commonly selected for experimental studies. In the latter, nerves have a simple fascicular structure, usually in the form of a single fasciculus. This arrangement favours fascicular apposition when the nerve ends are united, thereby greatly simplifying the repair and reducing the chances of axons growing into, and becoming lost in, the interfascicular epineurial tissue of the distal stump.

4. When evaluating the quality of the recovery after nerve repair, movements of the forepaws and hind limbs of experimental animals bear little, if any, relation to the human situation, where manual dexterity in particular and the refined elements of discriminative sensibility and the stereognostic sense, as we understand them, are peculiarly human attributes.

5. In experimental procedures, the repair of a transected nerve involves only the simple restoration of nerve trunk continuity with evaluations of functional recovery that, in the clinical context, are inadequate and of limited value.

Clinically, the ground rules are very different and far more demanding. The restoration of function is now the objective of the exercise and this requires a carefully planned and executed repair designed to minimise wasteful and abortive axon regeneration and to maximise useful regeneration, the re-establishment of functionally effective pathways, and the restoration of patterns of innervation that approximate as closely as possible to the original. The extent to which this is achieved determines the extent to which complex and delicately co-ordinated motor and sensory mechanisms are restored, and with them the efficient and effective performance of a wide range of normal daily activities. This scenario has no experimental counterpart.

6. In experimental studies on nerve grafting, the length of nerve excised to accommodate the interpositional graft is usually of the order of 10 mm or less and is rarely extended to 30 mm. However, it has been demonstrated experimentally that regenerating axons in large numbers are quite capable of crossing, independently and unaided,

defects in nerves of at least 30 mm and of then entering the distal nerve stump and continuing on to effectively reinnervate previously denervated muscles (Chapter 16). There is much supporting clinical evidence to this effect in the literature.

Experiments to study the relative merits of different grafting techniques and materials have rarely included controls in which a gap of corresponding length has been left unbridged in order to test the capacity of regenerating axons to cross the gap unaided in comparison with the effectiveness of the graft material as a bridging tissue. This adds to the difficulty of interpreting and evaluating the contribution that the graft has made to axon regeneration, reinnervation and functional recovery.

7. Experimental animals are usually small. This means that, regardless of the level of nerve repair, the distances to be travelled by regenerating axons in order to reach the periphery are short in comparison with the much greater distances in man. Consequently, in animals usually used in experiments, delays before the reinnervation of the periphery are much shorter than in man. In the latter the affected parts may remain denervated for considerable periods, particularly after high lesions, thereby introducing complications rarely seen in the experimental animal.

8. Axon length, and the distance of the growing axon tip from the cell body, are factors influencing the calculation of rates of axon regeneration after nerve injury. Measurements over the short distances obtaining in the experimental animal have been interpreted as demonstrating a constant rate of axon advance. However, when this feature was investigated in man, it became clear that regenerating axon tips advance down the nerve at a progressively diminishing rate, the rate declining as the distance from the parent cell body increases. The distances available in experimental animals were too short to reveal this feature of axon regeneration.

9. There is always the risk that species differences in the reaction to injury, and in the biological processes involved in axon regeneration and nerve repair, could invalidate the free transfer of data from one species to another, and particularly from animal to man. The size of an animal, and whether it is warm or cold-blooded,

are also factors of established significance and there are others. Cajal (1928) in his writings suggested that species, as well as age, influence the rate of regeneration following nerve section but he did not elaborate on this observation.

In a comprehensive study of the response to nerve injury in various species, Kline et al (1964) found that species differences in response to nerve crushing were minimal. On the other hand, the differences were more apparent after nerve transection and repair, and related to connective tissue proliferation, disorganisation of axonal growth at the suture site, remyelination of the distal segment and restoration of a functional threshold of conduction.

The potentially misleading effect of species differences should never be underestimated when transposing experimental data from the laboratory to the study of nerve injury and nerve repair in man.

10. Even among individuals within a given species, there is a range of variation in the nature of the response to injury, in the behaviour of axons during regeneration, and in the many factors that combine in an exceedingly complex manner to influence the outcome after nerve repair. This adds to the difficulty of correctly interpreting the results of experiments undertaken to determine the relative merits of different procedures and materials available for the repair of a severed nerve. This, of course, applies equally to both clinical and experimental investigations. However, whereas such a possible source of error is generally recognised in clinical practice, it is too often overlooked in animal experimentation.

11. Many electrophysiological methods used in experimental investigations reveal what the nervous system *can do* rather than what it *does do*.

12. It is common in laboratory procedures to select one particular feature of nerve injury and repair for study and, when analysing the results, to exclude from consideration those many other co-existing factors that influence axon regeneration and the quality of functional recovery. As FMR Walshe (1951) has reminded us:

The isolation of a phenomenon involves its abstraction from the total reality under study yet in nature all things are connected and nothing is isolated or torn from its context and in the hands of those who do not safeguard their abstractions by constant reference to what they are leaving out of immediate account, the results of experiments are capable of grave misinterpretation.

Though the experimental approach may tell us much about biological processes involved in nerve injury and nerve repair it tells us little about functional recovery as this relates to human needs. One should not, therefore, rely too heavily and uncritically on animal experimentation in the search for solutions to clinical problems. Clearly what is needed is an experimental model that approximates more closely, and has greater relevance, to the clinical situation. In this respect Kline and his associates have rightly stressed the importance of using higher primates in studies of nerve repair, although this still falls short of the ideal.

The concluding thought is that though animal experiments will not provide definitive answers to clinical problems they may provide important clues to their solution.

Finally, the clinician would do well to remember that valuable information is still to be obtained by the diligent and persistent clinical investigator with the capacity to recognise in unusual clinical situations those unique experiments by which nature reveals its secrets. As that distinguished and perceptive English surgeon James Paget wrote a century ago:

Receiving thankfully all the help that physiology or chemistry or any other sciences more advanced than our own can give us, and pursuing all our studies with the precision and circumspection that we may best learn from them, let us still hold that, within our range of study, that alone is true which is proved clinically, and that which is clinically proved needs no other evidence.

REFERENCES

Kline D G, Hayes G J, Morse A S 1964 A comparative study of response of species to peripheral nerve injury. I. Severance. Journal of Neurosurgery 21: 968

Kline D G, Hayes G J, Morse A S 1964 A comparative study of response of species to peripheral nerve injury. II. Crush and severance with primary suture. Journal of Neurosurgery 21: 980

Paget J 1908 Memoirs and letters of Sir James Paget. Longmans, Green & Co., London, p 244

Ramon Y, Cajal S 1928 Degeneration and regeneration of the nervous system. Vol. 1. Oxford University Press, London

Walshe F M R 1951 On the interpretation of experimental studies of cortical motor function: with special reference to the 'Operational view' of experimental procedures. Brain 74: 249

Anatomical considerations

4. Terms relating to the structure of nerve fibres and nerve trunks

NERVE AND NERVE FIBRE

Basic to any consideration of terminology is the need to draw a distinction between the terms nerve and nerve fibre.

Nerve is derived from the Latin 'nervus', meaning 'sinew' or 'tendon'. Nerves were identified as such and distinguished from tendons by Herophilus in the 3rd century BC. He also established the relationship of nerves to the spinal cord and separated them into motor and sensory components.

The term nerve has come to have a dual meaning and it is important to distinguish between the two definitions.

One defines a nerve as a composite structure made up of many nerve fibres and their supporting connective tissues. These different elements collectively form a cord-like structure to which a particular name is usually attached, e.g. median, ulnar, cutaneous, sciatic, sympathetic.

On the other hand, the term *nerve fibre*, which refers exclusively and solely to the conducting unit in a nerve, is often, for convenience, abbreviated to *nerve* e.g. sympathetic nerves, motor or efferent nerves, sensory or afferent nerves. Used in this sense, 'nerve' becomes synonymous with 'nerve fibre'. Hence the confusion.

Unless specified, nerve could refer to either a cord-like structure composed of several different elements or solely to the contained nerve fibres. Usually the nature of the text and the way in which the term 'nerve' is used provides the clue to the meaning attached to it. However, there could be occasions when confusion might occur and, to avoid this, the term nerve should be reserved for the macroscopic composite cord-like structure which contains, inter alia, nerve fibres.

EXTRANEURAL

Outside the nerve.

INTRANEURAL AND ENDONEURAL

Inside or within the nerve. The term endoneural should not be confused with endoneurial. These two terms differ significantly and should not be used synonymously. Intraneural is the preferred term.

NERVE FIBRE

This is the conducting unit of the nerve. It has a composite structure made up of the following elements: a central core, the axon, enveloped in a complex covering comprising a single layer of linked Schwann cells, external to which is a basement membrane and beyond this an outer limiting sheath of endoneurial tissue. In some nerve fibres there is an additional myelin component which establishes a complex relationship with the Schwann cells.

As mentioned above, nerve fibre is often misleadingly abbreviated to nerve.

MYELINATED NERVE FIBRE

A nerve fibre in which myelin is a conspicuous component of the complex sheath surrounding the axon. This term is preferable to medullated.

NONMYELINATED OR UNMYELINATED NERVE FIBRE

A nerve fibre in which myelin is absent. These terms are preferable to non- and unmedullated.

AXON OR AXIS CYLINDER

The central core of axoplasm that constitutes the conducting element of a nerve fibre. It is bounded by a surface membrane, the axolemma. 'Axon' is the preferred term. The axon is the elongated peripheral process of a motor neuron.

DENDRON OR DENDRITE

The elongated peripheral process of a posterior root ganglion neuron which forms the conducting core of a sensory nerve fibre. Because it has the essential structural features of an axon it is convenient to use the term axon for the central core of all peripheral nerve fibres.

AXOPLASMIC FLOW

A term introduced to describe the movement of axoplasm down the nerve fibre.

AXOPLASMIC TRANSPORT

This term refers to the intracellular movement of materials, both distally and centrally, within the axoplasm.

SCHWANN CELL SHEATH OR SCHWANN SHEATH

This is formed by Schwann cells and the basal lamina or basement membrane of those cells.

ENDONEURIUM

The connective tissue which forms the supporting framework for the nerve fibres and capillaries inside a fasciculus. It is sometimes referred to as intrafascicular connective tissue. Used as an adjective the word becomes *endoneurial* and *not endoneural*. Using these terms synonymously is a common error in the literature.

ENDONEURIAL SHEATH

The endoneurium applied to the outer surface of the Schwann cell basement membrane is organised to form an endoneurial sheath for the nerve fibre. This sheath is preserved during Wallerian degeneration. Other names given to this sheath are the Sheath of Key and Retzius and the Sheath of Plenk and Laidlaw.

ENDONEURIAL SPACES

These are tissue spaces within the nerve fascicle which contain endoneurial tissue fluid.

ENDONEURIAL TUBE

This is a misnomer because the endoneurial sheath never outlines a hollow tube. In the normal state the 'tube' is occupied by the axon, Schwann cells, and myelin if it is present. During Wallerian degeneration this column of tissue becomes represented solely by Schwann cells and macrophages as the axon and myelin disintegrate and the debris is removed. Endoneurial tube is a convenient term to describe the endoneurial sheath and the cylinder or column of tissue which it encloses.

NEURILEMMA OR NEUROLEMMA

This term has been variously used at different times and by different authors to refer to the Schwann cell layer, its basement membrane, the endoneurium, the perineurium and the epineurium. So much confusion surrounds its use that the term should be abandoned.

PERINEURIUM

This is the thin sheath of specialised perineurial or lamella cells arranged in concentric layers which encircles a bundle of nerve fibres. This sheath is also known as the gaine lamelleuse or lamellated sheath of Ranvier.

PERINEURIAL

Pertaining to the perineurium, e.g perineurial sheath. This term should not be used synonymously with perineural.

PERINEURAL

This term means around the nerve trunk.

EPINEURIUM

This is the connective tissue that envelops the nerve and extends internally to separate and enclose individual fasciculi so that they are embedded in it.

Superficial or outer epineurium. This is the epineurium at the surface of the nerve.

Epineurial sheath. This is the relative condensation of superficial epineurium at the surface of the nerve trunk that imparts a cord-like appearance and consistency to the nerve, so that it is readily distinguishable from the surrounding tissues in which it is free to move and from which it can be easily and readily separated.

Deep, inner or interfascicular epineurium. This is the epineurium in the interior of the nerve in which the fasciculi are embedded. Where the nerve is composed of a single fasciculus, the terms deep, inner or interfascicular no longer apply and the terms superficial epineurium and perifascicular epineurium become synonymous — the former remains the preferred term.

Perifascicular epineurium. This is the deep or interfascicular epineurial tissue that envelops, and is in direct contact with, the perineurial sheath of each fasciculus.

DEEP FASCIAL OR PARANEURAL CONNECTIVE TISSUE

For want of a more suitable term, this refers to the unnamed non-specialised loose meshwork of areolar connective tissue that fills the space between specialised structures such as muscles, nerves and vessels, connecting them loosely together and permitting the movement of one on the other. Though this tissue is associated in this way with nerve trunks, it is not regarded as a component of the nerve trunk, whose outer limits are clearly outlined by a definitive sheath of epineurial tissue. The significance of the relationship is discussed in Chapter 12.

MESONEURIUM

A mesentery of connective tissue outlined about nutrient vessels as they are conveyed to and from the nerve. The reasons for regarding this as a feature created artificially by scalpel and forceps are given on page 55.

EPINEURAL

This term has no place in peripheral nerve terminology. It means situated on a neural arch.

EPINEURIAL AND PERINEURIAL

It is again emphasised that these terms are not synonymous. The former refers to the epineurium and the latter to the perineurium, two components with strikingly different structural features and functional properties.

FASCICLE, FASCICULUS, FASCICULAR

(Derived from the Latin *fascis*, a bundle). Funiculus, funicular (derived from the Latin *funis*, a rope). These terms are synonymous. Both were introduced to describe a bundle of nerve fibres and their related endoneurial tissue, all of which are encircled by an outer limiting sheath of perineurium. Fasciculus is now used by the majority of authors and has become the preferred term.

Monofascicular. Composed of a single fasciculus (Fig. 4.1).

Polyfascicular. Composed of many fasciculi. An acceptable subdivision could be (Fig. 4.1).

1. Type 1. Few large fasciculi
2. Type 2. The fasciculi are small and of approximately the same size.
3. Type 3. Large and small fasciculi are combined.

FASCICULAR GROUP

This is a collection or group of several fasciculi observed in a transection of a nerve. The group is outlined by propinquity, by an encircling condensation of the epineurium around them or by arbitrary selection.

FASCICULAR PLEXUS

A complex of intercommunicating fasciculi formed by their repeated divisions and unions.

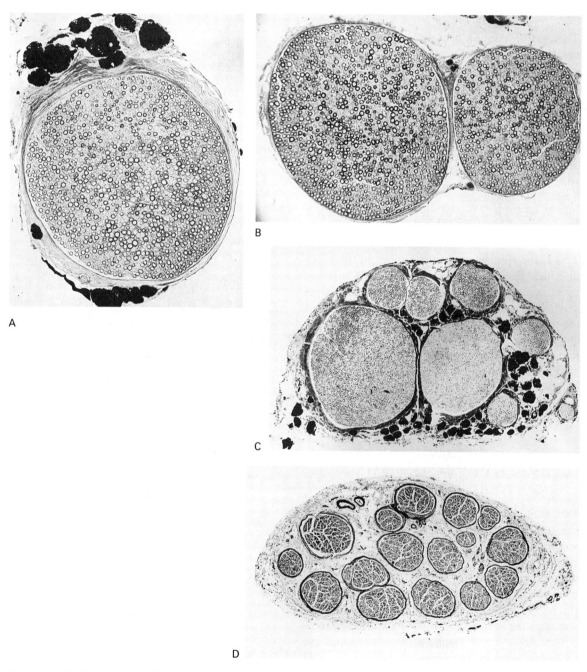

Fig. 4.1 Stained transverse sections of nerves illustrating examples of the mono- and poly- (types 1, 2 and 3) fascicular structure of nerves.

5. Nerve fibres

Nerve fibres are composed of an irregular cylindrical core of axoplasm, the axon, enclosed in an axolemmal membrane and surrounded by a complex sheath. This sheath varies in structure, according to the presence or absence of myelin, to give myelinated and nonmyelinated nerve fibres. In general, once axons reach a critical diameter of somewhere between 1 and 2 μm they acquire a covering of myelin that increases in thickness as the axon increases in size (Figs 5.1 and 5.2).

Where required, texts providing more detailed information than is provided here are those of Hubbard (1976), London (1976), Peters et al (1976) and Waxman (1978).

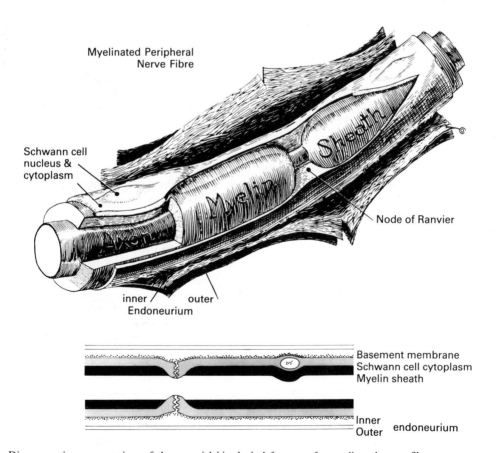

Myelinated Peripheral Nerve Fibre

Schwann cell nucleus & cytoplasm

Node of Ranvier

inner / outer
Endoneurium

Basement membrane
Schwann cell cytoplasm
Myelin sheath

Inner / Outer endoneurium

Fig. 5.1 Diagrammatic representations of the essential histological features of a myelinated nerve fibre.

17

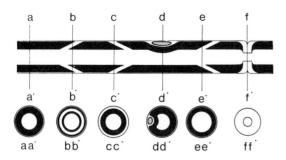

Fig. 5.2 Diagram of a longitudinal section of a nerve fibre, omitting all but the essential histological features, with transverse sections to illustrate variations in the cross-sectional appearance of the fibre.

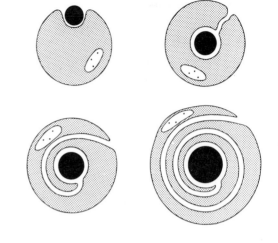

Fig. 5.3 Diagram to illustrate the changing axon-Schwann relationship leading to the development of a myelinated nerve fibre.

MYELINATED NERVE FIBRES

The axon

Axons vary from a few millimetres to somewhat more than a metre in length. They have the form of a cylinder that tapers gradually towards the periphery. On this are superimposed variations in diameter due to constriction at the nodes, indentations by the Schwann cell nuclei, reductions at the clefts of Schmidt-Lantermann and random variations elsewhere. Excluding these local variations, axons vary from about 0.5 μm to 10 μm in diameter.

The vital relationship that exists between the cell body and the axon is associated with an intracellular pressure that promotes a proximodistal flow from the cell body of materials that are essential for the survival and efficient functioning of the axon (see Axon transport systems p. 20).

The Schwann cell-myelin sheath

During development each Schwann cell gradually envelops an axon and finally surrounds it (Fig. 5.3). One lip of the Schwann cell cytoplasm then repeatedly wraps around the system so that a series of concentric cytoplasmic laminae are formed around the axon. The laminae are subsequently compressed together, the lipid protein membranes of the cytoplasmic surfaces collectively constituting the alternating layers of protein and lipid which, under high magnification, give the characteristic laminated structural organisation of the myelin sheath of the nerve fibre.

In the fully developed state this complex sheath presents the following appearance. Immediately surrounding the axon is the laminated layer of myelin, this is interrupted to outline the nodes and internodes of the fibre. The internodes vary in length, generally increasing with the thickness of the fibre. Internode length may, however, vary greatly in fibres of the same diameter while successive internodes may have different lengths.

Investing the myelin is the cytoplasm of a single layer of flattened Schwann cells, external to which is a basement membrane. Each internode has one Schwann cell nucleus situated approximately midway between adjacent nodes. At each node the Schwann cell layer reaches, embraces and constricts the axon. At this site each Schwann cell forms finger-like cellular processes that interlock with those of the next Schwann cell in the chain. The axon is more exposed to extracellular ions at the nodes where the myelin is absent. The incisures of Schmidt–Lantermann are conical clefts in the myelin. Their behaviour, when a nerve trunk is stretched, suggests that they function to prevent abnormal distortion and fracturing of myelin segments.

The endoneurial sheath

External to the Schwann cell layer is a thin, delicate, investment of intrafascicular connective tissue which is the endoneurium. This limiting layer outlines an endoneurial tube which is occupied by a cylinder of tissue composed of the axon and Schwann cells together with myelin when this is present.

General

1. Myelinated nerve fibres vary from about 1.5 μm to 20 μm in diameter. They are organised to become myelinated somewhere between 1 and 2 μm. Certainly by 2 μm they are mostly very finely myelinated. The diameters of the largest axons reported devoid of myelin range from 1.1 to 2.5 μm.
2. The belief that an axon has a constant diameter and a myelin sheath of uniform thickness along its length is without foundation.
3. Nerve fibres do not have the form of a simple rigid cylinder with a uniform structure along their length. In one study (Sunderland and Roche, 1958):

   a. the axon diameter along the same fibre varied from 3.25 to 11.75 μm and the total nerve fibre diameter from 6.5 to 16.0 μm;
   b. the total myelin thickness varied from 0.5 μm to 6.0 μm;
   c. the ratio of myelin area to axon area varied along the fibre from 0.66 to 1.44.

4. Though the myelin thickness is not constant for axons of the same diameter the absolute myelin thickness is generally greater in larger axons.

5. Despite the established variations in structure along the length of individual nerve fibres, it is reasonable to assume that these represent departures about a mean and that they contribute to an average arrangement in which a particular variation at one site is neutralised by changes at another level, the overall effect being to optimise nerve fibre function.
6. The nerve fibre calibre spectrum of individual fasciculi of cutaneous nerves varies from fasciculus to fasciculus. This means that the examination of a single fasciculus could give misleading information about the overall fibre composition of the nerve. The extent of these variations is shown in Table 5.1.

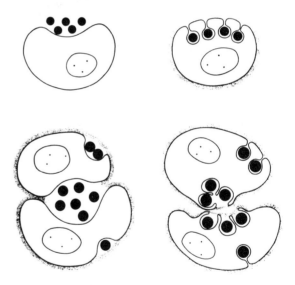

Fig. 5.4 Stages in the envelopment of several axons by a single Schwann cell.

Table 5.1 Nerve fibres of different sizes, expressed as a percentage of the total fascicular fibre count, in two fasciculi from the superficial radial nerve and the medial cutaneous nerve of the forearm of the same subject

Nerve	Less than 8 μm	8–15 μm	16–23 μm
Superficial radial			
Fasciculus 1	53.4	7.9	38.7
Fasciculus 2	67.7	16.0	16.3
Medial cutaneous of forearm			
Fasciculus 1	63.6	29.0	7.4
Fasciculus 2	82.4	9.7	7.9

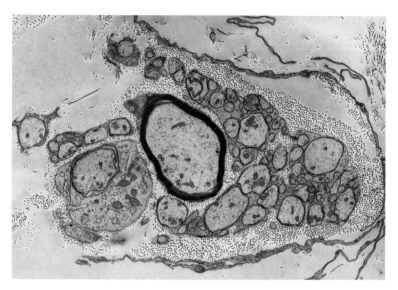

Fig. 5.5 A fasciculus containing one myelinated nerve fibre and many nonmyelinated axons enclosed in individual Schwann cells.

NON-MYELINATED NERVE FIBRES

The sheath of the axon consists of a single layer of Schwann cells, external to which is the endoneurium. The cytoplasm of individual Schwann cells surrounds, to a varying degree, one or more commonly several axons so that whereas the endoneurial tube of a myelinated fibre contains only one axon, those of non-myelinated fibres usually contain several axons (Figs 5.4 and 5.5).

AXON TRANSPORT SYSTEMS

Nerve impulses are not the only traffic travelling along nerve fibres, for the axon also represents a channel along which a great variety of cell constituents is continually on the move, using fast and slow centrifugal and retrograde transport systems to reach their destination and produce their effects. The survival and welfare of axons and the structures they innervate depend on these transport mechanisms.

These transport systems continue to be intensively investigated and have recently been the subject of numerous articles and reviews which should be consulted for details (Ochs and Worth 1978; Black and Lasek 1980; Grafstein and Forman 1980; Pleasure 1980; Sjöstrand et al 1980; Droz 1981; Griffin et al 1981; Brady 1982; Brady and Lasek 1982; Droz and Rambourg 1982; Gainer and Fink 1982; Lasek and Brady 1982; Weiss 1982; Weiss and Gross 1982; McLean et al 1983; Lasek et al 1984; Ochs 1984; Alvarez and Torres 1985; Blum and Reed 1985; Bray 1985; Gilbert et al 1985; Lasek and Brady 1985; Dahlin and McLean 1986; Dahlin et al 1986; Lynn et al 1986). Only those features that have some relevance to nerve injury and repair are included here.

1. A distinction should be drawn between bulk axoplasmic flow and axon transport in that the former implies movement of a column of axoplasm and the latter the transport of materials *within* a column of axoplasm.
2. The existence of fast and slow centrifugal and retrograde transport systems has now been amply documented.
3. Axon transport has been established as a universal property of all axons.
4. Fast and slow centrifugal and retrograde transport systems share the same axon.
5. Centrifugal axon transport systems convey a wide variety of materials, synthesised in the cell body, that are being continually transferred to, and transported down, the

axon to its remote terminals. These materials:

a. are required for maintenance of the axolemmal membrane and cytoskeletal elements of the axon such as microtubules and neurofilaments. The latter are believed to play an important role in determining axonal calibre (Hoffman et al 1984);

b. are required to maintain the integrity of the nerve fibre and its conducting properties;

c. are involved in neurotransmission across axon terminals;

d. on release from the axon terminals exert a trophic influence over innervated tissues.

6. Fast axon centrifugal transport rates have been described that cover a range of 40–500 mm per day.

7. Fast axon transport systems are involved in conveying a wide range of materials such as transmitter storage vesicles, lipids and glycoproteins.

8. Materials using the slow transport system differ from those carried down the axon by the fast system. These include materials associated with the cytoskeletal elements of the axon such as microtubules (tubulin and related proteins) neurofilaments (protein) and microfilaments (actin).

9. Slow transport rates vary from 1 to 8 mm per day.

10. The restriction of centrifugal transport systems to two general categories of fast and slow rates is obviously an oversimplification of a very complex process that almost certainly involves a spectrum of different rates for different materials.

11. The velocity of the slow component is significantly faster in young than in adult animals.

12. Retrograde axon transport operates at about half the descending rate, namely 100–200 mm per day, though there is some evidence of a slow component of 3–8 mm per day.

13. The retrograde transport system is presumed to convey materials centrally to the cell body where they participate in controlling the level of its activity.

14. There is much indirect evidence that neurotubules serve as the unit along which transport occurs.

THE BRANCHING OF NERVE FIBRES

Nerve fibres undergo repeated and extensive branching within the tissue innervated. They also branch where they are contained in the parent nerve trunk so that, in the latter, the total number of fibres is greater distally than proximally. This means that the territory served by a posterior root ganglion or anterior horn neuron is more extensive than is indicated by the penultimate branching of the fibre at the periphery and than is generally acknowledged to be the case.

Nerve fibre branching provides a mechanism whereby the action of relatively large masses of tissue, possibly of more than one kind, may be coordinated under the influence of a single neuron. This is also the basis of axon reflexes in which activity in one area may affect the physiological status of another.

Referred pain can also be explained on the basis of the branching of nociceptor fibres in which some of the branched fibres innervate the site of origin of the disturbance and others pass to the site of pain reference. Referred pain may originate in two ways. In one, nociceptor impulses originating from one branch are misinterpreted in the sensorium as originating from another. In the second, an axon reflex through branched axons provokes the liberation of some substance in the area of reference which sets up nociceptor impulses.

Unusual disturbances of function resulting from peripheral nerve injuries

Two puzzling features occasionally associated with severance of a major peripheral nerve are the impairment of cutaneous sensation in areas that are clearly not innervated by the injured nerve, and the recovery in certain muscles, initially paralysed as a result of the injury, that occurs long before this could be due to the regeneration of motor axons. A possible explanation to account for these phenomena is based on the branching of motor and sensory fibres at the root of the limb with the daughter divisions of a parent fibre travelling to the periphery by way of different named peripheral nerves. The mechanism by which this is brought about is discussed in Chapters 32 and 33.

PHYSIOLOGICAL TYPES OF NERVE FIBRES

Motor, sensory and sympathetic nerve fibres contribute to the formation of peripheral nerve trunks.

Motor fibres vary in diameter from 2 μm to 20 μm, the larger fibres innervating extrafusal muscle fibres and the smallest innervating the intrafusal muscle fibres of muscle spindles.

Sensory fibres are both non-myelinated and myelinated. The latter vary in diameter from 1.5 μm to 20 μm. The non-myelinated and finely myelinated variety predominate.

Sensory fibres terminate at the periphery either freely or in a variety of specialised end-organs or receptors. Cutaneous sensory fibres travel in the cutaneous nerves, terminate in the skin and tissues superficial to the deep fascia, and between them mediate sensations of touch, pressure, pain, warmth and cold. The deep sensory fibres travel in the deep branches of the main nerve trunks and terminate in muscles, tendons, articular and peri-articular structures, connective tissue and bone. These fibres mediate sensations of pressure, pain, temperature and stretch.

Sympathetic fibres are the postganglionic processes of the neurons of the ganglionated sympathetic trunk. They are non-myelinated and pass by way of cutaneous nerves to vessels, hair, muscles and glandular structures of the skin and to deeper structures via the deep branches of the main nerve trunks.

NERVE FIBRE STRUCTURE IN RELATION TO FUNCTION

Nerve fibre structure and the compound action potential

The compound nerve action potential elicited by electrical stimulation of a nerve trunk shows a series of elevations. When these characteristics of compound action potential records are compared with nerve fibre calibre histograms prepared from the same nerves, the comparisons furnish evidence that each of the elevations of the electrical record are associated with a particular nerve fibre group.

Three fundamental nerve fibre types, A, B, and C, have been identified in this way, with the first named being further divided into alpha, beta, gamma and delta categories.

Nerve fibre diameters, conduction velocities and the associated physiological functions assigned to these various nerve fibre types are shown in Table 5.2.

Nerve fibre structure and conduction velocity

1. To function efficiently each nerve fibre must transmit impulses at a certain speed and frequency.

Table 5.2 The relationship between nerve fibre types, diameters, conduction velocity and function

Nerve fibre		Nerve fibre Diameter in μm	Conduction velocity M/s	Function
A	Alpha	12–20	70–120	Motor. Extrafusal muscle fibres. Proprioceptors
	Beta	5–12	30–70	Touch. Pressure
	Gamma	3–6	15–30	Motor. Intrafusal muscle fibres
	Delta	2–5	10–30	Nociceptors. Touch. Temperature
B		1.5–3	3–15	Preganglionic sympathetic fibres
C		Less than 2.0	0.5–2	Nociceptors. Postganglionic sympathetic fibres

2. Factors influencing the conduction velocity of nerve fibres include, inter alia, the diameter of the axon, the thickness of its myelin sheath, the internodal distance and the condition of the axolemmal membrane.

3. The greater the diameter of a nerve fibre the faster the conduction velocity. Thus large fibres conduct faster than fine ones.

4. In myelinated nerve fibres the relationship between fibre diameter and conduction velocity is a linear one, whereas in non-myelinated fibres the conduction velocity is proportional to the square root of the diameter.

5. Fast conduction is also favoured by incorporation within the nerve sheath of increasing relative amounts of myelin.

6. Based on the work of Erlanger and Gasser (1937), a simple approximation of the relation between nerve fibre diameter and conduction velocity is:

   For myelinated nerve fibres the conduction velocity = the external diameter of the fibre in μm $\times$ 6.
   For non-myelinated nerve fibres the conduction velocity = the external diameter of the fibre in μm $\times$ 2.

7. Rates of conduction vary from 120 metres per second in the case of the largest fibres to <2 metres per second in the case of the finest (Table 5.2).

8. Because the diameter of a nerve fibre and the degree of myelination are factors influencing nerve conduction, any departure from the normal diameter and myelination of a fibre should disturb conduction along it.

Nerve fibre structure and physiological function

Attempts to establish a precise relationship between nerve fibre structure and nerve fibre function have met with only mixed success.

1. To function efficiently each nerve fibre must transmit impulses at a certain speed and frequency. Since the diameter of a nerve fibre and the degree of myelination are factors influencing nerve conduction, it might be expected that any departure from the normal diameter and myelination of a nerve fibre would be reflected in disturbances of motor and sensory functions. While this is generally true, there is evidence to the contrary in that, under certain circumstances, these two structural features may be grossly modified although peripheral functions are left undisturbed. Under these conditions, however, conduction velocity is slowed across the affected segment but not above or below it.

2. The structure of individual nerve fibres is constantly changing along their length while each fibre obviously retains the same function.

3. Though motor nerve fibres innervating extrafusal muscle fibres share a common function, they range in diameter from 3 μm to 20 μm. This morphological feature is most likely related to the size of the motor unit innervated by a nerve fibre; the greater the number of extrafusal fibres constituting the unit, the thicker the nerve fibre innervating it.

   While the intrafusal muscle fibres of the muscle spindles are known to be innervated by the finest of the motor nerve fibres there is as yet no proof that this is the sole destination of all such fibres.

4. Attempts to establish a relation between different somatic sensory functions and nerve fibre size in afferent nerves became indefensible when Gasser (1935, 1943) demonstrated that specific physiological functions are each served by nerve fibres having a wide range of fibre diameter. There is much other evidence confirming this view.

5. Collectively, the evidence demonstrates that:
   a. specific physiological functions are each served by nerve fibres with a considerable range of diameter:
   b. nerve fibres controlling different physiological functions may have similar diameters and conduction velocities.

6. *General*. Since the total nerve fibre diameter, myelin thickness, axon diameter and the internodal length vary along individual nerve

fibres, it is not surprising that attempts to establish precise mathematical relationships between a particular morphological feature, conduction velocity, and physiological function remain unsatisfactory. The data also throw doubt on the unqualified acceptance of the thesis that the physiological properties of nerve fibres are determined solely by their size and degree of myelination. Finally, if studies of such relationships are to have significance, they must avoid assumptions that an axon has the form of a simple cylinder of constant dimensions and a myelin sheath of uniform thickness.

It should be understood that the values listed in Table 5.2 are generalisations only.

THE FUNCTION OF NERVE FIBRES WHOSE STRUCTURE HAS BEEN DISORGANISED

The literature devoted to nerve fibre conduction contains many references to the relationship between the conducting properties of a nerve fibre and such morphological features as its calibre and degree of myelination, and modifications of the conducting properties that result from deviations from the normal structure of the fibre. Despite the general acceptance that such structural changes are associated with impairment of the functional efficiency of the fibre, there is experimental evidence that the architecture of nerve fibres may be grossly modified without destroying axonal continuity and the capacity of the axons to excite activity at the periphery.

Sunderland (1951) found that transfixing a nerve with chromic catgut created a reaction that obliterated the normal histological features of the nerve at that site, the principal change being the loss of myelin and the characteristic outlines of fasciculi and nerve fibres. However, that axonal continuity had been preserved was evidenced by two observations:

1. The normal structure and outlines of the nerve and nerve fibres were retained below the site of the inflammatory reaction to the catgut.

2. The behaviour of the animal, a study of movements and the use of the limb, and the histological examination of muscles innervated by the nerve were all consistent with the preservation of normal function.

This finding has been confirmed by others who have reported the same demyelinating effects with, however, three additional findings: electronmicroscopic evidence of axonal swelling and Schwann cell proliferation, a slowing of conduction across the transformed segment but not above or below it (Lehmann 1961; Lehmann and Ule 1963, 1964; Ule and Lehmann 1963; Lehmann and Pretschner 1966) while Burchiel (1980) has reported that the affected segment possesses abnormal impulse generation properties.

Clearly the intimate relationship claimed between fibre diameter and degree of myelination on the one hand, and fibre function on the other, requires further clarification.

The persistence of normal function in tissues innervated by nerves whose structure has been disorganised emphasises the need for caution when interpreting the findings based on an examination of biopsy material removed from the suture line after so-called 'failed repair', and from lesions in continuity in which inadequate time has been allowed for spontaneous recovery to reveal itself. Such an examination may give misleading information about the state of nerve fibres at the site of involvement. The fact that pathways possessing the characteristic morphological features of myelinated nerve fibres cannot be detected crossing the suture line, or in the traumatised section of a nerve in continuity, does not, in itself, exclude the presence of regenerating axons that, in time, would reach the periphery and function efficiently.

THE NUTRITION OF NERVE FIBRES

The survival and efficient functioning of nerve fibres depend on the state of the parent neuron. However, nerve trunks are also nourished by nutrient vessels which, in addition to supplying the supporting tissues of the nerve trunk, also contribute to the nutrition of nerve fibres and, in particular, the axons. This subject is discussed further in Chapter 10.

PATTERNS OF INNERVATION

In any sensory or motor event nerve fibres are activated not singly but in 'battalions'. This is because sensory receptors, which vary in their arrangement, distribution and threshold to stimulation do not, in the usual run of daily activities, receive single sharply localised punctate stimuli. On the contrary, they are subjected to more widely distributed multiple stimulations that simultaneously affect a wide variety of nerve endings in varying numbers and combinations and at different intensities. The sum total of the activity generated in this way is a complex signal pattern in which is encoded information relating to the nature, quality and intensity of the peripheral stimulus.

Though different sensory fibre terminals combine in intricate patterns to provide the peripheral basis for sensory perception, sensory discrimination and the stereognostic sense, this does not occur in any simple fashion but involves processes of great complexity, both peripherally and in the central nervous system as the signal pattern is transmitted through neural centres on its way to the sensory cortex.

Likewise, the control and precision of even simple voluntary movements require the combined and coordinated activity of many muscles involving large numbers of motor nerve fibres, some of which innervate extra- and infra-fusal muscle fibres while others subserve associated proprioceptor functions.

All this means that the restoration of function after nerve repair depends not only on axon regeneration but also, and importantly, on the restoration of complex patterns of innervation.

REFERENCES

Alvarez J, Torres J C 1985 Slow axoplasmic transport: a fiction? Journal of Theoretical Biology 112: 627

Black M M, Lasek R J 1980 Slow components of axonal transport to cytoskeletal networks. Journal of Cell Biology 85: 616

Blum J J, Reed M C 1985 A model for fast axonal transport. Cell Motility 5: 507

Brady S T 1982 Microtubules and the mechanisms of fast axonal transport. In: Weiss D G (ed) Axoplasmic transport. Springer-Verlag, Berlin, p 301

Brady S T, Lasek R J 1982 The slow components of axonal transport movements, compositions and organization. In: Weiss D G (ed) Axoplasmic transport. Springer-Verlag, Berlin, p 206

Bray D 1985 Fast axonal transport. Nature 315: 178

Burchiel K J 1980 Abnormal impulse generation in focally demyelinated trigeminal roots. Journal of Neurosurgery 53: 674

Dahlin L B, McLean W G 1986 Effects of graded experimental compression on slow and fast axonal transport in rabbit vagus nerve. Journal of Neurological Sciences 72: 19

Dahlin L B, Sjöstrand J, McLean W G 1986 Graded inhibition of retrograde axonal transport by compression of rabbit vagus nerve. Journal of Neurological Sciences 76: 221

Droz B 1981 Axonal transport in peripheral nerves. International Journal of Microsurgery 3: 93

Droz B, Rambourg A 1982 Axonal smooth endoplasmic reticulum and fast orthograde transport of membrane constituents. In: Weiss D G (ed) Axoplasmic transport. Springer-Verlag, Berlin, p 384

Erlanger J, Gasser H S 1937 Electrical signs of nervous activity. University of Pennsylvania Press, Philadelphia

Gainer H, Fink D J 1982 Covalent labelling techniques and axonal transport. In: Weiss D G (ed) Axoplasmic transport. Springer-Verlag, Berlin, p 464

Gasser H S 1935 Conduction in nerves in relation to fiber types. Chapter II in Sensation: its mechanisms and disturbances. Association For Research In Nervous and Mental Disease 15: 35. Williams and Wilkins, Baltimore

Gasser H S 1943 Pain-producing impulses in peripheral nerves. Chapter III in Pain. Association For Research In Nervous and Mental Disease 23: 44. Williams and Wilkins, Baltimore

Gilbert S P, Allen R D, Sloboda R D 1985 Translocation of vesicles in squid axoplasm on flagellar microtubules. Nature 315: 245

Grafstein B, Forman D 1980 Intracellular transport in neurons. Physiological Reviews 60: 1167

Griffin J W, Price D L, Drachman D B, Morris J 1981 Incorporation of axonally transported glycoproteins into axolemma during nerve regeneration. Journal of Cell Biology 88: 205

Hoffman P N, Griffin J W, Price D L 1984 Control of axonal calibre by neurofilament transport. Journal of Cell Biology 99: 705

Hubbard J J 1976 The peripheral nervous system. Plenum Press, New York

Landon D N 1976 The peripheral nerve. Chapman & Hall, London

Lasek R J, Brady S T 1982 The structural hypothesis of axonal transport: two classes of moving elements. In: Weiss D G (ed) Axoplasmic transport. Springer-Verlag, Berlin, p 397

Lasek R J, Brady S T 1985 Attachment of transported vesicles to microtubules in axoplasm is facilitated by ANP-PNP. Nature 316: 645

Lasek R J, Garner J A, Brady S T 1984 Axonal transport of the cytoplasmic matrix. Journal of Cell Biology 99: 212

Lehmann H J 1961 Erregbarkeit und Leitungsfähigkeit bei experimentell gesetzten Strukturveränderungen im peripheren Nerven. Pflügers Archiv für die gesamte Physiologie des Menschen und der Tiere 274: 29

Lehmann H J, Ule G 1963 Erregungsleitung in demyelinisierten Nervenfasern. Naturwissenschaften 4: 131

Lehmann H J, Ule G 1964 Electrophysiological findings and structural changes in circumscript inflammation of peripheral nerves. In: Bargmann W, Schade J P (eds) Progress in brain research. Elsevier, Amsterdam, 6: 169

Lehmann H J, Pretschner D P 1966 Experimentelle Untersuchungen zum Engpassyndrom peripherer Nerven. Deutsche Zeitschrift für Nervenheilkunde 188: 308

Lynn M P, Atkinson M B, Brener A C 1986 Influence of translocation track on the motion of intra-axonally transported organelles in human nerve. Cell Motility and Cytoskeleton 6: 339

McLean W G, McKay A L, Sjostrand J 1983 Electrophoretic analysis of axonally transported proteins in rabbit vagus nerve. Journal of Neurobiology 14: 227

Ochs S 1984 Basic properties of axoplasmic transport. In: Dyck P J, Thomas P K, Lambert E H, Bunge M B (eds) Peripheral neuropathy, 2nd edn. W B Saunders, Philadelphia, p 453

Ochs S, Worth R M 1978 Axoplasmic transport in normal and pathological systems. In: Waxman S G (ed) Physiology and pathology of axons. Raven Press, New York, p 251

Peters A, Palay S L, Webster H de F 1976 The fine structure of the nervous system: the neuron and supporting cells. Saunders, Philadelphia

Pleasure D 1980 Axoplasmic transport. In: Sumner A (ed) The physiology of peripheral nerve disease. W B Saunders, Philadelphia, p 221

Sjöstrand J, McLean G, Frizell M 1980 The application of axonal transport studies to peripheral nerve problems. In: Omer G, Spinner M (eds) Management of peripheral nerve problems. W B Saunders, Philadelphia, p 917

Sunderland S 1951 The function of nerve fibers whose structure has been disorganised. Anatomical Record 109: 503

Sunderland S, Roche A F 1958 Axon-myelin relationships in peripheral nerve fibres Acta Anatomica 33: 1

Ule G, Lehmann H J 1963 Ueber Ultrastrucktur und Function experimentell demyelinisierter Nervenfasern Pflügers Archiv für die gesamte Physiologie des Menschen und der Tiere 287: 74

Waxman S G 1978 Physiology and pathobiology of axons. Raven Press, New York

Weiss D G 1982 General properties of axoplasmic transport. In: Weiss D G (ed) Axoplasmic transport. Springer-Verlag, Berlin, p 1

Weiss D G, Gross G W 1982 The microstream hypothesis of axoplasmic transport: characteristics, predictions and compatibility with data. In: Weiss D G (ed) Axoplasmic transport. Springer-Verlag, Berlin, p 362

6. Nerve trunks

Anatomical and topographical features of peripheral nerve trunks of particular relevance to nerve injury and nerve repair fall into two groups. The first includes those macroscopic features revealed by gross dissection and the second comprises internal features that require some magnification for their study and special techniques to demonstrate them.

Those without a background knowledge of these features, and an appreciation of their clinical significance, should not assume responsibility for the management of nerve injuries.

THE MICROSTRUCTURE OF NERVE TRUNKS

The ground plan of a nerve trunk is best illustrated in a stained transverse section of a nerve (Fig. 6.1). This reveals that nerve fibres are collected into fasciculi each fasciculus being:

1. surrounded by a thin but distinctive lamellated sheath of perineurial cells interspersed with fine collagen fibrils;
2. occupied by a framework of endoneurial tissue which is specialised around each nerve fibre to form an outer endoneurial sheath;
3. the fasciculi are in turn set in an areolar connective tissue packing, the epineurium.

The internal structure of a nerve does not remain constant from level to level because its constituent fasciculi are repeatedly dividing and uniting to form complex fascicular plexuses that are found along the entire length of a nerve.

Features of the internal structure of nerves that have clinical significance concern:

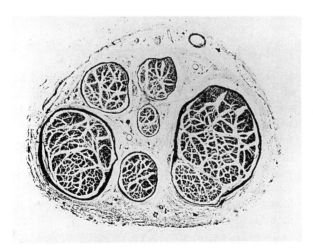 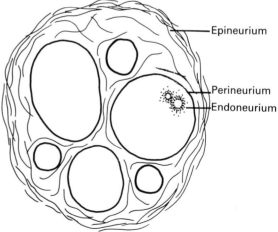

Fig. 6.1 A stained transverse section of a nerve illustrating its principal structural features, each of which is identified in the accompanying diagram.

27

1. Fascicular anatomy.
2. Numbers of nerve fibres representing individual branches.
3. Connective tissues.
4. Blood supply.
5. Lymphatics, endoneurial spaces and nervi nervorum.

These subjects are discussed in separate chapters.

THE GROSS ANATOMY OF NERVE TRUNKS

Of particular importance in this category are:

1. The relation of the nerve to its surroundings, including regional and surface anatomy, and the length and mobility of the nerve in its bed.
2. The origin, branch pattern and terminal distribution of branches and their variations.
3. Blood supply.

THE NERVE IN RELATION TO ITS SURROUNDINGS

Regional and surface anatomy

1. While a peripheral nerve may be injured by a penetrating or perforating object in any part of its course, it is more liable to damage from superficial injuries where it runs in subcutaneous tissues or approaches the surface. For example, the median and ulnar nerves in the upper arm and at the wrist are more prone to involvement in superficial injuries in these regions. Sites of maximal vulnerability in this respect should be noted.

2. The intimate relations that nerves establish with other structures may render them more susceptible to injury.

a. Bone

Where a nerve is in direct contact with bone, or there is little intervening soft tissue, the chances of its being damaged from fractures, or from com-
pression against the bone, are greatly increased. Examples illustrating this complication include: (i) damage to the axillary, musculocutaneous, radial, median and ulnar nerves from fractures of the humerus; (ii) damage to the posterior interosseous nerve from fractures of the upper third of the radius; (iii) damage to the sciatic nerve from fractures of the femur.

b. Bony abnormalities

Examples include: (i) the lower trunk of the brachial plexus and anomalous bony processes at the thoracic outlet; (ii) the median nerve in relation to a humeral supracondylar spur and ligament.

c. Joints

The intimate relation of a nerve to a joint, with little or no intervening soft tissue, exposes it to injury when the joint is dislocated in a direction that would stretch or compress the nerve. Examples are the axillary nerve and the shoulder joint, and the sciatic nerve and the hip joint.

d. Tendons

The intimate relationship of nerves to tendons may lead to errors of identification and the disaster of inadvertently suturing nerve to tendon or tendon to nerve — a costly error to both patient and surgeon.

e. Major vessels

In certain regions a nerve is intimately related to an artery with which it may share a common sheath to form a neurovascular bundle and to which it may be securely attached by short arteriae nervorum. Such an intimate relationship: (i) predisposes to combined neurovascular injuries; (ii) may result in the nerve being inadvertently crushed or ligated with the artery when controlling haemorrhage; and (iii) may add to the difficulty of mobilising the nerve.

f. Fibrous bands, arcades, septa and fascia

Where a free-running nerve crosses a fibrous band

or septum, or passes under a fibrous arcade or through fascia and ligamentous tissue, it may be injured by: (i) repeated friction; (ii) becoming attached by adhesions that fix the nerve at that site and expose it to further damage from traction; (iii) being compressed against a rigid septum.

Examples of this type of involvement abound and include: the ulnar nerve where it crosses the medial intermuscular septum and passes into the forearm under the humero-ulnar arcade at the elbow joint; cutaneous nerves where they pass through fascia; the lateral cutaneous nerve of the thigh where it passes through fibres of the inguinal ligament at the anterior superior iliac spine; the posterior interosseous nerve where it passes under the sharp musculotendinous upper edge of the superficial head of the supinator muscle.

g. Entrapment situations

Nerves are vulnerable to compression injury where they pass through a confined and crowded compartment bounded by unyielding walls and subject to space-occupying pathology. Examples are the median nerve in the carpal tunnel and the facial nerve in the facial canal.

LENGTH OF A NERVE IN ITS BED

The undulating course of a nerve trunk in its bed gives it a greater length than the distance between any two points along the limb; the difference is of the order of several centimetres. The undulations are a protective device in that the slack they provide is taken up during joint movements so that the nerve and nerve fibres normally remain tension free at all times.

The discrepancy between nerve trunk length and the distance between two fixed points on the limb should be taken into consideration when calculating nerve conduction velocities and the onset of recovery after nerve injury or nerve repair.

THE MOBILITY OF A NERVE IN ITS BED

Normally a nerve trunk is only loosely attached to surrounding structures by flimsy areolar connective tissue. This, and the undulating course

referred to above, means that the nerve normally enjoys considerable mobility in its bed.

The risk of a nerve sustaining a stretch or other injury is reduced when it is mobile and free to be displaced in its bed. On the other hand, the risk is increased when a nerve: (1) becomes firmly attached by adhesions to its bed or neighbouring structures; (2) is normally fixed at one or more sites along its course.

Examples are:

a. the lateral popliteal nerve at the neck of the fibula;
b. the entry of branches into muscles, particularly when they are short;
c. the passage of a cutaneous nerve through fascia or ligamentous tissue such as occurs with the lateral cutaneous nerve of the thigh where it passes into the thigh at the anterior superior iliac spine through fibres of the inguinal ligament.

ORIGIN BRANCH PATTERN AND TERMINAL DISTRIBUTION OF THE BRANCHES AND THEIR VARIATIONS

Though the general form of the branch pattern and the distribution of branches is constant for any particular nerve, variations in both features are common. In this respect:

1. A nerve may extend its field of supply by sending branches to structures not normally innervated by it. On the other hand, certain branches may be absent, or have a reduced distribution, in which case the structure concerned is innervated from another source. Common and notoriously misleading variations of this type involve the median and ulnar nerves with particular regard to: (a) the cutaneous innervation of the hand; (b) the motor innervation of the flexor digitorum profundus and the intrinsic muscles of the hand.
2. A muscle or cutaneous area may be innervated from more than one source.
3. Muscles may be supplied by widely spaced multiple branches and the first branch does not necessarily carry the shortest fibres into the muscle.

4. Information about these features is essential for:

    a. localising the site of a nerve injury;

    b. recognising departures from what are regarded as the normal order of reinnervation of structures during recovery;

    c. studying rates of regeneration;

    d. estimating, using accepted rates of regeneration and a knowledge of the level of the injury, when the onset of recovery is to be expected.

Intercommunicating branches

Intercommunicating branches of clinical significance exist between nerves, in particular the median and musculocutaneous nerves in the upper arm and the median and ulnar nerves in the forearm and hand.

VASA NERVORUM

A knowledge of the arteriae nervorum is essential to an understanding of the importance of their contribution to the nutrition and survival of nerve fibres and to the manner in which they should, for example, be treated in order to preserve the blood supply to the nerve when mobilising it over considerable distances. Because of its importance the blood supply to nerves is discussed separately in Chapter 10.

7. Fascicular anatomy

UNDULATIONS IN FASCICULI AND NERVE FIBRES

In addition to the undulating course taken by a nerve trunk in its bed, the fasciculi also pursue an undulating course within the nerve and nerve fibres do the same inside the fasciculi (Fig. 7.1). The slack in the nerve trunk, fasciculi and nerve fibres provided in this way ensures that traction forces generated by joint movements are normally

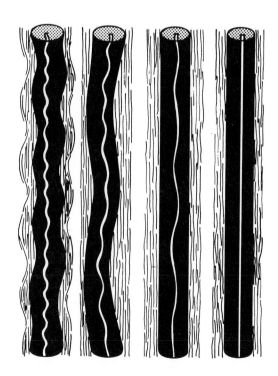

Fig. 7.1 Undulations in the nerve trunk, of the fasciculi within the nerve and nerve fibres within the fasciculi. Only one fasciculus is shown.

fully spent taking up the slack in the system so that the contained nerve fibres are not in jeopardy until deformation reaches pathological levels. The significance of this feature in the genesis of stretch injury is discussed in Chapter 18.

FASCICULI AND FASCICULAR PLEXUSES

Details of the fascicular anatomy of the major peripheral nerves originally provided by Sunderland and his coworkers (1945, 1948, 1959, 1978) have since been confirmed by others (Wintsch 1966; Tamura 1969; Bonnel et al 1978, 1980; Jabaley et al 1980; Shi-Zhen Zhong et al 1980, 1981, 1983; Bonnel 1981, 1985; Chang-Man Zhou 1984; Terzis et al 1984; Chow et al 1985, 1986; Yun-Sho He 1985; Williams and Jabaley 1986; Zhen Han et al 1986; Bartolaminelli 1988; Battiston et al 1988; Di Rosa et al 1988; Guizzi et al 1988; Jäger et al 1988; Libassi 1988). Features of the fascicular anatomy of nerves are:

1. The fasciculi are not arranged as parallel uninterrupted strands along the length of a nerve trunk. On the contrary, they repeatedly divide and unite to form fascicular plexuses that are a key feature of their anatomy (Fig. 7.2).
2. The plexuses are found along the entire length of a nerve, though they are more complex and a more prominent feature in some regions than in others. Even terminal branches such as digital nerves have fascicular plexuses.
3. Not all fasciculi participate in plexus formations at any given level. Some fasciculi or groups of fasciculi run quite long

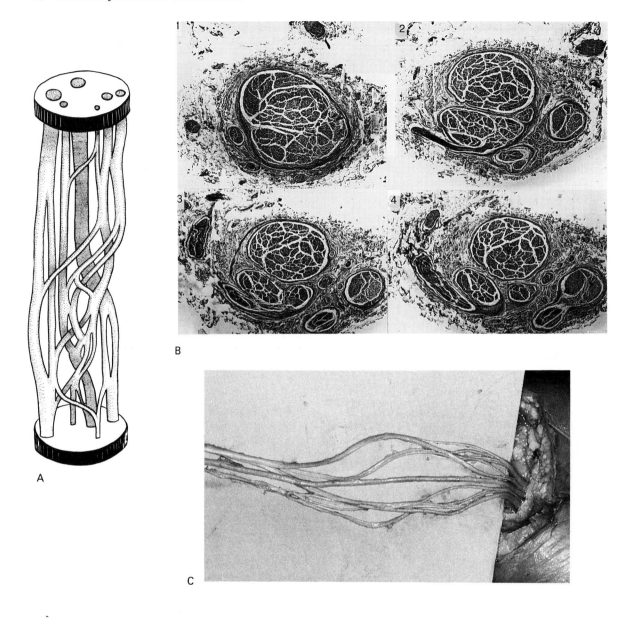

Fig. 7.2   Preparations demonstrating the fascicular structure of nerves. **a** A reconstruction from serial transverse sections of the fascicular structure of a 3 cm length of the musculocutaneous nerve of the arm. **b** Four equidistant transverse sections from a 2 mm length of the facial nerve to illustrate the changes brought about by fascicular divisions and unions. **c** The fascicular plexus in a specimen of the median nerve at and just above the wrist.

distances before engaging in plexus formations.

4. No fasciculus runs an independent unaltered course along the entire length of a nerve. This excludes the possibility of a group of fibres retaining its identity within

the same fasciculus throughout its entire course in the nerve.

5. The precise form of the plexus varies from nerve to nerve, level to level, side to side, and individual to individual.

6. For variable distances above the site of

branching, the fasciculi of that branch are segregated from the others by slight thickenings in the epineurium that allow them to be identified in transverse sections of the nerve.

7. Fascicular plexuses are responsible for producing repeated changes in the size, number, arrangement and branch fibre content of the fasciculi at successive levels along the nerve (Tables 7.1 and 7.2, Fig. 7.3).

8. The size and number of fasciculi are inversely related at any level. The number varies from 1 to more than 100 depending on the nerve and the level.

9. The diameters of most fasciculi range from 0.04 to 2 mm with an occasional fasciculus reaching 4.0 mm.

10. The fasciculi are smaller and more numerous where a nerve crosses a joint.

Table 7.1 The smallest and greatest number of fasciculi observed, regardless of the level and the specimen, in transverse sections from a large series of different peripheral nerves

Nerve	Number
Median	3/37
Radial. Ulnar. Common peroneal division	1/36
Tibial division	11/93
Sciatic nerve in the gluteal region	43/137

Table 7.2 Range of variation in fascicular numbers along the length of four specimens of each major nerve

Nerve	Range of fascicular numbers			
Median	3–22	5–16	4–13	15–36
Ulnar	1–8	1–18	3–8	12–36
Radial	1–20	2–13	2–36	8–29
Tibial division	11–27	16–33	28–93	32–83
Common peroneal division	1–15	1–21	5–20	8–24

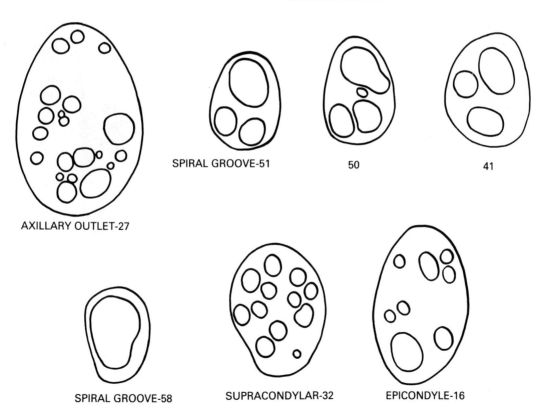

Fig. 7.3 Variations in the size, number and arrangement of the fasciculi in a specimen of the radial nerve between the axilla and the elbow. The figures given are the percentage cross-sectional areas of the nerve devoted to fasciculi.

11. Generalising, the fasciculi in the median and ulnar nerves are larger and fewer in number above the elbow compared with the forearm.

12. For a given total fascicular area, the tensile strength of a nerve increases with the number of fasciculi. Cables of the same size are stronger and more flexible if composed of many strands.

13. In some regions of certain nerves the nerve fibres may be collected into a single fasciculus for a short distance. Examples are the ulnar nerve behind the medial humeral epicondyle, the radial nerve in the spiral groove, the axillary nerve beneath the shoulder joint and the common peroneal (lateral popliteal) nerve in the lower part of the thigh.

14. The examination of successive transverse sections of a nerve reveals rapid and repeated changes in the fascicular pattern so that sections taken more than a few millimetres apart fail to present fascicular patterns that are identical in every respect

(Fig. 7.4). The greatest length of a major nerve with an unchanged fascicular pattern will be about 15–20 mm. However, it is worth repeating that every fasciculus is not involved at the same level, so that some individual fasciculi or fascicular groups run unchanged for much greater distances (Fig. 7.6).

15. The fasciculi are more closely packed in some regions than in others. This is a feature that favours the apposition of fascicular tissue when nerve ends are brought together, thereby offsetting the fascicular mismatching illustrated in Fig. 7.4.

16. The cross-sectional area of a nerve trunk devoted to fascicular tissue varies from nerve to nerve, from level to level along the same nerve and from individual to individual. In general, values range from 25 to 70 per cent. The sciatic nerve in the gluteal region is an exception in that the fascicular tissue in most of these nerves occupies only 20–30 per cent of the cross-sectional area of the nerve. In one specimen examined this area was as low as 12 per cent. This anatomical feature influences:

   a. the susceptibility of nerves to compression (p. 131);
   b. the mismatching of fascicular tissue and epineurial tissue at the nerve ends during nerve repair (p. 398);
   c. the degree to which the distal stump of a transected nerve atrophies (p. 85).

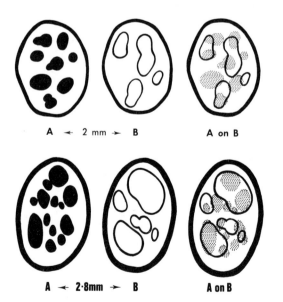

A ← 2 mm → B   A on B

A ← 2·8mm → B   A on B

Fig. 7.4 Tracings of transverse sections from two specimens of the radial nerve, taken 2 mm and 2.8 mm apart, to illustrate: **a** the rapidity of changes in the fascicular pattern (see also Fig. 7.1 b) and **b** the mismatching of fascicular tissue when the sections are brought together.

THE FASCICULAR DISTRIBUTION OF DIFFERENT BRANCH FIBRES

1. Fascicular plexuses bring about the fascicular redistribution, dispersal and intermingling of different branch fibre systems as they are traced along the nerve (Figs 7.5, 7.6, 7.7). Despite the changing fascicular pattern, a particular distal branch fibre system initially pursues a localised course in the nerve for variable, though often considerable, distances above the site of branching. Fascicular plexuses along the nerve then effect a

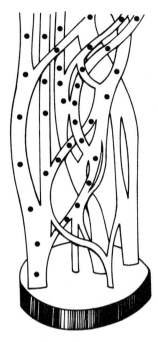

gradual mixing of these fibres with those from other branches, though the combined fibres remain confined to fasciculi in the same quadrant of the nerve for long distances. Further scattering and mixing of the different branch fibre systems gradually continues as the intercommunications are repeated at successive levels until, finally at the root of the limb, the fibres of the different distal branches are widely dispersed through the nerve, each fasciculus containing representatives of many, if not all, of the different branches in varying combinations and proportions.

Thus the arrangement, considered from distal to proximal, is one in which the localisation of any particular branch system is at first discrete, then discrete in combination with other fibres and finally a predominant one only until fibre scattering ultimately reaches a degree at the root of the limb where it cannot be claimed that there is any segregation or localisation of the branch fibre system.

Fig. 7.5 Diagrammatic representation of the fascicular redistribution and dispersal of a branch fibre system brought about by fascicular plexuses.

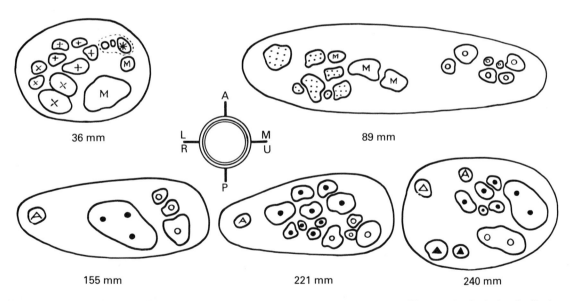

Fig. 7.6 Selected transverse sections of a serially-sectioned specimen of an ulnar nerve to illustrate the fascicular distribution of branch fibre systems in the forearm (not to scale). They illustrate the long course of the dorsal cutaneous branch fascicular group as an independent system within the nerve though the fasciculi comprising the group engage in plexus formations among themselves. Levels are in mm above the tip of the radial styloid process. M, deep (muscular) division fibres; ∗, cutaneous fibres from the hypothenar eminence; +, cutaneous fibres from the ulnar side of the little finger; ×, cutaneous fibres from the fourth digital interspace; fine dots, combined terminal cutaneous fibres; heavy dots, combined terminal motor and cutaneous fibres; ○, dorsal cutaneous fibres of the hand; △, flexor carpi ulnaris fibres; A, branch fibres to the ulnar artery; ▲, flexor digitorum profundus fibres.

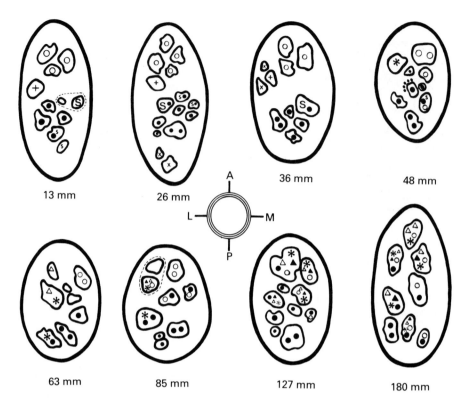

Fig. 7.7 Selected transverse sections from a serially-sectioned radial nerve illustrating the fascicular redistribution of the different branch fibre systems brought about by fascicular plexuses. The levels are in mm above the lateral humeral epicondyle. The code for the fibres of the different branches is: ○, superficial radial; ●●, posterior interosseous; S, supinator; +, X, extensor carpi radialis brevis and longus, respectively; ★, combined radial wrist-extensors; △, brachioradialis; ▲, brachialis.

However, in the case of branches leaving the nerve at the root of the limb, their fibres, though localised in the nerve above the site of branching, will occupy fasciculi that also contain fibres representing more distal branches.

Expressed in another way, this means that, at the root of the limb, the nerve fibres representing all distal branches are intermingled and widely distributed through the fasciculi of the nerve. On the other hand, the fibres of proximal branches are concentrated in that sector of the nerve from which branching is about to occur, though the fibres will be mixed with those for distally destined branches. As the nerve proceeds distally, the fascicular plexuses effect a sorting out of the different branch fibre systems until, finally, the fibres for a particular branch are collected into their own fasciculus or group of fasciculi which then leaves the nerve as a definitive branch.

2. The fascicular composition of the fibres representing any particular branch can be expressed in terms of three levels:

a. At the root of the limb the fibres of branches at and below the elbow and knee are widely distributed over many, if not all, of the fasciculi, and are mixed with the fibres of other more distal branches in varying combinations and proportions, though each fasciculus does not necessarily contain fibres from every branch. The fibres of high branches, though mixed with those from distal sources, are relatively localised and superficially placed because they are shortly to leave the nerve.

b. An intermediate zone where the fibres are contained in fasciculi which, though not devoted exclusively to them, occupy a

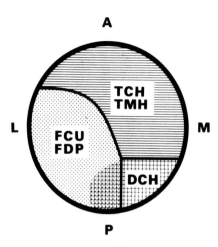

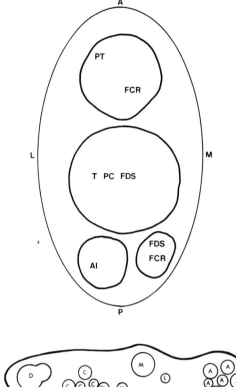

Fig. 7.8 Diagram of a transverse section of an ulnar nerve at the elbow showing a predominant localisation of the different branch fibres in the nerve at that level. TCH and TMH: the terminal sensory and motor divisions respectively of the ulnar nerve at the wrist; DCH: dorsal cutaneous fibres of the hand; FCU: flexor carpi ulnaris; FDP: flexor digitorum profundus; A.P.M.L. Anterior, posterior, medial and lateral, respectively.

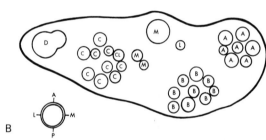

relatively localised position in the nerve (Figs 7.8, 7.9).

c. A distal zone where, for a variable but usually short distance above the site of branching, the fibres of a branch are contained in a fasciculus or group of fasciculi devoted exclusively to them, and are sharply localised and superficially placed in the nerve.

3. A fasciculus or fascicular group representing a particular branch may, while retaining its identity in the nerve, migrate from one sector to another before engaging in plexus formations with other fasciculi. This often leads to a considerable translocation of one or other fascicular systems before union is effected. This occurs, for example:

a. where multiple branches from a muscle enter different aspects of a nerve at different levels. The fasciculi representing one branch may migrate considerable distances through or over the surface of the nerve in order to reach and unite with fasciculi representing the other branch. Multiple branches serving the flexor digitorum sublimis are a case in point. Though the fasciculi of different

Fig. 7.9 Diagrams of transverse sections of: **a** a median nerve at the elbow showing the branch fibre sharing of fasciculi but with some degree of localisation retained. The circles represent groups of fasciculi and not a single fasciculus. T, Terminal motor and sensory fibres for the hand; P, Palmar cutaneous; FDS, Flexor digitorum superficialis (sublimis); FCR, Flexor carpi radialis; AI, Anterior interosseous; PT, Pronator teres; A.P.M.L., Anterior, posterior, medial and lateral, respectively. **b** at the wrist where the localisation is now precise in terms of the individual branches of the median nerve in the hand, each circle now representing a single fasciculus: A.B.C., cutaneous nerve fibres from the branches to the third, second and first interdigital areas; D, cutaneous fibres to the radial side of the thumb; M, thenar motor fibres; L, lumbrical fibres.

branches join different aspects of the median nerve, some later migrate to reach and combine with others to form a common flexor sublimis fascicular group.

b. where fasciculi representing different muscles having similar actions come together and fuse before participating in further fascicular intercommunications. Thus the extensor carpi radialis longus fascicular group migrates some distance round the radial nerve in order to reach and later fuse with the extensor carpi radialis brevis fascicular group (Fig. 7.7).

Finally, a nerve trunk may undergo a change in shape or partial rotation during its course.

All this means that, in transverse sections of a nerve a few centimetres apart, a bundle group representing a particular branch system may occupy different sectors. Alignment of the nerve ends to correct for this would only throw other fascicular groups out of alignment.

4. As regards branch fibre composition, fasciculi are of two types (Figs 7.6 and 7.7):

a. simple fasciculi that are composed of fibres from the same source. These are found at distal levels.
b. compound fasciculi that are composed of fibres from different sources in varying numbers, combinations and proportions. These are found at proximal levels.

COMMENT

Recent work by Schady et al (1983) on the peripheral projections of fascicles in the human median nerve has cast doubt on some features of the fascicular redistribution of peripheral branch nerve fibre systems as described here. They write 'Our results suggest that despite the changing anatomical fascicular pattern, a degree of segregation of muscle and skin nerve fibres is present in the proximal segments of the median nerve'. This claim is based on the results of a study of the responses to intrafascicular microstimulation in alert human subjects employed to study the degree of mixing of muscle and skin nerve fibres at two levels in the median nerve. Sixty-six experiments were conducted on 4 subjects and the median nerve was stimulated at the wrist and 5–13 cm above the medial humeral epicondyle. Because of its importance their paper calls for the following comment:

1. The use of the term 'upper arm' in their paper is misleading in that the recordings were made 5–13 cm above the medial humeral epicondyle without any reference as to whether or not there was a bias towards the 5 cm or the 13 cm level. A more appropriate term would have been 'lower half of the upper arm'. As regards fascicular fibre redistribution there is a significant difference between 'upper arm' and lower half of upper arm because, in the case of the latter, the fascicular translocation of nerve fibres is far from complete. Even at the root of the limb, some branch fibres, particularly those of proximal branches, may remain concentrated in certain fasciculi though in combination with others.

2. Nerve fibre segregation is expressed solely in terms of 'skin' and muscle fibres as opposed to branch fibre systems. In this respect the choice of the median nerve for study was, perhaps, unfortunate in that 'skin' nerve fibres predominate in this nerve, outnumbering motor fibres by 9 to 1 at the wrist and by about 2 to 1 above the elbow. This means that unqualified 'skin' nerve fibres will not only include several different sensory branches but will also dominate the fibre composition of some fasciculi at all levels.

3. The number of fascicles in the median nerve at the wrist varies from 11 to 37 and in the lower half of the upper arm from 4 to 26. In their experiments there was no way of knowing precisely how many fasciculi there were at any given test level. Nor is the number of fasciculi subjected to intrafascicular stimulation at any one level in any one experiment given, though it is unlikely, in view of their numbers, that every fasciculus at the test level would have been subjected to intrafascicular stimulation. This, of course, leaves unanswered the branch fibre composition of the many other untested fasciculi at that level. In such a situation the conclusions drawn from the observations could be in error.

4. The concept of segregation at central levels relates to 'skin' fibres on the one hand and motor fibres on the other, without reference to individual branch fibre systems. However, within each group (skin and motor) there was evidence of the fascicular redistribution and mixing of fibres at proximal levels, e.g. 'territories of upper arm fascicles often appeared to cover three or four fingers

and much of the palm'; fascicular fields were 'considerably smaller when recording at the wrist than in the upper arm'.

There are also references to motor fibres for different muscles being located in the same fasciculus and a reduction of 'strictly pure skin fascicles' in the upper arm compared with their numbers at the wrist.

5. The claim that most of the rearrangements of spinal root fibres into terminal branch groupings occur at brachial plexus level is not disputed, since the word *most* relates to a question of degree that defies measurement. What is emphasised in reply is that a fascicular rearrangement of branch fibre systems continues into and down the arm.

6. That some segregation of some branch fibre systems may exist in the lower half of the upper arm is not denied but there are many factors that could account for this without jeopardising the general concept of a gradual fascicular redistribution and mixing of the different branch fibres as they course centrally or distally in the nerve.

7. Stimulation of the exposed nerve ends at operation in the conscious patient and the histochemical analysis of biopsy sections from nerve ends confirm the mixing of motor and sensory fibres at levels distal to the brachial plexus (Chapter 42).

8. The lesson is that morphological conclusions should not be drawn from physiological evidence alone. An examination of the reported findings of Schady and his associates reveals that it is the extent to which branch fibre mixing occurs that is in dispute. However, with the techniques currently available, it is not possible to quantify this feature so that the nature and extent of fibre mixing in human nerves can be expressed only in general terms. Their findings do not disprove the existence of a high percentage of fasciculi in the upper arm bearing fibres from different branches, that is from different peripheral sources. Nor do they in any respect weaken the claim that fascicular intercommunications, traced along the nerve from distal to proximal, are responsible for effecting the gradual mixing of the fibres representing different branches.

In conclusion, as an addendum to the aforesaid, it should be stressed again that:

a. the fascicular redistribution of branch fibres brought about by fascicular plexuses occurs gradually over successive levels;

b. the precise manner in which fasciculi divide and fuse, and the manner in which these changes bring about the mixing and fascicular redistribution of different branch fibres are subject to considerable individual variation;

c. the branch fibre content and composition of fasciculi will naturally be affected by variations in the number of branches, in the level at which these enter or leave the nerve, and in their distribution. For example, common variations in the motor innervation of thenar muscles vis à vis the relative contributions from median and ulnar sources, as well as in the cutaneous distribution of these two nerves, will be reflected in the branch fibre composition of fasciculi and in their fascicular redistribution in the nerve.

d. The concentration of fibres representing a particular branch in individual fasciculi at any given level will vary depending on the level in question, individual variations in the pattern of branching, and in the distribution of individual branches as well as in the manner in which fascicular intercommunications take place.

CLINICAL SIGNIFICANCE

These features of fascicular anatomy have particular relevance to:

1. The consequences of partial injury.
2. The pathology and classification of nerve injuries.
3. Nerve repair. In this respect they emphasise the importance of:

   a. maintaining correct axial alignment of the nerve ends during repair in order to take advantage of any branch fibre localisation obtaining at that level;

   b. the need to maximise fascicular apposition during nerve repair and to minimise the wasteful regeneration of axons into the interfascicular epineurial tissue occasioned by dissimilarities in the fascicular patterns at the nerve ends. This can be achieved by grouping the fasciculi not only to improve fascicular apposition but also arranging them in a manner designed to take advantage of any persisting concentration of branch fibre systems at that level;

c. the distance for which a branch may be safely stripped from the nerve trunk, when mobilising the nerve, without damaging the remaining fasciculi. This is determined by the intraneural length over which the branch fasciculi retain their individuality before engaging in plexus formations with other fasciculi composed of fibres from other branches.

REFERENCES

Bartolaminelli P 1988 Femoral nerve: anatomy and fascicular arrangement In: Brunelli G (ed) Textbook of Microsurgery. Masson, Milano, p 591

Battiston B, Guizzi P, Di Rosa F 1988 Median nerve: anatomy and fascicular arrangement. In: Brunelli G (ed) Textbook of Microsugery. Masson, Milano, p 567

Bonnel F 1981 Fascicular organisation of the peripheral nerves. International Journal of Microsurgery 3: 85

Bonnel F 1985 Histologic structure of the ulnar nerve in the hand. Journal of Hand Surgery 10A: 264

Bonnel F, Durand Y, Blotman F, Godebout 1978 Anatomie et systematisation fasciculaire du nerf médian. Masson, Paris

Bonnel F, Mailhe P, Allieu Y, Rabischong P 1980 Bases anatomiques de la chirurgie fasciculaire du nerf médian. Annales Chirurgie 34: 707

Chang-Man Zhou 1984 A study of the microsurgical anatomy of the sciatic nerve. Acta Anatomica Sinica 15: 118

Chow J, van Beek A, Meyer D L, Johnson M C 1985 Surgical significance of the motor fascicular group of the ulnar nerve in the forearm. Journal of Hand Surgery 10A: 867

Chow J, van Beek A, Bilos Z J, Meyer D L, Johnson M C 1986 Anatomical basis for repair of ulnar and median nerves in the distal part of the forearm by group fascicular suture and nerve grafting. Journal of Bone and Joint Surgery 68A: 273

Di Rosa F, Guizzi P, Battiston B 1988 Radial nerve: anatomy and fascicular arrangement. In: Brunelli G (ed) Textbook of Microsurgery. Masson, Milano, p 571

Guizzi P, Battiston B, Di Rosa F 1988 Musculocutaneous nerve: anatomy and fascicular arrangement. In: Brunelli G (ed) Textbook of Microsurgery. Masson, Milano, p 579

Jabaley M E, Wallace W H, Heckler F R 1980 Internal topography of major nerves of the forearm and hand: a current view. Journal of Hand Surgery 5: 1

Jäger C, Guizzi P, Di Rosa F 1988 Ulnar nerve: anatomy and fascicular arrangement. In: Brunelli G (ed) Textbook of Microsurgery. Masson, Milano, p 575

Libassi G, Vigasio A 1988 Sciatic nerve: anatomy and fascicular arrangement. In: Brunelli G (ed) Textbook of Microsurgery. Masson, Milano, p 583

Schady W, Ochoa J L, Torebjork H E et al 1983 Peripheral projections of fascicles in the human median nerve. Brain 106: 745

Shi-Zhen Zhong, Mu-Zhi Liu, Jia-Kai Zhu 1980 A study of the microsurgical anatomy of the median nerve. Acta Anatomica Sinica 11: 337

Shi-Zhen Zhong, Mu-Zhi Liu, Yong-Song Tao 1981 A study of the microsurgical anatomy of the ulnar nerve. Acta Anatomica Sinica 12: 346

Shi-Zhen Zhong, Mu-Zhi Liu, Chang-Man Zhou et al 1983 A study of the microsurgical anatomy of the radial nerve. Acta Anatomica Sinica 14: 1

Sunderland S 1945 The intraneural topography of the radial, median and ulnar nerves. Brain 68: 243

Sunderland S 1978 Nerves and nerve injuries. 2nd edn. Churchill Livingstone, Edinburgh

Sunderland S, Ray L J 1948 The intraneural topography of the sciatic nerve and its popliteal divisions in man. Brain 71:242

Sunderland S, Marshall R D, Swaney W E 1959 The intraneural topography of the circumflex musculocutaneous and obturator nerves. Brain 82: 116

Tamura K 1969 The funicular pattern of Japanese peripheral nerves. Archivum Japonicum Chirurgicum 38: 35

Terzis J K, Feeker B L, Sismour E N 1984 A computerized study of the intraneural organisation of the median nerve. Journal of Hand Surgery 9A: 605

Williams H B, Jabaley M E 1986 The importance of internal anatomy of the peripheral nerves to nerve repair in the forearm and hand. Hand Clinics 2: 689

Wintsch K 1966 Die Topographie des medianus — querschnittes. Chirurgie: Zeitschrift für aller Gebiete der Operativen Medizin 37: 268

Yun-Sho He 1985 Applied anatomical study on radial nerve using histochemical method for acetylcholine esterase. Chinese Journal of Clinical Anatomy 3: 135

Zhen Han, Shi-Zhen Zhong, Bo Sun et al 1986 Anatomical study of the natural fasciculi of radial, ulnar and median nerves and the clinical significance. Chinese Journal of Surgery 24: 23

8. Numbers of nerve fibres for individual branches

In the absence of any known influence directing a regenerating axon back into its original endoneurial tube in the distal stump after nerve transection and repair, the entry of axons into the endoneurial tubes becomes largely a matter of chance. Under these circumstances the numbers of axons representing a particular branch in the nerve at the level of the repair becomes a factor influencing the restoration of functionally useful connections at the periphery.

Where, for example, a particular branch system is represented by large numbers of axons then the chances of at least some of these entering the corresponding, or a functionally related, endoneurial tube in the distal stump are greatly enhanced. On the other hand, these chances are greatly reduced when the axons of a branch system are, in comparison, much fewer in number. This factor is of particular relevance at levels in the nerve where the nerve fibres of various branches are widely dispersed and intermingled. It is in this way that branch fibre numbers become a factor influencing the quality of recovery after nerve repair.

Counting the number of fibres in every branch of a major peripheral nerve would be a formidable task and, to the knowledge of the author, has not yet been attempted. However, it is possible to obtain some estimate of this feature by measuring the cross-sectional area of the fasciculi devoted solely to individual branches. Admittedly this method has its limitations, because the relationship between area and numbers is affected by such factors as the size of individual nerve fibres and the amount of intrafascicular endoneurial tissue. With this proviso the cross-sectional area of the fasciculi devoted to individual branches may be accepted as a rough estimate of the numbers of fibres in a nerve representing individual branches. Such area data for the median, ulnar, radial and sciatic nerves are provided in Tables 8.1–8.7. They are abbreviations from more detailed information available elsewhere (Sunderland & Bedbrook 1949, Sunderland 1978).

In the tables the term muscular is used to refer to the branches entering a muscle. The term motor has not been used because the branch also contains proprioceptor and other sensory nerve fibres.

In expressing branch fibre numbers in this way it should be noted that such estimates are also influenced by variations in the number of branches, the level of branching and the distribution of those branches.

The percentage cross-sectional area of fasciculi composed of fibres representing individual branches also depends on the level at which the measurement is made. This is illustrated by reference to the percentage cross-sectional fascicular areas of a median and an ulnar nerve trunk occupied by cutaneous and 'muscle' nerve fibres *from the hand*, measured at the wrist and above the elbow (see p. 45)

At the wrist

	Muscle	*Cutaneous*
Median	6	94
Ulnar	44	56

Data provided by Bonnel (1985) for the ulnar nerve at the wrist, based on myelinated nerve fibre counts in 20 specimens, give the fibres of the superficial (sensory) division outnumbering those of the deep (muscular) division by about 2 to 1.

Table 8.1 Median nerve. The percentage fascicular cross-sectional area occupied by the fibres of different branches. Ten specimens

Branch	Maximal	Minimal	Mean
Pronator teres	7	4	6
Flexor carpi radialis	6	3	4
Flexor digitorum sublimis	12	5	7
Anterior interosseous	14	9	11
Palmar cutaneous	2	1	2
Terminal muscular	6	1	4
Terminal cutaneous	74	61	66
Total muscular	39	26	33
Total cutaneous	74	61	67

Table 8.2 Ulnar nerve. The percentage fascicular cross-sectional area occupied by the fibres of different branches. Twelve specimens

Branch	Maximal	Minimal	Mean
Flexor carpi ulnaris	14	7	11
Flexor digitorum profundus	9	2	6
Palmar cutaneous	6	1	2
Dorsal cutaneous of hand	26	11	18
Terminal cutaneous (superficial division)	43	29	35
Terminal muscular (deep division)	36	22	28
Total muscular	56	40	46
Total cutaneous	60	44	54

Table 8.3 Radial nerve. The percentage fascicular cross-sectional area occupied by the fibres of different branches. Eleven specimens

Branch	Maximal	Minimal	Mean
Superficial radial	37	23	29
Brachialis	5	1	2
Brachioradialis	12	3	6
Extensor carpi radialis longus	12	5	9
Extensor carpi radialis brevis	10	6	7
Posterior interosseous	57	38	47
Branches of the posterior interosseous (four specimens only)			
Supinator	14	3	
Extensor carpi ulnaris } Extensor digiti quinti } Extensor digitorum communis }	20	7	
Extensor indicis proprius	5	2	
Abductor pollicis longus	8	3	
Extensor pollicis brevis	6	3	
Extensor pollicis longus	10	4	
Total muscular	77	63	71
Total cutaneous	37	23	29

Table 8.4 Tibial (medial popliteal) nerve in the gluteal region. The percentage fascicular cross-sectional area occupied by the fibres of different branches. Ten specimens

Branch	Maximal	Minimal	Mean
Semimembranosus	7	2	4
Semitendinosus	7	2	4
Biceps	8	4	6
Adductor magnus	6	3	4
Medial gastrocnemius	7	3	5
Lateral gastrocnemius	5	2	3
Soleus	12	6	8
Popliteus	7	2	3
Tibialis posterior	6	2	3
Flexor digitorum longus	3	1	2
Flexor hallucis longus	2	1	2
Sural	8	3	5
Medial calcaneal	10	2	6
Articular	7	0.5	3
Total muscular	52	38	44
Total sensory (cutaneous and articular)	18	7	14
Total plantars	52	35	41
Total arterial	1	0.2	1

Table 8.5 Tibial (medial popliteal) nerve in the popliteal fossa. The percentage fascicular cross-sectional area occupied by the fibres of different branches. Ten specimens

Branch	Maximal	Minimal	Mean
Medial gastrocnemius	8	4	6
Lateral gastrocnemius	7	3	4
Soleus	14	7	10
Popliteus	8	2	4
Tibialis posterior	7	2	4
Flexor digitorum longus	4	1	2
Flexor hallucis longus	3	2	2
Sural	9	4	6
Medial calcaneal	12	3	7
Articular	8	1	4
Total muscular	40	27	32
Total sensory (cutaneous and articular)	22	10	17
Total plantars	62	43	50
Total arterial	1	0.3	1

Table 8.6 Common peroneal (lateral popliteal) nerve in the gluteal region. The percentage fascicular cross-sectional area occupied by the fibres of different branches. Ten specimens

Branch	Maximal	Minimal	Mean
Biceps femoris	9	4	7
Peroneus longus	13	8	9
Peroneus brevis	6	3	5
Tibialis anterior	10	5	8
Extensor digitorum longus	8	3	5
Extensor hallucis longus	5	2	3
Extensor digitorum brevis	2	1	1
Sural communicating	19	3	9
Lateral cutaneous of calf	17	6	11
Superficial peroneal (musculocutaneous)	39	16	25
Arterial	3	1	2
Articular	9	3	6
Total muscular	44	32	38
Total sensory (cutaneous and articular)	66	56	60
Total arterial	3	1	2

Table 8.7 Common peroneal (lateral popliteal) nerve in the popliteal fossa. The percentage fascicular cross-sectional area occupied by the fibres of different branches. Ten specimens

Branch	Maximal	Minimal	Mean
Peroneus longus	14	8	11
Peroneus brevis	7	3	5
Total peronei	20	13	16
Tibialis anterior	11	5	9
Extensor digitorum longus	9	3	5
Extensor hallucis longus	5	2	3
Extensor digitorum brevis	2	1	1
Sural communicating	20	4	10
Lateral cutaneous of calf	18	6	12
Superficial peroneal (musculocutaneous)	41	19	26
Arterial	3	1	2
Articular	10	3	6
Total muscular	39	26	34
Total sensory (cutaneous and articular)	72	61	64
Total arterial	3	1	2

Above the elbow

The same nerve fibres from the hand are here combined with the fibres of the remaining branches of the nerves, and collectively they now occupy a reduced percentage cross-sectional area of the nerve.

	Muscle	*Cutaneous*
Median	4	66
Ulnar	28	35

REFERENCES

Bonnel F 1985 Histologic structure of the ulnar nerve in the hand. Journal of Hand Surgery 10A: 264
Sunderland S 1978 Nerves and nerve injuries, 2nd edn. Churchill Livingstone, Edinburgh
Sunderland S, Bedbrook G M 1949 The cross-sectional area of peripheral nerve trunks occupied by the fibres representing individual muscular and cutaneous branches. Brain 72: 613

9. Connective tissues of nerve trunks

The epineurium, endoneurium and perineurium constitute the connective tissues of peripheral nerves and each has its own special structural characteristics and functional properties. Terminology relating to this component is given in Chapter 4.

THE EPINEURIUM

Key features of this tissue are:

1. The epineurium provides a supporting and protective framework for the fasciculi embedded in it (Fig. 6.1 see p. 27).
2. It is composed of areolar connective tissue with the usual varieties of cells, a loose meshwork of collagen fibres and an occasional elastic fibre.
3. When elastic fibres are seen they occur singly and branch in an irregular manner. In contrast, the collagen fibres predominate, are unbranched, and are arranged singly or are collected into longitudinal bundles that interlace in all directions to outline an irregular lattice pattern.
4. The collagen fibres of the epineurium are thicker than those of the perineurium and endoneurium (Fig. 9.1).
5. Adipose tissue may be present in the epineurium of some nerves, varying in amount from individual to individual and at different levels along the same nerve. The sciatic nerve usually contains appreciable quantities of adipose tissue in the gluteal region, the lateral popliteal division usually containing less adipose tissue than the medial (Sunderland 1945).

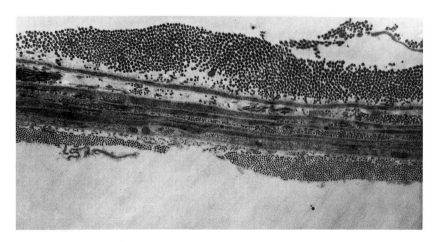

Fig. 9.1 Transverse section across the epineurial (*top*), perineurial (*centre*) and endoneurial (*lower*) tissue interfaces. The collagen fibres of the epineurium are thicker than those of the perineurium and endoneurium. Elastin is present in the inner layers of the perineurium.

6. Other constituents of the epineurium are nerves, lymphatics and the largest nutrient vessels together with the vascular networks formed from them. Venae nervorum outnumber the arteriae nervorum.

7 The epineurium is generally of the same consistency throughout the nerve trunk but shows condensations:

    a. at the surface to give the nerve a circumscribed and distinctive cord-like structure and consistency that clearly demarcate it from surrounding tissues;

    b. around a group of fasciculi that are about to leave the nerve as a branch.

8. Though collagen fibres are relatively inextensible and inelastic their lattice arrangement imparts an element of extensibility and elasticity to the system that maintains the undulations in the nerve trunk.

9. The capacity of the epineurium to resist tensile loading is limited. Once the undulations in the nerve trunk are eliminated, and the nerve fully straightened, continued stretching involves the fasciculi which resist and control further extension until the elastic limit is reached.

10. The main function of the epineurium is to protect the fasciculi and their contained nerve fibres from compression forces.

11. The amount of this tissue varies not only from nerve to nerve and person to person but also from level to level along the same nerve.

12. In general the cross-sectional area of a nerve trunk devoted to epineurial tissue varies from 30 to 75 per cent. An exception is the sciatic nerve in the gluteal region where the nerve consistently contains large amounts of epineurium, most sciatic nerves being composed of from 70 to 88 per cent of this tissue. Information on this feature is available for each of the peripheral nerves (Sunderland and Bradley 1949; Sunderland 1978).

13. The cross-sectional area of a nerve occupied by epineurium is related to the size and number of the fasciculi. There is usually more epineurium where the fasciculi are small and numerous compared with where they are large and few in number.

14. Regardless of their number, the fasciculi are more closely packed with less epineurial tissue in some regions, and in some nerves, than in others.

15. Generally speaking, where nerves cross joints they are composed of numerous small fasciculi widely separated by large amounts of epineurial tissue. This arrangement provides a greater degree of protection for the fasciculi and their contained nerve fibres during limb movements.

16. Solutions diffuse widely and freely through the loose epineurium where adipose tissue, when present, may absorb and fix fat soluble agents.

17. The relative cross-sectional areas of a nerve devoted to epineurial and fascicular tissues vary from nerve to nerve, and level to level along individual nerves. This feature has special relevance to:

    a. the susceptibility of nerves to compression and stretch injury (p. 131);

    b. the apposition of fascicular to epineurial tissue at the nerve end during nerve repair (p. 398);

    c. the degree to which the denervated distal stump of a severed nerve atrophies (p. 85).

THE PERINEURIUM

The perineurium is the thin but dense and distinctive tissue sheath investing each fasciculus (Fig. 6.1). It is composed of three readily identifiable layers.

1. *An internal layer*. This is composed of a single layer of flattened mesothelial cells presenting a smooth inner surface with tight junctions at cell boundaries. This layer is separated from the endoneurium by a potential subperineurial space which is crossed by septa passing from the perineurium to blend with the endoneurium. These septa represent the recent union of

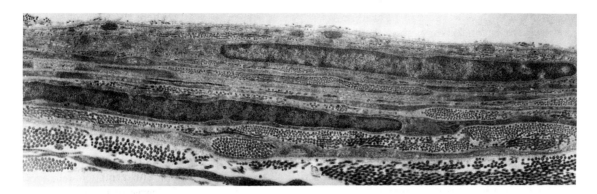

Fig. 9.2 Transverse section of the perineurial sheath of a fasciculus, illustrating the perineurial cells and collagen fibres interposed between the lamellae.

two fasciculi, the impending division of a single fasciculus, or the passage of nutrient vessels into the fasciculus.

2. *An external layer.* This merges with the epineurium and marks a gradual transition from perineurium to epineurium, perineurial cells being replaced by fibroblasts and the collagen fibres becoming thicker and losing their somewhat orderly arrangement in favour of that characteristic of the epineurium.

3. *A middle layer.* This is composed of flattened perineurial cells arranged in a series of 3–15 concentric lamellae depending on the size of the fasciculus (Fig. 9.2). The lamellae are separated by clefts that are crossed by the processes of perineurial cells and contain collagen fibres, most of which are longitudinally aligned. Others are arranged circularly and obliquely to outline a compact network. The collagen fibres are about half the thickness of those in the epineurium. The clefts contain only an occasional elastic fibre. The perineurial cells have features that suggest that they may have contractile properties. They possess a basement membrane, have tight cell junctions and collectively constitute a diffusion barrier to the passage of a wide range of macromolecular substances.

Key features of the perineurium are:

1. It forms a tubular sheath for the contents of the fasciculus from which it may be easily separated and within which nerve fibres have some freedom of movement.

2. The perineurium varies in thickness from 1.3 μm to 100 μm, a linear relationship existing between the diameter of a fasciculus and the thickness of its perineurial sheath. This applies to all nerves at all levels but the ratio varies slightly.

3. The structural properties of the perineurium give the fasciculi an undulating course in the epineurium, smaller fasciculi having finer undulations than larger fasciculi.

4. The function of the perineurium is to protect the nerve fibres in the fasciculus.

5. The perineurium resists and maintains an intrafascicular pressure. Evidence for this is provided by the following sets of observations:

   a. The direct measurement of endoneurial fluid pressure by micropipette techniques (Low and Dyck 1977, Low et al 1977, Myers et al 1978; Lundborg et al 1983).

   b. Any breach in the perineurium is immediately followed by the herniation of the contents of the fasciculus through the opening (Sunderland 1946).

   c. In order to maintain the same circumferential tension to resist a given internal pressure, the relationship between the diameter of a thin walled tube and the thickness of its wall must be a linear one. This is the relationship that obtains between the diameter of a fasciculus and the thickness of its perineurial sheath (Sunderland & Bradley 1952).

d. The manner in which endoneurial tubes shrink and the fascicular area is reduced, following Wallerian degeneration and the removal of the axon and myelin debris, is consistent with the existence of an intrafascicular pressure maintained by a contractile elastic perineurium (Chapter 14).

6. The tensile strength and elasticity of nerve trunks depend largely on fascicular tissue, the perineurium playing the major role in maintaining the integrity of a nerve under tension.

7. The denervated distal segment of a nerve has the same tensile strength and elasticity as the normal proximal segment.

8. The elasticity and integrity of a nerve under elongation are retained as long as the perineurium remains intact (Chapter 12).

9. For a given total fascicular area, the total perineurial circumference will increase as the total number of fasciculi increases. This explains why the strength of a nerve increases as the number of its component fasciculi increases. Cables of the same size are stronger when they are composed of many strands.

10. The perineurium has considerable tensile strength and elasticity. The intrafascicular pressure can be raised experimentally to 750 mm Hg before the perineurium ruptures (Selander & Sjöstrand 1978).

11. The perineurium functions as a bidirectional diffusion barrier (Martin 1964, Olsson & Reese 1969, Söderfeldt et al 1973, Oldfors & Sourander 1978, Oldfors & Johansson 1979, Oldfors 1981). Where a nerve is composed of one or a few large fasciculi, the thicker perineurium reduces and slows the movement of diffusible agents across it. On the other hand, where the nerve is composed of many small fasciculi the perineurium is not only thinner but its surface area is also greatly increased. Both features increase the accessibility of a greater number of nerve fibres to diffusible agents.

12. The diffusion barrier properties of the perineurium are resistant to ischaemia of at least 24 hours duration (Lundborg et al 1973; Soderfeldt et al 1973).

13. The perineurium is a barrier to the spread of infection and the inflammatory reaction associated with it. Providing this sheath remains intact a nerve may traverse, and be surrounded by, an infected field without the fasciculi being invaded, though the infection may spread through the epineurium. If the perineurium is breached or a fasciculus severed, the damaged fasciculus becomes involved in a rapidly spreading neuritis.

14. Spinal nerve roots do not possess epineurial or perineurial tissue which (a) increases their susceptibility to stretch and compression injury, and (b) increases their exposure to chemical and other agents.

THE ENDONEURIUM

The endoneurium is the intrafascicular connective tissue packing that provides a framework for the support and protection of the nerve fibres that are embedded in it (Fig. 6.1). Key features of this tissue are:

1. Collagen fibres predominate and are about half the thickness of those in the epineurium. The majority are arranged longitudinally and the remainder obliquely. There is considerable doubt surrounding the presence of elastin fibres. They are certainly not a conspicuous feature of the endoneurium.

2. There is some evidence to suggest that the collagen fibres of the endoneurium are a product of the activity of Schwann cells rather than of endoneurial fibroblasts.

3. Condensations of the endoneurium form fine septa that subdivide the nerve fibres into small groupings.

4. The endoneurium contains tissue spaces occupied by tissue fluid. There are no intrafascicular lymphatics.
5. With few exceptions the only vessels found in the endoneurium are capillaries.
6. The endoneurium has a special relationship to individual nerve fibres, around which it forms a thin bilaminar sheath which is applied to the basement membrane of the Schwann cell layer.
The inner of the two layers is composed of a fine reticulum of argyrophilic material. It is more delicate than the outer of the two layers, which is composed of closely packed collagen fibres. This bilaminar sheath forms the wall of what is conveniently referred to as an endoneurial tube that contains the axon, the Schwann cell layer and myelin when it is present. When the Schwann cells become active during Wallerian degeneration they separate readily from this sheath.
7. The endoneurium of cutaneous nerves contains more collagen fibres than deeply placed nerves, presumably reflecting the greater protection required for the nerve fibres of the more vulnerable superficial nerves.
8. Nerve fibres run an undulating course inside the fasciculi. When nerve trunks are stretched nerve fibres do not commence to share the load until these undulations have been eliminated.
9. The endoneurial sheath of a nerve fibre is not a rigid structure but has extensibility and elasticity. With Wallerian degeneration, and the removal of axon and myelin debris from the tube, the wall of the latter contracts around the surviving Schwann cells to give a thinner endoneurial tube. During axon regeneration the elasticity and extensibility of the endoneurial sheath allow it to yield to the forces generated by the new axon as its diameter increases.
10. The collagen fibres of the endoneurial tissue of spinal nerve roots are fewer and finer than those of the endoneurium of peripheral nerves.
11. That the endoneurium has some tensile strength and elasticity is revealed by mechanically testing spinal nerve roots where endoneurial tissue is present but epi- and perineurial tissues are absent. However, values for these two properties are well below those for the perineurium.
12. In the case of spinal nerve roots, where epineurial tissue is absent, the effects of compression appear earlier and are more severe than is the case with peripheral nerves where the fasciculi, and indirectly their contained nerve fibres, are well protected by epineurial tissue.

REFERENCES

Low P A, Dyck P 1977 Increased endoneurial fluid pressure in experimental lead neuropathy. Nature 269: 427
Low P, Marchand G, Knox F, Dyck P 1977 Measurement of endoneurial fluid pressure with polyethylene matrix capsules. Brain Research 122: 373
Lundborg G, Nordborg C, Rydevik B, Olsson Y 1973 The effect of ischaemia on the permeability of the perineurium to protein tracers in rabbit tibial nerve. Acta Neurologica Scandinavica 49: 287
Lundborg G, Myers R, Powell H 1983 Nerve compression injury and increase in endoneurial fluid pressure. 'A miniature compartment syndrome'. Journal of Neurology, Neurosurgery and Psychiatry 46: 1119
Martin K H 1964 Untersuchungen über die perineurale Diffusionsbarriäre an gefriergetrockneten Nerven. Zeitschrift für Zellforschung 64: 404

Myers R R, Powell H C, Costello M L, Lambert P W, Zwërfach B W 1978 Endoneurial fluid pressure: direct measurement with micropipettes. Brain Research 148: 510
Oldfors A 1981 Permeability of the perineurium of small nerve fascicles; an ultrastructural study using ferritin in rats. Neuropathology and Applied Neurobiology 7: 183
Oldfors A, Sourander P 1978 Barriers of peripheral nerve towards exogenous peroxidase in normal and protein deprived rats. Acta Neuropathologica Berlin 43: 129
Oldfors A, Johansson B R 1979 Barriers and transport properties of the perineurium. An ultrastructural study with ^{125}I-labelled albumin and horse-radish peroxidase in normal and protein deprived rats. Acta Neuropathologica Berlin 47: 139
Olsson Y, Reese T S 1969 Inaccessibility of the endoneurium of mouse sciatic nerve to exogenous proteins. Anatomical Record 63: 722
Selander D, Sjöstrand J 1978 Longitudinal spread of

intraneurally injected local anaesthetics. Acta
Anaesthesiologica Scandinavica 22: 622

Söderfeldt B, Olsson Y, Kristensson K 1973 The
perineurium as a diffusion barrier to protein tracers in
human peripheral nerve. Acta Neuropathologica 25: 120

Sunderland S 1945 The adipose tissue of peripheral nerves.
Brain 68: 118

Sunderland S 1946 The effect of rupture of the perineurium
on the contained nerve fibres. Brain 69: 149

Sunderland S 1978 Nerves and nerve injuries 2nd edn.
Churchill Livingstone, Edinburgh

Sunderland S, Bradley K C 1949 The cross-sectional area of
peripheral nerve trunks devoted to nerve fibres. Brain
96: 865

Sunderland S, Bradley K C 1952 The perineurium of
peripheral nerves. Anatomical Record 113: 125

10. Blood supply of nerves

Detailed information on the origin, number and distribution of the nutrient arteries to the major peripheral nerves is available (see Sunderland 1945a,b, 1978). The histological features of intraneural vascular patterns and the dynamics of the intraneural-microcirculation in a variety of conditions have received considerable attention in recent years (Smith 1966a,b, Lundborg & Brånemark 1968; Lundborg 1970a,b, 1975, 1979, 1980, 1988; Lundborg & Rydevik 1973; Miyamoto et al 1979; Bell & Weddell 1984a,b; Ogata & Naito 1986).

The following are the more general features of the blood supply that have relevance to nerve injury and nerve repair (Figs 10.1–10.4).

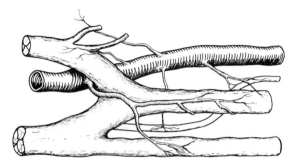

Fig. 10.2 Diagram from a dissected specimen of the axillary artery and related nerves in the axilla to illustrate one large nutrient artery supplying more than one nerve.

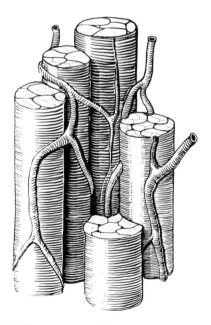

Fig. 10.3 Diagram prepared from a dissected injected specimen of a nerve to illustrate the branchings of the major nutrient arteries that occur in the interfascicular tissues. it will be seen from these branchings that the size, number and location of the intraneural nutrient arteries vary from level to level.

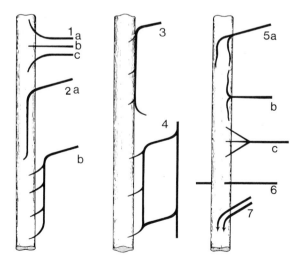

Fig. 10.1 Diagram illustrating the behaviour of the major nutrient arteries as they approach and enter a nerve.

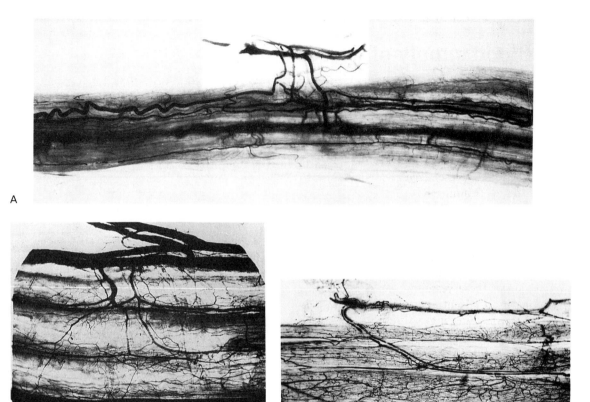

Fig. 10.4   Injected specimens of peripheral nerves to illustrate gross features of their distribution on reaching the nerve: the relation of arterioles to venules, tortuosities in the vessels to allow for nerve stretching and the fine vascular plexuses formed within the nerve.

1. Arteriae nervorum are vessels that enter the nerve, terminate there and supply the tissues of the nerve trunk exclusively. They are derived in an irregular and inconstant manner from neighbouring arteries. Since gross neurovascular relations in the limb are reasonably constant, each nerve comes to be supplied from arteries that are favourably placed to send branches to the nerve. These include the main arteries of the limb, their named branches and unnamed muscular and cutaneous branches.

2. Each nerve is nourished along its course by a succession of nutrient arteries. These vary in size and number and enter the nerve at irregular intervals. By their repeated branching and anastomosis on the surface of and within the nerve, these vessels form continuous longitudinal arterial channels and networks along the nerve.

3. The size of the first nutrient artery, or group of nutrient vessels, to enter a nerve appears to determine the subsequent size and number of the remaining branches.

4. A nerve may run a considerable distance without receiving an entering nutrient vessel, the circulation then being maintained by a major nutrient vessel that provides long ascending and descending branches to a considerable length of the nerve. Where, however, a small nutrient artery enters the nerve, the process must be repeated at short

intervals in order to achieve the same result.

5. Nutrient arteries show tortuosities that provide a reserve in length to accommodate any displacement of the nerve that occurs during joint movement (Fig. 10.4).

6. Sites on the surface of the nerve where the nutrient vessels enter have a random distribution, though they usually join that aspect of the nerve facing the parent artery. Nutrient vessels certainly enter nerves at sites other than the alleged attachment of any mesoneurium.

7. Where a nerve and major artery share a common neurovascular sheath, short, stout and numerous nutrient arteries may so securely anchor the nerve to the vessel that it is impossible to free the nerve without sacrificing these vessels.

8. Though a nutrient artery may enter a nerve before branching into its main ascending and descending branches, it usually does so either on the surface of the nerve or a little distance from it. These primary branches, of which the descending is the larger, anastomose with similar branches from the nutrient artery above and below. This arrangement is repeated at irregular intervals by newly entering nutrient arteries, so that unbroken longitudinal channels are formed that extend the full length of the nerve.

9. The superficial longitudinal arterial chains send branches into the nerve which also divide into ascending and descending branches. These in turn branch and rebranch in the interfascicular epineurial tissue where they anastomose with similarly disposed interfascicular vessels from nutrient arteries above and below to form a deep longitudinal anastomotic system.

   Thus there are two major longitudinal arterial systems, linked by anastomoses, one superficially on the surface of the nerve and another deeply located in the interfascicular epineurium. A third, though less obvious, unbroken longitudinal system is provided by the intrafascicular capillary network of the endoneurium.

10. The repeated branching of these longitudinally aligned nutrient vessels, the entry of new vessels and changes to the fascicular patterns imposed by plexus formations, all combine to vary the number, location and size of nutrient vessels from one level to another.

11. Despite this general arrangement, the *major superficial* longitudinal vessels often, but not invariably, maintain a constant position on the surface of the nerve as they travel along it.

12. A distinctive feature of this pattern is the overlap in the distribution of nutrient arteries entering the nerve at different levels. No single vessel dominates the pattern over the entire length of a nerve. Sometimes, however, the blood supply to a considerable length of it is provided by a single nutrient artery. Thus the median nerve in the forearm may receive its sole arterial supply from the arteria nervi medianes which accompanies the nerve down the forearm, often to the wrist and sometimes even into the hand. The sciatic nerve always receives its major arterial supply in the gluteal region from the arteria comitans ischiadici which enters and descends in the substance of the nerve. The dependence of a significant length of a nerve from a single nutrient source increases its susceptibility to ischaemic damage.

13. Branches emerge from the deep longitudinal interfascicular vessels that form the finer vascular networks of the intraneural vascular pattern. These vascular nets are at first openly arranged and then become progressively finer until intrafascicular capillary networks are reached that are very fine meshed.

14. The arteriae nervorum are not end arteries, the entire vascular pattern being structured to ensure that the blood supply to the various components of the nerve trunk will not be threatened should one or more serving nutrient arteries be interrupted. Even when a single vessel supplies a long stretch of the nerve, the anastomoses at the peripheral limits of the solitary channel are

usually of such dimensions as to exclude segmental ischaemia following the ligation of such a single vessel.

15. The capacity of nerve trunks to tolerate gross interference with their regional blood supply is an indication of the rapidity with which the longitudinal systems provide an effective collateral circulation to the nerve.

16. So effective are these longitudinal anastomotic systems that, under certain circumstances, they may contribute to the development of a collateral circulation to the limb when the major arterial channel to the limb has been interrupted.

17. However, the simultaneous destruction or obliteration of regional nutrient arteries serving a length of a nerve and the longitudinal anastomotic channels in the epineurium to which they give rise deprives that length of the nerve of a blood supply and leads to ischaemic changes.

18. The largest nutrient vessels are found in the epineurium, either on the surface of the nerve or deeply between the fasciculi. The perineurial and intrafascicular vessels are all capillaries with an occasional precapillary arteriole. The latter, when present inside a fasciculus, are located in septal tissue that marks the site of impending division of a fasciculus or the recent fusion of two fasciculi.

19. Vessels entering and leaving a fasciculus take an oblique course as they pass through the perineurium. As a consequence, any swelling of the fasciculus could embarrass blood flow through these vessels.

20. Nutrient veins outnumber arteries. Each nutrient artery is often accompanied on each side by a venous channel.

21. The manner in which the intraneural vascular pattern is established is fundamentally the same for all nerves while the terminal intrafascicular capillary network is of approximately the same density throughout. On the anatomical evidence alone it would appear that no nerve, or part thereof, receives a better or a poorer blood supply than any other.

22. Intraneural vessels have a sympathetic innervation, stimulation of which reduces blood flow through them (Lundborg 1970a,b; Appenzeller et al 1984; Selander et al 1985).

23. Capillary permeability and the blood-nerve barrier. This subject has been studied and reported on in considerable detail (Waksman 1961; Olsson 1966a–c, 1968 a,b, 1984; Mellick & Cavanagh 1967; Lundborg 1970a,b, 1988; Lundborg & Schildt 1971; Olsson & Reese 1971; Olsson et al 1971; Rydevik & Lundborg 1977; Bell & Weddell 1984a,b).

The following key features of relevance to nerve injury have been extracted from the mass of information available.

a. Endoneurial capillaries have the structural and functional features of the capillaries of the central nervous system to give a blood-nerve barrier analogous to the blood-brain barrier.

b. The endothelial cells of the capillaries of the endoneurium have particularly tight junctions to give a system that is normally impermeable to a broad range of macromolecular substances, particularly proteins.

c. The diffusion barrier property of the capillary endothelium is impaired by ischaemia, trauma and some toxic agents.

d. Capillary permeability is increased by the liberation of histamine and serotonin from mast cells that are found in the endoneurium and epineurium.

e. The junctions of the endothelial cells of capillaries in the epineurium are not as secure as those of the endoneurium and fail earlier under unfavourable conditions.

FUNCTIONAL CONSIDERATIONS

It has been known for a very long time, and repeatedly confirmed that the survival and well-being of the peripheral processes of nerve cells depend on the state of the cell body. It is also well established that nerve trunks receive a succession of nutrient arteries along their course. The question is whether peripheral axons, particularly those of considerable length, are solely dependent on intracellular transport mechanisms or whether they also require a continuing blood supply along their length. In other words, do the arteriae nervorum play any part in satisfying the nutritional requirements of long axons or is their usefulness entirely spent providing for the needs of the non-conducting elements of the nerve trunk?

The finding that considerable lengths of a nerve trunk could be deprived of a blood supply from arteriae nervorum without any disturbance or loss of function was at first interpreted as evidence that the integrity of peripheral axons was not dependent on a peripheral blood supply. Even when damage to nerve fibres was reported, this was attributed not to any interference with their blood supply but to direct injury caused during the devascularisation.

Such a conclusion was, however, shown to be unacceptable when it was revealed that the procedure adopted to devascularise the nerve, namely one dividing the nutrient arteries to a considerable length of a nerve, failed to deprive its components of a blood supply (Adams 1943). This was because of the anastomotic efficiency of the intraneural vascular pattern which ensured a continuing blood supply to all components of the nerve, including the axons, from nutrient arteries entering the nerve well above and well below the length deprived of entering nutrient arteries.

The results of devascularising nerves by dividing the nutrient arteries passing to them reflect more on the effectiveness of the collateral circulatory mechanisms built into the intraneural vascular pattern, and the considerable margin of safety that they provide, than they do on the capacity of peripheral axons to survive after the elimination of a blood supply.

Are there limits to the distances over which the longitudinal intraneural system of vessels will maintain an adequate blood supply to the nerve after reinforcing regional nutrient arteries have been interrupted? This determines the distance for which a nerve can be mobilised by sacrificing the nutrient arteries attaching it to neighbouring arteries.

The capacity of nerves and their contained axons to survive after the regional nutrient arteries servicing considerable lengths of the nerve have

been sacrificed is well established experimentally and clinically. Thus the ulnar nerve has been mobilised by sacrificing the nutrient arteries to the nerve between the axilla and the wrist without impairing its blood supply. In this regard, however, care should be taken, when freeing the nerve from the nutrient vessels anchoring it to its bed, to do this well away from the nerve in order to avoid interfering with and interrupting the major superficial longitudinal arterial chains upon which the maintenance of an effective collateral circulation depends (see Chapter 38).

More importantly, in view of the necessity of providing a good blood supply to the site of nerve repair and of meeting the additional nutritional requirements of regenerating axons, it would be unwise to make unreasonable demands on intraneural anastomotic arterial systems. Ogata and Naito (1986) have shown in experimental animals (primates) that mobilising and transposing a 2–3 cm segment of the ulnar nerve anterior to the medial humeral epicondyle temporarily reduced the intraneural blood flow for 3 days. Accordingly, mobilising the proximal and distal segments of a nerve to facilitate end-to-end union should not be extended beyond a critical limit of about 8 cm (Smith 1966a,b).

There is a considerable body of indirect evidence to the effect that the blood supply to peripheral nerves does play a critical role in the well-being of peripheral axons.

1. The nature of the intraneural vascular pattern, and in particular the density of the intrafascicular capillary network appear, from comparisons with the blood supply to supporting tissues elsewhere in the body, to provide a blood supply in excess of that required for the exclusive needs of the supporting connective tissue of peripheral nerves (Fig.10.4).

2. Generalised sclerosing pathology that narrows or occludes nutrient arteries introduces two complications:

   a. the capacity of the neural arterial system to provide for the development of effective collateral circulations is greatly reduced or even eliminated;

   b. the nutrition of nerve fibres is impaired,

which results in the disturbances and even the loss of function.

3. The importance of the blood supply is illustrated by the finding that, for the first 6–8 hours after section of a nerve, the metabolic activities associated with the recovery from fatigue induced by stimulation are more dependent on the blood supply than on its connection with the cell body (Causey & Schoepfle 1951; Causey & Stratmann 1953).

4. Experimental and clinical studies relating to the relative merits of vascularised and conventional nerve grafts have produced conflicting results. Most reports have favoured the vascularised variety on the basis that axons regenerate faster and more successfully through them (Taylor & Ham 1976; Taylor 1978; Starkweather et al 1978; Koshima & Harii 1981, 1985; Koshima et al 1981; Hunt 1983; Breidenbach & Terzis 1984; Townsend & Taylor 1984; Lux et al 1986; Shibata et al 1986; Boorman & Sykes 1987). Others, however, found no significant difference between the two (McCullough et al 1984; Pho et al 1985; Seckel et al 1986; Comtet 1988) while according to a third group, the conventional method of grafting proved to be superior (Settergen & Wood 1984; Daly & Wood 1985). Free neurovascular nerve grafting is discussed in Chapter 43 (p. 483).

Kline et al (1972) crushed or lacerated the sciatic nerve (rhesus monkey) and destroyed the *extrinsic* blood supply over a 12 cm distal segment of the nerve. Studying nerve regeneration by nerve conduction and light microscopy, they concluded that there was no functional difference whether the blood supply was intact or had been eliminated. Revascularisation from the nerve bed and an undisturbed intrinsic system fed from below could account for this finding.

Clearly, in these studies much depends on the length of the graft and the nature of the graft bed. With long grafts and particularly those occupying an extensively scarred bed, the vascularised graft has an advantage, a finding that endorses the importance of the blood supply to the graft and to axon regeneration through it.

5. When a major nerve and its accompanying artery are both transected, for example the ulnar nerve and artery at the wrist, the results are claimed to be better when the nerve and the artery are repaired at the same operation rather than when the artery is ligated and the nerve alone repaired (Starkweather et al 1978; Leclercq et al 1985; Merle et al 1988).

6. Porter & Wharton (1949) have shown that when nerve fibres are subjected to ischaemia they become hyperexcitable and commence to discharge spontaneously. In this respect large myelinated fibres suffer earlier than fine fibres.

7. The neurological signs and symptoms associated with the early stages of localised nerve compression, e.g. the median nerve in the carpal tunnel, are due not to physical deformation of nerve fibres but to an impaired intrafascicular capillary circulation (see Chapter 17).

8. Internal iliac artery embolisation by microspheres has been used to control pelvic haemorrhage in a variety of pelvic conditions (Miller et al 1978; Hare & Holland 1983). The lower limb paresis reported following this procedure has been attributed to an impaired blood supply to the femoral and sciatic nerves resulting from the obliteration of the vessels providing the nutrient blood supply to those nerves. These lesions illustrate the importance of an adequate blood supply to peripheral axons.

CONCLUSIONS

1. Nerve trunks have an abundant blood supply along their entire length.
2. The peripheral blood supply to nerve trunks has an important role in maintaining the structural and functional integrity of peripheral axons and every attempt should be made to preserve it during surgical procedures on the nerve.
3. An impoverished blood supply to a nerve

trunk, regardless of its cause, adversely affects axon conduction but whether this is a direct effect on axon mechanisms or an indirect effect through involvement of the Schwann cell remains unclear.

4. Each nerve is nourished along its course by a succession of nutrient arteries which vary in size and number and enter the nerve at irregular intervals.

5. By their repeated branching on the surface of, and within, the nerve these vessels form a series of continuous longitudinal arterial channels and networks along the nerve. A distinctive feature of this pattern is the overlap in the distribution of nutrient arteries entering at different levels.

6. The capacity of nerve trunks to tolerate gross interference with the regional nutrient arteries passing to them is an indication of the rapidity with which the longitudinal systems provide an effective collateral circulation to the nerve.

7. Details relating to the blood supply of peripheral nerves are worthy of the most careful consideration.

8. The blood supply of nerves in relation to their mobilisation, compression, traction and friction injury, intraneural fibrosis, nerve repair and nerve grafting is discussed in the relevant chapters devoted to those subjects.

REFERENCES

Adams W E 1943 The blood supply of nerves. II. The effects of exclusion of its regional sources of supply on the sciatic nerve of the rabbit. Journal of Anatomy 77: 243

Appenzeller O, Dithal K K, Cowen T, Burnstock G 1984 The nerves to blood vessels supplying blood nerves: the innervation of vasa nervorum. Brain Research 304: 383

Bell M A, Weddell A G M 1984a A morphometric study of intrafascicular vessels of mammalian sciatic nerve. Muscle and Nerve 7: 524

Bell M S, Weddell A G M 1984b A descriptive study of the blood vessels of the sciatic nerve in the rat, man and other mammals. Brain 107: 871

Boorman J G, Sykes P J 1987 Vascularised versus conventional nerve grafting:, a case report. Journal of Hand Surgery 12B: 218

Breidenbach W B, Terzis J K 1984 The anatomy of free vascularized nerve grafts. Clinics in Plastic Surgery 11: 65

Causey G, Schoepfle G M 1951 Fatigue of mammalian nerve in relation to the cell body and vascular supply. Journal of Physiology, London 115: 143

Causey G, Stratmann C J 1953 The relative importance of the blood supply and the continuity of the axon in recovery after prolonged stimulation of mammalian nerve. Journal of Physiology (London) 120, 373

Comtet J-J 1988 Vascularized nerve grafts. In: Tubiana R(ed) The Hand. Saunders, Philadelphia, p 587

Daly P J, Wood M B 1985 Endoneural and epineural blood flow evaluation with free vascularised and conventional nerve graft in the canine. Journal of Reconstructive Microsurgery 2: 51

Hare W S C, Holland C J 1983 Paresis following internal iliac artery embolization. Radiology 146: 47

Hunt D M 1983 A model for the study of free vascularised nerve graft. Journal of Bone and Joint Surgery. 65B: 659

Kline D G, Hackett E R, Davis G D, Myers M B 1972 Effects of mobilization and the blood supply and regeneration of injured nerves. Journal of Surgical Research 12: 254

Koshima I, Harii K 1981 Experimental studies on vascularised nerve grafts in rats. Journal of Microsurgery 2: 225

Koshima I, Harii K 1985 Experimental study of vascularized nerve grafts. Multifactorial analyses of axonal regeneration of nerves transplanted into an acute burn wound. Journal of Hand Surgery 10A: 64

Koshima I, Okabe K, Harii K 1981 Comparative study of free and vascularised nerve grafts transplanted in the scar tissue in rats. Journal of Microsurgery 3: 126

Leclercq D C, Cartier A J, Khuc T, Depierreux L, Lejeune G N 1985 Improvement in the results in sixty-four ulnar nerve sections associated with arterial repair. Journal of Hand Surgery 10A: 997

Lundborg G 1970a A method for long term in vivo studies on the microcirculation of peripheral nerve. Advances in Microcirculation 3: 91

Lundborg G 1970b Ischemic nerve injury. Experimental studies on intraneural microvascular pathophysiology and nerve function in a limb subjected to temporary circulatory arrest. Scandinavian Journal of Plastic Reconstructive Surgery Supplement 6

Lundborg G 1975 Structure and function of the intraneural microvessels as related to trauma, edema formation and nerve function. Journal of Bone and Joint Surgery 57A: 938

Lundborg G 1979 The intrinsic vascularization of human peripheral nerves. Structural and functional aspects. Journal of Hand Surgery 4: 34

Lundborg G 1980 Intraneural microcirculation and peripheral nerve barriers. In: Omer G, Spinner M (eds) Management of peripheral nerve problems. Saunders, Philadelphia, p 903

Lundborg G 1988 Nerve injury and repair. Churchill Livingstone, Edinburgh

Lundborg G, Branemark P I 1968 Microvascular structure and function of peripheral nerves. Vital microscopic studies of the tibial nerve in the rabbit. Advances in Microcirculation 1: 66

Lundborg G, Schildt B 1971 Microvascular permeability in irradiated rabbits. Acta Radiologica 10: 311

Lundborg G, Rydevik B 1973 Effects of stretching the tibial nerve of the rabbit. A preliminary study of the intraneural circulation and the barrier function of the perineurium. Journal of Bone Joint Surgery 55-B: 390

Lux P S, Breidenbach W C, Firrell J 1986 Determination

of temporal changes in blood flow in vascularised and nonvascularised nerve grafts in the dog. Journal of Hand Surgery 11A: 768

McCullough C J, Gagey O, Higginson D W, Sandin B M, Crow J C, Sebille A 1984 Axon regeneration and vascularisation of nerve grafts. An experimental study. Journal of Hand Surgery 9B: 323

Mellick R S, Cavanagh J B 1967 Longitudinal movement of radio-ionated albumin within extravascular spaces of peripheral nerves following three systems of experimental trauma. Journal of Neurology, Neurosurgery and Psychiatry 30: 458

Merle M, Amend P, Michon J 1988 Microsurgical repair in 150 patients with lesions of the median and ulnar nerves. In: Tubiana R (ed) The Hand. Saunders, Philadelphia, p 595

Miller F J, Rankin R S, Gliedman J B 1978 Experimental internal iliac artery embolization. Evaluation of low viscosity silicone rubber, isobutyl-2-cyanoacrylate and carbon microspheres. Radiology 129: 51

Miyamoto Y, Watari S, Tsuge K 1979 Experimental studies on the effects of tension in intraneural microcirculation in sutured peripheral nerves. Plastic and Reconstructive Surgery 63: 398

Ogata K, Naito M 1986 Blood flow of peripheral nerve. Effects of dissection, stretching and compression. Journal of Hand Surgery 11B: 10

Olsson Y 1966a Studies on vascular permeability in peripheral nerves. I. Distribution of circulating fluorescent serum albumin in normal, crushed and sectioned rat sciatic nerve. Acta Neuropathologica (Berlin) 7: 1

Olsson Y 1966b Studies on vascular permeability in peripheral nerves. 2. Distribution of circulating fluorescent serum albumin in rat sciatic nerve after local injection of 5-hydroxy-tryptamine, histamine and compound 48/80. Acta Physiologica Scandinavica 69, Supplement 284

Olsson Y 1966c The effect of the histamine liberator compound 48/80 on mast cells in normal peripheral nerves. Acta Pathologica, Microbiologica et Immunologica Scandinavica 68: 565

Olsson Y 1968a Topographical differences in the vascular permeability of the peripheral nervous system. Acta Neuropathologica (Berlin) 10: 26

Olsson Y 1968b, Mast cells in the nervous system. International Review of Cytology 24: 27

Olsson Y 1984 Vascular permeability in the peripheral nervous system. In: Dyck P J, Thomas P K, Lambert E H, Bunge M B (eds) Peripheral neuropathy Vol 1, 2nd edn. Saunders, Philadelphia, p 579

Olsson Y, Reese T S 1971 Permeability of vasa nervorum and perineurium in mouse sciatic nerve studied by fluorescence and electron microscopy. Journal of Neuropathology and Experimental Neurology 30: 105

Olsson Y, Kristensson K, Klatzo I 1971 Permeability of blood vessels and connective tissue sheaths in the peripheral nervous system to exogenous proteins. Acta Neuropathologica (Berlin) Suppl V: 61

Pho R W H, Lee Y S, Rujiwetpongstorn V, Pang M 1985 Histological studies of vascularised nerve graft and conventional nerve graft. Journal of Hand Surgery 10B: 45

Porter E L, Wharton P S 1949 Irritability of mammalian nerve following ischaemia. Journal of Neurophysiology 12: 109

Rydevik B, Lundborg G 1977 Permeability of intraneural microvessels and perineurium following acute, graded experimental nerve compression. Scandinavian Journal of Plastic and Reconstructive Surgery 11: 179

Seckel B R, Ryan S E, Simons J E, Gagne R G, Watkins E 1986 Vascularised versus non-vascularised nerve grafts. An experimental structural comparison. Plastic and Reconstructive Surgery 78: 211

Selander D, Mansson L G, Karlsson L, Svanvik J 1985 Adrenergic vasoconstriction in peripheral nerves of the rabbit. Anesthesiology 62: 6

Settergren C R, Wood M B 1984 Comparison of blood flow in free vascularised versus nonvascularised nerve grafts. Journal of Reconstructive Microsurgery 1: 95

Shibata M, Breidenbach W C, Tsai T-M 1986 Comparison of functional results following vascularized and nonvascularized nerve grafting of the rabbit median nerve. Journal of Hand Surgery 11A: 765

Smith J W 1966a Factors influencing nerve repair. I. Blood supply of peripheral nerves. Archives of Surgery 93: 335

Smith J W 1966b Factors influencing nerve repair. II. Collateral circulation of peripheral nerves. Archives of Surgery 93: 433

Starkweather R J, Nerviaser R J, Adams J P, Parsons D B 1978 The effect of devascularization on the regeneration of lacerated peripheral nerves: an experimental study. Journal of Hand Surgery 3: 163

Sunderland S 1945a Blood supply of the nerves of the upper limb in man. Archives of Neurology and Psychiatry 53: 91

Sunderland 1945b, Blood supply of the sciatic nerve and its popliteal divisions in man. Archives of Neurology and Psychiatry 54: 283

Sunderland S 1978 Nerves and nerve injuries, 2nd edn. Churchill Livingstone, Edinburgh

Taylor G I 1978 Nerve grafting with simultaneous microvascular reconstruction. Clinical Orthopaedics 133: 56

Taylor G I, Ham F J 1976 The free vascularized nerve graft. A further experimental and clinical application of microvascular techniques. Plastic Reconstructive Surgery 57: 413

Townsend P L G, Taylor G I 1984 Vascularised nerve grafts using composite arterialised neurovenous systems. British Journal of Plastic Surgery 37: 1

Waksman B H 1961 Experimental study of diphtheric polyneuritis in rabbit and guinea pig. III The blood-nerve barrier in the rabbit. Journal of Neuropathology and Experimental Neurology 21: 35

11. Lymphatics. Endoneurial spaces. Nervi nervorum

There is a lymphatic capillary network in the epineurium that drains to regional lymph nodes. There are no lymphatic capillaries inside fasciculi. These are replaced by endoneurial spaces between the nerve fibres, and spaces between the lamellae of the perineurial sheath. Fluid flow in the intrafascicular tissue spaces occurs both distally and centrally within the fasciculi.

The perineurium provides an effective barrier between these spaces and the extra-fascicular epineurial lymphatics so that a nerve may pass through a grossly infected area without the contents of the fasciculus being affected. Once the perineurium is breached, however, the infection invades the fasciculus and spreads easily and rapidly in all directions within it.

Nervi nervorum. Not much can be written about the nervi nervorum because so little is known about them. They originate from nerve fibres within the nerve and from perivascular plexuses from which they are distributed to the epineurium, where they form plexuses, the perineurium and the endoneurium. They comprise sympathetic and sensory fibres. Stimulating the sympathetic chain results in constriction of the intraneural vessels and a slowing of the intraneural blood flow (Lundborg 1970, Appenzeller et al 1984, Selander et al 1985). The sensory fibres are nonmyelinated or very finely myelinated and appear to function solely as nociceptors.

REFERENCES

Appenzeller O, Dithal K K, Cowen T, Burnstock G 1984 The nerves to blood vessels supplying blood to nerves: the innervation of the vasa nervorum. Brain Research 304: 383

Lundborg G 1970 Ischemic nerve injury. Experimental studies on intraneural microvascular pathophysiology and nerve function in a limb, subjected to temporary circulatory arrest. Scandinavian Journal of Plastic and Reconstructive Surgery Supplement 6: 1

Selander D, Mänsson L G, Karlsson L, Svanik J 1985 Adrenergetic vasoconstriction in peripheral nerves of the rabbit. Anaesthesiology 62: 6

12. Features of nerves that protect them from injury during normal daily activities

Normally joint movements can be freely carried out over a wide range, both actively and passively, during which nerves are subjected to stresses and strains that are tolerated without pain or any disturbance of neurological function. This chapter is devoted to a consideration of those features of nerve trunks that protect the contained nerve fibres from traction deformation and compression during normal daily activities. A knowledge of these features is essential for an understanding of the genesis of stretch and compression nerve injury. These features include the mechanical properties of nerve trunks, the slack provided by undulations in the nerve trunk, fasciculi and nerve fibres, the nerve in relation to its bed, the course taken by nerves in relation to joints, the cushioning effect of the epineurium, and muscle tone.

THE MECHANICAL PROPERTIES OF NERVE TRUNKS

For the purposes of this account, mechanical properties will be defined as those that enable a nerve to respond to physical forces by undergoing changes that do not threaten its survival and that are fully reversible, until deformation finally reaches a point where structural failure occurs. These mechanical properties are revealed by subjecting a nerve to progressively increasing traction or compression up to and beyond the point of structural failure.

The investigation of these properties is complicated by the fact that nerves are not homogeneous but heterogeneous structures composed of several different components with differing properties that are combined in such a way as to make it impossible to isolate each com-ponent for separate study. Furthermore, the arrangement is one which means that the internal stresses and strains set up in a nerve by the application of an external force are not uniformly distributed through the nerve. From this it follows that:

1. such stresses will vary in degree at different points in the nerve, some sites being affected to a greater degree than others;
2. with deforming forces of the same magnitude such stresses will also vary from nerve to nerve according to variations in their microstructure.

It is against such a background that the tensile strength of nerves and their behaviour under tensile loading should be examined.

The tensile strength of nerves and their behaviour under tensile loading

Details of the test method used to study these properties in human peripheral nerves (24 ulnar, 24 median, 13 medial popliteal and 15 lateral popliteal), the results, and the reasons for variations in the stress-strain values for different specimens of the same nerve, are available (Sunderland and Bradley 1961a–c, Sunderland 1978). In this connection it is important to note that the rate of application of the deforming force is an important factor influencing the behaviour of a nerve under tensile loading. The data provided in the accompanying tables are based on a rate of elongation of 7.5 cm/minute.

The results may be summarised as follows:

1. Peripheral nerves have tensile strength and elasticity.

Table 12.1 The range of maximum loads (kg) taken by nerves irrespective of size. Rate of elongation 7.5 cm/minute

Ulnar	6.5–15.5
Median	7.3–22.3
Medial popliteal	20.6–33.6
Lateral popliteal	11.8–21.4
Anterior spinal nerve root	0.2–2.2
Posterior spinal nerve root	0.5–3.3

2. Information relating to stress-strain values for different peripheral nerves is given in Tables 12.1 and 12.2.

3 When a nerve is subjected to a gradually increasing tensile load there is a linear relationship between load and elongation over a certain range beyond which proportionality no longer holds and the nerve ceases to behave as an elastic material. Providing the elastic limit is not exceeded, the nerve regains its original length and retains its elastic properties when the load is removed. The elastic range is of the order of 6–20 per cent (Table 12.2).

4. For some nerves the elongation at the elastic limit may be as low as 6 per cent.

5. Regarding the contribution of the component tissues to the mechanical properties of a nerve, elasticity and tensile strength reside in the fascicular tissue and in particular the perineurium. This conclusion is supported by the following observations:

   a. The tensile strength and elasticity of a nerve are retained as long as the perineurium remains intact.

   b. The tensile strength of a nerve increases with increasing amounts of fascicular tissue but not with increasing amounts of epineurial tissue.

   c. The maximum load taken by a nerve increases with increasing thickness and, in particular, with increasing fascicular cross-sectional area.

   d. The tensile strength of a nerve increases as the number of fasciculi increases.

   e. Though the epineurium has some elasticity, which assists in maintaining the undulations in the nerve trunk, it lacks both the tensile strength and elasticity of the perineurium.

   f. The endoneurium contributes in a small measure to the tensile strength and elasticity of a nerve. This is revealed by studying the behaviour of spinal nerve roots as they are being stretched, for these lack epineurial and perineurial tissue (Sunderland & Bradley 1961a–c). Reference to Table 12.2 shows that nerve roots have some tensile strength and elasticity despite the fact that they lack epineurial and perineurial tissue.

   g. That axons do not contribute to the physical properties of nerve trunks is suggested by the observation that the denervated distal segment of a severed nerve has the same tensile strength and elasticity as the normal proximal segment (Sunderland & Bradley 1961a–c)

6. Fascicular plexuses add to the tensile strength of nerves.

7. Nerves are stronger where they are

Table 12.2 Percentage elongation of human nerve trunks under tensile loading. Rate of elongation 7.5 cm/minute

Nerve	At the elastic limit		At mechanical failure	
	Range	Mean	Range	Mean
Ulnar	8–21	15	9–26	18
Median	6–22	14	7–30	19
Medial polpliteal	7–21	17	8–32	23
Lateral popliteal	9–22	15	10–32	20
Anterior spinal roots	9–15	11	9–21	15
Posterior spinal roots	8–16	12	8–28	19

composed of numerous small fasciculi; cables of the same thickness are stronger and more flexible if composed of many strands.

8. Nerve fibres are more vulnerable to mechanical deformation where they are collected into a single fasciculus or a small number of large closely packed fasciculi.

9. The rate of application, as well as the severity of a deforming force acting on a nerve is important. Nerves tolerate greater degrees of stretch when deformation occurs slowly. Providing a nerve is strectched sufficiently slowly, involving time scales of months or even years, remarkable increases in its length may occur without any disturbance of function. Such increases greatly exceed those at which structural failure would have occurred had the deforming force been abruptly applied.

10. Though nerve roots have some tensile strength and elasticity they are more vulnerable to traction and compression injury than peripheral nerves because:

   a. they lack both epineurial and perineurial tissue;
   b. nerve root fibres are arranged in parallel non-plexiform bundles;
   c. the collagen fibres of the endoneurium are fewer and finer than elsewhere.

Changes occurring in nerves as they are stretched to the point of structural failure

The initial effect of stretching the nerve is to take out the undulations in the nerve trunk. With continued stretching the undulations in the fasciculi are eliminated and finally the undulations in the nerve fibres, at which point the latter are then subjected to tension.

As the elastic limit of the nerve is approached with progressively increasing traction, nerve fibres rupture inside the fasciculi despite which the nerve continues to behave as an elastic material. Later fractures appear in the perineurium and with the structural failure of this tissue the nerve trunk loses its elasticity and the entire system elongates as a plastic structure (see Chapter 18).

As the nerve is being stretched, the cross-sectional area of fasciculi is steadily reduced. This introduces a compression factor that results in the further deformation of nerve fibres as well as impairing their blood supply. This compression factor has also been reported by Orf (1978).

In their experimental studies Lundborg & Rydevik (1973) and Lundborg (1975) found that nerves tolerated an elongation of about 8% before the intraneural microvascular flow was impaired. With elongations of 11–18% the vessels were totally occluded and the nerve tissue suffered complete ischaemia. Following relaxation the circulation recovered well.

Features of this pattern of structural failure are:

1. nerve fibres rupture inside fasciculi before breaks appear in the perineurium and while the nerve is still behaving as an elastic structure;

2. the extensive longitudinal distribution of lesions as the elastic limit of the nerve is exceeded;

3. the concurrent compression of the contents of the fasciculi and the impairment of the intrafascicular circulation;

4. the tensile strength and elasticity of a nerve are retained as long as the perineurium remains intact;

5. the range of elasticity is of the order of 6–20% but for some nerves the critical limit is as low as 6%;

6. the evidence suggests that conduction failure would occur before the elastic limit is reached. Orf's (1978) detailed studies on nerve stretching (rabbit) put functional failure occurring at elongations of 5–8% (see Chapter 18);

7. Orf (1978) reports that both the epineurium and perineurium rupture at elongations of less than 8%, the nerve fibres being more vulnerable than the supporting connective tissue elements. Nauck (1931) gives the physiological limit of elongation being reached as soon as the undulations are eliminated. In his experiments (mice, sciatic) this occurred with elongations of 5–6%. In Orf's (1978) experiments (rabbit, sciatic) the breaking point of nerve fibres was 2–4%.

THE SLACK PROVIDED BY UNDULATIONS IN THE NERVE TRUNK, FASCICULI AND NERVE FIBRES

A nerve trunk runs an undulating course in its bed, the fasciculi run an undulating course in the epineurium and the nerve fibres run an undulating course inside the fasciculi. This means that the length of a nerve trunk and its contained nerve fibres between any two fixed points on the limb is greater than a straight line joining those points.

The initial effect of stretching a nerve is to take out the undulations in the nerve trunk. With continued stretching this is followed by the elimination of the undulations in the fasciculi and finally the undulations in the nerve fibres. It is only at this last point that the nerve fibres are subjected to tension (Fig. 12.1).

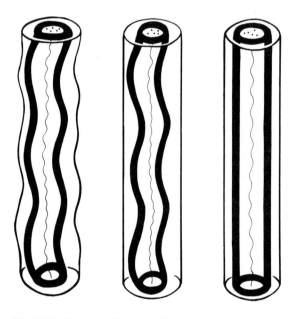

Fig. 12.1 Diagrams illustrating the undulations in nerves, fasciculi and nerve fibres that protect nerve fibres when nerves are stretched during a full range of limb movements.

The slack provided in the system in this way absorbs and neutralises traction forces generated during limb movements so that the contained nerve fibres are at all times protected from being overstretched.

THE NERVE IN RELATION TO ITS BED

Reference has been made elsewhere (Chapter 4) to the non-specialised, unnamed fascial connective tissue, of gossamer-like consistency, that is left over as packing between the specialised, differentiated structures of the limbs. Nerves travel through this tissue which separates them from neighbouring structures to which they are loosely attached.

Two simple but important roles are fulfilled by this connective tissue:

1. It provides a loose framework in which the nerve can readily slide, and move sideways, so that throughout its course it can move freely in relation to other structures. Wilgis & Murphy (1986) have measured the extent of this sliding movement and their results are reported in Table 12.3.

Table 12.3 Excursions (in mm) occurring during a full range of joint movement of the upper limb (Wilgis & Murphy 1986)

Brachial plexus During full abduction at the shoulder from a position of adduction		15.3	
	Arm	Forearm	Hand
Median nerve	7.3	14.5	6.8
Ulnar nerve	9.8	13.8	6.5

2. Those familiar with injection techniques know that pressure on the skin overlying a nerve often causes the nerve to slip away from the point of pressure. It is the cord-like consistency of the nerve and the mobility conferred on it by virtue of this connective tissue that permit the nerve to do this.

   This feature also allows a nerve to slip out of the way and so escape involvement from a penetrating injury or the near passage of a high velocity bullet passing through the limb in the immediate vicinity.

THE COURSE TAKEN BY NERVES IN RELATION TO JOINTS

Nerves crossing joints are subjected to deforming forces during limb movements. These forces are normally dissipated as the slack in the nerve is taken up. However, the relationship of a nerve to a joint it crosses is an additional factor influencing the effect on the nerve of traction forces introduced during limb movements.

The significance of a routing across the flexor aspect of joints is illustrated following transection of the median and ulnar nerves in the mid-upper arm. When the forearm is fully extended the median nerve ends are slightly drawn apart but remain unchanged when the forearm is flexed. On the other hand, the ulnar nerve ends are drawn much further apart when the elbow is fully flexed but remain unchanged when the forearm is fully extended.

Thus a nerve crossing the flexor aspect of a joint remains relaxed during flexion and is only slightly stretched during extension, whereas a nerve crossing the extensor aspect of a joint is relaxed during extension but is put under considerable tension during flexion.

Because the range of joint flexion is much greater than that of extension, it is clear that nerves crossing the extensor aspect of a joint are at a disadvantage as regards exposure to forces generated during limb movements. This explains the advantages of crossing the flexor aspect of a joint and why most nerves do so. The only two notable exceptions to this rule are the ulnar nerve, which crosses the extensor aspect of the elbow joint, and the sciatic nerve where it crosses the extensor aspect of the hip joint. As a result, both nerves are repeatedly stretched during full joint flexion.

It is of interest that where nerves cross joints they are also composed of many small fasciculi separated by large amounts of epineurial tissue. This is particularly so where the sciatic nerve crosses the extensor aspect of the hip joint, the epineurial tissue representing as much as 88 per cent of the cross-sectional area of the nerve in this situation. This is probably a special protective feature, for much time is spent squatting or sitting on the sciatic nerves with the thighs flexed.

THE CUSHIONING ROLE OF THE EPINEURIUM

1. A special feature of peripheral nerves is the often large amount of epineurial connective tissue that separates the fasciculi and holds them together.

2. When pressure is applied to a nerve the epineurium functions as a shock-absorber which dissipates the stresses set up in the nerve, thereby cushioning the fasciculi and their contained nerve fibres and in this way protecting them from damage.

3. On the basis of established variations in the relative amounts of fascicular and epineurial tissue, it is conceivable that where nerves are composed of large and closely packed fasciculi with little supporting epineurial tissue they would be more vulnerable to mechanical injury than where the fasciculi are smaller and more widely separated by a greater amount of epineurial tissue. With the former arrangement, forces would fall maximally on the main component of the nerve trunk which is fascicular tissue and, therefore, nerve fibres. In the latter, the damaging forces would be dissipated and cushioned by the epineurial tissue packing and the fasciculi would be more easily displaced within the nerve and so would tend to escape (Fig. 12.2). An additional advantage is also enjoyed by a nerve composed of numerous small fasciculi when it is subjected to mechanical trauma that falls unevenly across the nerve. Under these circumstances the tendency is for some fasciculi to escape damage, while only those in the direct path of the deforming force suffer. The tendency then is for such

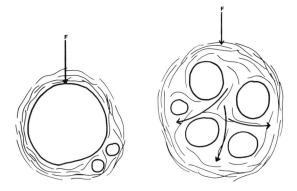

Fig. 12.2 Diagram illustrating **a** the role of the epineurium in protecting the fasciculi from the stresses set up in a nerve by the application of an external force, and **b** the greater vulnerability of nerves where they are composed of a large fasciculi with little supporting epineurial tissue.

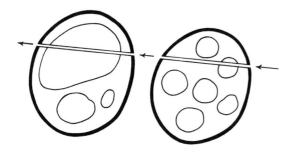

Fig. 12.3 Diagram illustrating the influence of intraneural fascicular structure on the extent of the damage following partial nerve injury.

lesions to be self-limiting. On the other hand, where the fasciculi are few in number and large in size the effects are concentrated on all or the majority of the fibres comprising the nerve (Fig. 12.3).

The significance of this feature is illustrated by reference to the well-established clinical finding that, in injuries of the sciatic nerve, the common peroneal division is known to be more frequently injured and more often suffers greater damage than the tibial (Sunderland 1953, 1978).

An investigation of the cross-sectional area of the sciatic nerve and its common peroneal and tibial divisions devoted to fasciculi and to epineurial tissue has revealed that the fascicular pattern of the common peroneal does present features that render this nerve more susceptible to injury than the associated tibial division (Fig.12.4). The peroneal division, particularly in the distal half of the thigh, is composed of fewer and larger fasciculi with less epineurial tissue than is the corresponding tibial division. This morphological difference would, as we have seen, be a significant factor increasing the susceptibility of the common peroneal nerve to stretch and compression injury.

It has also been shown that the common peroneal division usually contains much less adipose tissue in the epineurium than does the tibial (Sunderland 1945).

MUSCLE TONE

The role of muscle tone in protecting nerves and nerve fibres is well illustrated by reference to the

brachial plexus at the root of the upper limb (See Chapters 18 and 19).

Nerve fibres in the brachial plexus are particularly at risk for the following reasons:

1. On emerging from an intervertebral foramen the fibres of each spinal nerve are collected into a single fasciculus.
2. The protective undulations in the fasciculi and nerve trunks have been eliminated by the weight of the limb. In other words the plexus is an already tautly drawn structure.
3. There are regional features at the thoracic outlet that predispose to friction and compression trauma such as:

   i. The intervertebral foramen.
   ii. The posterior firm edge of Sibson's fascia across which the lower trunk of the plexus rides, and particularly first thoracic fibres.
   iii. The slope of the first rib and the angulation of the lower trunk of the plexus against the posterior tendinous attachment of the scalenus anterior to the rib.

Compensatory arrangements to offset the unfavourable features include:

1. attachment of the fifth, sixth and seventh cervical spinal nerves to corresponding cervical transverse processes. This does not apply to the eighth cervical and first thoracic spinal nerves, which means that traction on these nerves is transmitted directly to the corresponding nerve roots. This feature explains why severe traction injuries of the plexus commonly result in rupture of C5, 6 and 7 at the transverse processes but nerve root avulsion of C8 and T1;
2. on emerging from the intervertebral foramina the spinal nerves immediately engage in plexus formations that add to the tensile strength of the system;
3. muscle tone in the elevators of the shoulder girdle relieves the plexus of the deforming influence of gravity and the weight of the limb;
4. muscle tone in the scalene muscles reduces the slope of the first rib and the tendency of the lower trunk of the plexus to: (a) slide downwards against the posterior tendinous

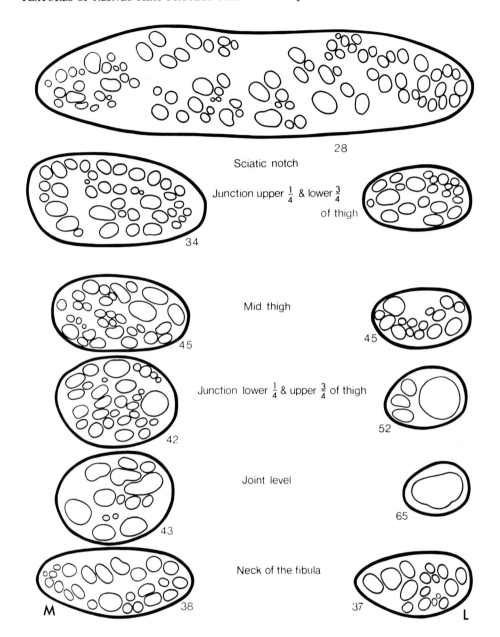

Fig. 12.4 Transverse sections from a specimen of the sciatic nerve and its medial (*M*) and lateral (*L*) popliteal divisions, illustrating the relationship between the amount of epineurium and the number of fasciculi. The figures given are the percentage cross-sectional areas of the nerve devoted to fasciculi (not to scale).

edge of the scalenus anterior and (b) become still further angulated against the posterior edge of Sibson's fascia. The lower trunk of the plexus is particularly susceptible to friction trauma at these two sites.

These several complications are aggravated by the loss of tone in the shoulder girdle elevators which allows the shoulder girdle to sag and move forwards on the thoracic wall, with the following two consequences:

1. traction on the plexus is considerably increased by the now unrelieved weight of the limb, and
2. the risk of trauma to the lower trunk from friction against the sharp edge of Sibson's fascia and the tendinous attachment of scalenus anterior is greatly increased as the nerve is drawn downwards and forwards on the rib.

CONCLUDING COMMENT

All in all, nerves are normally well protected from injury during the course of normal daily activities. However there is always a point at which a traumatic incident is sufficient to overcome those protective devices and when this occurs traction and/or compression nerve injuries are the result.

REFERENCES

Lundborg G 1975 Structure and function of the intraneural microvessels as related to trauma, edema formation, and nerve function. Journal of Bone and Joint Surgery 57A: 938

Lundborg G & Rydevik B 1973 Effects of stretching the tibial nerve of the rabbit. A preliminary study of the intraneural circulation and the barrier function of the perineurium. Journal of Bone and Joint Surgery 55B: 390

Nauck E T 1931 Bemerkungen über den mechanisch-funktionellen Bau der Nerven. Anatomische Anzeiger 72: 260

Orf G 1978 Critical resection length and gap distance in peripheral nerves. Acta Neurochirurgica Supplementum 26: 1

Sunderland S 1945 The adipose tissue of peripheral nerves. Brain 68: 118

Sunderland S 1953 The relative susceptibility to injury of the medial and lateral popliteal divisions of the sciatic nerve. British Journal of Surgery 41: 300

Sunderland S 1978 Nerves and nerve injuries, 2nd edn. Churchill Livingstone, Edinburgh

Sunderland S & Bradley K C 1961a Stress-strain phenomena in human peripheral nerve trunks. Brain 84: 102

Sunderland S & Bradley K C 1961b Stress-strain phenomena in human spinal nerve roots. Brain 84: 120

Sunderland S & Bradley K C 1961c Stress-strain phenomena in denervated peripheral nerve trunks. Brain 84: 125

Wilgis S & Murphy R 1986 The significance of longitudinal excursion in the peripheral nerves. Hand Clinics 2: 761

The pathology of nerve injury

13. Introduction. Nerve conduction block injury

Because of the limited availability of relevant human material for histological examination we are forced to rely on the findings of animal experiments for much of the information relating to the pathology of nerve injury.

Such experimental work has shown that these changes do not develop in a constant or uniform manner but vary according to the conditions of the experiment, species, age, nerve fibre calibre, temperature, nature and severity of the injury and its proximity to the cell body. All this makes extrapolation to the human situation difficult and sometimes unreliable.

With this reservation in mind, an attempt has been made to extract from the morass of detail available a coherent account of what may be accepted as a reasonably close approximation of what happens in the clinical situation.

Localised nerve injuries fall into two main categories, each of which presents special and distinctive features.

1. Those causing a temporary block of nerve conduction at the site of the injury without loss of axon continuity.
2. Those in which axons are severed or damaged to a degree that results in their disintegration at the site of the injury, and their degeneration below, and for a variable distance above, that level. In this category there are three subgroups, each requiring separate consideration.

   a. Nerve injury in which axons alone are involved, the endoneurial sheath being preserved.
   b. Nerve injury in which nerve fibres, including their endoneurial sheaths, are severed or so damaged that their normal structure is destroyed. However, fascicular continuity is preserved.
   c. Nerve injury in which the entire nerve trunk is severed.

The reaction to the injury in each of the three subgroups proceeds in two phases. The first involves the disintegration of the axon and its myelin sheath along the entire length of the nerve fibre below the injury and for a variable distance above it. These changes, known as Wallerian degeneration, lead to the separation of the end organ from its corresponding neuron. The parent cell and its connections may also react to the peripheral injury and, if this retrograde neuronal reaction proceeds to the degeneration of the cell, then the entire axon pathway perishes.

The second phase of the reaction involves the regeneration of the surviving portion of the axon and, hopefully, the restoration of axon continuity with the periphery. Whether or not this occurs depends on the state of the endoneurial sheath of each nerve fibre. When this is preserved the growing axon is confined to the endoneurial tube originally occupied by it and so is inevitably directed back to the end organ that it originally innervated. This is *uncomplicated axon regeneration*, the inevitable result of which is the restoration of the original pattern of innervation and so the complete restoration of function.

Transection or the disorganisation of the nerve fibre, including its endoneurial sheath, complicates regeneration by introducing conditions that threaten the return of the axon to its original terminal ending. This is because axons are now free to enter foreign endoneurial tubes as they regenerate. In doing so they are often misdirected in their growth so that the restored pattern of innervation is both imperfect and incomplete in comparison with the original and function suffers accordingly. This is *complicated axon regeneration*.

NERVE CONDUCTION BLOCK INJURY

In this type of injury, both continuity of the axon and the overall microstructure of nerve fibres are preserved. Providing relief occurs before the critical point is reached at which disintegration of the axon sets in, the changes responsible for blocking conduction are fully reversible and recovery is rapid and complete.

Aetiology

Though conduction block injury can be caused in many ways, most cases seen clinically are the result of compression and ischaemia. This explains why these agents have attracted and received particular attention, both experimentally and clinically. The literature on this subject is extensive (see Sunderland 1978). Only recent key references are given here (Lundborg 1970, 1975, Aguayo et al 1971, Ochoa et al 1972, Rydevik & Lundborg 1977, Gilliatt 1980, Ochoa 1980, Rydevik & Nordborg 1980, Rydevik et al 1980, 1981, Lundborg et al 1983). There are also references to this subject in Chapters 10 and 20.

What little evidence is available about cold conduction blockade suggests that the effects on nerve fibres of compression and cooling are fundamentally different. These differences are not fully understood.

Pathogenesis

Because this condition is inevitably and invariably followed by complete and rapid recovery, human material rarely becomes available for histological examination. When it has, pathological changes have been conspicuous by their absence. We are therefore forced to rely on experimental studies for information on the pathology of conduction block nerve injury.

The severity of the conduction block lesion as measured by its duration is influenced by the magnitude of the deforming force, its rate of application, the time for which it acts, and the manner in which it is applied.

Using the duration of the block as a criterion, these lesions fall into three groups: brief, moderate and severe. However, there is no sharp line of separation between them and the three groups have three features in common.

1. They are localised lesions.
2. Continuity of the axon is preserved.
3. All changes are fully reversible providing the offending agent ceases to operate.

The transient conduction block lesion. This is of a few minutes' or hours' duration, is without overt pathological changes and is primarily vascular in origin.

The moderately severe lesion. Here conduction block persists for up to 4 weeks. Pathological changes are now present in the injured segment which is oedematous, hyperaemic, and infiltrated with macrophages and· lymphocytes. There is swelling, notching, vacuolation and thinning of axons and a change in their staining qualities. The myelin is granulated, fissured and vacuolated, particularly in the vicinity of nodes. Finally, thinned axons are left with only a thin coating of myelin, the overall picture being one of segmental and paranodal demyelination. There is no Schwann cell activity.

The severe conduction block lesion. In these the block persists for several months.

In the experimental studies the pathological changes were maximal at the margins of the compressed segment, with the thicker myelinated fibres being the principal sufferers. Conspicuous pathological features were again axon thinning and segmental demyelination, but with an additional distinctive deformity in the form of nodal dislocations in which nodes were telescoped into a neighbouring paranode. This caused gross distortion and fracturing of the paranodal myelin. The direction of the nodal displacement was always away from the compressed segment of the nerve. The form and distribution of these displacements are consistent with the view that the pathological changes associated with prolonged conduction block are caused by the direct action of deforming forces on nerve fibres.

It is worth noting that the forces required experimentally to produce these advanced structural changes were of considerable magnitude and were abruptly applied.

THE ROLE OF ISCHAEMIA IN THE PRODUCTION OF THE CONDUCTION BLOCK LESION

1. The structural integrity, conducting properties and survival of nerve fibres depend on a continuing and adequate blood supply.
2. Compression ischaemia, measured in minutes rather than hours, may be all that is required to block conduction.
3. The transition from a conduction block injury to the onset of axon degeneration is reached when ischaemia is unrelieved for about 6 hours.
4. Experiments on human nerves have revealed that function is rapidly restored following release from pressure that has rendered a limb ischaemic for 30–40 minutes.
5. As the capillary blood flow through a compressed nerve segment slows ischaemia ultimately reaches a level where:

    a. nerve fibres become hyperexcitable and commence to discharge spontaneously. In this respect thick, myelinated nerve fibres are more vulnerable than nonmyelinated and thinly myelinated fibres;
    b. the epineurial capillaries, that are more sensitive to ischaemia than the intrafascicular vessels, begin to leak and lead to an epineurial oedema.

    With further slowing of the blood flow, and the consequent deepening ischaemia, the intrafascicular capillaries begin to leak with the development of an intrafascicular oedema that raises the intrafascicular pressure. This alters the environment and nutrition of nerve fibres in such a way and to such a degree that conduction failure occurs.

    If the pressure is relieved the circulation through the compressed segment improves and with this the changes are reversed and recovery follows. Failing this, the changes in the compressed segment proceed to the point where axons break down and Wallerian degeneration occurs.

6. There is an ischaemic element in every compression injury, because it is impossible to compress a segment of a nerve without at the same time involving the intraneural vessels, impairing the circulation and adversely affecting the nutrition of nerve fibres. This interrelationship makes it difficult at times to determine the role of each in blocking conduction and the relative contribution of each to the associated pathological changes which should, therefore, be regarded as a combination of those caused by mechanical trauma and those due to an impaired blood supply.
7. Transient conduction block lesions caused by low pressure compression are primarily ischaemic lesions. On the other hand, the distinctive structural changes at the nodes in nerve fibres associated with prolonged conduction block are produced by the direct action of the deforming force on nerve fibres.

INTERFERENCE WITH AXON TRANSPORT MECHANISMS AS A POSSIBLE CAUSE OF THE CONDUCTION BLOCK

Bearing in mind the importance of transport mechanisms in maintaining the well-being of axons, it is tempting to speculate on the possibility that interference with these mechanisms in the affected nerve segment might be responsible for blocking nerve conduction (see Chapter 15).

However, this is an unlikely explanation because axons below the site of injury not only survive but also retain their electrical excitability, which would be unlikely if interference with transport mechanisms was depriving them of the essential materials on which their survival and functional integrity depended. Whatever the nature of the disturbance responsible for the conduction block, it remains confined to the affected segment of the nerve.

CHANGES IN THE AXON AND MYELIN

The importance of axon diameter, the axolemmal membrane, the myelin sheath, and particularly the nodes, in the transmission of the nerve impulse, is well established. It is conceivable that compression ischaemia could so disturb the physical, chemical and electrical properties of these components that the affected nerve fibres cease to conduct across the injured segment of the nerve trunk.

Axon thinning and demyelination could well account for the early failure and slower recovery of thick, heavily myelinated fibres. However, in brief transient conduction block, the same fibre selectivity obtains and yet such advanced structural changes are absent.

In the present incomplete state of our knowledge we must be content with the explanation that in conduction block injury the structure of the axon, the properties of its axolemmal membrane and/or its myelin sheath are temporarily deranged by compression and ischaemia to a point where conduction through the affected segments is blocked.

Regardless of the nature of the mechanism responsible for the block, providing the offending agent ceases to act before the critical point is reached at which disintegration of the axon sets in, the changes responsible for the block are, whatever their nature, fully reversible and function is rapidly and completely restored.

CLINICAL FEATURES

From clinical observation, the study of aetiological factors and the examination of pathological data provided from experimental studies, it is possible to identify the following distinguishing clinical features of conduction block injury.

1. The block is localised to a segment of the nerve.
2. There is no Wallerian degeneration.
3. Axonal continuity between the cell body and end organ is preserved.
4. Conduction across the affected segment is impaired or completely blocked.
5. Nerve fibres continue to respond to electrical stimulation both above and below the affected segment, though the amplitude of the action potential may be reduced and nerve conduction velocity slowed.
6. The disturbance responsible for blocking conduction is fully reversible.
7. After a delay of variable duration the affected nerve segment recovers and the conducting properties of the entire nerve fibre are fully and rapidly restored.
8. On the basis of the duration of the block, the severity of the injury can be arbitrarily expressed in terms of three grades:

   a. Brief.   The duration of the block is measured in minutes or hours.
   b. Moderate. The block persists for up to 4 weeks.
   c. Severe.   The block is prolonged for several months.

9. This type of injury is the basis of a first degree nerve injury when a nerve trunk is involved (Chapter 25).
10. Large myelinated nerve fibres are the most susceptible to compression and ischaemia, and finely myelinated and non-myelinated nerve fibres the most resistant.
11. Motor and sensory fibres behave differently, though the precise manner in which they do so requires clarification. In general, clinical findings point to motor fibres being more susceptible to compression than sensory fibres.
12. During the development of, and recovery from, compression nerve block, the different sensory modalities fail sequentially in the following order and recover in the reverse order: proprioception, touch, temperature and nociception. This is only another way of saying that large myelinated nerve fibres fail earlier and recover more slowly than fine and non-myelinated fibres.
13. There is no agreement on the question of whether, in a nerve trunk, long nerve fibres are more, or less, susceptible to compression and ischaemia than short fibres. Thick fibres are certainly more vulnerable than fine fibres.
14. Some nerve fibres are clearly more susceptible to conduction block damage

than others. The basis of this selectivity remains unknown, but it is probably based on physical and/or chemical differences in the fibres themselves, differing nutritional requirements, and even local extrinsic and intrinsic anatomical features of the nerve

trunk that render some fibres more susceptible to compression ischaemia than others.

15. The disturbance responsible for blocking conduction is not fully understood.

REFERENCES

Aguayo A, Nair C P V, Midgely R 1971 Experimental progressive compression neuropathy in the rabbit. Archives of Neurology 24: 358

Gilliatt R W 1980 Acute compression block. In: Sumner A J (ed) The physiology of peripheral nerve disease. Saunders, Philadelphia, p 287

Lundborg G 1970 Ischemic nerve injury. Experimental studies on intraneural microvascular pathophysiology and nerve function in a limb, subjected to temporary circulatory arrest. Scandinavian Journal of Plastic and Reconstructive Surgery Supplement 1

Lundborg G 1975 Structure and function of the intraneural microvessels as related to trauma, edema formation and nerve function. Journal of Bone and Joint Surgery 57A: 938

Lundborg G, Myers R, Powell H 1983 Nerve compression injury and increase in endoneurial fluid pressure: a 'miniature compartment syndrome'. Journal of Neurology, Neurosurgery and Psychiatry 46: 1119

Ochoa J 1980 Nerve fibre pathology in acute and chronic compression In: Omer G E, Spinner M (eds) Management of peripheral nerve problems. Saunders, Philadelphia, p 487

Ochoa J, Fowler T J, Gilliatt R W 1972 Anatomical changes in peripheral nerves compressed by a pneumatic tourniquet. Journal of Anatomy 113: 433

Rydevik B, Lundborg G 1977 Permeability of intraneural microvessels and perineurium following acute, graded experimental nerve compression. Scandinavian Journal of Plastic and Reconstructive Surgery 11: 179

Rydevik B, Nordborg C 1980 Changes in nerve function and nerve fibre structure induced by acute, graded compression. Journal of Neurology, Neurosurgery and Psychiatry 43: 1070

Rydevik B, MacLean W G, Sjöstrand J, Lundborg G 1980 Blockage of axonal transport induced by acute graded compression of the rabbit vagus nerve. Journal of Neurology, Neurosurgery and Psychiatry 43: 690

Rydevik B, Lundborg G, Bagge U 1981 Effects of graded compression on intraneural blood flow. Journal of Hand Surgery 6: 3

Sunderland S 1978 Interruption of conduction with preservation of continuity of the axon. In: Nerves and nerve injuries, 2nd edn. Churchill Livingstone, Edinburgh, p 70

14. Axon degeneration

For details of the extensive literature on axon degeneration the reader is referred to *Nerves and Nerve Injuries* (Sunderland 1978). The position outlined at that time has not changed significantly in the past 10 years and the following account covers the essential features of the subject.

NERVE INJURY IN WHICH CONTINUITY OF AXONS IS LOST BUT THE ENDONEURIAL SHEATH OF THE NERVE FIBRE IS PRESERVED — WALLERIAN DEGENERATION

This is the simplest and mildest form of a localised nerve injury that is sufficiently severe to cause the breakdown of axons but not severe enough to threaten the integrity and continuity of its endoneurial sheath. It introduces the classic phenomenon of Wallerian degeneration in which the essential change is the degeneration of the axon and myelin along the entire length of the nerve fibre below the injury, the proliferation of Schwann cells, and the removal of the axon-myelin debris so that the surviving endoneurial sheath is finally left enclosing only a column of Schwann cells. The related histological and biochemical changes through which the parent cell body passes, and the proliferation of Schwann cells, are but the forerunners of regenerative processes that are to restore the lost axon.

This type of nerve lesion is usually caused by compression. However, to ensure that the basal lamina and integrity of the endoneurial sheath of the nerve fibres are left undisturbed, the most reliable method of causing this type of lesion experimentally is localised freezing of the nerve.

This technique has been effectively used by Mira (1971, 1972, 1979, 1981) in a series of experimental investigations using a liquid nitrogen cryode at $-180°C$ applied for 30–40 seconds to a 2–3 mm segment of the sciatic nerve in the rat. With this technique the axon, myelin and Schwann cells are destroyed but the blood vessels, basal laminae and connective tissue elements of the nerve are left unaffected.

The method is now used clinically for creating a lesion from which spontaneous recovery is complete in every respect.

With localised freezing the lesion passes through a conduction block phase and then one resulting in loss of continuity of the axon, the reaction depending on such factors as the temperature, the duration of exposure and the number of applications.

The changes in the nerve favouring this type of injury have followed the same pattern as those seen when mechanical trauma is the offending causal agent.

Reaction at the site of injury

There is little local reaction and most of this is in response to the disintegration of the axon rather than to the trauma.

The histological features of the lesion are an extension of those producing the conduction block lesion described in the previous chapter, the essential difference being the disintegration of axons and their myelin. The affected segment of the nerve trunk is mildly hyperaemic and there is some intrafascicular oedema which follows the increased permeability of damaged capillaries.

Reaction and changes in nerve fibres below the injury — Wallerian degeneration

The axon and myelin

Changes appear in the axon before they do in the myelin but the two soon overlap.

The first signs of axon degeneration appear within hours of the injury, when neurotubules and neurofilaments become disorganised and fragment so that the axoplasm becomes filled with granular material that collects into irregular clumps. Swelling of the axon is followed by the appearance of irregularities in contour and staining until the axon soon has a varicose appearance. Axon continuity is lost about 48–96 hours after the injury when the axon breaks into twisted fragments along its length. The ability of the fibre to conduct impulses then ceases. All traces of the axon debris are usually lost by the end of the 2nd week but isolated remnants may persist for longer periods.

The earliest signs of the disintegration of myelin are also seen within hours of the injury and myelin breakdown is well advanced by 36–48 hours, the paranodal regions and incisures acting as foci for physical disintegration. By the 3rd day myelin fragments are collecting into ovoids that may enclose axon debris, and the removal of myelin debris by phagocytosis is commencing.

The primary changes in Wallerian degeneration are physical fragmentation unaccompanied by chemical change. The former is completed by about the 8th day and the latter follows at the end of the 2nd week.

The final stage is one in which the interior of the nerve fibre is occupied by an amorphous mass of axon and myelin debris which is removed by the phagocytic action of macrophages and Schwann cells. The disposal of the myelin debris takes from 1 week to 3 months, most of it having gone by the 2nd to the 4th week.

Whether or not Wallerian degeneration takes place simultaneously along the length of the fibre is unclear because the degenerative changes proceed so rapidly that a distal or proximal progression could go undetected unless examinations were conducted at sufficiently short intervals. However, there is some evidence supporting a centrifugal course (Lubinska 1977, Mira 1981).

Schwann cells

Schwann cells are already hyperactive within 24 hours of the injury. They become discrete, their nuclei enlarge and the cytoplasm increases in amount. These changes are followed by increased mitotic activity and cell proliferation that peaks during the 1st week and then sharply declines. The factors controlling the proliferation of Schwann cells are not fully understood. The height of Schwann cell activity appears to coincide with the period when Wallerian degeneration and the removal of axon and myelin debris is occurring most rapidly. There is some evidence that metaplastic transformations occur between the Schwann cells, perineurial cells and endoneurial fibroblasts.

Macrophages

Macrophages accumulate in large numbers by the 3rd day and are most actively phagocytic in the traumatised zone where the capillary permeability aids their passage into the tissues. Elsewhere along the degenerating nerve fibre resorption of the products of degeneration is effected by the phagocytic action of macrophages and Schwann cells.

The bulk of phagocytes is accounted for by haematogenous cells migrating into degenerating nerve fibres through the walls of the endoneurial vessels. Both Schwann cells and macrophages participate in eliminating the debris from the endoneurial tubes, the former ingesting the debris and passing it on to the latter.

Mast cells

These are well authenticated components of the connective tissues of peripheral nerves. They undergo the following two important changes in a nerve undergoing Wallerian degeneration.

1. Their numbers are greatly increased, the increase being maximal in the endoneurium. This increase peaks at about the 4th day and persists until the 15th day when their numbers decline so that 4 weeks after the injury their numbers are within the normal range.

2. Rapid degranulation occurs which liberates histamine and serotonin. Both increase capillary permeability which aids the passage of macrophages through the capillary wall and leads to capillary leakage and oedema.

The endoneurium

In this type of injury, the early reoccupation of endoneurial tubes by regenerating axons arrests the increase in new collagen that would otherwise occur if the reinnervation of endoneurial tubes were delayed.

Endoneurial capillary bed

The blood vessels and vascular pattern in the nerve below the injury are unchanged.

Endoneurial tube shrinkage

Initially there is a preliminary swelling of the tube, but by the 12th day the lumen is already becoming smaller. Developments, contributing to the continuing reduction in the diameter of the endoneurial tubes are:

a. the disintegration of the axon and myelin and the removal of the resulting debris reduces the contents of the tube;
b. the intracellular pressure transmitted along a normal axon is lost as it disintegrates.

With these changes, tension is reduced in the endoneurial wall of the fibre, which slowly contracts down on the remaining contents of the tube so that its calibre is gradually reduced. This reduction increases with the duration of denervation, rapidly over the first 3 months, beyond which there is little further change. The fibres are affected in proportion to their size, so that the largest are ultimately reduced to tubes $2–3\,\mu m$ in diameter.

At the end of 4 months most tubes are less than $3\,\mu m$ in diameter with only an occasional tube $4–5\,\mu m$ (Figs 14.1 and 14.2).

In the early stages the progressive reduction in calibre of the endoneurial tubes is due to shrinkage and not to a thickening of the tube wall at the expense of the lumen. If the reduction in calibre were due to an increase in endoneurial collagen

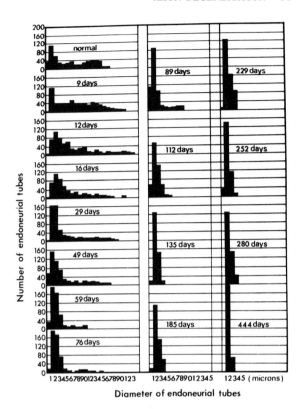

Fig. 14.1 Histograms illustrating the distribution of endoneurial tube diameters in a normal median nerve and in nerves which have been denervated for various periods. (Australian marsupial *Trichosurus vulpecula*)

then the fascicular area would remain unchanged over the period of denervation. There is, on the contrary, a progressive decrease in the fascicular area corresponding in time and degree to the reduction in the lumen of the endoneurial tubes. With shrinkage of the latter tension is also relieved in the perineurium, the circular and oblique fibres of which shorten to reduce the cross-sectional area of the fasciculus.

The reaction in non-myelinated nerve fibres

Here there is no myelin to degenerate but axon disintegration and degeneration follow the same course as for myelinated fibres. However, at least some non-myelinated axons survive section of the axon for longer periods than myelinated.

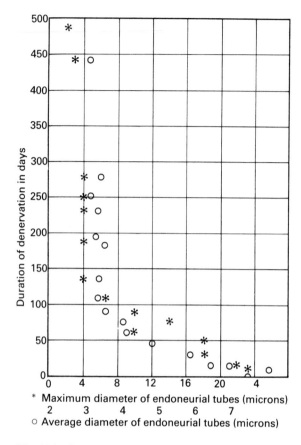

* Maximum diameter of endoneurial tubes (microns)
○ Average diameter of endoneurial tubes (microns)

Fig. 14.2 Graph to illustrate the effect of increasing periods of denervation on the maximum and average endoneurial tube diameters of denervated nerves. Note that the scale of the abscissa for the maximum tube diameter is not the same as that for the average tube diameter. (Australian marsupial *Trichosurus vulpecula*)

The reaction in nerve fibres and nerve cells above the injury

Human material is not available for examination in this type of nerve injury because axon regeneration proceeds without interruption to the restoration of the original pattern of innervation and recovery is complete in every respect. Under these conditions it is assumed that the retrograde reaction in nerve fibres and nerve cells must be minimal and rapidly reversible. At most, the nerve fibre reaction is confined to a few millimetres above the site of the injury and is but an extension of the local reaction at that site. The retrograde neuronal reaction only becomes a significant feature when the injury is sufficiently severe to destroy nerve fibres. This

reaction is described in the section devoted to a consideration of nerve injuries in which continuity of the entire nerve trunk is lost.

Factors influencing the onset and rate of degeneration

Species, age, fibre size and degree of myelination, level of the lesion, temperature, and general body nutrition are said to influence the onset and rate of Wallerian degeneration but there is no agreement on precisely how and in what way they do so.

Concluding comments

Generalising, the hallmarks of Wallerian degeneration appear within 24 hours of the injury in the axon, myelin and Schwann cells and these changes are well established during the early part of the 1st week after injury. The 1st week is occupied by the physical disintegration of axons and myelin, accompanied by a proliferation of Schwann cells and endoneurial mast cells, and the appearance of macrophages in large numbers in the endoneurial spaces. Chemical degradation of the myelin and axon debris commences towards the end of the 1st week and continues through the 2nd, and perhaps the 3rd, week, which is a period of intense phagocytic activity. Towards the end of this period Schwann and other cell activity declines as the debris is progressively removed. Finally, and usually by the end of weeks 5–8, the endoneurial tube is emptied of debris, except for the odd persisting remnant, and the nerve fibre is then composed of a central core of Schwann cells, enclosed in a sheath of endoneurium.

Changes in the endoneurial tissue are minimal throughout and though there is a reduction in the calibre of the endoneurial tubes as the axon and myelin debris is removed, the shrinkage must be a reversible process because, in this type of injury, functional recovery proceeds smoothly and is complete in every respect. Alternatively, regenerated axons that have been prevented from enlarging to their original diameters, because of permanent shrinkage of the endoneurial tubes, can function as efficiently as the original occupants.

NERVE INJURY IN WHICH NERVE FIBRE CONTINUITY IS LOST BUT FASCICULAR CONTINUITY IS PRESERVED

Local reaction at the site of injury

In these intrafascicular lesions the reaction is more severe. The ends of nerve fibres retract under the influence of an elastic endoneurium and the traumatised region becomes the site of an early inflammatory reaction. Capillaries suffer along with nerve fibres. Haemorrhage and capillary leakage lead to oedema and the formation of an exudate that accumulates between and around the nerve fibre ends. Macrophages invade the region in large numbers and Schwann cells, escaping from the ends of nerve fibres, and fibroblasts multiply in the exudate to increase the endoneurial matrix containing capillaries, collagen fibres and macrophages. With time this reactionary tissue settles into dense fibrous scar tissue. The involved fasciculi in the injured segment are swollen and hyperaemic and are finally left with a firm permanent fusiform swelling.

In injuries of this severity the epineurium is usually damaged as well. This, and the haemorrhage occurring in the interfascicular tissue, is followed by the usual inflammatory reaction and terminal fibrosis. As a consequence fasciculi become surrounded by interfascicular scar tissue, the end result being a local enlargement not only of the affected fasciculi but also of the entire nerve trunk. If surrounding structures have also been damaged the injured nerve trunk, which is left in continuity, may become embedded in scar tissue and/or fixed to neighbouring structures by adhesions.

The reaction and changes in nerve fibres below the injury

These follow the same pattern as that described in the preceding section but with one important difference. In intrafascicular injuries the endoneurial tubes may remain denervated for unduly long periods, or even permanently, because of the obstacles to axon growth imposed by intrafascicular fibrosis with consequences that are identical with those described later in this chapter.

The retrograde changes in nerve fibres and parent cell bodies and related trans-synaptic changes

The retrograde reaction is identical with that which follows loss of continuity of the entire nerve trunk (p. 86).

NERVE INJURY IN WHICH CONTINUITY OF THE ENTIRE NERVE TRUNK IS LOST

When a nerve trunk is severed, the simple pattern of Wallerian degeneration outlined earlier is complicated by a number of additional changes. There is a marked reaction at the ends of the severed nerve, the retrograde changes affecting nerve fibres and nerve cells are more severe, and the endoneurial tubes and fasciculi below the transection undergo further changes if, for any one of a number of reasons, the former fail to become occupied within a reasonable time by a regenerating axon.

Local reaction at the site of injury

When a nerve is severed, or a section of it is destroyed, the nerve ends retract and become separated. The distance between them and the condition of the intervening tissues depend on the severity of the injury and the length of nerve destroyed. Importantly, proliferating Schwann cells and, later, regenerating axons are no longer confined to endoneurial tubes and fasciculi.

Proliferating epineurial fibroblasts are present at the nerve ends as early as the 1st day. These are joined within the next few days by proliferating Schwann cells, and perineurial and endoneurial fibroblasts. The greatest increase in cell numbers occurs during the 1st week. Cellular activity then declines though the increase in epineurial fibroblasts, which are the major contributors to the formation of scar tissue in the region, continues for long periods.

The cellular outgrowths appearing at the nerve ends may or may not meet depending on the distance separating the nerve ends.

At the site of the injury there is an increase in capillary permeability within 24 hours which reaches a peak between days 7 and 14. This is probably the result of mast cell activity and the degranulation that liberates histamine and serotonin.

The end result of this activity is the formation of a swelling at each nerve end which is composed of a disorganised oedematous matrix of Schwann cells and fibroblasts along with capillaries, macrophages, other connective tissue cells and collagen fibres. Initially, capillaries enter the injury site from the nerve ends and from intraneural rather than extraneural sources. In the absence of the protective perineurial barrier, infection may contribute to the reaction and to the formation of scar tissue.

Later, regenerating axon tips appear at the end of the proximal stump and enter the swelling that has developed at that site. There, many are arrested, forming whorls, spirals and other abnormal endings and branchings all of which add to the size of the bulb. Some axons are deflected back along the nerve or into surrounding tissues. Some successfully weave their way through this tissue obstacle and enter the strand of tissue linking the two bulbs, along which they continue to grow distally. Whether or not regenerating axons reach and enter the distal stump depends on many factors such as the vigour of the regenerative process, the distance between the nerve ends and the nature of the intervening tissue. With the passage of time the traumatised zone is converted into scar tissue.

Schwann cell activity, at and between the nerve ends, is at its height when proliferation within the tubes is at its peak. The capacity of Schwann cells to act in this way is retained for long periods. If the ends of the tubes are freshened, as is done when a nerve trunk is repaired, the neighbouring Schwann cells become active again. Clinically, there is good reason for believing that the capacity to respond in this way is retained for several years after the original injury.

The characteristic zoning of the tissue reaction at the end of the proximal nerve stump and neuroma formation is described in Chapter 23.

Injuries that are sufficiently severe to sever a nerve usually damage neighbouring tissues as well, so that the pathology of the traumatised bed of the nerve is then added to the pathology of the nerve ends. The reaction to this added injury may result in the nerve ends becoming buried in scar tissue or fixed by adhesions to surrounding structures.

Reaction and changes in nerve fibres below the injury

These follow the same pattern as that described for axon degeneration and the related changes when axon continuity alone is lost as the result of the injury (p. 80).

When continuity of the entire nerve trunk is destroyed there are additional problems to consider. One relates to the fate of endoneurial tubes that are either not reinnervated or that remain denervated for unduly long periods. Another concerns the effect of this on the cross-sectional areas of the fascicular tissue and the nerve trunk.

Further changes in denervated endoneurial tubes

The progressive shrinkage of denervated endoneurial tubes that occurs with increasing periods of denervation has already been described (p. 81). This shrinkage continues until the endoneurial tubes present are 2–3 μm in diameter with an occasional tube of 4 μm. This occurs over the first 4 months, beyond which there is little further shrinkage.

Over this period the endoneurial collagen has been slowly increasing, new collagen being added to the outer surface of the basement membrane of the Schwann cells so that the endoneurial sheath thickens. With the passage of time the new collagen fibres become coarse and densely packed and the Schwann cells become thinned until finally the original denervated nerve fibre persists only as a fine strand of tissue.

Endoneurial fibrosis after prolonged denervation of the nerve below a transection is not an inflammatory process but is simply a replacement fibrosis to make up for the atrophy of nerve fibres.

The effect of these advanced changes on axon regeneration and the restoration of the structural features and physiological properties of nerve fibres is discussed in Chapter 15.

Endoneurial tubes left unoccupied by a regenerating axon are finally obliterated by the deposit of collagen fibres. Schwann cells atrophy and appear to contribute to the formation of collagen fibres that complete the obliteration, Schwann cells then reverting to a more primitive type indistinguishable from fibroblasts.

Changes in the fasciculi and nerve trunk below the injury

When preparing the ends of a severed nerve for repair it will often be found that their cross-sectional areas do not correspond, the size of the distal stump varying in an apparently unpredictable manner that is not always related to the time for which it has been denervated. Closer examination of this phenomenon reveals that it is based on variations in the relative cross-sectional areas of nerves devoted to fascicular and epineurial tissue respectively.

The reduction in the contents of the endoneurial tubes consequent on the degeneration of the axon and myelin, and the removal of the debris, are followed by shrinkage of the endoneurial tubes. These changes in turn result in a corresponding atrophy of the fasciculi which, with increasing periods of denervation, follows a pattern similar to that traced by the endoneurial tubes. Thus the cross-sectional fascicular area is reduced by about 40–50 per cent at 2 months, 50–60 per cent at 3 months and 60–70 per cent at 4.5 months, beyond which there is no further significant reduction (Fig. 14.3).

On the other hand, epineurial tissue undergoes little change except for some oedematous swelling at the nerve end. This tissue is excised at the time of the repair.

Because the fasciculi and epineurial tissue react so differently to denervation it follows that the extent of the shrinkage of the nerve trunk will be influenced, not only by the duration of denervation, but also by the percentage cross-sectional

Table 14.1 Comparison between the amount of nerve trunk and fascicular atrophy after different periods of denervation

Nerve	Duration of denervation in days	Percentage fascicular atrophy	Percentage nerve trunk atrophy
Median	9	0	+16
Median	12	12	12
Ulnar	16	37	6
Median	16	17	+ 2
Median	29	21	+27
Ulnar	44	64	49
Median	49	54	10
Ulnar	59	67	28
Median	59	50	31
Ulnar	68	61	56
Median	76	50	13
Median	76	54	58
Ulnar	76	50	59
Ulnar	89	68	35
Median	89	56	43
Median	112	56	32
Ulnar	112	73	37
Median	135	62	34
Median	135	70	43
Ulnar	140	61	30
Median	140	68	26
Median	185	62	25
Median	196	60	+12
Ulnar	196	54	45
Ulnar	224	63	54
Median	224	54	45
Median	229	59	33
Ulnar	229	69	54
Median	252	68	42
Ulnar	254	62	53
Ulnar	254	67	52
Ulnar	280	74	55
Ulnar	335	72	22
Ulnar	335	74	42
Ulnar	444	88	86
Ulnar	444	67	61
Ulnar	485	72	48
Ulnar	485	66	56

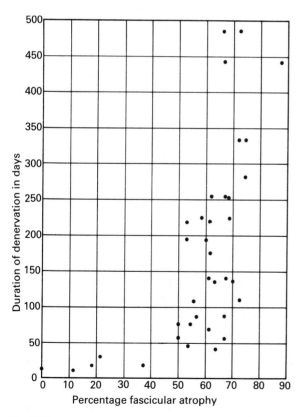

Fig. 14.3

area of the nerve occupied by fascicular tissue. Thus the reduction will be greater when the fasciculi are closely packed and occupy most of the cross-sectional area of the nerve than where the fasciculi are small and widely separated by a large amount of epineurial tissue.

Consequently, the reduction in the cross-sectional area of the distal nerve end below the reactionary zone, that will be excised when the nerve ends are prepared for repair, does not follow the fascicular atrophy. On the contrary it will, for a given period of denervation, vary irregularly depending on fascicular-epineurial tissue ratios. This is illustrated in Table 14.1.

The endoneurial capillary bed. With prolonged denervation and increasing fascicular shrinkage, many of the capillaries become thickened and finally obliterated, thereby promoting the fibrosis that will steadily replace the neural contents of the fasciculus. The density of the interfascicular vascular network is reduced but the larger intraneural vessels appear to survive indefinitely.

RETROGRADE CHANGES IN NERVE FIBRES PARENT CELL BODIES AND RELATED TRANS-SYNAPTIC CHANGES

Injuries that are sufficiently severe to sever nerve fibres are invariably followed by retrograde changes involving the nerve fibres, the parent cell bodies and their trans-synaptic connections. The nature, extent and magnitude of these changes depend not only on the severity of the injury but also on other factors to be discussed.

Changes in nerve fibres above the site of the injury. The changes described for nerve fibres below the injury extend centrally for one or several centimetres depending on the severity of the injury. Schwann cells are lost for a few millimetres but not as far centrally as the loss of the axon and myelin. The end result is one in which the endoneurial tubes of the last centimetre or so of the proximal nerve end are left occupied by Schwann cells only. Above this histologically modified segment of the nerve the surviving axon undergoes further changes.

The fate of nerve fibres above the injury depends on whether the parent cell survives and recovers to regenerate a new axon, is left with a residual defect, or degenerates. As long ago as 1903 van Gehucten stressed the significance of this factor in determining the calibre of nerve fibres in the proximal segment of a severed nerve and all subsequent work has only served to confirm his earlier observations.

Should the parent cell degenerate, the entire surviving length of the nerve fibre above the injury then undergoes Wallerian degeneration, though a little later than the onset and progress of Wallerian degeneration in the fibres below the injury.

Short of this extreme event, however, the surviving axons undergo a reduction in diameter that is greater if the regenerating axon is unable to re-establish functional connections with the periphery. Both axon diameter and myelin thickness are affected. As regeneration proceeds the axon diameter increases but is left with a permanent deficit. This reduction is accompanied by a slowing of conduction velocity and a reduction in axon transport, though the rate of transport remains essentially unchanged.

As regards these retrograde fibre effects in response to axotomy, Hoffer et al (1979, 1980) have reported that myelinated sensory fibres are more severely affected than motor fibres.

The reduction in calibre of nerve fibres above the injury has been attributed to the escape of axoplasm from the end of the severed endoneurial tube, to an outflow of axoplasm associated with axon regeneration, and to the failure of the regenerating axon to re-establish a functional connection with the periphery.

However, just as the re-establishment of functional connections by the regenerating axon is essential for the complete recovery of the cell body, so does the condition of the latter influence the final calibre of the regenerated nerve fibre.

Neurons may survive indefinitely in a modified state that can support correspondingly atrophied nerve fibres. These retrograde changes in nerve fibres will only result in significant reductions in the fascicular and nerve trunk cross-sectional areas when nerve cell degeneration results in the total loss of nerve fibres.

Changes in parent cell bodies. The development of tracer techniques and the availability of electron microscopy for the ultrastructural study of the changes taking place in the parent cell body following severance of its axon have greatly extended our knowledge of this subject.

The retrograde neuronal changes are concerned firstly with the survival of the cell, secondly with the restoration of its structural, chemical and functional properties and thirdly with the additional burden of replacing the axon that has perished as the result of the injury.

The retrograde neuronal reaction involves changes in the structure, biochemistry and function of the cell. The end result of this reaction may be complete recovery, cell death, or the persistence of a residual defect that adversely affects the function of the cell.

The fate of the cell body is, therefore, of crucial importance in any consideration of the consequences of the traumatic injury of a peripheral nerve.

Histological changes. Section of an axon does not invariably result in retrograde changes in the parent cell body. Why some should suffer and others escape is not fully understood.

On the basis of the histological changes through which the cell body passes, the reaction may be divided into a reactive or chromatolytic phase, a recovery phase and a degenerative phase.

Reactive phase. Changes are present within 6 hours, develop rapidly and peak towards the end of the 1st week. The most conspicuous initial changes are those affecting the nucleus and the Nissl material. The nucleus is displaced to the periphery, and the Nissl granules break into fine, dust-like particles that are dispersed through the cytoplasm, which becomes diffusely and weakly basophilic.

All compact Nissl material has disappeared by about the 4th day, though a narrow rim of fine particles may be left around the cell membrane. The changes collectively constitute chromatolysis, which is the most sensitive morphological indicator of the retrograde neuronal reaction. These changes have ultrastructural counterparts but these are not the concern of this text. This phase may be followed by the complete or incomplete recovery of the cell or its degeneration.

It is conceivable that the function of the neuron may be temporarily depressed or arrested by disturbances of cell mechanisms that have yet to be detected by any of the methods currently available for the study of cell function.

The perineuronal glial reaction. This has assumed special significance in retrograde phenomena in recent years. During the reactive phase, the perineuronal glial cells are greatly increased in size and numbers, proliferation commencing within 24–48 hours and reaching a peak within the 1st week. There is evidence that the glial proliferation is induced by agents liberated from chromatolytic neurons. The processes from glial cells extend to loosen and then displace the synaptic terminals from the surface membrane of the neuron. This activity results in synaptic stripping and lamellar cladding of the neuron, both of which isolate the neuron from surrounding influences and synaptic activity, thereby leaving it undisturbed to recover and regenerate a new axon. This synaptic stripping does not appear to adversely affect axon regeneration.

Another possibility is that the microglia may be activated in preparation for a phagocytic role should the neuron degenerate. Should the cell recover, however, this need does not arise, glial activity declines and the perineuronal satellites slowly return to their original state, taking about 4 months to do so.

Recovery phase. The delay before the onset of recovery, if it is to occur, depends on many factors, such as the severity of the injury, but it usually occurs in 2–3 weeks. Recovery then continues to completion through weeks 3–10, though the normal state may not be reached until many months after the injury. The earliest signs of recovery are the return of the nucleus to the centre of the cell and the reappearance of compact Nissl material.

Degenerative phase. During the 1st week neurons that are destined to degenerate react in the same way as those that are to recover. Degeneration may then proceed rapidly or be delayed for several months. Only degenerated neurons are attacked by microglial phagocytes, the sequence being degeneration — disintegration — phagocytosis.

The number of neurons perishing after nerve section varies from 15 to 80 per cent.

Chemical component of the retrograde reaction. The injury to the axon triggers an increased metabolic activity that is required to satisfy the needs of the recovering neuron and this is reflected in the early appearance of a high rate of protein synthesis and certain enzyme activity.

Detailed information continues to accumulate regarding the chemical changes and mechanisms involved in these processes, but the part they play in nerve injury and nerve repair in the actualities of the clinical situation remains obscure.

The residual defect. Finally, retrograde neuronal degeneration represents more than a reduction in the number of neurons. It also, and more importantly, means their removal from an integrated system. Additionally, the incomplete recovery of other neurons affects not only their capacity to provide new axon pathways to the periphery but also their capacity to contribute effectively to complex patterns of activity. As a result of the loss of some neurons and the incomplete recovery of others, complex patterns of activity are disorganised and thrown into disarray.

The signal for chromatolysis

While accepting that the injury, which detaches a variable amount of cytoplasm from the parent cell, triggers those retrograde changes through which the cell passes, this leaves unanswered the perplexing question of precisely how this triggering or signalling mechanism operates. There is considerable speculation on this point, the favoured explanation being the interruption of some trophic influence from the periphery, though this fails to explain the finding that repeated transection of the nerve induces a retrograde reaction on each occasion despite the absence of any contact with the periphery and, therefore, any signalling mechanism from that source.

The effects of repeated nerve transection on the retrograde neuronal reaction

Repeated nerve fibre transection induces a retrograde neuronal reaction on each occasion that resembles that occurring at the time of the first injury.

Related trans-synaptic changes. The retrograde reaction may extend beyond the nerve cells originally involved by inducing trans-synaptic effects in related neurons. Depression and failure of synaptic transmission, abnormalities in the pattern of synaptic activity and unfavourable effects on integrated functions have all been described for neurons during chromatolysis. As a result of these changes the functions of whole groups of neurons may be impaired and even their existence jeopardised. These changes are reversible providing the affected nerve cells recover.

Factors influencing the severity of the retrograde reaction. Many factors influence the severity of the retrograde reaction following the loss of continuity of a nerve trunk. These were identified by Marinesco (1901, 1909) at the turn of the century. The following account is based on his observations that have stood the test of time.

1. *The severity of the injury.* The greater the violence to the axon the more intense the retrograde reaction. It is more intense when the nerve is ruptured than when it is cleanly transected. Stretching a nerve experimentally, by applying graded degrees of traction, revealed the retrograde reaction to be proportional to the magnitude of the deforming force. The intensity of the reaction also increases with the length of the nerve destroyed.

2. *The level of the injury with reference to the parent cell.* The intensity of the retrograde reaction varies inversely with the site of the injury from the cell and so is related to the amount of axoplasm that is lost as the result of the injury.

3. *The type and size of the neuron.* The reaction often occurs more rapidly and to a greater degree in sensory than in motor neurons; this is especially so for the small cells of spinal ganglia. Consistent with this finding is the observation that, following transection of the sciatic nerve in kittens, the neurons of nonmyelinated fibres are more susceptible to retrograde cell necrosis than those of myelinated fibres (Aldskogius & Risling 1981, 1983).

4. *The restoration of functional connections with the periphery.* Failure to do this results in prolongation of the reaction.

5. *Miscellaneous.* The intensity of the reaction varies from species to species and from individual to individual. It is more severe in the young than in the adult but the young possess greater recuperative powers.

REFERENCES

Aldskogius H, Risling M 1981 Effect of sciatic neurectomy on neural number and size distribution in the L7 ganglion of kittens. Experimental Neurology 74: 597

Aldskogius H, Risling M 1983 Preferential loss of unmyelinated L7 dorsal root axons following sciatic nerve resection in kittens. Brain Research 289: 358

Hoffer J A, Stein R B, Gordon T 1979 Differential atrophy of sensory and motor fibers following section of cat peripheral nerves. Brain Research 178: 347

Hoffer J A, Gordon T, Stein R B 1980 Differential atrophy of sensory and motor fibers following ligation or resuture of cat hindlimb nerves In: Jewett D L, McCarroll H R (eds) Nerve repair and regeneration: its clinical and experimental basis. Mosby, St Louis, p 163

Lubinska L 1977 Early course of Wallerian degeneration in myelinated fibres of the rat phrenic nerve. Brain Research 130: 47

Marinesco G 1901 Sur les lésions des centres nerveux consécutives à l'elongation des nerfs périphériques et craniens. Comptes rendus des Séances de la Société de Biologie et de ses filiales 53: 324

Marinesco G 1909 La cellule nerveuse. Doin, Paris

Mira J C 1972 Maintien de la continuité de la lame basale des fibres nerveuses myelinisées après une congelation localisée. Compte rendus de l'Academie des Sciences, serie D273, 1836

Mira J C 1972 Effets d'une congelation localisée sur la structure des fibres nerveuses myelinisées et leur régéneration. Journal de Microscopie 14: 155

Mira J C 1979 Quantitative studies of the regeneration of rat myelinated nerve fibres: variations in the number and size of regenerating fibres after repeated localized freezings. Journal of Anatomy 129: 77

Mira J C 1981 Degeneration and regeneration of peripheral nerves: ultrastructural and electrophysiological observations, quantitative aspects and muscle changes during reinnervation. International Journal of Microsurgery 3: 102

Sunderland S 1978 Degeneration of the axon and associated changes. In: Nerves and nerve injuries, 2nd edn. Churchill Livingstone, Edinburgh, p 82

Van Gehuchten A 1903 La dégénérescence dite retrograde ou dégénérescence Wallérienne indirecte. Névraxe, 5: 1

15. Axon regeneration and related changes

When a nerve suffers an injury that leads to the degeneration of axons below the site of the injury, that part of the axon that survives regenerates to replace the part that has perished. This chapter is devoted to a consideration of the complicated and uncomplicated regeneration of axons, their conversion into mature functioning nerve fibres, the manner in which, and the rate at which, regeneration occurs and factors influencing these processes.

This subject is reviewed and discussed in some detail in Chapter 8 of *Nerves and Nerve Injuries* (Sunderland 1978), which also covers the literature up until 1976.

AXON REGENERATION AND THE FUNCTIONAL RECOVERY OF REINNERVATED TISSUES

At the outset it is necessary to emphasise the importance of carefully distinguishing between axon regeneration and the functional outcome of that regeneration.

The recovery of function requires far more than the regeneration of axons to replace the part lost below the injury. Of even more importance is the final destination of those axons because, for regeneration to be functionally effective, each axon must reach and reinnervate its old, or at least a functionally related, end organ. Failure to do this represents abortive and wasteful regeneration which leaves recovery incomplete and impaired.

Thus axon regeneration per se does not necessarily guarantee functional recovery and, because it is possible to have good axon regeneration and yet little functional recovery, it is necessary at all times to keep in mind that axon regeneration and func-tionally effective axon regeneration are two very different events in the regenerative process.

In determining the outcome of axon regeneration, the condition of the endoneurial sheath is critical.

Uncomplicated axon regeneration. When the wall of the endoneurial tube is undamaged, the regenerating axon is confined throughout its growth to the tube that originally contained it, regeneration proceeds smoothly and uninterruptedly, and the growing axon inevitably reaches the end organ originally innervated by it. This is uncomplicated regeneration.

Under these conditions, nerve fibres recover their normal structural features and physiological properties, the restored pattern of innervation is precisely the same as the original and recovery is complete in every respect.

Complicated axon regeneration. This occurs when the endoneurial sheath has been ruptured or severed. Regenerating axons are then free, on emerging from the cut end of the fibre, to wander in the tissue separating the nerve ends. As a result, many fail to reach and establish appropriate connections with functionally related end organs so that the restored pattern of innervation is left both imperfect and incomplete in comparison with the original and function suffers accordingly.

The course of regeneration differs so significantly in these two types of injury that a separate account is required for each.

Functionally effective regeneration involves a series of processes of great complexity, that include:

1. The recovery of the parent cell body and the onset of regeneration at the axon tip.

2. The growth of the axon tip to the site of the injury.
3. The passage of the axon tip through the injured region.
4. The growth of the axon down an endoneurial tube below the injury.
5. The restoration of appropriate end organ relationships.
6. Further changes to newly created axons leading to the restoration of their original structural features and physiological properties.
7. The recovery of sufficient numbers of nerve fibres, and in appropriate combinations, to provide a relevant response to voluntary effort or to a sensory stimulus.
8. The recovery from those changes that have developed in denervated structures that will enable them to function efficiently following reinnervation.

The time taken to complete this sequence of events is divisible into four periods.

1. *The initial delay.* This is the time taken by the neuron to recover, for axon growth to commence, and for the axon to reach the damaged zone. It is influenced by the severity of the injury and its proximity to the cell body.

2. *The site delay.* This is the time taken by growing axons to traverse the damaged zone. It is often included in the initial delay, which then represents the time before a regenerating axon enters an endoneurial tube below the site of the injury.

3. *The period of axon growth below the site of injury.* This is the time required for the axon tip to reach its peripheral termination. It is influenced by the distance to be travelled, the rate of advance of the axon tip, and any delays that occur en route.

4. *The period of functional recovery.* This is the time required:

a. to complete those changes in the restored axonal pathway that determine the normal conduction properties of individual nerve fibres, and for their recovery in sufficient numbers and in appropriate combinations to recreate those patterns of activity on which normal function depends;

b. for the reinnervated tissues to recover from a period of denervation and enforced disuse.

This sequence of events may be delayed or arrested at any stage during, or after, the restoration of axonal continuity with the periphery. This introduces wide variations in the interval between injury and recovery, and makes it exceedingly difficult to predict with any degree of accuracy the precise time course of regeneration in any individual patient.

RECOVERY OF THE NEURON AND THE ONSET OF REGENERATION

Recovery of the neuron from retrograde effects that depress or arrest its activity is marked by the correction of disorganised physicochemical processes, reversal of the transient depression of protein synthesis and the associated chromatolysis, and the accumulation of nucleoproteins that are re-formed into the characteristic pattern of Nissl material. Coincident with these are regenerative activities at the axon tip. At a later stage the rapid elongation of the regenerating axon makes demands on the protein-manufacturing apparatus of the nucleus, which becomes intensely active.

The relative roles of the cell body and the axon tip during regeneration are not fully understood. Changes in the nerve fibre proximal to the injury favour the latter rather than readjustments occurring further centrally in the nerve cell. Observations, based on changing fibre diameters, suggest that the axoplasm for the regenerating axon tip is provided exclusively from axoplasm proximal to the injury, and that it is the properties of the axon itself that provide the processes involved in regeneration. At the same time there is much evidence indicating that the rate of growth and final calibre of the axon must be influenced by complex physicochemical processes in the cell body that result in the production of substances that are transported down the new axon to participate in its growth and organisation.

The precise role that the parent neuron plays in the maturation, as opposed to the growth, of the regenerated axon is still obscure. Regenerating axons apparently derive their mature characteristics from the parent cells as well as from their peripheral connections, and there is also evidence that the volume of surviving neurons increases as a consequence of peripheral overloading introduced by axon branching.

Of decisive importance following severe injuries is the capacity of the neuron to send a new axon to the periphery and, on re-establishing continuity with an appropriate end organ, to induce satisfactory function in the reinnervated tissue. This alone can be accepted as an expression of its full regenerative power.

After emerging from the proximal end of a severed nerve, regenerating axons may terminate blindly in surrounding scar tissue. It is possible to restart the regenerative process by freshening the nerve end. This gives the axon another opportunity under more favourable conditions to grow and reach endoneurial tubes in the distal nerve end. This raises the question of for how long does a neuron retain the capacity, after repeated insults, to regenerate a new axon? There is much clinical evidence to indicate that, in human nerves, the capacity of some neurons to regenerate functionally efficient pathways is fully retained for at least 12 months and there is some presumptive clinical evidence that this capacity is retained for longer periods, but whether it is retained indefinitely is not known.

It has also been shown experimentally that nerve cells will tolerate repeated nerve transections without the vigour of axon outgrowth being arrested or seriously impaired, though these recuperative powers may be reduced with time (Duncan & Jarvis 1943, Mira 1979, 1981).

AXON REGENERATION ABOVE THE SITE OF THE INJURY

Owing to retrograde fibre degeneration, the axon tip is situated some distance above the site of injury, the distance varying from millimetres to centimetres depending on the severity of the injury. With the onset of regeneration, the advancing axon tip is initially confined in its endoneurial tube until it reaches the injury site, where its subsequent behaviour depends on the nature of the injury. The first signs of the onset of axon growth are present in this section 24

hours after the injury but may be delayed for days, or even weeks, depending on the severity of the injury and the extent of the retrograde changes. Here the first signs of axon branching may also be evident, though this does not usually become a feature of the process until the injured zone is reached.

AXON REGENERATION THROUGH AND BELOW THE INJURED SEGMENT

From this point onwards the fate of regenerating axons depends on whether there is loss of continuity of:

1. axons with their endoneurial sheaths left intact;
2. the entire nerve fibre, including its endoneurial sheath, with fascicular continuity preserved;
3. the entire nerve trunk.

The subsequent progress of the axon tip down the endoneurial tube below the lesion is the resultant of the combined action of three forces:

1. Central changes in the cell that propel the axon tip distally.
2. The activity of an especially organised growth cone, constituting the axon tip which, as it descends, leads to the elongation of the axoplasm. This activity requires dynamic impulses from the cell body for its effective control.
3. The tissue through which the axon must pass constitutes the peripheral resistance that must be overcome by the intrinsic forces of growth.

Axon regeneration when the endoneurial sheath has been preserved

The reaction at the site of an injury that does not destroy the continuity of the endoneurial tube presents no obstacle to the regenerating axon, though it is here that its advance may be temporarily slowed and some axon branching may occur. Regarding the fate of multiple axon sprouts confined within the original endoneurial tube, it is not clear whether only one or more survives to re-establish continuity with the periphery.

This type of lesion is best produced experimentally by freezing, and Mira (1976, 1979, 1981) in a study of axon regeneration under these conditions has reported a large increase in the number of myelinated fibres in branches of the sciatic nerve below the lesion but an accompanying reduction in their size. The ultimate fate of the excess myelinated fibres in terms of long-term survival and terminal connections is not known. However, Lugnegård et al (1984) report a reduction in the excess of myelinated fibres between 26 and 52 weeks postoperatively. Since multiple myelinated axons are not seen sharing the same endoneurial sheath at the periphery, this suggests a resculpturing of these fibres during regeneration.

Endoneurial tubes with Schwann cells appropriately aligned to minimise resistance to the advancing axon tips provide ideal conditions for their subsequent growth.

From a comparison of the times given for the onset of regeneration, and the time scale of the processes of degeneration, it is clear that, in this type of injury, axon tips must reach the affected portion of the endoneurial tubes when the latter are still occupied by the products of degeneration. However, neither this debris, nor the reaction associated with its removal, obstruct the advance of the axon. Further distally, depending on the level of the injury and the time when axons reach such levels, the endoneurial tubes will be free of debris.

With high lesions the endoneurial tubes at distal levels will be reduced in calibre by the time regenerating axons reach them. This, however, does not restrict their advance, though it may contribute to the slowing in the rate that obtains at distal levels.

The observation that Wallerian degeneration must reach a certain stage before a regenerating axon will occupy an endoneurial tube would, if confirmed, be an additional factor contributing to the delay in the onset of regeneration.

Because uncomplicated axon regeneration leads to the complete restoration of function, it follows that any endoneurial and fascicular shrinkage that has occurred during degeneration must be reversible, the regenerating axon having the capacity, as it enlarges, to inflate the atrophied tube into which

it has grown. This interpretation is consistent with the elastic properties of the endoneurium and perineurium.

The effect on uncomplicated axon regeneration of interfering with the blood supply to the nerve

Providing the longitudinal nutrient channels within the nerve are not interfered with, considerable lengths of a nerve may be deprived of entering nutrient arteries without affecting the regeneration of axons. However, this observation needs to be subjected to a more critical evaluation than has so far been the case.

Further changes in the regenerated axon and nerve fibre

The growth of the axon and the restoration of the axonal pathway to its original state, on which the functional efficiency of the new fibre depends, occur as two separate but related events during regeneration. Both proceed down the fibre but the complex morphological changes that constitute maturation advance at a slower rate than does the axon tip, and they continue long after the axon has been reconstituted.

The first of these is the alignment of Schwann cells, each forming a mesaxon which encircles the regenerating axon by repeated turns to form a multilamellated sheath. In this way remyelination of the new fibre proceeds as it does for the developing nerve fibre.

New myelin is obtained from at least three sources: (1) the synthesis of molecules in situ; (2) the incorporation of cholesterol molecules from the blood stream by Schwann cells; and (3) the reutilisation of cholesterol from myelin debris. Myelin is present 7–15 days after the onset of regeneration and remyelination proceeds down the nerve fibre in a manner that is not unduly delayed in comparison with the advance of the axon.

With segmentation of the myelin, the Schwann cells become reorientated so that there is one Schwann cell to each myelin segment. In this way the nodal arrangement is restored with, however, one curious departure from the original arrangement in that the internodes are now all shorter than before and are of approximately the same length.

Growth in the diameter of the axon continues after the appearance of the myelin sheath, the fibre enlarging until its original dimensions and axon-myelin relationships have been restored. This final stage is delayed until end-organ connections and functional relationships have been re-established. Such peripheral connections are essential for the full development of regenerated nerve fibres. However, this is inevitable when regenerating axons are inevitably directed back to the end organs that they originally innervated. Furthermore, early reinnervation of the endoneurial tube prevents the development of complications that would inhibit and delay the maturation of the new fibre.

Because complete recovery is inevitable in these injuries it is difficult, on account of the unavailability of human material for histological examination at critical stages during regeneration and recovery, to relate morphology to function. The assumption is that, since function is fully restored, the morphology of the reconstituted fibre is identical with that obtaining before the injury.

Further changes are undoubtedly required for the conversion of regenerated axons into functionally efficient systems but the precise nature of these changes remains obscure. The following are known to be involved but there could well be others:

1. Changes in the nerve fibre leading to its functional maturation. Nerve fibre diameter and degree of myelination are two features that are known to influence conduction properties.
2. Analogous changes at motor and sensory end organs leading to functionally effective connections.
3. Several thousand medium sized fibres with some evidence of myelination are necessary to permit the electrical recording of nerve action potentials (Kline et al 1981).
4. A minimum number of nerve fibres must be present before muscles will respond in a meaningful way to voluntary effort and sensory endings to a stimulus.

AXON REGENERATION WHEN CONTINUITY OF ENDONEURIAL TUBES HAS BEEN LOST BUT FASCICULAR CONTINUITY HAS NOT BEEN DISTURBED

Regenerating axons now escape from the ends of ruptured endoneurial tubes into the scar tissue that marks the site of the intrafascicular injury. This scar tissue obstructs the advance of some axons while others are misdirected into foreign endoneurial tubes, their subsequent fate depending on the branch fibre composition of the fasciculi at the level of the injury (see Chapters 28 and 42). Those that are successful in traversing the scar and entering an endoneurial tube below the lesion regenerate along it in a manner described in the next section.

AXON REGENERATION WHEN CONTINUITY OF THE NERVE TRUNK HAS BEEN LOST

As regenerating axons emerge from the free end of the severed nerve they escape into, and wander freely in, the tissues separating the nerve ends. This tissue must be traversed if axons are to reach the distal nerve stump. In this new environment the advancing axon tips are faced with hazards that delay or prevent them doing this, or misdirect them into foreign endoneurial tubes that conduct them to functionally unrelated end organs.

Axon regeneration through the bridging tissue or interface between the nerve ends

When continuity of a nerve trunk has been destroyed the nerve ends are either left separated by a gap or are reunited surgically. In either event the tissue that develops between them is essentially the same, except that the bridging tissue between separated nerve ends is more extensive and usually denser and more disorganised than is the interface tissue that develops as healing occurs between reunited nerve ends. The barrier to the passage of axons created by bridging and interface tissue is therefore one of degree. Special consideration is given to the latter in Chapter 42.

The capacity of regenerating axons to bridge long gaps between nerve ends

That regenerating axons may, unaided, bridge long gaps in injured nerves, find their way into the distal stump, and reach the periphery is well established (see Chapter 16). Though such regeneration sometimes gives a surprising degree of recovery, this is not usual because of the many hazards that, under these conditions, reduce the functional effectiveness of regeneration, firstly by preventing axons reaching the periphery in appropriate numbers, and secondly by distorting the pattern of reinnervation. The spontaneous recovery occurring when the ends of a severed nerve are left widely separated is far inferior to that obtainable after a good nerve repair. Mira (1981) reported only about 20% of the myelinated fibres crossing a 10 mm gap in a rat sciatic nerve.

The bridging tissue becomes composed of Schwann cell columns and groups, proliferating fibroblasts from the endoneurium, perineurium and epineurium, perineurial cells, collagen fibres and the usual capillaries. It is never as suitable a medium for the growth of the axon as is the endoneurial tube. Though varying in density, arrangement and amount, it usually obstructs, delays and misdirects axons in their passage distally.

The movement of axon sprouts through the tissue is determined by resistance gradients, the sprout that meets with the least resistance advancing more easily and rapidly than the others. Thus the direction taken by each axon tip as it grows is influenced by the structural organisation of the medium through which it is regenerating. Resistance to the advancing axons is minimal where the collagen fibres are arranged in open parallel strands. There is also good evidence that axons are attracted to the distal stump and to Schwann cells in preference to all others (see Chapter 16).

As they grow, some axons have a tendency to collect into groups or minifascicles, each of which becomes surrounded by cells that later develop into perineurial cells. These minifascicules may fuse to form larger collections. Axons that reach the distal stump may do so as early as the 3rd day or their entry may be delayed for much longer periods, depending on the nature, consistency and extent of the tissue separating the ends of the severed nerve. Consequently, the site delay is subject to considerable individual variation.

Under favourable conditions regenerating axons may cross a suture line and enter the distal stump as rapidly as after a simple crush injury, that is within 3–20 days of the suture. Generally speaking, however, the site delay in any single individual case will be greater when the nerve has been severed and later repaired.

An axon, having forced its way through the junctional tissue between the nerve ends, may continue to be impeded in its subsequent growth down an endoneurial tube. This is because the unfavourable junctional tissue could, by constricting axons passing through it, exert a local throttling effect on their growth. If the advance of the axon is due to central influences forcing it distally, then such a constriction would operate continuously throughout the growth of the axon and in this way slow its advance. It is of interest that the rate of regeneration is usually faster when the endoneurial tube escapes injury than when it is severed; scarring at the site of injury is absent or minimal in the former but is significant in the latter.

The resistance which the axon tip meets in its advance through the junctional scar tissue also results in the formation of multiple sprouts, a single axon giving rise to as many as 50 sprouts. The daughter axons produced in this way have diameters that are less than that of the parent axon. Such multiple axons do not all reach the diameter of the parent nerve fibre as they develop and the persistence of fine axons may contribute to the failure to achieve full restoration of the conduction properties of the nerve.

Several axon sprouts may enter and descend along the same endoneurial tube. On the other hand, a single regenerating axon may, by branching, reinnervate more than one endoneurial tube. Horsch & Lisney (1981) have reported that, one and a half years after transecting but not suturing cat cutaneous nerves, regenerating neurons supported multiple sprouts in the distal stump of the nerve, some of which innervated split receptive fields in the skin.

The manner in which such sprouting may complicate, reduce, or improve the chances of useful regeneration remains the subject of speculation.

Not only does the junctional tissue act as a barrier to regenerating axons, but the disorganised growth imposed on others results in some axons failing to enter endoneurial tubes while others are misdirected into tubes that differ from those they originally occupied. These foreign tubes may, or may not, lead them back to functionally related end organs. This is because, in their growth through the bridging tissue, axon tips are not subjected to any known neurotropic influences that would guide them into their old endoneurial tubes, thereby ensuring that neurons would be reconnected to the structures they originally innervated (Chapter 16). There is the further interesting observation that the axons of non-myelinated fibres enter and grow down the endoneurial tubes of myelinated fibres in preference to their original pathway. This is related to the Schwann cell population, which increases markedly in the endoneurial tubes of denervated myelinated fibres but undergoes little change in the tubes of non-myelinated fibres.

The overall effect of unfavourable scar tissue between the nerve ends is to:

1. obstruct the advance of some regenerating axons thereby reducing the nerve fibre population;
2. delay the advance of some regenerating axons and, in doing so, constrict them;
3. retard the subsequent development of those that have regenerated by delaying and limiting their maturation so that the structural features and physiological properties of nerve fibres below the injury are never fully restored, even when the severed nerve is repaired;
4. misdirect axons into functionally unrelated endoneurial tubes.

Collectively, these complications mean that the restored pattern of innervation is grossly disorganised and functionally impaired in comparison with the original. Under such adverse circumstances recovery is negligible unless regenerative processes are assisted by some form of nerve repair.

As we have seen, the combined initial and site delays may vary from a few days to weeks.

Governing factors are the severity of the injury, the length of the gap between the nerve ends, the nature and extent of the intervening tissue, and the extent and degree of retrograde changes in the system.

Axon regeneration in the endoneurial tube below the injury

After section of a nerve trunk the reoccupation of endoneurial tubes may be considerably delayed and may not occur until endoneurial tube shrinkage is maximal. Despite this, there is much clinical evidence to indicate that, once regenerating axons have entered endoneurial tubes then, given reasonable conditions, regeneration follows much the same course regardless of the period of denervation, at least within 1–2 years following the injury.

The new axon regenerates down the endoneurial tube at a slower rate than is the case when continuity of the tube has not been destroyed.

Providing a favourable terminal connection is made, the structure of the fibre is restored in much the same way as has been described for uncomplicated regeneration. If, on the other hand, the terminal connection is with a functionally unrelated tissue then further development of the axon and myelin is aborted.

It is generally believed that, when more than one axon enters an endoneurial tube, only one eventually survives and only a single fibre is left when myelination is well advanced. However, an increase in the number of regenerated myelinated fibres below a transected and repaired nerve has been reported on several occasions (Aitken et al 1947, Evans & Murray 1956, O'Daly & Imaeda 1967, Mira 1976, 1981, Orgel & Terzis 1977, Miyamoto 1979, Jenq & Coggeshall 1984a,b, Lugnegård et al 1984). This suggests that other early occupants of an endoneurial tube can survive, myelinate and acquire a separate identity.

In respect of this increase, Mira (1981) has described simple and compound myelinated fibres below the lesion. In the former the single occupant was the original reconstituted axon. The latter were complex temporary structures, each consisting of several myelinated and nonmyelinated axons enclosed in a common basal lamina. Each unit was shown to have originated as multiple sprouts from a single regenerating axon. The basal lamina subsequently disintegrated to release new fibres into the fasciculus. However, all the new fibres did not reach the periphery, though the overall effect was to leave an increase in the number of restored fibres. How this is related to terminal connections is not known, while the survival of multiple axon sprouts raises the question of the effect of overloading parent neurons.

The growth of axons that fail to enter an endoneurial tube is soon aborted.

As in uncomplicated regeneration, myelination proceeds centrifugally along the fibre somewhat later than the advance of the axon tip. A delay of about 1–2 weeks separates the two processes near the lesion, but the delay is somewhat greater at the periphery. The onset of myelination appears to be determined by the size of the axon, myelination commencing when axons reach a diameter of about 2 μm, just as occurs during the normal development of nerve fibres. Maturation of the fibre is a slower process requiring about 1 year for completion, but it may be further delayed or arrested by complications operating central to, at, and/or peripheral to the lesion. Reference has already been made to the first two.

Importantly, the maturation of the restored fibre proceeds to completion only when appropriate functional connections are restored. If, during regeneration, an axon is directed into a tube that conducts it to a functionally unrelated end organ, the axon does not regain its original size or degree of myelination. Even when an axon reoccupies its original tube, its development into a mature fibre will be incomplete if it is prevented from reinnervating the end organ because of changes that have developed in the peripheral tissue as the result of prolonged denervation.

Other important factors influencing the maturation of regenerating nerve fibres are changes that develop in nerve fibres subjected to prolonged denervation. There is as yet no firm data on when atrophy of the tubes and collagenisation of the endoneurial sheath reach a degree that prevents; (a) the entry of axons into, and their growth down, endoneurial tubes and (b) the enlargement of regenerating axons as they grow and their conversion into functionally mature nerve fibres.

Four months after nerve severance, the largest endoneurial tubes available for regenerating axons will rarely exceed 3 μm in diameter. If such atrophied tubes prevent large fibres from regaining their original diameters then nerve repair, delayed for more than 4 months, should result in a permanent reduction in the diameters and myelination of many of the regenerated fibres, and consequently a significant residual functional disability.

That the conduction properties of regenerated nerve fibres never return to normal after nerve repair and that the rate of axon advance is slower under these conditions would suggest that this could be so.

While, in general, the quality of the recovery after nerve repair declines as the preoperative delay increases, this can be explained on the grounds that many factors contribute to this, of which the state of the endoneurial tubes is only one possible element.

At the same time, there is considerable clinical evidence that, following nerve repairs that have been unavoidably delayed for at least 12 months and even longer, the endoneurial tubes will convey regenerating axons to the periphery in a manner that does not differ significantly from that observed after immediate nerve repair. Furthermore, some reinnervated muscles may recover completely under these conditions.

Clearly endoneurial tube atrophy does not necessarily impair axon regeneration, nor does it prevent those changes in restored axonal pathways that convert them into functionally efficient nerve fibres. The precise morphological nature of the changes occurring under these conditions remains unknown. If it represents the restoration of original fibre diameters then endoneurial tube shrinkage must be a reversible process, the tube presumably responding to pressures generated by an enlarging axon. This conclusion is in keeping with the elastic properties of the endoneurial wall. On the other hand, there is also evidence that the restoration of the normal architecture of nerve fibres may not be necessary for the recovery of function.

Providing a regenerating axon enters an endoneurial tube that will guide it to a functionally related end organ, the course and end result of regeneration are essentially the same, at least within the first 12 months after injury.

The changes due to prolonged denervation that do impair recovery are those that either prevent regenerating axons from entering appropriate endoneurial tubes, or make it impossible for peripheral tissues to respond satisfactorily when they have been reinnervated.

THE REGENERATION OF NONMYELINATED NERVE FIBRES

The axons of nonmyelinated nerve fibres regenerate in much the same way as the myelinated variety and, like the latter, do not fully recover if they fail to make functional connections. Regenerating 'nonmyelinated' axons will also enter endoneurial tubes previously occupied by myelinated fibres.

Of interest is the curious finding of Jenq & Coggeshall (1984a,b, 1985a,b) that, after transection and repair of the sciatic nerve in the rat, there was an excess of both myelinated and nonmyelinated axons in the branch to the medial head of gastrocnemius, and an increase in myelinated but decrease in nonmyelinated axons in the sural nerve.

THE MANNER AND RATE OF AXON REGENERATION

The rate at which regenerating axons advance is of interest, firstly as a feature of a growth process with general biological implications, and secondly for calculating when the first signs of recovery are to be expected. An estimate of the latter is an essential part of the clinical management of the injury, the object being to avoid interfering prematurely with an injured, or repaired nerve, that would recover if left undisturbed, while at the same time recognising 'failed recovery' with the least possible delay so that appropriate remedial procedures can be instituted.

Despite the difficulties implied in equating functional recovery with maturation, there is some justification for regarding the progress of motor and sensory recovery as at least an expression of the advance of maturation down the fibre.

The manner in which axons tips advance down the nerve

The manner in which axon tips advance down endoneurial tubes, the rate at which they do so and the factors influencing these events are summarised in the following statements.

1. Is the rate at which an axon regenerates constant or not and, in the event of the latter, how and in what way does it vary?

Experimental investigations of rates of regeneration led to the conclusion that the rate was constant, and this was generally held to be true for man for whom a rate of 1 mm per day was commonly quoted in the literature. The lengths of nerve fibres available for the study of this problem in experimental animals are, however, too short to reveal any possible decline in the rate.

Furthermore, the unqualified acceptance of a constant rate, and the practice of averaging this over the much greater distances covered by regenerating axons in man, obscures some important features of the growth process.

More carefully planned clinical studies of the course of recovery in suitable cases of nerve injuries have shown that the rate of advance of the axon tip, gradually declines over the whole period of recovery (Sunderland 1978). This is not surprising, for a steadily diminishing rate is characteristic of most growth processes.

2. Another feature is the relationship between the distance of the axon tip from the cell body and its rate of advance. The rate is faster the closer the axon tip is to the cell body. The rate then gradually slows as the distance of the advancing axon tip from the cell increases. The rate over a given section of the nerve fibre at a given distance from the cell body is therefore always the same regardless of the level of the lesion. Thus the rate of regeneration over the section X of the nerve fibre shown in Fig. 15.1 is the same whether the lesion is lo-

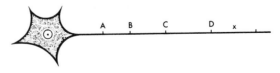

Fig. 15.1

cated, and regeneration commences, at A, B, C, or D.

3. While the level of the lesion, and therefore the level at which regeneration commences, does not affect the rate over any given section of the nerve, it does determine the initial velocity. Thus the commencing rate of regeneration is greater at A than at B, at B than at C and at C than at D. An axon commencing to regenerate after a lesion at A will grow at a rate that gradually declines until, at B, its rate corresponds to what would be the commencing rate if the lesion had been at B. Finally, concerning the time factor, an axon advancing along the section X has been growing for a longer time after a lesion at A than after a lesion at D, and yet the rate over this section is the same for both lesions.

4. Regeneration proceeds at a progressively diminishing rate regardless of the nature of the lesion.

5. Because the rate of axon growth is not uniform along the nerve fibre, the distance as well as the level over which it is calculated becomes important. Thus a single calculation based on the total length of a nerve fibre gives misleading information about the process because the influence of factors that operate locally to affect the rate is spread over the full length of the fibre. On the other hand, calculations for successive sections, though they assume a constant rate for each section, nevertheless collectively reveal a progressively diminishing rate for the entire fibre. It would, however, be unwise to assume that growth proceeds without any delays or that the progressive slowing necessarily takes place without irregularities. The rate measured for any particular section merely represents the sum total of the change occurring within that section over a certain time interval; it also has the advantage of confining the effect of factors that influence the rate to the particular section of the nerve in which they operate.

6. The velocity of regeneration is the resultant of central forces provided by the cell body and the peripheral resistance against which the central growth forces act. The progressively diminishing rate is principally the result of waning central forces that are reduced as the distance of the actively growing axon tip from the cell lengthens, and as the cytoplasmic load increases with the restoration of the axon. There appears to be no significant contribution to that decline from a peripheral resistance gradient along the endoneurial tube created by tubal shrinkage.

7. Two factors should always be taken into account when calculating rates of axon regeneration, the distance over which the rate is measured, and the level, with reference to the parent neuron, at which the measurements are made.

8. Finally, the rate of axon advance at any given level need not necessarily be the same for every regenerating fibre in the nerve.

9. Regeneration rates vary from individual to individual and species to species. Furthermore, the different methods employed for calculating rates may give different results because they do not always measure the same event. It is these variables that account for the wide variations reported in the literature for rates of regeneration.

Rate of axon regeneration

1. In uncomplicated regeneration. Most of the information on rates of axon regeneration is experimentally based with values varying from 1 to 4.8 mm per day. More recent measurements give rates of the order of 4.4 mm/day (Berenberg et al 1977, Legrain 1977, McQuarrie et al 1977, Forman & Berenberg 1978, Mira 1979, 1981, Forman 1980).

The little information available on rates in man gives overall values varying from 1 to 4.5 mm/day, without reference to the level of the injury or the distance over which the rate was calculated.

The data concerning this question shown in Table 5.1 are from the author's limited records. Clearly much more information is needed on this feature of axon regeneration.

Table 5.1 Rates of uncomplicated axon regeneration

Root of the limb	6.0 mm/day
Elbow	4–5.0 mm/day
Wrist	1–2.0 mm/day
Hand	1–1.5 mm/day
Lower leg	1–2.0 mm/day
Ankle	1.0 mm/day

Table 5.2 Rates of axon regeneration after nerve suture

Lower forearm	2.0 mm/day
Wrist and hand	1.0 mm/day
Upper leg	2.0 mm/day
Lower leg	1.5 mm/day
Ankle	1.0 mm/day

2. After nerve suture. The reservations expressed in the previous section in relation to rates of regeneration also apply to the rates recorded after nerve suture. Clinical data, limited and inadequate though they may be, give overall rates of from 1 to 5 mm/day and declining rates as shown in Table 5.2. The best that can be said, comparing data available for the two types of injury, is that the rate is slower after nerve suture, a view shared by others (Forman and Berenberg 1978, Forman et al 1979, Danielson et al 1986a).

Rates based on the advance of functional recovery

Regeneration of the axon and the later conversion of the newly reconstituted axon pathway into a functionally mature nerve fibre occur as separate but closely related events during regeneration. Both progress in a proximo-distal direction, though maturation lags behind the advancing axon tip.

The course of the maturation process can only be traced with any degree of accuracy by using histological techniques and such a study is not possible in man. What then can be done to obtain some estimate of the rate at which the maturation of regenerating nerve fibres occurs in man?

Because motor recovery is dependent on the restoration of the normal structural features and physiological properties of motor nerve fibres, there is some justification for using the progress of motor recovery as a rough measure of the progress of motor nerve fibre maturation during regeneration. This can be done in cases of second degree injury (uncomplicated regeneration) by using:

1. differences in the onset of recovery in two muscles innervated at different levels, and
2. the difference in the distances to the same two muscles based on measurements made on cadaver material.

Values for time and distance obtained in this way are then used to estimate a rate. Clearly there are obvious sources of error in proceeding in this way.

1. Motor recovery involves more than the conversion of motor axons into mature motor nerve fibres. The inability of a patient to contract muscles in response to voluntary effort after they have been reinnervated is a case in point.
2. Distances are based on the average of measurements made on cadavers, where branch patterns for the same nerve vary from individual to individual as do the distances to muscles measured from a fixed point along the nerve and its branches. In any particular patient the true distances are, therefore, concealed and unknown.
3. The true distance from the lesion to the structure in which recovery is being studied is greater, by an unknown amount, than the distance measured along the nerve trunk and the branch to the structure concerned. This is because:

   a. The undulations of a nerve trunk in its bed, of fasciculi within the nerve, and of nerve fibres within the fasciculi, invalidate by an unknown amount all measurements relating to distance.
   b. The intramuscular length of nerve fibres between their point of entry into the muscle and their neuromuscular terminations is not known. The ramifications of sensory nerve fibres in the cutaneous plexuses likewise increase the distance to terminal connections by an unknown but probably significant amount.

Obviously no great reliance should be put on maturation rates calculated from such shaky data. However, providing these sources of error are kept in mind, the manner and rate at which motor and sensory functions recover could be regarded as some measure of those changes in the new axon that result in the restoration of its calibre, degree of myelination, and conducting properties.

Mindful of these reservations, the findings are

consistent with the general conclusion that, in man, the maturation of reconstituted nerve fibres takes place more slowly than axon regeneration.

Rates calculated in this way vary considerably but do not exceed 3–4 mm per day with a bias towards even lower ranges. The only available values for a declining rate are: arm and thigh, 3 mm/day; wrist and ankle, 0.5 mm/day. Once again the rate after nerve suture is slower by about 0.5–1 mm per day; the difference is greater proximally but over the terminal portion of the nerve in the hand and foot there is little difference between the two.

Sympathetic fibres

The regeneration of sympathetic nerve fibres has not been subjected to the same intensive study as have somatic nerve fibres, and little confirmation is available relating to the rates at which pre- and post-ganglionic axons advance during regeneration. It is sometimes assumed that they regenerate more rapidly than somatic axons but, in the absence of any adequate comparative studies, there can be no certainty on this point.

THE CONDUCTION VELOCITY IN REGENERATED NERVE FIBRES

Following uncomplicated axon regeneration, the conduction velocity in regenerated nerve fibres slowly improves but takes at least 6–15 months to reach normal limits depending on the level of the lesion.

After nerve suture the conduction velocity in regenerated nerve fibres improves very slowly indeed and is never fully restored as is shown in Table 5.3.

AXON TRANSPORT SYSTEMS IN REGENERATING NERVE FIBRES

Axon transport systems operate in regenerating axons conveying organelles, proteins and other essential materials to and from the growing axon tip. However, they are all modified in a manner that is the subject of uncertainty and disagreement. There are reports to the effect that:

1. During axon regeneration the needs of the

Table 5.3 Conduction velocities in regenerated nerve fibres

Hodes et al 1948	40% at 42 months
Struppler & Huckauf 1962	4–29% (average 14.8%) at 17 years
Kline & de Jonge 1968	10% at 12 months
Kline et al 1972	40% at 12 months
Ballantyne & Campbell 1973	20–30% at 15 months

regenerating segment do not require dramatic changes in axon transport systems within which however there are some discrete adjustments (Frizell & Sjöstrand 1974a–c, Lasek & Hoffman 1976, Droz 1981).

2. Transport rates are unchanged (Kreutzberg & Schubert 1971), though there are changes in the nature and amounts of the transported material.

3. Fast and slow axon transport are increased (Grafstein & Murray 1969, Frizell & Sjöstrand 1974a–c, Grafstein & McQuarrie 1978).

4. Transport rates are slowed (Carlsson et al 1971).

5. There is an increase in the amount of proteins carried by the slow transport system (Frizell & Sjöstrand 1974a–c, Grafstein & McQuarrie 1978).

6. Neurofilament protein transport is selectively reduced in regenerating axons (Hoffman & Lasek 1980, Droz 1981, Hoffman et al 1984).

7. During regeneration the flow rate of acetylcholinesterase is reduced (Couraud & Di Giamberardino 1981).

8. The amount of rapidly transported proteins remains high (Danielsen et al 1986b).

9. Membrane proteins are conveyed at a normal rate in increased or decreased amounts 'according to the molecular species' whereas other proteins 'would be transported at a higher velocity or in larger amounts' (Droz 1981).

10. Axonal constituents that are normally destined for release at the terminal endings are returned to the cell from the regenerating axon segment by retrograde transport (Droz 1981).

From this confusion it is not possible at this time to extract any information of relevance to axon regeneration in the clinical sense.

FACTORS INFLUENCING AXON REGENERATION

Because several factors operate concurrently to influence the rate of regeneration in any individual patient, it is difficult, and often impossible, to isolate and determine the role of any one specific factor.

Type of nerve fibre

All other things being equal, rates of axon regeneration appear to be the same for all somatic nerve fibres. So far as the maturation of the new axon is concerned, this could be expected to take place more slowly in thicker, more heavily myelinated nerve fibres compared with non-myelinated fibres, and there is some evidence to support this.

Type of nerve injury

The balance of the evidence favours a slower rate after nerve suture than after lesions in which the integrity of the endoneurial tube is preserved. This could be due to factors operating proximal, at, and distal to the site of damage.

Retrograde neuronal disturbances increase with the severity of the injury and its proximity to the cell body, and are known to be more marked after nerve section. Residual disturbances of this nature could reduce the capacity of the neuron to propel the axon tip distally.

Scar tissue, that develops at the site of nerve repair but not when the wall of the tube is undamaged, could contribute to the slower rates recorded after nerve suture.

It could be argued that severe shrinkage of the endoneurial tubes consequent on the delayed arrival of axons following nerve repair, could contribute to a slower rate by retarding the advance of the axon. After immediate suture, however, regenerating axons reoccupy endoneurial tubes under conditions not significantly different from those obtaining when regeneration is uncomplicated. Despite the fact that endoneurial tube shrinkage has not had time to develop to a degree that might be expected to impair regeneration, the rate after immediate suture is slower than that recorded for uncomplicated regeneration.

A comparison of the progress of regeneration after immediate suture at a distal level and after a lesion in continuity at a much higher level is also of interest. In the former, the new axon reaches its destination after a relatively short delay, and at a time when the changes that develop in the system as the result of denervation are still of relatively short duration. On the other hand, the axon regenerating spontaneously from a higher level has a much greater distance to cover, so that its arrival at the corresponding peripheral level is greatly delayed in comparison. This means that the changes due to denervation will be of longer duration and, consequently, more advanced. Despite this, the rate of axon growth, when calculated over a corresponding distal section of the nerve, is faster after a second degree injury than after immediate suture. This clinical finding suggests that, within the conditions set by the clinical situation, neither the duration of denervation nor the state of the peripheral tissues is responsible for the slower rate of regeneration after suture.

Of greater significance are factors operating at and central to the site of injury. Among these, the role of weaker forces of growth consequent on more severe retrograde neuronal effects, and of constricting scar tissue at the repair site, appear to be established.

The level of the lesion

For reasons outlined earlier in this chapter the rate declines as the distance of the growing axon tip from its cell body increases. This explains why the level of the injury determines the initial velocity, which is faster the closer the lesion is to the cell.

Duration of the period of denervation

The capacity of the central stump for sprouting is retained for long periods, though no information is available on rates of regeneration that follow after such delays.

It is possible that after very long delays the

capacity of the neuron to propel the axon distally may wane, with a consequent reduction in the velocity of growth, but there is no evidence to support this. The slower rate after nerve suture is more directly related to the severity of the retrograde neuronal disturbances and to scar tissue at the suture site that constricts growing axons.

Different nerve trunks

It is not known for certain whether there are different rates for different nerves, though there are some interesting clinical observations suggesting that this could be the case.

Age

Young patients have significantly better results following nerve repair, but whether the rate of regeneration is faster in the young remains to be answered.

Temperature

Increased regenerative activity in experimental animals has been reported with a rise in temperature, but it is difficult to test this concept in patients. Thermal variations between summer and winter appear to be without effect.

Individual variations

While, in any given case, the rate diminishes progressively as the axon advances down the nerve, the rate is subject to individual variation. Furthermore, different methods of measuring the rate do not always measure the same event in what is an exceedingly complex process. After excluding differences introduced in this way and those which are due to factors that are known to influence the rate, there remain differences that appear to be due to properties of the growth process that are specific to the individual.

ENHANCEMENT OF AXON REGENERATION

In the search for potentially effective axon growth accelerators it should be remembered that severed axons have a natural and remarkable capacity to regenerate. In fact, a continuing problem is to prevent them from doing so, as those involved with the treatment of painful neuromas will readily testify.

Despite the natural propensity of axons to regenerate, the availability of agents that would accelerate this process would have the special advantage of reducing the time for which muscles and skin are denervated, the overall effect being to hasten their reinnervation and the onset and quality of motor and sensory recovery. Always providing, of course, that the now more rapidly growing axons find their way back to functionally related endings. Such agents would have a particular value following nerve repair at high levels in the limbs where regenerating axons have much greater distances to grow.

Nerve growth factor

In the early 1950s Levi-Montalcini and her co-workers (1951, 1953) isolated an active factor from mouse tumour that stimulated the growth of sensory and sympathetic nerve cells in cultures of embryonic neural tissue. This factor was called 'nerve growth factor' shortened to NGF. This factor was later isolated from snake venom and finally from the salivary glands of mice which proved to be the richest source. This pioneering work and subsequent studies have been reviewed by Levi-Montalcini (1966, 1976, 1983) and Levi-Montalcini & Angeletti (1968).

A number of growth stimulating and regulating agents has since been isolated from mouse submaxillary gland (Hoffman & McDougall 1968) but by far the most extensively studied has been NGF.

There is now a rapidly expanding literature on this subject which is not reviewed here because, though NGF is of considerable neurobiological interest, its relevance to axon regeneration and nerve repair in the adult has yet to be demonstrated. However, the following features of NGF that could be of significance have been extracted from key references, additional to those mentioned above, that should be consulted for details (Angeletti et al 1971, Campenot 1977, 1982, Gundersen & Barrett 1979, 1980, Kessler & Black 1980, Varon & Adler 1980, Johnson 1983,

Korsching & Thoenen 1983a,b, Politis 1986, Rich et al 1987).

1. NGF is a polypeptide which when administered to an embryonic tissue culture of sympathetic and sensory neurons induces a prolific sprouting of cell processes.
2. NGF is required for the maintenance and survival of sympathetic and dorsal root ganglion neurons.
3. NGF appears to have no effect on motor neurons.
4. NGF stimulates protein synthesis in immature sympathetic and dorsal root ganglion neurons. Under its influence the neurons increase in size with a dramatic proliferation of their processes.
5. NGF is believed to be present in many different tissues from which it is transported to the cell body by the retrograde transport system.
6. There is presumptive evidence that Schwann cells are a source of NGF.
7. NGFs extracted from different sources differ in their chemical properties but produce the same biological effects.
8. The preferential outgrowth of neurites towards a source of NGF, and to foci of higher concentrations, is interpreted as evidence of a neurotropic role for this agent (Gundersen and Barrett 1979, 1980).
9. Knowledge of the manner in which the NGF regulates the growth, development and maintenance of nerve cells is far from complete.

Gangliosides

Gangliosides are glycolipids that are a constituent of the outer membrane surface of neurons. Preparations of gangliosides promote neurite regeneration in vitro (Roisen et al 1981, Skaper & Varon 1985). When administered daily in vivo they are said to increase neuron sprouting and to improve the reinnervation of muscle without necessarily accelerating the rate of axon regeneration (Cecarelli et al 1976, Caccia et al 1979, Gorio et al 1980, 1981, 1983, Gorio & Carmignoto 1981, 1984, Kleinbeckel 1982, Sparrow & Grafstein 1982).

Other neurite promoting factors

Of particular interest in this group are laminin and acidic fibroblast growth factor.

Laminin. This glycoprotein is an important component of basement membranes. It has been found in culture media of Schwann cells. It is known to promote and enhance the growth of neurites in vitro (Manthorpe et al 1983, Rogers et al 1983, Davis et al 1985, Hammarback et al 1985) and in vivo (Da Silva et al 1985, Madison et al 1985, 1987, Politis 1988). In the latter, the influence of the growth factor on axon regeneration was studied by using nerve guide tubes filled with a laminin-containing gel for the passage of regenerating axons across the gap between the nerve ends.

Acidic fibroblast growth factor. Cordeiro et al (1989a,b) bridged a 5 mm gap between the ends of a transected sciatic nerve in the rat with a tube guide containing a purified acidic fibroblastic growth factor. They found that this significantly increased the number of myelinated axons crossing the gap. This increase was not due to axon branching but involved an increase in the number of primary axons from sensory and motor neurons with a bias in favour of sensory fibres. The exact mechanism by which this beneficial effect is produced is not known. It could be by a direct action on regenerating axons, indirectly through Schwann cells or by improving the blood supply.

Comment

It is now clear that axonal growth is influenced by a complicated system of chemical regulatory mechanisms though much more remains to be done to unravel the mechanisms involved. The introduction of chamber models by Lundborg and his co-workers and others will greatly facilitate this work (see Chapter 16, p. 118).

In the reports the word enhancement is the operative word and this is based on axon structure and numbers. The question of accelerating axon regeneration is left unanswered, nor is there any reference to the problem of directing regenerating axons into fascicular as opposed to interfascicular tissue, or of promoting their entry into their original, or at least functionally related, endoneurial tubes in the distal stump. And that is what nerve repair is all about.

Despite these reservations, work on nerve growth factors in relation to regeneration is unquestionably promising but for the time being should be confined to the laboratory and be directed more specifically to meeting the requirements for *useful* regeneration.

Other agents

The vitality of axons is influenced by deficiencies of vitamins and other essential factors in the body fluids and by the presence of toxins. However, whether such agents and the physical well-being of an individual in any way influence post-traumatic axon regeneration remains a matter of speculation.

Pyrogenic complexes. Several studies indicate that the administration of a pyrogenic bacterial polysaccharide complex (pyrogens, Piromen), when given in sufficient dosage to elevate the peripheral temperature, has a stimulating effect on nerve regeneration by accelerating the growth and maturation of new axons, possibly because of the inhibitory action of this drug both on fibrosis and the formation of collagen in scar tissue (Hoffman 1952, 1954, Bammer & Martini 1953, Gamble 1958, Gamble & Jha 1959). Others, however, claim that pyrogenous substances are without effect on nerve fibres (Arteta 1956, McCullough 1959).

Thyroid hormone. Cockett & Kiernan (1973) found that the administration of triiodothyronine to rats dramatically increased axon outgrowth following a crush lesion. Acting on this information, McQuarrie (1975) administered dessicated thyroid to a patient following suture of a severed ulnar nerve and, using the Hoffmann–Tinel sign as an indicator of axon advance, found rates over successive segments of the nerve of 1.4, 5.0 and 1.6 mm per day. The isolated reading of 5.0 mm per day, did appear to coincide with the administration of the thyroid therapy.

Berenberg et al (1977) reported accelerated motor recovery, after crushing the sciatic nerve (rat), from the administration of triiodothyronine which they attributed to an effect on the maturation of the regenerating axon rather than on

axonal outgrowth. Others have also reported enhancement of axon growth (Stelmack & Kiernan 1977, Danielson et al 1986c) and recovery of muscle function (McIsaac & Kiernan 1975, Berenberg et al 1977). On the other hand, Cotrufo et al (1979) Frizell & McLean (1979) and Forman (1980) have reported that experimental hyperthyroidism is without effect on axon regeneration.

In view of these discrepancies clinical trials of thyroid hormone therapy to accelerate axon regeneration are not justified.

Steroid therapy. Lytton and Murray (1954) found that the adminstration of cortisone, which is known to inhibit the normal increase in the number of Schwann cells during Wallerian degeneration, also significantly decreased the rate of growth of regenerating axons in rabbits. They suggested that the altered metabolism of the dividing Schwann cells leads to the elaboration of a chemical agent that affects the physical state of the growing axon tips and facilitates their regeneration. On the other hand, Bijlsma et al (1983a,b) have reported an increase in the number of regenerating axons following the administration of ACTH.

Cyclic AMP. Pichichero et al (1973) have reported that dibutyryl cyclic AMP improved regeneration whereas McQuarrie et al (1977), in a more careful study, found that this substance had no effect on the rate of axonal outgrowth measured by the pinch test.

PULSED ELECTROMAGNETIC FIELD AND DIRECT CURRENT STIMULATION

The use of electromagnetism to promote the healing of tissues goes back to the 18th century but along the way the method acquired a dubious reputation, largely because of the absence of any scientific support. Today the method is emerging as a subject of serious study, based as it now is on the knowledge that cells are complex electrical systems that are sensitive to electrical field changes. This has rekindled interest in the possibility of controlling cell function and the healing of tissues by electrical stimulation.

Extensive clinical studies have recently directed attention to the potential of both direct and pulsating currents for healing recalcitrant bone fractures (Becker & Murray 1970, Bassett et al 1971, 1974, Spadaro 1977, de Haas et al 1980, Mulier & Spaas 1980, Brighton 1981, Sharrard et al 1982). That there is a good correlation between the use of pulsed electromagnetic therapy and an improved rate at which a non-united bone fracture heals is now generally accepted.

Experimentally it has also been shown that pulsed electromagnetic and direct current stimulation enhances dermal and epidermal repair in superficial wounds, ligament healing and joint arthrodesis with increased activity of fibroblasts and a significant increase in collagen formation (Cameron 1961, Young 1966, Alvarez et al 1983, Bigliani et al 1983, Frank et al 1983). A contrary view has been expressed by Wu et al (1967), who found direct current to be without effect on wound healing.

Regarding the increase in collagen in these studies, it is not certain whether this is due to a local increase in the number of collagen producing cells or to an increase in the ability of existing cells to synthesise collagen.

The use of pulsed electromagnetic and direct currents to enhance axon regeneration is a relatively new concept that is attracting considerable experimental attention.

In vitro studies exposing embryonic neural tissue to electromagnetic and direct currents have demonstrated a marked enhancement of neurite outgrowth and an influence on the direction followed by these neurites. However, these in vitro studies are not the concern of this text. Of more immediate interest are the in vivo studies on the effects of such stimulation on axon regeneration.

Despite variations in such parameters as local or whole body exposure, type of field created, pulse frequency, duration of pulses and the duration of treatment, there appears to be general agreement on the beneficial effects on axon regeneration of direct current stimulation and exposure to pulsing electromagnetic fields (Bassett et al 1974, 1982, Wilson et al 1974, Wilson & Jagadeesh 1976, Kort & Bassett 1980, Raji & Bowden 1982, 1983, Ito & Bassett 1983, Nix & Hope 1983, Parker et al 1983, Pomeranz et al 1984, Raji 1984, Pocket & Philip 1986, Politis et al 1988, Beveridge & Politis 1988).

These studies are the basis of claims that these methods:

1. increase the numbers of axons regenerating below a suture line or down a guide tube joining the stumps of a severed nerve;
2. increase the rate of axon regeneration;
3. increase the numbers of motor axons that are claimed to have re-established appropriate connections with muscles;
4. accelerate the recovery of nerve conduction;
5. enhance functional recovery;

The most supportive report is one by Raji & Bowden, which describes dramatic effects not only on axon regeneration but also as regards a reduction in the development of intraneural fibrosis and adhesions with an overall improvement in limb function.

The mechanism by which the alleged beneficial effects are brought about is not known. It could involve a direct effect on the regenerating axon itself, or an indirect effect by way of suture line healing, blood flow to the affected region, the activity of Schwann cells and fibroblasts, collagen formation and orientation, or by influencing other cellular mechanisms as yet unidentified.

Contrary views have been expressed by Orgel et al (1984) and Murray et al (1984), who found the method to be without effect on axon regeneration, though this conclusion carried the reservation that such treatment can increase the numbers of motor neurons re-establishing connections with their target organs after nerve repair.

In their study Cordeiro et al (1989) found that exposing rat sciatic regenerating axons to a high intensity static magnetic field was without a statistically significant effect.

The claims that direct current and pulsed electromagnetic field stimulation enhance axon regeneration are open to the following objections:

1. The course of axon regeneration and the recovery of function after nerve repair are subject to many influences, each of which varies from subject to subject and incident to incident, and in a manner calculated to complicate the evaluation of any innovatory procedure introduced to aid axon regeneration and functional recovery.

Preoccupation with only one factor, in this case pulsed electromagnetic or direct current stimulation, to the exclusion of other variables that might have been of greater significance in determining the end result, introduces the danger of assigning merit to a particular method or procedure to which it is not entitled.

While some factors influencing axon regeneration and functional recovery may have been taken into consideration in these investigations, others appear to have been overlooked.

2. Evaluation of the response of regenerating axons to electrical field stimulation has been largely based on morphological and morphometric data, any reference to function failing to meet the demanding standards required for the evaluation of motor and sensory recovery in a clinical situation. In this respect the walking gait and crude limb movements of experimental animals are in no way comparable to the skilled and dexterous movements of the hand and digits that require more than the simple regeneration of axons, based as they are on the restoration of exceedingly intricate and complex reinnervation patterns.

It could well be that what is interpreted as a plus in an experimental situation could turn out to be a definite minus in a clinical setting.

3. From the data provided it is impossible to decide, with any confidence, whether or not the results attributed to electrical stimulation were consistently and significantly better than those recorded for the controls.

4. In some studies the number of experimental animals used was inadequate for the purpose of unravelling complex phenomena to which many variable factors are contributing.

5. A disturbing observation from the study on bone repair and wound healing is that pulsed electromagnetic stimulation results in a significant increase in collagen. A similar effect at the suture line following nerve repair would seriously prejudice axon regeneration. There is no reference to this possibility in the reports reviewed.

6. The value of these electrical methods for enhancing functional recovery has not been proven beyond all reasonable doubt. Moreover, one study involved exposing cats to electrical field stimulation for 10 hours per day, for 6 days a week, for 12 weeks in order to achieve a result of functionally doubtful value, namely an improvement in the numbers of regenerating motor neurons re-

establishing connections with their target organs (Murray et al 1984, Orgel et al 1984).

Adopting such a routine clinically would be unacceptable on the grounds that the time and effort required would make unreasonable demands on both patient and therapist while the costs involved would be prohibitive; and all for a benefit that is only questionably better than is already obtainable.

Electromagnetic field and direct current interactions with regenerating nerve and allied tissues, particularly fibroblasts, await further study. Both have a long way to go before becoming established as a worthwhile adjunct to nerve repair.

THE EFFECT OF A CONDITIONING LESION ON AXON REGENERATION

From a study of the metabolic background of nerve regeneration, Ducker et al (1969) suggested that axon growth would proceed more rapidly after a second lesion, 2–3 weeks later, than after an original lesion.

This suggestion has been tested in a series of experiments on the sciatic nerve in rodents in which the animals received two nerve lesions (McQuarrie & Grafstein 1973, McQuarrie et al 1977, Grafstein & McQuarrie 1978, McQuarrie 1978, 1979, 1981). The tibial nerve was first crushed at the knee as a conditioning lesion. Two weeks later a test lesion was created by crushing the sciatic nerve at the level of the hip joint. The results showed that the rate of regeneration for both motor and sensory axons following a test lesion preceded by a conditioning lesion was faster than after a high sciatic lesion alone. In the case of adrenergic axons, however, the rate of regeneration was impaired by the conditioning lesion (McQuarrie et al 1978).

The favoured interpretation of these findings is that the conditioning lesion induces a retrograde neuronal reaction to prepare for the additional metabolic requirements that will be needed to regenerate a new axon after the test lesion, the assumption being that this would take about 2 weeks.

These findings are related to the perennial problem of the optimal time for repairing a severed nerve, the results being advanced as evidence favouring nerve repair being delayed for 2 weeks (see Chapter 40).

These experiments pose a number of problems.

1. The selection of a delay of 2 weeks between the conditioning and test lesions was presumably based on Ducker et al's (1969) claim that the neuron is in an optimal state for regenerating a new axon at that time. However, the time course of the retrograde neuronal response to peripheral injury is by no means clear and there is good evidence that axon sprouting can commence earlier than 2 weeks.

There is no way of knowing what the regeneration rates would have been had the interval between the two lesions in these experiments been shortened. In this respect it is interesting that in Forman et al's (1980) experiments an accelerated axon rate was present with only a 2-day interval between the lesions.

2. There is no reference to the effect of the second or test lesion on the parent nerve cells, the inference being that there is no further disturbance to neurons now primed for the task of regenerating new axons. This is an unjustifiable assumption.

3. There could well be species differences in these matters, while the distances involved in rodents are trivial in comparison with the considerable distances obtaining in man. The question of whether or not the benefits conferred by a conditioning lesion in rodents would apply in man remains unanswered.

4. The difference between the rates over the distances involved is hardly significant and could be due to factors other than a central priming effect.

5. 'To what extent the acceleration is due to a shorter initial delay rather than an increased outgrowth rate remains to be determined' (McQuarrie 1978).

6. Sebille & Bondoux-Jahan (1980) were unable to confirm the beneficial effects claimed for a conditioning lesion. In a related investigation Hunt et al (1983) produced a second degree cryogenic lesion proximal to a suture repair and found that a priming lesion produced in this way brought no benefit to the repair.

Despite what has been said, the overall concept of

a potential role for a conditioning lesion in axon regeneration is worthy of further study.

REFERENCES

Aitken J T, Scharman M, Young J Z 1947 Maturation of regenerating nerve fibres with various peripheral connexions. Journal of Anatomy 81: 1

Alvarez U M, Mertz P M, Smerreck R V, Eaglestein W H 1983 The healing of superficial skin wounds is stimulated by external electric current. Journal of Investigative Dermatology 81: 144

Angeletti P U, Levi-Montalcini R, Carminia F 1971 Ultrastructural changes in sympathetic neurons of newborn and adult mice treated with nerve growth factor. Journal of Ultrastructure Research 36: 24

Arteta J L 1956 Action of the pyrogenous substances (5 or 3895) on the regeneration of the peripheral nerve. Journal of Comparative Neurology 105: 185

Ballantyne J P, Campbell M J 1973 Electrophysiological study after surgical repair of sectioned human peripheral nerves. Journal of Neurology, Neurosurgery and Psychiatry 36: 797

Bammer H, Martini V 1953 Neurogenerative Wirkung von Pyrogenen. Pflügers Archiv für die gesamte Physiologie 257: 308

Bassett C A L, Pawluk R J, Pilla A A 1971 Augmentation of bone repair by inductively coupled electromagnetic fields. Science 184: 575

Bassett C A L, Pawluk R J, Pilla A A 1974 Acceleration of fracture repair by electromagnetic fields: a surgically noninvasive method. Annals of the New York Academy of Sciences 238: 242

Bassett C A L, Mitchell S N, Gaston S R 1981 Treatment of ununited tibial diaphyseal fractures with pulsing electromagnetic fields. Journal of Bone and Joint Surgery 63A: 511

Bassett C A L, Mitchell S N, Gaston S R 1982 Pulsing electromagnetic field treatment in ununited fractures and failed arthrodeses. Journal of the American Medical Association 247: 623

Becker R O, Murray D G 1970 The electrical control system regulating fracture healing in amphibians. Clinical Orthopaedics and Related Research 73: 169

Berenberg R A, Forman D S, Wood D K, da Silva A, Demarre J 1977 Recovery of peripheral nerve function after axotomy: effect of triiodothyronine. Experimental Neurology 57: 349

Beveridge J A, Politis M J 1988 Use of exogenous electrical current in treatment of delayed lesions in peripheral nerves. Plastic and Reconstructive Surgery 82: 573

Bigliani L U, Rosenwasser M P, Caulo N, Schink M M, Bassett C A L 1983 The use of pulsing electromagnetic fields to achieve arthrodesis of the knee following failed total knee arthroplasty. A preliminary report. Journal of Bone and Joint Surgery 65B: 480

Bijlsma W A, Jennekens F G I, Schotman P, Gispen W H 1983a Stimulation by ACTH 4–10 of nerve fibre regeneration following sciatic nerve crush. Muscle and Nerve 6: 104

Bijlsma W A, van Asselt E, Veldman H, Jennekens F G I, Schotman P, Gispen W H 1983b Ultrastructural study of the effect of ACTH 4–10 on nerve regeneration: outgrowing axons become larger in number and smaller in diameter. Acta Neuropathologica (Berlin) 62: 24

Brighton C T 1981 Treatment of nonunion of the tibia with constant direct current. Journal Trauma 21: 189

Caccia M R, Meola G, Cerri C, Frattola L, Scarlato S, Aporti F 1979 Treatment of denervated muscle by gangliosides. Muscle and Nerve 2: 382

Cameron B M 1961 Experimental acceleration of wound healing. American Journal of Orthopaedics 53: 336

Campenot R B 1977 Local control of neurite development by nerve growth factor. Proceedings of the National Academy of Sciences USA 74: 4516

Campenot R B 1982 Development of sympathetic neurite growth by nerve growth factor I. Local control of neurite growth by nerve growth factor II. Local control of neurite survival by nerve growth factor. Developmental Biology 93: 1

Carlsson C A, Bolander P, Sjöstrand J 1971 Changes in axonal transport during regeneration of feline ventral roots. Journal of Neurological Science 14: 75

Ceccarelli B, Aportic F, Finesso M 1976 Effects of brain gangliosides on functional recovery in experimental regeneration and reinnervation. In: Porcellati G, Ceccarelli B, Tettamantic G (eds) Ganglioside function. Plenum Press, London, p 275

Cockett S A, Kiernan J A 1973 Acceleration of peripheral nervous regeneration in the rat by exogenous triiodothyronine. Experimental Neurology 39: 389

Cordeiro P G, Seckel B R, Lipton S A, D'Amore P A, Wagner J, Madison R 1989a Acidic fibroblast growth factor enhances peripheral nerve regeneration in vivo. Plastic and Reconstructive Surgery 83: 301

Cordeiro P G, Seckel B R, Miller C D, Gross P T, Wise R E 1989b Effect of high-intensity static magnetic field on sciatic nerve regeneration in the rat. Plastic and Reconstructive Surgery 83: 307

Cotrufo R R, Dattola R, Deotato M, Pisani F, Messina C 1979 Experimental hyperthyroidism fails to expedite reinnervation of muscles denervated by crush in sciatic nerves in rabbits. Experimental Neurology 65: 271

Couraud J Y, Di Giamberardino L 1981 Axonal transport of the molecular forms of acetylcholinesterase in normal and regenerating peripheral nerves. International Journal of Microsurgery 3: 133

Danielson N, Lundborg G, Frizell M 1986a Nerve repair and axonal transport: outgrowth delay and regeneration rate after transection and repair of rabbit hypoglossal nerve. Brain Research 376: 125

Danielson N, Lundborg G, Frizell M 1986b Nerve repair and axonal transport: distribution of axonally transported proteins during maturation period in regenerating rabbit hypoglossal nerve. Journal of Neurological Sciences 73: 269

Danielson N, Dahlin L B, Ericsson L E, Crenshaw A, Lundborg G 1986c Experimental hyperthyroidism stimulates axonal growth in mesothelial chambers. Experimental Neurology 94: 54

Da Silva C F, Madison R, Dikkes P, Chiu T H, Sidman R L 1985 An in vivo model to quantify motor and sensory peripheral nerve regeneration using bioresorbable nerve guide tubes. Brain Research 342: 307

Davis G E, Manthorpe M, Varon S 1985 Parameters of neuritic growth from ciliary ganglion neurons in vitro: influence of laminin, Schwannoma polyornithine-binding neurite promoting factor and ciliary neuronotrophic factor. Developmental Brain Research 17: 75

de Haas W G, Watson J, Morrison D M 1980 Non-invasive treatment of ununited fractures of the tibia using electrical stimulation. Journal of Bone and Joint Surgery 62B: 465

Droz B 1981 Axonal transport in peripheral nerves. International Journal of Microsurgery 3: 93

Duncan D, Jarvis W H 1943 Observations on repeated regeneration of the facial nerve in cats. Journal of Comparative Neurology 79: 315

Ducker T B, Kempe I G, Hayes G J 1969 The metabolic background for peripheral nerve surgery. Journal of Neurosurgery 30: 270

Evans D H L, Murray J G 1956 A study of regeneration in a motor nerve with a unimodal fiber diameter distribution. Anatomical Record 126: 311

Forman D S 1980 The use of axonally transported radioactive proteins as markers of axonal regeneration following crush or suture. In: Jewett D L, McCarroll H R (eds) Nerve repair and regeneration. Mosby, St Louis, p 95

Forman D S, Berenberg R A 1978 Regeneration of motor axons in the rat sciatic nerve studied by labelling with axonally transported radioactive proteins. Brain Research 156: 213

Forman D S, Wood D K, Desilva S 1979 Rate of regeneration of sensory axons in rat transected sciatic nerve repaired with epineurial sutures. Journal of Neurological Sciences 44: 55

Forman D S, McQuarrie I G, Labore F W et al 1980 Time course of the conditioning lesion effect on axonal regeneration. Brain Research 182: 180

Frank C, Schachar N, Dittrich, Shrive N, de Haas W, Edwards G 1983 Electromagnetic stimulation of ligament healing in rabbits. Clinical Orthopaedics 175: 263

Frizell M, McLean W G 1979 The effect of triiodothyronine on axonal transport in regenerating peripheral nerves. Experimental Neurology 64: 225

Frizell M, Sjöstrand J 1974a Transport of proteins, glycoproteins and cholinergic enzymes in regenerating hypoglossal neurons. Journal of Neurochemistry 22: 845

Frizell M, Sjostrand J 1974b The axonal transport of ^{3}H-labelled glycoproteins in normal and regenerating peripheral nerves. Brain Research 78: 109

Frizell M, Sjöstrand J 1974c The axonal transport of slowly migrating ^{3}H-leucine labelled proteins and the regeneration rate in regenerating hypoglossal and vagus nerves of the rabbit. Brain Research 81: 267

Gamble H J 1958 Effect of a raised peripheral temperature upon rate of regeneration in a mammalian peripheral nerve. Nature London 182: 287

Gamble H J, Jha B D 1959 An effect of pyronin upon the rate of maturation of injured peripheral nerve fibres. Journal of Anatomy 93: 195

Gorio A, Carmignoto G 1981 Reformation maturation and stabilization of neuromuscular functions in peripheral nerve regeneration: the possible role of exogenous gangliosides on determining motoneuron sprouting. In: Gorio A, Millesi H, Mingrino S (eds) Post-traumatic peripheral nerve regeneration: experimental basis and clinical implications. Raven Press, New York, p 481

Gorio A, Carmignoto G 1984 Enhancing reinnervation of muscle by ganglioside treatment. In: Serratrice G (ed) Neuromuscular disease. Raven Press, New York, p 287

Gorio A, Carmignoto G, Facci L, Finesso M 1980 Motor nerve sprouting induced by ganglioside treatment. Possible implications for gangliosides on neuronal growth. Brain Research 197: 236

Gorio A, Carmignoto G, Ferrari G 1981 Axon sprouting stimulated by gangliosides: a new model for elongation and sprouting. In: Rapport M M, Gorio A (eds) Gangliosides in neurological and neuromuscular function: development and repair. Raven Press, New York, p 177

Gorio A Marini P, Zanoni R 1983 Muscle reinnervation III Motoneuron sprouting capacity, enhancement by exogenous gangliosides. Neuroscience 8: 417

Grafstein B, McQuarrie I G 1978 Role of the nerve cell body in axon regeneration. In: Cotman C W (ed) Neuronal plasticity. Raven Press, New York, p 155

Grafstein B, Murray M 1969 Transport of proteins in goldfish optic nerve during regeneration. Experimental Neurology 25: 494

Gundersen R W, Barrett J N 1979 Neuronal chemotaxis: chick dorsal root axons turn toward high concentrations of nerve growth factor. Science 206: 1079

Gundersen R W, Barrett J N 1980 Characterization of the turning response of dorsal root neurites towards nerve growth factor. Journal of Cell Biology 87: 546

Hammarback J A, Palm S L, Furcht L T, Letourneau P C 1985 Guidance of neuritic outgrowth by pathways of substratum — adsorbed laminin. Journal of Neuroscience Research 13: 213

Hoffman H 1952 Acceleration and retardation of the process of axon sprouting in partially denervated muscles. Australian Journal of Experimental Biology and Medical Science 30: 541

Hoffman H 1954 Effects of a fibrosis-inhibiting substance on the innervation of muscles by nerve implants. Journal of Comparative Neurology 100: 441

Hoffman H, McDougall J 1968 Some biological properties of proteins of the mouse submaxillary gland as revealed by growth of tissues on electrophoretic acrylamide gels. Experimental Cell Research 51: 485

Hoffman P N Lasek R J 1980 Axonal transport of the cytoskeleton in regenerating motor neurons: constancy and change. Brain Research 202: 317

Hoffman P N, Griffin J W, Price D L 1984 Control of axonal caliber by neurofilament transport. Journal of Cell Biology 99: 705

Hodes R, Larrabee M G, German W 1948 The human electromyogram in response to nerve stimulation and the conduction velocity of motor axons. Archives of Neurology and Psychiatry, Chicago 60: 340

Horsch K W, Lisney S J W 1981 On the number and nature of regenerating myelinated axons after lesions of cutaneous nerve in the cat. Journal of Physiology, London 313: 275

Hunt D M, McCarthy R, Green C J 1983 The effect of freezing on peripheral nerve repair. The Hand 15: 317

Ito H, Bassett C A L 1983 Effect of weak, pulsing electromagnetic fields on neural regeneration in rat. Clinical Orthopaedics and Related Research 181: 283

Jenq C B, Coggeshall R E 1984a Effects of sciatic nerve regeneration on axonal populations in tributary nerves. Brain Research 295: 91

Jenq C B, Coggeshall R E 1984b Regeneration of axons in tributary nerves. Brain Research 310: 107

Jenq C B, Coggeshall R E 1985a Numbers of regenerating

axons in parent and tributary peripheral nerves in the rat. Brain Research 326: 27

Jenq C B, Coggeshall R E 1985b Nerve regeneration through holey silicon tubes. Brain Research 361: 233

Johnson E M 1983 An autoimmune approach to the study of nerve growth factor and other factors. In: Guroff G (ed) Growth and maturation factors, Vol 1. Wiley, New York, p 55

Kessler J A, Black I B 1980 The effects of nerve growth factor NGF and antiserum to NGF on the development of embryonic sympathetic neurons in vivo. Brain Research 189: 157

Kleinbeckel D 1982 Acceleration of muscle reinnervation in rats by ganglioside treatment: an electromyographic study. European Journal of Pharmacology 80: 243

Kline D G, De Jonge B R 1968 Evoked potentials to evaluate peripheral nerve injuries. Surgery Gynaecology and Obstetrics 127: 1239

Kline D G, Hackett E R, Davis G D, Myers M B 1972 Effect of mobilisation on the blood supply and regeneration of injured nerves. Journal of Surgical Research 12: 254

Kline D G, Hackett E R, Happel L R 1981 Function of the regenerating distal segment of nerve. In: Gorio A, Millesi H, Mingrino S (eds) Post traumatic peripheral nerve regeneration. Experimental basis and clinical implications. Raven Press, New York, p 445

Korsching S, Thoenen H 1983a Nerve growth factor in sympathetic ganglia and corresponding target organs of the rat: correlation with density of sympathetic innervation. Proceedings of the National Academy of Sciences USA 80: 3513

Korsching S, Thoenen H 1983b Quantitative demonstration of retrograde axonal transport of endogenous nerve growth factor. Neuroscience Letters 39: 1

Kort J, Bassett C A L 1980 Effect of pulsing electromagnetic fields (PEMFs) on peripheral nerve regeneration (abstract). Orthopaedic Research Society, Atlanta, Georgia, Feb 5

Kreutzberg G W, Schubert P 1971 Changes in axonal flow during regeneration of mammalian motor nerves. Acta Neuropathologica (Berlin) Supplement 5.70

Lasek R J, Hoffman P N 1976 The neuronal cytoskeleton, axonal transport. In: Goldman R, Pollard J, Rosenbaum J (eds) Cell motility. Cold Spring Harbor Laboratory, p 1021

Legrain Y 1977 Méthode de comparaison de la vitesse de régénération des fibres du nerf sciatique de rat. Journal de Physiologie Paris 73: 13

Levi-Montalcini R 1966 The nerve growth factor: its mode of action on sensory and sympathetic nerve cells. Academic Press, New York, Harvey Lectures 60: 217

Levi-Montalcini R 1976 The nerve growth factor: its role in growth, differentiation, and function of the sympathetic axon. Progress in Brain Research 45: 235

Levi-Montalcini R 1983 The nerve growth factor-target cell interactions: a model system for the study of directed axonal growth and regeneration. Birth Defects Original Article Series 19: 3

Levi-Montalcini R, Angeletti P V 1968 Nerve growth factor. Physiological Reviews 48: 534

Levi-Montalcini R, Hamburger V 1951 Selective growth-stimulating effects of mouse sarcoma on the sensory and sympathetic nervous system of the chick embryo. Journal of Experimental Zoology 116: 321

Levi-Montalcini R, Hamburger V 1953 A diffusible agent of

mouse sarcoma producing hyperplasia of sympathetic ganglia and hyper-neurotization of the chick embryo. Journal of Experimental Zoology 123: 233

Lugnegård C, Berthold H, Rydmark M, Andersson M 1984 Ultrastructure morphometric studies on regeneration of the lateral sural cutaneous nerve in the white rat after transection of the sciatic nerve. II Regeneration after nerve suture and nerve grafting. Scandinavian Journal of Plastic and Reconstructive Surgery. Supplementum 20, p 27

Lytton B, Murray J G 1954 Effects of the peripheral pathway on the regeneration of nerve fibres. Journal of Physiology London 126: 627

McCullough A W 1959 Studies on peripheral nerve regeneration I Peripheral nerve regeneration in white rats at various ages when treated with a pyrogenic bacterial polysaccharide complex in various dosage. Journal of Comparative Neurology 113: 471

McIsaac G, Kiernan J A 1975 Acceleration of neuromuscular reinnervation by triiodothyronine. Journal of Anatomy 120: 551

McIsaac G, Kiernan J A 1975 Accelerated recovery from peripheral nerve injury in experimental hyperthyroidism. Experimental Neurology 48: 88

McQuarrie I G 1975 Nerve regeneration and thyroid hormone treatment. Journal of Neurological Science 26: 499

McQuarrie I G 1978 The effect of a conditioning lesion on the regeneration of motor axons. Brain Research 152: 597

McQuarrie I G 1979 Accelerated axonal sprouting after nerve transection. Brain Research 167: 185

McQuarrie I G 1981 Acceleration of axonal regeneration in rat somatic motoneurons by using a conditioning lesion. In: Gorio A, Millest H, Mingrino S (eds) Post-traumatic nerve regeneration. Raven Press New York, p 49

McQuarrie I G, Grafstein B 1973 Axon outgrowth enhanced by a previous nerve injury. Archives of Neurology 29: 53

McQuarrie I G, Graftstein B, Gershon M D 1977 Axonal regeneration in rat sciatic nerve: effect of a conditioning lesion and of dcb — AMP. Brain Research 132: 443

McQuarrie I G, Graftstein B, Dreyfus C F, Gershon M D 1978 Regeneration of adrenergic axons in rat sciatic nerve: effect of a conditioning lesion. Brain Research 141: 21

Madison R, Da Silva C F, Dikkes P, Chiu T H, Sidman R L 1985 Increased rate of peripheral nerve regeneration using bioresorbable nerve guides and a laminin containing gel. Experimental Neurology 88: 767

Madison R, Da Silva C F, Dikkes P, Chiu T H, Sidman R L 1987 Peripheral nerve regeneration with entubulation repair: comparison of biodegradable nerve guides as polyethylene tubes and the effects of a laminin containing gel. Experimental Neurology 95: 378

Manthorpe M, Engvall E, Rouslathi E, Longo F M, Davies G E, Varon S 1983 Laminin promotes neurite regeneration from cultured peripheral and central neurons. Journal of Cell Biology 97: 1882

Mira J C 1976 Etudes quantitatives sur la régénération des fibres nerveuses myélinisées II Variations du nombre et du calibre des fibres régénérées après un écrasement ou une section du nerf. Archives d'anatomie microscopique et de morphologie expérimentale 65: 255

Mira J C 1979 Quantitative studies of the regeneration of rat myelinated nerve fibres: variations in the number and size of regenerating fibres after repeated localised freezings. Journal of Anatomy 129: 77

Mira J C 1981 Degeneration and regeneration of peripheral nerves: ultrastructural and electrophysiological observations, quantitative aspects and muscle changes during reinnervation. International Journal of Microsurgery 3: 102

Miyamoto Y 1979 Experimental study of results of nerve suture under tension vs nerve grafting. Plastic and Reconstructive Surgery 64: 540

Mulier J C, Spaas F 1980 Out-patient treatment of surgically resistant non-unions by induced pulsing current. Clinical results. Archives of Orthopaedic and Traumatic Surgery 97: 293

Murray H M, O'Brien W J, Orgel M G 1984 Pulsed electromagnetic fields and peripheral nerve regeneration in cat. Journal of Bioelectricity 3: 19

Nix W A, Hope H C 1983 Electrical stimulation of regenerating nerve and its effect on motor recovery. Brain Research 272: 21

O'Daly J A, Imaeda T 1967 Electron microscopic study of Wallerian degeneration in cutaneous nerves caused by mechanical injury. Laboratory Investigation 17: 744

Orgel M G, Terzis J K 1977 Epineurial vs perineurial repair. Plastic and Reconstructive Surgery 60: 80

Orgel M G, O'Brien W J, Murray H M 1984 Pulsing electromagnetic field therapy in nerve regeneration. An experimental study in the cat. Plastic and Reconstructive Surgery 73: 173

Parker B, Bryant C, Apesos J, Sisken B F, Nickell T 1983 The effects of pulsed electromagnetic fields (PEMF) on rat sciatic nerve regeneration. Bioelectrical Repair and Growth Society 3: 19

Pichichero M, Beer B, Clody D E 1973 Effects of dibutyryl cyclic AMP on restoration of function of damaged sciatic nerves in rats. Science 182: 724

Politis M J 1986 Retina-derived growth promoting extracts supports axonal regeneration in vivo. Brain Research 364: 369

Politis M J 1989 Exogenous laminin induces regenerative changes in traumatized sciatic and optic nerve. Plastic and Reconstructive Surgery 83: 228

Politis M J, Zanakis M F, Albala B J 1988 Facilitated regeneration in the rat peripheral nerve system using applied electric fields. Journal Trauma 28: 1375

Pomeranz B, Mullen M, Markus H 1984 Effect of applied electrical fields on sprouting of intact saphenous nerve in adult rat. Brain Research 303: 331

Pocket S, Philip B A 1986 Electric stimulation accelerates peripheral nerve regeneration. Proceedings International Union of the Physiological Sciences, Vancouver Canada July 13–18, p 463

Raji A R M 1978 Effects of pulsed electromagnetic field energy (Diapulse) on the normal common peroneal nerve in rats. Journal of Anatomy 127: 667

Raji A R M 1984 An experimental study of the effects of pulsed electromagnetic field (Diapulse) on nerve repair. Journal of Hand Surgery 9B: 105

Raji A R M, Bowden R E M 1982 Effects of high peak pulsed electromagnetic fields on degeneration and regeneration of the common peroneal nerve in rats. Lancet 2: 444

Raji A R M, Bowden R E M 1983 Effects of high-peak pulsed electromagnetic field on the degeneration and regeneration of the common peroneal nerve in rat. Journal of Bone and Joint Surgery 65B: 478

Rich K M, Luszczynski J R, Osborne P A, Johnson E M

1987 Nerve growth factor protects adult sensory neurons from cell death and atrophy caused by nerve injury. Journal of Neurocytology 16: 261

Rogers S L, Letourneau P C, Palm S L, Furcht L T 1983 Neurite extension by peripheral and central nervous system neurons in response to substratum-bound fibronectin and laminin. Developmental Biology 98: 212

Roisen F J, Bartfield H, Nagele R, Yorke G 1981 Ganglioside stimulation of axonal sprouting in vitro. Science 214: 577

Sebille A, Bondoux-Jahan M 1980 Effects of electric stimulation and previous nerve injury on motor function recovery in rats. Brain Research 193: 562

Sharrard W J W, Sutcliff M L, Robson M J, MacEachern A G 1982 The treatment of fibrous non-union of fractures by pulsing electromagnetic stimulation. Journal of Bone and Joint Surgery 64B: 189

Skaper S D, Varon S 1985 Ganglioside GMI overcomes serum inhibition of neuritic outgrowth. International Journal of Developmental Neuroscience 3: 187

Spadaro J A 1977 Electrically stimulated bone growth in animals and man: review of the literature. Clinical Orthopaedics 122: 325

Sparrow J R, Grafstein B 1982 Sciatic nerve regeneration in ganglioside treated rats. Experimental Neurology 77: 230

Stelmack B M, Kiernan J A 1977 Effects of triiodothyronine on the normal and regenerating facial nerve of the rat. Acta Neuropathologica 40: 151

Struppler A, Huckauf H 1962 Propagation velocity in regenerated motor nerve fibres. Electromyography Electroencephalography Clinical Neurophysiology Supplement 22: 58

Sunderland S 1978 Regeneration of the axon and related changes. In: Nerves and nerve injuries. Churchill Livingstone, Edinburgh, p 108.

Varon S, Adler R 1980 Nerve growth factor and control of nerve growth. Current Topics in Developmental Biology 16: 207

Wilson D H, Jagadeesh P 1976 Experimental regeneration in peripheral nerves and the spinal cord in laboratory animals exposed to a pulsed electromagnetic field. Paraplegia 14: 12

Wilson D H, Jagadeesh P, Newman P P, Harriman D G 1974 The effects of pulsed electromagnetic energy on peripheral nerve regeneration. Annals New York Academy of Sciences 238: 575

Wu D T, Go N, Dennis C, Enquist L, Sawyer P N 1967 Effects of electrical currents and interfacial potentials on wound healing. Journal of Surgical Research 7: 122

Young G H 1966 Electrical impulse therapy aids wound healing. Modern Veterinary Practice 47: 60

16. Neurotropism in axon regeneration and nerve repair

We shall not cease exploration
And the end of all exploring
Will be to arrive where we started
And know the place for the first time.
                    T. S. Eliot

A question of crucial importance to nerve repair is whether or not the distal stump of a severed nerve is the source of neurotropic influences that attract regenerating axons to that site where each regenerating axon is then directed into its old endoneurial tube or one functionally related to it.

If such neurotropic influences do not exist then the surgeon, when repairing a nerve, is faced with the additional responsibility of devising methods to minimise the loss of axons during their regeneration and to maximise the restoration of functionally useful pathways.

Axon growth in tissue culture and during embryonic development have only a fringe relationship to nerve repair and will not be discussed. The main thrust of the discussion is directed to a consideration of factors influencing the direction and course taken by regenerating axons after they have emerged from the proximal end of a severed nerve.

TERMINOLOGY

Some preliminary remarks on terminology are necessary in order to avoid any misunderstanding on the part of the reader.

Nerve repair. In this chapter nerve repair is used in the wider sense to mean any procedure or method designed to unite the nerve ends and to maintain the repaired system in continuity.

Trophism. This relates to nutrition and should not be confused with tropism.

Tropism. This is the purposeful movement of a motile cell, or part thereof, towards another cell or tissue under the influence of some attractant stimulus emanating from that source and in this way determining the direction taken by the moving part. There are various types of tropism depending on the nature of the attractant stimulus, e.g. chemotropism, galvanotropism, stereotropism, phototropism, neurotropism.

Throughout the text these terms will be used with specific reference to nerve tissue, the source of the attractant stimulus being the distal stump of the severed nerve, and the moving part attracted to it being the regenerating axon tip.

Chemotactism. Chemotaxis and chemotropism. At the close of the 19th century Cajal, in his compelling writings on the developing nervous system, advanced the hypothesis that, during development, the course taken by growing axon sprouts and their final destination are influenced by chemical substances elaborated by the target tissues. He referred to this influence as chemotactism, or chemotropism as it later came to be called.

Cajal soon extended his studies to include the regeneration of axons following nerve transection and he again concluded that regenerating axons were attracted towards the distal nerve stump in response to chemical concentration gradients created by chemical stimuli emanating from that site.

Neurotropism. This term was introduced by Forssman (1898, 1900) to describe the same phenomenon that Cajal had previously referred to as chemotactism. Though neurotropism and chemotropism are usually regarded as synonymous, the former is preferred because it specifies an association with nerve tissue and includes all forms of tropism.

Galvanotropism. This refers to the bioelectrical fields created by an injury that determine the path taken by advancing axon tips.

Stereotropism. This is the capacity of a solid or rigid object to influence the direction taken by a regenerating axon that establishes contact with it.

Odogenesis. This term was introduced by Dustin (1910) to describe the property of young connective tissue cells to outline spaces and paths between the nerve ends that facilitate the passage of regenerating axons to the distal stump.

INTRODUCTION

Reference is made in Chapter 36 to the comment in mediaeval writings on the treatment of wounds that occasionally some recovery of motor and sensory function occurred in the absence of any attempt to suture a severed nerve. The reason for this was not appreciated at the time, but the finding could have been responsible for the general belief that nerve suture was an unnecessary procedure. This attitude prevailed for 5 centuries, receiving support as late as 1846 from Virchow's observation that gaps exceeding 10 cm in length between nerve ends could be followed by remarkable recovery, though there could have been another explanation to account for these 'unbelievable' recoveries (see Chapters 32 and 33).

This negative attitude to the treatment of nerve wounds persisted until it was convincingly demonstrated, in the 19th century, that transection of a nerve was followed by, inter alia, the degeneration of the severed axons below the lesion, and that recovery depended on the growth of the surviving tip of severed axons to re-establish a new pathway to the tissues denervated as the result of the original nerve injury.

This new information on nerve healing established the need to unite the nerve ends in order to facilitate the entry of regenerating axons into the distal nerve stump. At the turn of the century nerve repair was confined to the simple restoration of nerve trunk continuity by nerve suture in the belief that axon regeneration would then attend to the restoration of function. This practice was consistent with the general belief at the time that,

once some form of mechanical repair of severed tissues and structures had been effected, natural healing processes would attend to the restoration of function.

However, a continuing uncertain, unpredictable and too often disappointing outcome of nerve repair was finally subjected to a searching critical examination in the 1940s. This revealed that nerve trunks are not simple cord-like structures but have an internal structure of considerable complexity with features that exert a profound effect on the destination of those regenerating axons that enter the distal stump of a repaired nerve. These structural features have been identified and the manner in which they affect the functional outcome of axon regeneration has been established.

For axon regeneration to be functionally effective, each axon must reach and re-establish its original terminal relationships with peripheral tissues. Failure to do this represents wasteful regeneration.

Of the many complex structural arrangements now known to influence the course taken by regenerating axons, some have the potential to so misdirect them in their growth that many fail to re-establish their original, or even functionally related, terminal connections in peripheral tissues. This leaves the restored pattern of innervation both incomplete and imperfect in comparison with the original. Function suffers accordingly. This means that:

1. The final destination of a regenerating axon is as important as axon growth itself.
2. Despite active axon regeneration, it is possible to finish up with little in the way of functional recovery.
3. A careful distinction should be drawn between axon regeneration and functional recovery (Chapter 15).

The question to be settled is whether or not there are neurotropic influences that attract and guide axons to the distal stump and in doing so confer an element of specificity on their further growth so that each axon is attracted into its original, or a functionally related, endoneurial tube that will inevitably guide it back to a functionally useful terminal connection.

Because of the intense competition for endoneurial tubes in the distal stump during regeneration, such neurotropic influences would also need to include a provision for rejecting 'foreign' axons as well as attracting those that are functionally related.

Such neurotropic influences would lighten the surgeon's task and if they do not exist then he must rely solely on his own resources and initiative when devising methods to maximise the useful regeneration of axons and to minimise their loss by misdirection during regeneration.

NEUROTROPISM IN RELATION TO THE DISTAL STUMP OF A SEVERED NERVE

The pioneer studies of Ramon Y Cajal (1928) did so much to establish chemotropism as an influential force in axon regeneration following nerve transection that it is important to keep in mind precisely what he did have to say on that subject. This is necessary in order to avoid any misunderstanding when reference is made to his work. The relevant points made by Cajal on chemotropism (neurotropism) are:

1. He interpreted his findings as demonstrating 'the great influence that the proximity of the peripheral nerve stump has on the growth and orientation of the outgrowing newly formed fibres due to stimulating substances formed by the rejuvenating cells of Schwann of the distal stump'.
2. Endoneurial tubes in the distal stump will receive axon sprouts even if they become 'insensitive and degenerate through physiological uselessness'.
3. The difficulty experienced by axons in orienting themselves at a distance from the peripheral stump suggests that the orienting enzymes have only a small diffusive power.
4. Illustrations accompanying Cajal's text show that not all axons growing from the proximal nerve stump converge on the distal stump. Many take a direction that will deny them entry.
5. The mechanism of chemotropic action remains unknown. It probably does not operate through attraction but creates a

region or environment that is favourable for axon growth.
6. Cajal originally implicated the cells of Schwann as the source of chemotropic substances, and, though he later noted that these cells were not necessary for the genesis and growth of axons, he finally returned to his original claim in their favour. Forssman thought that the chemotropic substance was produced by the disintegration of the myelin sheath, but this was denied by Cajal. According to Tello (1911, 1923a,b) the mesodermal cells of the scar and even the fusiform cells of the endoneurium participate in the production of the chemotropic factor. The source of this factor remains a controversial subject.
7. When the axon is in conflict with its environment it makes a purely utilitarian choice.

Significant points that emerge from the work of Cajal and his contemporaries are:

1. Chemotropic substances are elaborated by the distal nerve stump that cause growing axons to converge on it.
2. The cone of axon growth is extremely sensitive to both physical and chemical influences in its surroundings. Cajal, the great advocate of chemotropism, was well aware of the significance of physical factors as a cause of the arrest and deviation of regenerating axons.
3. The source of chemotropic factors elaborated by the distal stump appears to be broadly based in terms of the various tissue components of the nerve.

Returning briefly to clinical thinking around the turn of the century, it would appear that clinicians were unduly impressed by the general concept of neurotropism and completely failed to appreciate the significance of the finer qualifying details of the mechanism. Looked at in this light it is possible to understand the clinicians' conviction that their only task was to restore continuity of the severed nerve trunk, neurotropic influences then effecting the necessary sorting out of axon growth at the suture site in a manner calculated to restore the original pattern of innervation. A more careful reading of Cajal's findings would have discouraged them from reaching this conclusion.

The saga of neurotropism and its role in axon regeneration and the reinnervation of the distal nerve stump was by no means finished with the convincing and authoritative work of Cajal, Forssman and others. An opposing view at the time, and one that carried considerable weight, was based on the claim that the growth of axons is extremely sensitive to structural features of their environment and that chance physical influences outlining paths of least resistance are the principal determinants of the course and direction taken by axons regenerating in crossing the gap between the nerve ends.

Forty years later Weiss with his co-workers (Weiss & Taylor 1944, Weiss 1950) re-opened the chemotropism controversy by designing an experimental model to test the validity of this concept.

Briefly, the experimental design involved using the aorta and its bifurcation into common iliac arteries in one rat as a graft for another. The sciatic nerve was transected and the proximal end inserted into the aorta while the distal nerve end was inserted into one iliac vessel, the other being treated in a variety of ways as a control. This Y shaped device, filled with blood, provided regenerating axons growing down the aorta with a choice of entering one or the other or both common iliac arteries. In the event, the path taken by axons suggested a random distribution between the available channels, and certainly not one preferentially favouring entry into the vessel containing the distal nerve end with its alleged source of neurotropic stimuli.

The experimental design and methods employed by Weiss have been criticised on the grounds that due attention was not paid to:

1. The local reaction to implanted foreign tissue.
2. The effect of distance on diffusible chemical agents in a foreign environment. In these experiments the nerve ends were approximately 15 mm apart, which recalls the earlier warnings by Cajal and Tello that orienting chemical stimuli have only a limited diffusive power and act only over short distances.
3. Ultrastructural differences in the blood clot filling the channels might have influenced the direction taken by regenerating axons.
4. The methods employed for evaluating axon growth could have been inadequate for the task.

Despite these objections, the influence of Weiss and his teachings has been so great that few remained unconvinced of his claim to have conclusively demonstrated that chemotropism as enunciated by Cajal is a non-event in axon regeneration. Active interest in this subject consequently lapsed and it was not until many years later that Weiss' claim to have negated chemotropism as an aid to axon regeneration was challenged.

Mindful of the shortcomings in Weiss' experiments, steps were taken later by others to correct them by substituting a variety of improved nerve guides in place of the aorta graft. The latter included silastic tubes and implant devices, ingeniously constructed mesothelial tubes and complex silicone chamber systems (Lundborg & Hansson 1979, 1980, 1981, Lundborg et al 1981, 1982a–c, 1986, Politis et al 1982, Ochi 1983, Politis & Spencer 1983, Williams et al 1983, 1984, Mackinnon et al 1984, 1986, Politis 1985, Politis & Steiss 1985, Nachemson & Lundborg 1986, Williams 1987).

The improved experimental methods and a more critical approach to the problem led to completely different conclusions, the new findings now clearly demonstrating:

1. a preferential growth of axons towards the distal stump of a severed nerve as opposed to other tissues;
2. the existence of a neurotropic factor liberated from the distal nerve stump that, by diffusion, attracts regenerating axons to that site;
3. a link between the neurotropic factor and Schwann cell activity, as was originally suggested by Cajal, with some indication of a protein or protein dependent structure.

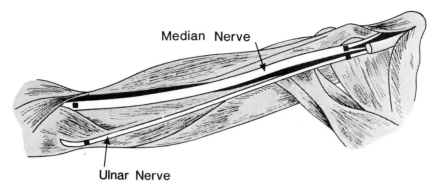

Fig. 16.1 Diagram illustrating the median and ulnar nerves and the brachial artery in the upper arm. The nerves were resected between the axilla and the elbow at the sites indicated.

These findings have received additional support from tissue culture studies on nerve growth factors (Charlwood et al 1972; Ebendal & Jacobson 1977; Letourneau 1978; Gundersen & Barret 1979; Varon & Adler 1980: Richardson & Ebendal 1982).

Regarding the source of the neurotropic factor, more than Schwann cells appear to be implicated because these cells are as abundant at the proximal as at the distal nerve end, unless, of course, the Schwann cells at the two sites have different properties. It would also be interesting to know if the laminin concentration in the distal stump is greater than in the proximal, having in mind the nerve growth promoting properties of laminin (Chapter 15) and the accumulation of laminin material as the result of Wallerian degeneration. However, these changes also occur in the proximal stump, though probably not to the same degree.

The precise mechanism by which neurotropic factors achieve their effect remains a matter of conjecture. It could be by means of chemical concentration gradients acting directly on axon tips, or the effect could be on Schwann cells themselves which are attracted from the proximal nerve-end and which are later followed by axons (Politis & Spencer 1983; Williams et al 1983). In this respect it should be remembered that Cajal, from his usually reliable studies, reported that in the initial stages new axons in the union scar are bare, the Schwann cell covering coming later.

Some interesting observations relating to this subject were contained in a paper by Sunderland (1953) on the capacity of regenerating axons to bridge long gaps in nerves. The investigation, of which this paper was a by-product, was directed to a study of the changes in striated muscle due to prolonged denervation (Sunderland and Ray 1950). In 34 of these experiments, which were conducted on adult specimens of the Australian opossum (*Trichosurus vulpecula*), the median and ulnar nerves were removed on one side between the elbow and the axilla, the nerve ends retracting to leave a gap between them of approximately 30–35 mm (Fig. 16.1). The nerve-ends were crushed and treated to prevent regenerating axons from reaching the distal nerve stumps or the denervated muscles directly. The duration of the shortest experiment was 9 days and of the longest 485 days.

Despite the precautions taken to prevent the reinnervation of the distal nerve stumps, the postoperative behaviour of the animal and the condition and use of the affected limb indicated that some recovery had occurred in 8 of the 34 animals studied. Subsequently, histological examination of the involved muscles and nerve segments confirmed that the precautions taken to prevent reinnervation had failed in these 8 animals but had been effective in the remaining 26. The findings in these 8 specimens are the subject of the following comment.

When the tissues of the upper forelimb were exposed at the termination of each experiment a gap of 30–35 mm still separated the proximal and distal nerve stumps but in four of the eight specimens these were joined by a thin but clearly visible

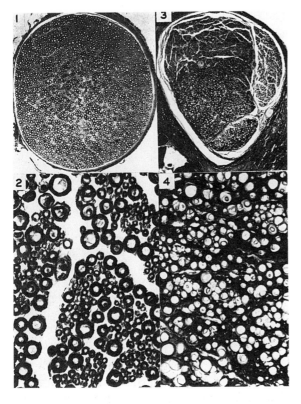

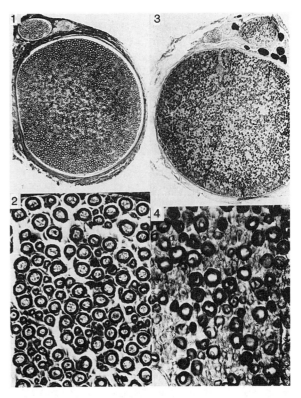

Fig. 16.2 Histological preparations from the right and left median nerves in which one had been resected 432 days before. Sections *1* and *2* are from the contralateral normal nerve at a level corresponding to the distal stump of the resected nerve. Sections *3* and *4* are from the distal stump of the resected nerve.

Fig. 16.3 Histological preparations from the right and left ulnar nerves in which one had been resected 426 days previously. Sections *1* and *2* are from the contralateral normal nerve at a level corresponding to the distal stump of the resected nerve, sections from which are shown in Sections *3* and *4*. The regeneration was sufficient to limit atrophy of the flexor carpi ulnaris to 12%.

strand of tissue. No such bridging strand could be seen in the remaining four specimens. Of particular significance was the finding that the bridging strands joined the ends of corresponding nerves. No cross-unions between the ulnar and the median nerves were seen, though this does not exclude the existence of fine communications not visible to the naked eye.

The essential points emerging from the histological study were:

1. Quite long gaps between nerve ends were successfully crossed by regenerating axons. The experimental and clinical implication of this finding in relation to the evaluation of various forms and methods of nerve grafting require no elaboration. This finding is also a vindication of

observations, repeatedly reported over the last 500 years and as recently as 1947 by Pollock et al that some recovery, inadequate though it be, can occur when a severed nerve is not repaired.

2. Sections taken from the distal stump, and from the corresponding nerve at the same level on the opposite side, are provided for comparison (Figs 16.2 & 16.3). Myelinated fibres were numerous in the distal stump and, though the majority did not exceed 7μm in diameter, some specimens provided representatives of the largest fibres present in the corresponding normal nerve. This indicates that maturation of at least some of the larger regenerated fibres had been completed. The bridging strand was composed of minifascicles of regenerated nerve fibres in a framework of dense connective tissue. Figure 16.4 illustrates the

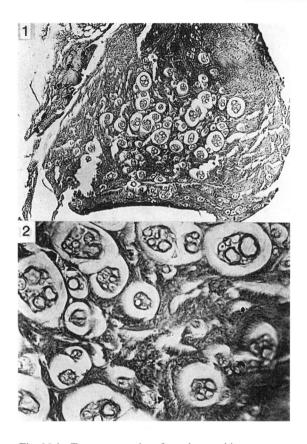

Fig. 16.4 Transverse sections from the transition zone between the distal stump of the ulnar nerve and the strand of tissue linking it to the proximal stump, 426 days after resecting the ulnar nerve segment. Scattered through a dense connective tissue framework are small clusters of regenerated nerve fibres arranged in minifascicles and showing a wide range of fibre diameters.

histology of the transition zone between the strand and the distal nerve stump.

3. In the axilla, the median and ulnar nerves and the brachial artery are intimately related. In the case of the median nerve, the brachial vessels form a favourable path along which regenerating axons could track to the elbow and so to the distal stump of the median nerve. No such pre-existing pathway is available for the guidance of regenerating ulnar axons. The ulnar nerve accompanies the brachial artery only as far as the mid-upper arm, beyond which it continues obliquely downwards and backwards across the arm to pass behind the medial humeral epicondyle. Following the resection of the ulnar nerve the tissues forming its bed became scarred. When this area was examined at the conclusion of the experiments it was clear that, for regenerating axons to reach the distal stump of the ulnar nerve, they could only have done so by overcoming formidable obstacles. Surprisingly they were successful in doing this in six specimens.

In four specimens regenerating axons were present in the distal stump of the ulnar nerve but not in that of the median nerve (see Table 16.1). Though both proximal nerve stumps were together in the axilla, and the brachial artery provided a favourable path distally for regenerating axons from both nerves, those from the ulnar elected to grow along the track originally taken by the nerve despite the unfavourable nature of the terrain (Fig 16.5).

Table 16.1   Capacity of regenerating axons to cross unaided, a 35 mm gap separating the nerve ends

Subject	Duration in days	Regenerated Axons	
		Ulnar nerve	Median nerve
1	68	+	−
2	76	+	−
3	252	+	−
4	335	−	+
5	426	+*	−
6	432	−	+*
7	447	+*	+*
8	449	+	+*

* Visible strand of bridging tissue joining the ends of corresponding nerves
Regeneration: Present +; Absent −

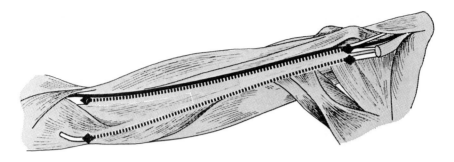

Fig. 16.5 Diagram illustrating the course taken by regenerating axons (interrupted lines).

In a further two experiments, regenerating axons were not present in the distal stump of the ulnar nerve but had followed the brachial artery to the elbow to enter the distal stump of the median nerve.

In two other specimens regenerated nerve fibres were present in the distal stumps of both nerves. Some axons had followed the old course of the ulnar nerve to reach the distal stump behind the medial epicondyle, while others had continued distally along the brachial artery to reach the median stump at the elbow.

Thus, on at least six occasions, regenerating axons had managed to reach their corresponding distal stumps without the apparent cross-passage of axons occurring from one nerve to the other.

4. Though regenerating ulnar axons were obliged to negotiate unfavourable scar tissue in order to reach the distal ulnar stump, they followed this route in preference to the more direct and favourable route provided by the brachial vessels which would have taken them to the distal stump of the median nerve.

These findings collectively provide evidence supporting the thesis that the distal nerve end is the source of a neurotropic factor that influences the direction taken by regenerating axons by attracting them to that site. The findings also show that:

a. this influence can operate over a distance of at least 35 mm;
b. the neurotropic factor has a preferential effect on axons regenerating from the proximal stump of the same nerve;

c. this pattern of axon regeneration occurs in the absence of any artificial device interposed between the nerve ends to provide regenerating axons with a circumscribed pathway to the distal stump.

NEUROTROPISM AND THE ENTRY OF REGENERATING AXONS INTO THE ENDONEURIAL TUBES OF THE DISTAL STUMP OF A SEVERED NERVE

A more complex and controversial question is whether or not regenerating axons, on reaching the distal nerve stump, are directed by neurotropic influences into their original or even functionally related endoneurial tubes, thereby leading to the restoration of the original pattern of innervation in the first instance and to at least some functional recovery in the second.

Cajal is clear on this point when he wrote that, though the distal stump exerts an attractive influence on regenerating axons, those which reach it do so in great disorder. He further emphasised that 'The observed facts compel us to reject the supposition of those authors who believe that the newly formed fibre infallibly ends in the old sheath of the peripheral stump and unerringly restores the old terminal arborisation thus preserving the anatomical and physiological individuality of the pre-existent conductor.' Again, quoting Cajal, 'the action exercised by the peripheral stump on the growth of the young fibres is not individual and specific, that is from tube to tube, but is general and collective.'

Later Weiss was to express similar views when he reported that endoneurial tubes admitted regenerating motor and sensory axons indiscriminately regardless of their former contents, and that he could find no evidence of path specificity in the distal stump by which a regenerating axon selected one pathway to the exclusion of others.

Horsch (1979) concluded from his studies of axon guidance after transection of cutaneous nerves, that:

1. if neurotropic factors exist they are not sufficient to ensure that cutaneous sensory axons select the appropriate fascicle in the distal stump, and
2. the return of regenerating cutaneous sensory axons to wrong areas of the skin and the aberrant receptor innervation found after recovery indicate that the regenerated axons are somatotopically disarrayed.

In the case of motor axon regeneration Brushart et al (1983) have demonstrated the inappropriate reinnervation of peroneal muscles by tibial motor neurons following transection and suture of the rat sciatic nerve.

A contrary point of view to that just outlined has now been reported on a number of occasions (Politis et al 1982, Seckel et al 1984, 1986, Politis 1985, Politis & Steiss 1985). It is based on the findings of experiments using silastic Y-shaped devices and transected peroneal and tibial divisions of the sciatic nerve. The source of regenerating axons was provided by the proximal stump of either the peroneal or the tibial division which was inserted into the single inlet of the device (Fig. 16. 6(a)). The distal stump of the peroneal nerve was inserted into one outlet of the device and the distal tibial stump into the other. The results showed a preferential growth of regenerating axons to the distal stump of their own nerve as opposed to the 'alien' nerve.

Likewise, when the proximal tibial stump was made the source of regenerating axons the latter selected that fork of the device containing its own distal stump.

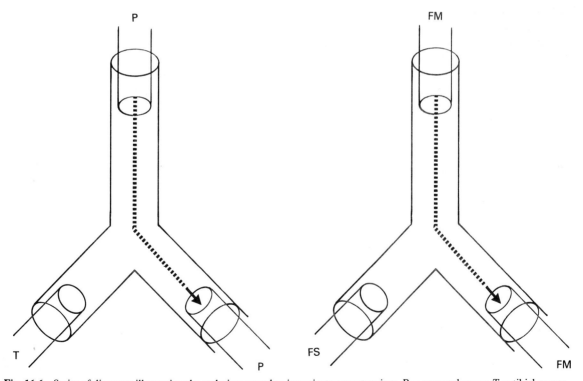

Fig. 16.6 Series of diagrams illustrating the techniques used to investigate neurotropism. P = peroneal nerva; T = tibial nerve; F = femoral nerve; M = motor division of the femoral nerve; S = sensory division of the femoral nerve.

The results of Brushart & Seiler's (1987) experiments are even more interesting. Here the motor part of a transected femoral nerve became the source of the regenerating axons at the inlet of the device, with one outlet containing the distal stump of the same motor part of the femoral nerve and the other the distal stump of the sensory part of the femoral nerve (Fig.16.6(b)). Motor regenerating axons followed the path to the motor target, though this selective reinnervation of the motor distal stump in preference to the sensory was not absolute. In seeking an explanation for this specificity the authors point out that there are known differences between motor and sensory fibres, the former, for example, characteristically containing acetylcholinesterase and acetylcholinetransferase, and that there could well be other differences that would account for the specificity revealed in their experiments.

All contemporary investigators are agreed that the distal nerve stump is the source of a neurotropic factor that attracts regenerating axon tips to that site. However, it is difficult to reconcile the findings relating to axon and endoneurial tube specificity with the usually reliable observations of Cajal, ardent advocate as he was of neurotropism, and others reporting a disorderly and random entry of regenerating axons into the endoneurial tubes of the distal stump.

On this matter, the clinical evidence comes down strongly in support of the conclusion that neurotropic influences that direct the entry of regenerating axons into functionally appropriate endoneurial tubes do not exist.

1. A study of neuroma formation at suture lines provides incontrovertible evidence that regenerating axons grow just as readily into the interfascicular epineurial connective tissue as they do into fascicular tissue with its endoneurial tubes. This is consistent with Tello's observation that the supporting mesodermal tissue at the distal nerve end contributes to the production of a neurotropic factor.
2. Suturing motor to cutaneous nerves reveals that motor regenerating axons will occupy and grow down sensory endoneurial tubes. This finding confirms Cajal's observation

that 'a central motor stump can innervate a sensory peripheral stump'. At the same time one should be mindful of Nageotte & Guyon's (1918) observation that regenerating motor axons fare better if they find the distal stump of their own nerve than if they are directed to the distal end of a sensory nerve.
3. Regenerating sensory processes readily reinnervate endoneurial tubes previously occupied by motor axons (Gutmann 1945; Weiss & Edds 1945; Weiss & Hoag 1946).
4. Nerve grafts prepared from cutaneous nerves receive regenerating motor axons and transmit them to the distal stump.
5. Failed nerve repair is not unknown even when the severed nerve has been repaired under favourable conditions by a skilled and experienced surgeon. If neurotropism were a potent and reliable force directing regenerating axons into functionally appropriate endoneurial tubes then nerve repairs should never be complete failures.

GALVANOTROPISM

That the direction taken by regenerating axons might be influenced by differences in electric potentials generated by the nerve injury has never received the attention devoted to chemotropism. Consequently, the case for galvanotropism as a factor influencing axon growth between the ends of a severed nerve remains inconclusive.

Most of the work relating to the genesis of bioelectric potentials and their influence on the formation, growth and orientation of the processes of nerve cells relates to normal neurogenesis and not to the regeneration of axons following severance of a peripheral nerve. This is particularly so with the extensive studies on neurobiotaxis carried out by Ariëns Kappers (1921).

In 1910, at the height of activity directed to the study of axon regeneration, Scaffidi (1910) showed that, in the regenerating central end of a severed nerve, the sprouting growth cones carried a positive charge generating what he called a regeneration or growth current. In 1920 Ingvar's experiments on tissue cultures of neuroblasts revealed that weak galvanic currents can affect the formation and direction taken by developing cell processes. According to Tello (1923) neurotropic substances originating in the distal stump have only a small diffusive power, and so are effective only over short distances, whereas bioelectrical activity has a much wider influence.

Since that time the subject appears to have been neglected until recently, when some have been encouraged to explore the effect of artificially applied electromagnetic and direct current stimulation on axon regeneration. This subject is discussed in Chapter 15. However, this is not quite the same as galvanotropism which is a naturally occurring process introduced by nerve injury. There is currently no evidence to suggest that galvanotropism plays any part in directing regenerating axons into the fasciculi of the distal stump, let alone into their corresponding endoneurial tubes.

PHYSICAL FACTORS INFLUENCING THE DIRECTION AND COURSE TAKEN BY REGENERATING AXONS

Physical factors that influence the direction and course taken by regenerating axons in their passage through the bridging tissue joining the nerve ends include: stereotropism, odogenesis, contact guidance, tactile adherence, and adhesive attraction. These all have one feature in common in that all are intimately associated with the physical structure of the supporting tissue between the nerve ends, some features of which introduce barriers to axon growth whereas others facilitate their ready passage to the distal nerve end. The part played by such factors as osmotic pressure and surface tension has yet to be determined.

The concept that the direction of growth of newly formed axons between the nerve ends is determined solely by the physical state and properties of the environment we owe to Ranvier (1878) and Vanlair (1885, 1894). They believed that axons grew blindly through the bridging tissue, following paths of least resistance and arriving at the distal nerve stump only by chance. They were supported in these views by Stroebe (1893) and later by Dustin (1910) with his hypothesis of odogenesis which was based on the belief that regenerating axons followed spaces and tracks formed by young connective tissue cells that facilitated their passage to the distal nerve stump.

That axon growth is influenced solely by such physical factors was disputed by Cajal and Forssman, who assigned the primary role in the process to chemotropism. However, both were prepared to concede that such factors do play a secondary role. Cajal is quite clear on this point when he comments as follows.

1. Mechanical factors affect the passage of axons through scar tissue. Even single cells will deflect them. He also writes that 'This strange propensity of the nerve sprouts to adhere to supports or pre-established paths constitutes in many cases a serious resistance to the trophic and orientating influences and is a frequent cause of arrests and deviations.'
2. The cone of axon growth is extremely sensitive to mechanical as well as chemical variations in its surroundings.
3. During the first phases of regeneration bare axon sprouts grow freely in the bridging tissue by virtue of stereotropism.
4. Axon sprouts become intimately applied to the cells of scar tissue and follow their processes if these in any way have the general direction of axon growth (tactile adhesion or stereotropism).
5. Axons become aggregated as a result of reciprocal stereotropism. Elsewhere Cajal refers to a Law of Reciprocal Homotropism which 'is the property that axon sprouts possess of congregating in bundles in order to pass with the greatest economy of effort through mesodermal tissue.'
6. Newly formed fibres have a tendency to adhere to obstacles and especially to those which have smooth surfaces along which they slide rapidly — adhesive attraction or stereotropism.

Cajal's views have been given at some length because it is often inferred that he was preoccupied with the case for neurotropism and was unaware of other factors influencing axon growth.

In recent times the most active advocate for the dominant role of physical factors in axon growth has been Weiss, whose extensive studies were also directed to rejecting neurotropism as originally expressed by Cajal. According to Weiss axon growth proceeds initially in a random fashion until some axons establish a chance encounter with the distal nerve-end. Having outlined a path of least resistance in this way, these 'pathfinder' axons undergo further changes that provide them with a surface to which succeeding axons attach and along which they grow by a process of tactile adherence, contact guidance and chemical guidance that, however, involve contact affinity or local attraction and not attraction from a distance as was originally implied in chemotropism. In this respect there is no preferential growth of axons towards the distal nerve end, directed axon growth being the end result of random axon growth. Thus 'nerve fibres are definitely guided to their destination rather that attracted by them' (Weiss 1944).

While much of the reasoning behind Weiss' conclusions remains speculative it is clear that the main thrust of his concept of contact guidance is in many respects reminiscent of the views collectively expressed by Cajal and his contemporaries at the turn of the century, the only point of difference being to the existence or non-existence of neurotropic stimuli originating in the distal nerve stump. However, Weiss' contributions have done much to clarify the way in which physical factors influence the growth of axons between the nerve ends and, importantly, those structural features of the bridging tissue that determine the direction and course taken by regenerating axons. Neurotropism, whatever its role, will not overcome the obstacles to axon advance created by unfavourable tissue at a suture line.

CONCLUDING COMMENTS

This review of neurotropism has revealed data that are of special relevance to the surgical repair of severed nerves.

1. It is remarkable how much ground was covered by Cajal and his contemporaries and how wide ranging were their ideas and thoughts on the subject of axon regeneration. A study of contemporary literature on the subject raises the question of just how much further ahead are we today, despite the availability of modern methods and techniques.

2. The surgical literature between the middle ages and the present century contains references to the surprising degree of spontaneous recovery that sometimes occurs despite the loss of nerve trunk continuity. Such spontaneous recovery is more likely to occur when the nerve ends are close together.

3. Regenerating axons will bridge considerable gaps in nerves to reach and reinnervate the corresponding distal nerve stump.

4. The passage of regenerating axons to the distal nerve stump is under the influence of neurotropic factors generated in and operating from the distal stump of the severed nerve.

5. The nature of this neurotropic factor is not known, though there is evidence to suggest that it has a complex protein structure and a limited diffusive power.

6. The source of the neurotropic factor appears to be widely distributed throughout the tissues of the distal nerve stump. It is not confined to Schwann cells as was originally believed.

7. The influence on axon growth of galvanotropism, based on bioelectrical field effects and potential gradients introduced by nerve injury, awaits further study.

8. Chance physical influences outlining paths of least resistance through the tissue between the nerve ends are the principal determinants of the direction taken by regenerating axons after they leave the proximal nerve end.

9. Axon growth between the nerve ends follows a random pattern and entry into the distal stump occurs as a matter of chance.

10. Regenerating axons show no preference for fascicular tissue and will grow just as readily into the interfascicular epineurial connective tissues.

11. The endoneurial tubes of the distal stump admit axons indiscriminately. There is no neurotropic influence to impart a matching specificity to the process whereby each regenerating axon is attracted into the endoneurial tube that it originally occupied or to which it is even functionally related.

12. On reaching the distal stump regenerating axons compete for endoneurial tubes, entry

favouring the axons of those branch fibre systems that are numerically greater.

13. The only contribution of neurotropism to axon growth is to assist regenerating axons to reach the distal stump.

14. Spontaneous recovery, consequent on axon regeneration occurring across the gap between the ends of a severed nerve, is far inferior to that obtainable by nerve repair.

15. When nerve ends are brought together and maintained in apposition, any consideration of neurotropism no longer applies. Regenerating axons are then at the face of the distal nerve stump when they emerge from the proximal nerve end and there are no neurotropic influences to direct growing axons either into fasciculi or matching endoneurial tubes.

16. The nature of the union scar after nerve repair becomes of critical importance in determining the destination of regenerating axons (Chapters 39, 41 & 42).

17. In the absence of any neurotropic influences to assist him the surgeon is forced to rely solely on his own resources and initiative when devising methods to satisfy the four essential objectives of nerve repair:

   a. to obtain and preserve correct axial alignment of the nerve ends;
   b. to maximise the entry of regenerating axons into the fasciculi of the distal nerve end;
   c. to minimise the loss of regenerating axons that occurs at the suture line when:

      i. they are arrested by unfavourable junctional tissue, and
      ii. they enter interfascicular epineurial tissue and foreign functionally unrelated endoneurial tubes.

   d. to take advantage of any branch fibre localisation in the nerve at the level of the repair with the intention of facilitating the entry of axons into functionally related endoneurial tubes.

18. With a clean transection injury these objectives can be met with a simple epineurial repair. Where, however, the injury involves the loss of a length of the nerve, the repair calls for some form of

group fascicular repair. The reasons for this are discussed in Chapters 42 and 43.

19. In nerve repair there are no neurotropic influences to rescue the surgeon from ignorance or incompetence.

REFERENCES

Ariëns Kappers C U 1921 On structural laws in the nervous system: The principles of neurobiotaxis. Brain 44: 125

Brushart T M, Tarlov E C, Mesulam M-M 1983 Specificity of muscle reinnervation after epineurial and individual fascicular suture of the rat sciatic nerve. Journal of Hand Surgery 8: 248

Brushart T M, Seiler W A 1987 Selective reinnervation of distal motor stumps by peripheral motor axons. Experimental Neurology 97: 289

Charlwood K A, Lamont D M, Banks B E C 1972 Apparent orienting effects produced by nerve growth factor. In: Zaimis E, Knight J (eds) Nerve growth factor and its antiserum. Athlone Press, University of London, p 102

Dustin A P 1910 La rôle des tropisme et de l'odogenèse dans la régénération du systeme nerveux. Archives Biologie 25: 269

Ebendal T, Jacobson C O 1977 Tissue explants affecting extension and orientation of axons in cultured chick embryo ganglia. Experimental Cell Research 105: 379

Forssman J 1898 Über die Ursachen welche die Wachstumrichtung der peripheren Nerven fasern beri der Regeneration bestimmen. Ziegler's Beiträge zur Pathologische Anatomie 24: 56

Forssman J 1900 Zur Kenntniss des Neurotropismus. Ziegler's Beiträge zur Pathologische Anatomie 27: 407

Gundersen R W, Barret J N 1979 Neuronal chemotaxis: chick dorsal root axons turn towards high concentrations of nerve growth factor. Science 206: 1079

Gutmann E 1945 The reinnervation of muscle by sensory fibres. Journal of Anatomy 79: 1

Horsch K W 1979 Guidance of regrowing sensory axons after cutaneous nerve lesions in the cat. Journal of Neurophysiology 42: 1437

Ingvar S 1920 Reactions of cells to the galvanic current in tissue cultures. Proceedings of the American Society of Experimental Biology and Medicine 17: 198

Le Tourneau P C 1978 Chemotactic responé of nerve fibre elongation to nerve growth factor. Developmental Biology 66: 183

Lundborg G, Hansson H A 1979 Regeneration of nerve through a preformed tissue space. Preliminary observations on the reorganisation of regenerating nerve fibers and perineurium. Brain Research 178: 573

Lundborg G, Hansson H A 1980 Nerve regeneration through pre-formed pseudosynovial tubes. A preliminary report of a new experimental model for studying the regeneration and reorganisation capacity of peripheral nerve tissue. Journal of Hand Surgery 5: 35

Lundborg G, Hansson H A 1981 Nerve lesions with interruption of continuity. Studies on the growth pattern of regenerating axons in the gap between the proximal and distal nerve ends. In: Gorio A, Millest H, Mingrino S (eds) Post-traumatic nerve regeneration. Raven Press, New York, p 229

Lundborg G, Dahlin L B, Danielsen N, Hansson H A, Larsson K 1981 Reorganization and orientation of regenerating nerve fibers, perineurium and epineurium in preformed mesothelial tubes — an experimental study on the sciatic nerve of rats. Journal of Neuroscience Research 6: 265

Lundborg G, Dahlin L B, Danielsen N 1982a Nerve regeneration across an extended gap: a neurobiological view of nerve repair and the possible involvement of neurotrophic factors. Journal of Hand Surgery 7: 580

Lundborg G, Longo F, Varon S 1982b Nerve regeneration model and neuronotrophic factors in vivo. Brain Research 232: 157

Lundborg G, Dahlin L B, Danielsen N, Johannesson A, Hansson H A 1982c Regeneration of nerve fibres in preformed mesothelial tubes — influence of distal nerve segment of a transected nerve on growth and direction. In: Lee A J C, Albrektsson T, Branemark P I (eds) Clinical applications of biomaterials. Advances in Biomaterials vol 4, John Wiley, Chichester, p 323

Lundborg G, Dahlin L B, Danielsen N, Nachemson A 1986 Tissue specificity in nerve regeneration. Scandinavian Journal of Plastic and Reconstructive Surgery 20: 279

Mackinnon S, Dellon L, Hudson A, Hunter D 1984 Nerve regeneration through a pseudosynovial sheath in a primate model. Plastic and Reconstructive Surgery 75: 833

Mackinnon S E, Dellon A L, Lundborg G, Hudson A R, Hunter D A 1986 A study of neurotropism in a primate model. Journal of Hand Surgery 11A: 888

Nachemson A, Lundborg G 1986 A study of neurotropism in a primate model. Journal of Hand Surgery Proceedings 11A: 766

Nageotte J, Guyon L 1918 Différences physiologiques entre la néuroglie des fibres motrices et celle des fibres sensitives, dans les nerfs périphériques, mises en evidence par la régénération. Compte Rendue Société de Biologie 81: 571

Ochi M 1983 Experimental study on orientation of regenerating fibres in severed peripheral nerve. Hiroshima Journal of Medical Sciences 31: 389

Politis M J 1985 Specificity in mammalian peripheral nerve regeneration at the level of the nerve trunk. Brain Research 328: 271

Politis M J, Spencer P 1983 An in vivo assay of neurotropic activity. Brain Research 278: 229

Politis M J, Steiss J E 1985 Electromyographic evaluation of a novel surgical preparation to enhance nerve-muscle specificity that follows mammalian peripheral nerve transection. Experimental Neurology 87: 326

Politis M J, Ederle K, Spencer P 1982 Tropism nerve regeneration in vivo. Attraction of regenerating axons by diffusible factors derived from cells in distal stumps of transected peripheral nerves. Brain Research 253: 1

Pollock L J, Golseth J G, Mayfield F, Arieff A J, Liebert E, Oester Y T 1947 Spontaneous regeneration of severed nerves. Journal of the American Medical Association 134: 330

Ramon Y Cajal S 1928 Degeneration and regeneration of the nervous system, Vol 1. Oxford University Press, London

Ranvier M L 1878 Leçons sur l'histologie du système nerveux. F. Savy, Paris

Richardson P, Ebendal T 1982 Nerve growth activities in rat peripheral nerve. Brain Research 246: 57

Scaffidi F V 1910 Sulle correnti di demarcasione dei nervi

duronte la degenerazione Walleriana e la regenerazione. Zeitschrift für Allgemeine Physiologie 11: 339

Seckel B R, Chiu T H, Nyalis E, Sidman R L 1984 Nerve regeneration through synthetic biodegradable nerve guides: regulation by a target organ. Plastic and Reconstructive Surgery 74: 173

Seckel B R, Ryan S E, Gagne R G, Chiu T H, Watkins E 1986 Target — specific nerve regeneration through a nerve guide in the rat. Plastic and Reconstructive Surgery 78: 793

Stroebe H 1893 Experimentelle Untersuchungen über Degeneration und Regeneration peripherer Nerven nach Verletzungen. Zeiglers Beitrage zur pathologische Anatomie 13: 160

Sunderland S 1953 The capacity of regenerating axons to bridge long gaps in nerves. Journal of Comparative Neurology 99: 481

Sunderland S, Ray L J 1950 Denervation changes in mammalian striated muscle. Journal of Neurology, Neurosurgery and Psychiatry 13: 159

Tello J F 1911 La influencia del neurotropismo en la regeneracion de los centros nerviosos. Instituto de investigaciones biologicas Universite de Madrid Trabajos Travaux 9: 123

Tello J F 1923a Discurso de ingreso en la Academia de Medicina de Madrid. Ideas actuales sobre el neurotropismo

Tello J F 1923b Gegenwärtige Anschauungen über den Neurotropismus. Vorträge und Aufsätze über Entwicklungsmechanik der Organismen 33: 1. Springer, Berlin

Vanlair C 1885 Nouvelles recherches expérimentales sur la régénération des nerfs. Archives de Biologie 6: 127

Vanlair C 1894 Recherches chronometriques sur la régénération des nerfs. Archives de Physiologie Normale et Pathologique 6: 217

Varon S, Adler R 1980 Nerve growth factor and control of nerve growth. Current Topics in Developmental Biology 16: 207

Virchow R 1846 Die krankhaften Geschwülste. A. Hirschwold, Berlin

Weiss P 1944 The technology of nerve regeneration. A review. Sutureless tubulation and related methods of nerve repair. Journal of Neurosurgery 1: 400

Weiss P 1950 An introduction to genetic neurology. In: Weiss P (ed) Genetic neurology. University of Chicago Press, Chicago, p 1

Weiss P, Taylor A C 1944 Further experimental evidence against "neurotropism" in nerve regeneration. Journal of Experimental Zoology 95: 233

Weiss P, Edds M V 1945 Sensory — motor nerve crosses in the rat. Journal of Neurophysiology 8: 173

Weiss P, Hoag A 1946 Competitive reinnervation of rat muscles by their own and foreign nerves. Journal of Neurophysiology 9: 413

Williams L R 1987 Rat aorta isografts possess nerve-regeneration promoting properties in silicone Y-chambers. Experimental Neurology 97: 555

Williams L R, Longo F, Powell H C, Lundborg G, Varon S 1983 Spatio-temporal progress of peripheral nerve regeneration within a silicone chamber: parameters for a bioassay. Journal of Comparative Neurology 218: 460

Williams L R, Powell H C, Lundborg G, Varon S 1984 Competence of nerve tissue as distal insert promoting nerve regeneration in a silicone chamber. Brain Research 293: 201

17. Causes of nerve injury. Terminology. Compression nerve injury

TERMINOLOGY

Trauma. An injury caused by a physical agent.

Nerve injury. In the text this term is applied to the damage caused by a force applied to the nerve either from outside the body or generated from within the body.

Nerve lesion. This term has a somewhat wider connotation in that it also includes any damage to the nerve regardless of the mechanism by which it was produced. The terms nerve injury and nerve lesion are used synonymously in this text.

Traumatic nerve lesion. One caused by physical injury.

Neuropathy. This term is usually applied to those nerve lesions that are not caused by physical injury but are a consequence of, for example, toxic and metabolic disturbances and primary vascular disease. They do not fall within the scope of this text other than to include those in which vascular complication secondary to mechanical trauma play a role in the production of the lesion.

Compression. This is introduced when a force, regardless of its source, is applied to the surface of a nerve and alters its cross-sectional dimensions.

Traction. This term refers to the application of a deforming force applied along the long axis of the nerve and increasing its length.

Friction. This is introduced when a nerve rubs across a roughened surface or structure.

Rupture and avulsion. These are the extreme consequences of traction injury. They are not interchangeable terms and it is important to distinguish between the two.

Avulsion. This means torn from, and refers to the tearing of nerve fibres from the surface of the spinal cord or from a muscle.

Rupture. This implies a break in continuity of the nerve with clearly defined proximal and distal nerve stumps.

Laceration. This term refers to a jagged, ragged or mangled tear in which there is partial or complete loss of continuity of the nerve. There is no such injury as a clean laceration unless it refers to the absence of infection.

Ischaemia. This refers to the reduction in the blood supply to tissues from constriction or obstruction of a blood vessel.

PRIMARY CAUSES OF NERVE INJURY

The primary causes of nerve injury considered in this text are:

Physical trauma. This takes the form of compression, stretch or friction. With compression and stretch the wounding may be closed or open, the injured nerve being penetrated by a sharp object or fragment of bone, partially or completely but cleanly severed, ruptured, crushed, contused or lacerated. Though compression and stretch are usually associated in the production of any nerve injury, it is convenient to consider the effects of each on the nerve as separate events.

Friction based injuries are closed injuries, the most common being the entrapment nerve lesion.

Ischaemia. Only those ischaemic nerve lesions due to physical trauma are considered.

The action of sclerosing and toxic agents. These nerve injuries may be caused by therapeutic agents being inadvertently injected into a nerve or to the planned injection of a destructive sclerosing agent with the intention of silencing abnormal activity in nerve fibres.

Cooling, freezing, ionising radiation.
Special miscellaneous causes of nerve injury involving one or a combination of the primary causes:

1. Compression nerve injuries caused during anaesthesia, coma, drug narcosis and the undisturbed sleep of the fatigued and wasted individual.
2. Nerve injuries associated with dislocations and closed and open fractures.
3. Nerve injuries caused by high velocity and other missile wounding.
4. Obstetrical, birth and neonatal nerve injuries.
5. Sports injuries.

COMPRESSION NERVE INJURY

General comment

1. Two major categories of compression nerve injury are:
   a. the acute injury of immediate onset and
   b. the chronic injury of delayed and gradual onset.

   In both, the deforming force responsible for injuring the nerve originates in two ways, one from some external source delivered from outside the body and the other from a source within the body.
2. The role of ischaemia as a contributory factor in nerve compression injury calls for comment. In acute nerve compression injury, the deforming force may be applied so rapidly and be of such severity that the involvement of a vascular factor in the production of the lesion becomes irrelevant because nerve fibres have either failed functionally or been destroyed before ischaemia would have had time to produce its harmful effect on the nerve. The role of a vascular factor then shifts to the development of post-traumatic complications.

   On the other hand, a vascular component is inevitably introduced when the nerve is slowly compressed, as in the development of chronic lesions, because it is impossible under these conditions to compress a segment of a nerve without simultaneously impairing the flow of blood to and through it. Thus a nerve segment may be compressed so slowly and under such conditions, that the blood supply to nerve fibres is impaired to a degree that results in conduction failure and compromises their survival long before they are threatened by physical deformation, which is a later event. Such lesions are therefore more appropriately classified as compression-ischaemic nerve lesions.

Factors influencing the extent and severity of the compression nerve lesion

The extent and severity of the damage due to compression are determined by such factors as:

1. The magnitude of the deforming force which can be arbitrarily assigned to one of three grades of severity — mild, intermediate and severe. Mild compression produces first degree and second degree damage, the intermediate causes structural changes representing a third degree injury, and deforming forces of considerable magnitude cause fourth degree and fifth degree damage with widespread bruising, laceration and severance.
2. The rate of application of the deforming force and the time for which it operates. Nerves tolerate greater degrees of compression when deformation occurs so slowly as to be measured in months and years rather than in milliseconds or seconds. When a deforming force is gradually applied and slowly increases over long periods of time, nerves can be compressed to a remarkable degree with little, if any, disturbance of function. On the other hand, the nerve may be compressed so rapidly and violently that conduction failure and the appearance of structural damage are instantaneous.
3. The manner in which the deforming force is applied to the nerve. The force may be localised to a point on the surface of the nerve leading to a penetrating or puncture injury by a sharp object, it may slice

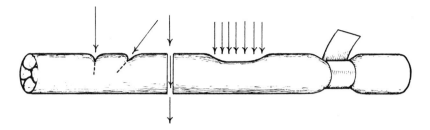

Fig. 17.1.

obliquely or transversely across the nerve or it may be applied to a length of the nerve and crush or lacerate that segment (Fig. 17.1).

Features that increase the vulnerability of a nerve to compression injury

Thousands of sedentary workers sit with elbows on tables for hours every day. Why should one and not others develop an ulnar nerve palsy?

Features of nerves that protect nerve fibres from physical deformation are outlined in Chapter 12. Here we are concerned only with those that render them more susceptible to compression.

The microstructure of nerves and nerve roots

1. Nerve fibres are more susceptible to injury where they are collected into a single or a few large closely packed fasciculi with little

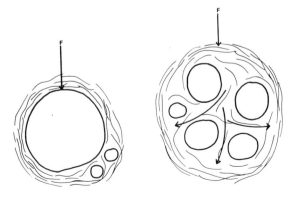

Fig. 17.2 The dispersal of compression forces through the epineurium.

supporting epineurial tissue. Forces then fall maximally on the main component of the nerve which is fascicular tissue and, therefore, on nerve fibres. The rupture of intrafascicular vessels also leads to complications that still further embarrass large collections of nerve fibres. On the other hand, the effects of compression are minimised where a nerve is composed of small fasciculi widely separated by a large amount of epineural tissue. The damaging forces are then dispersed and cushioned by the epineurial tissue, while the fasciculi are more easily displaced within the nerve, all of which reduces the damaging effects of the deforming force (Fig. 17.2).

2. Nerve roots differ structurally from peripheral nerves in certain important respects (Table 17.1; Fig. 17.3).

    a. The perineurium is absent. Nerve roots accordingly lack the tensile strength of peripheral nerves and so are more vulnerable to traction injury.
    b. The epineurium is absent so that nerve roots are more susceptible to compression.
    c. The protective undulations in nerve trunks, fasciculi and nerve fibres, that are such a characteristic feature of peripheral nerves, are not a prominent feature of nerve roots.
    d. The nerve root entry zone at the cord is a transition zone where axons are more exposed to chronic irritation.
    e. Large vessels are more directly related to nerve root fibres than in peripheral nerves.

Table 17.1 Some significant differences in the microstructure of peripheral nerves and nerve roots and their consequences

Associated tissues	Peripheral nerve trunk	Nerve root	Consequences
Epineurium	Present	Absent	Nerve root fibres are more vulnerable to compression injury than their peripheral counterparts
Perineurium	Present	Absent	Nerve roots lack the tensile strength of their peripheral counterparts and so are more liable to traction injury
Endoneurium	Present	Present: Collagen fibrils fewer and finer	The greater accessibility of pharmacological and other agents

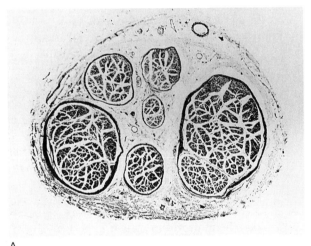

A

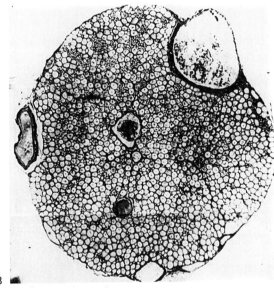

B

Fig. 17.3 Transverse sections of a peripheral nerve (**a**) and nerve root (**b**), illustrating the structural differences between them.

Regional features of nerves that increase their susceptibility to compression

A nerve is particularly at risk where:

1. it is in direct contact with an unyielding surface against which it can be compressed, e.g. the ulnar nerve behind the medial humeral epicondyle, the radial nerve in the musculospiral groove of the humerus and the lateral popliteal nerve at the neck of the fibula;
2. it passes through, or is contained within, a compartment with unyielding walls such as:
   i. the median nerve in the carpal tunnel;
   ii. the lumbar plexus in the psoas compartment.
3. it is intimately related to a structure, enlargement of which would stretch and compress the nerve, e.g. an aneurysmal swelling of a vessel in contact with the nerve.

Pre-existing damage to the nerve in the form of a clinically silent lesion

Normal nerve fibres possess a remarkable tolerance to physical deformation but once they are damaged they become particularly sensitive to further compression and ischaemia.

1. A clinically silent lesion increases the susceptibility to further injury at another level, the two lesions together creating a situation that is incompatible with normal function. The double lesion, or double crush syndrome as it is often called, is discussed in the section on the entrapment nerve lesion (see Chapter 19).
2. A similar condition to the double entrapment lesion is one in which a latent subclinical toxic-metabolic neuropathy renders a nerve more susceptible to compression injury. Such covert pre-existing pathology only becomes clinically evident when its latent effects are intensified by compression ischaemia. Examples are the association between Bell's palsy and diabetes and a greater incidence of carpal tunnel compression in patients with diabetes.
3. Some febrile conditions of viral or other origin may lower the threshold at which compression damages the nerve.

The general health of the patient

Nerves are less well protected by surrounding tissues in the wasted limbs of the debilitated.

Categories and causes of compression nerve injury

The major categories of compression nerve injury are:

1. The acute injury caused by an abruptly applied exogenous force.
2. The acute injury caused by an endogenous force.
3. The chronic injury caused by forces that:

   a. are applied intermittently;
   b. fluctuate in intensity;
   c. gradually increase.

THE ACUTE COMPRESSION NERVE INJURY

In the severe acute compression injury the mechanical deformation of nerve fibres dominates the pathology of the lesion. In the chronic com-pression nerve lesion, ischaemia becomes a significant factor in the genesis of the lesion.

Delayed secondary effects that may contribute to the pathology of the lesion include spreading oedema, haemorrhage, infection, neural fibrosis and the formation of adhesions that fix the nerve to its bed.

The wound may be open or closed, the nerve injury may be partial or complete, localised or in-volve a length of the nerve, be uniform in degree or vary throughout the thickness of the nerve.

The mildest type of compression injury to have clinical significance is the prolonged conduction block or first degree injury (see Chapter 25). These lesions may, in turn, be classified as transient, moderately severe or severe depending on the duration of the conduction block and the time taken to attain complete recovery, with intervals measured in hours, weeks and months res-pectively (see Chapter 13).

With rapidly increasing and unrelieved com-pression the lesion is converted into one of second degree severity. With further compression the af-fected segment of the nerve is crushed, its fascicular structure disorganised, and it is finally converted into a cord or ribbon of fibrous tissue in which all trace of endoneurial tubes is lost and through which regenerating axons are unable to find their way (third and fourth degree injury, see Chapter 25). With some severe compression injuries nerve trunk continuity is lost.

The course of regeneration and the quality of the recovery following Wallerian degeneration depend on the extent to which pressure and is-chaemia have disorganised the structure of the nerve trunk.

1. Provided the endoneurial sheath of nerve fibres is preserved, regeneration results in the full restoration of the original pattern of innervation. Recovery, though delayed, proceeds to completion, the various structures recovering in the order in which they are innervated. This represents a second degree nerve injury.
2. Destruction of the endoneurium with disorganisation of the intrafascicular tissues and, finally, the disorganisation of the internal architecture of the nerve trunk represent third and fourth degree injuries

respectively, in which extensive fibrosis and marked collagenisation of the endoneurium are added complications. Under these adverse conditions regeneration is so seriously affected that recovery is incomplete or negligible.

Acute compression nerve injury caused by exogenous forces

With these lesions the nerve is abruptly and severely compressed by a force that is transient or persists until relieved. Examples are legion but common ones are:

1. A sharp severe blow from a blunt object with the deforming force transmitted transcutaneously to the nerve, particularly when the nerve is forced against an unyielding surface such as bone, e.g. a rifle butt forcibly driven against the outer aspect of the upper arm, injuring the radial nerve.
2. Unrelieved pressure on a nerve as in the case of the radial nerve in Saturday night paralysis.
3. Inadvertently clamping a nerve with artery forceps or including it in a ligature.
4. Pressure on a nerve from a too tightly applied bandage, a tourniquet or an ill-fitting splint or plaster cast, e.g. compressing the radial nerve against the humerus and the common peroneal nerve against the neck of the fibula.
   Tourniquet compression. This is a good example of this type of injury. Features of tourniquet paralysis are:

   a. They are more common in the upper limb than in the lower owing to the exposed position of the major nerves above the elbow compared with the protected course run by the sciatic nerve in the thigh.
   b. The radial nerve is the most commonly affected in the upper limb. This is explained by its relationship to the humerus against which it is compressed, and where it is frequently composed of a single or a few large fasciculi with relatively little supporting epineural tissue.
   c. The nerve injury varies in severity from first to third degree involvement. However, the compression may be sufficiently severe and prolonged to cause pressure necrosis of the nerve trunk with marked intraneural scarring and neuroma formation.
   d. Motor nerve fibres are the first to fail, the last to recover, and, in the mildest lesions, may be the only ones to suffer.
   e. Only the exceptional case fails to recover spontaneously and completely. Recovery is usually complete or well advanced by the 3rd month but may be delayed for 6.
   f. There is no constant relationship between the length of time for which the tourniquet is applied and involvement of the nerve. Variations are probably due to differences in the magnitude of the deforming force and in the internal structure of the nerve trunk at the site of compression.

5. Secondary involvement from:

   a. the displaced fragment of a fracture;
   b. a dislocated bone such as the dislocated head of the humerus impinging on the axillary nerve, and the semilunar bone dislocated into the carpal tunnel and compressing the median nerve.
6. Prolonged unrelieved pressure on a nerve during anaesthesia, drug-induced coma, unconsciousness and the deep undisturbed sleep of the grossly fatigued and debilitated person;
7. Pressure on a nerve in the mother during pregnancy or delivery and in the baby during birth.

Acute compression nerve injury caused by endogenous forces

Here the offending force is generated internally, develops abruptly and persists until relieved or the pathology responsible resolves. An example is haemorrhage into a confined compartment containing a nerve or nerves, e.g. compression of the median nerve in the carpal tunnel and of the lumbar plexus in the psoas compartment.

THE NERVE INJURY CAUSED BY CHRONIC COMPRESSION

In these injuries the damaging force:

1. originates either externally or internally;
2. develops slowly and irregularly;
3. is progressive or intermittent. In some instances it is clear that one insult is insufficient to damage the nerve, repeated physical deformation over a period being required before functional and structural failure finally occur;
4. is accompanied by slow progressive deterioration of function, sometimes with remissions;
5. produces effects on nerve fibres in three ways:

   a. by physical trauma;
   b. by impairing the blood supply to and through the compressed segment of the nerve;
   c. by constriction as the result of the fibrosis developing in and around the fasciculi and about the entire nerve trunk in response to trauma and ischaemia.

Initially the lesion is one of first degree severity which, if unrelieved, progresses through second to third and even fourth degree damage. Unless the deforming force is corrected or the nerve is decompressed nerve fibres are finally destroyed and the nerve trunk is converted into fibrous tissue, the terminal pathology being identical with that resulting from acute unrelieved compression. Clinically, this group includes the important chronic compression and entrapment lesions that call for special consideration (see Chapter 19).

The signs and symptoms associated with these lesions are often subject to irregular remissions and exacerbations that, presumably, reflect irregular fluctuations in the pathology of a lesion that is delicately balanced between blocking conduction and allowing recovery. Fluctuations in both the offending pressure and in the intraneural circulation could be responsible for at one time aggravating symptoms and at another of alleviating them. An illustrative example is the fluctuating symptomatology in the carpal tunnel syndrome.

Intermittent repetitive compression trauma from some external source

1. Involvement of the brachial plexus between the clavicle and a normal or abnormal first rib during limb movements;
2. The position in which a part of the limb is habitually held or used during work is the basis of occupational compression nerve injury, examples of which are:

   a. squatting, crouching, kneeling and sitting for long periods with knees crossed, resulting in compression palsy of the common peroneal nerve;
   b. constantly positioning the forearm and elbow against a hard surface which gives compression ulnar lesions;
   c. the day-to-day use of tools that are repeatedly and firmly grasped or forced into the palm of the hand. A variant of this type of injury is the lesion caused by repetitive percussion, the most common being involvement of the ulnar nerve at the wrist from using a pneumatic drill or driving a tractor.

3. The radial nerve at the axillary outlet in crutch palsy.

Internal causes of chronic nerve compression

A nerve may be gradually compressed by:

1. callus surrounding and encasing a nerve;
2. the formation of a constricting collar or band of scar tissue around a nerve that constricts it and blocks conduction. Conduction across the affected segment returns immediately the injured nerve is freed from constrictive scar tissue (Chapters 25 & 38).
3. an enlarging aneurysm;
4. a slowly enlarging tumour or ganglion. These commonly involve the median and ulnar nerves at the wrist, the ulnar nerve at the elbow and the common peroneal nerve at the knee joint;
5. increasing pressure introduced as a haematoma enlarges beneath the deep fascia;
6. increasing pressure developing from any cause in a compartment traversed by a

nerve. The classical compression nerve injury in this group is the median nerve lesion in the carpal tunnel syndrome. However, the same applies to any nerve occupying a compartment with unyielding walls. The pathogenesis of this compression-ischaemic lesion is discussed in the next section.

PATHOGENESIS OF CHRONIC COMPRESSION NERVE INJURY

The pathogenesis of chronic compression nerve lesions, particularly in an entrapment situation, remains a controversial issue. There are those who insist that the primary pathology is the result of the physical deformation of nerve fibres. The opposing point of view claims that the primary pathology in the initial stages of the development of the lesion is based on vascular complications introduced by compression.

In examining these two propositions it is important to keep constantly in mind that the deforming force in chronic compression develops very slowly and may operate only intermittently.

Physical deformation as the primary cause of chronic compression nerve injury

The revived interest in the physical deformation of nerve fibres as the primary cause of the lesion in chronic nerve compression is based on four sets of observations:

1. The case for direct mechanical damage in chronic compression lesions was reawakened with the important studies of Gilliatt and his group on pressure and entrapment neuropathies based on the fortuitous finding of these spontaneous lesions in the plantar and median nerves of the guinea pig (Fullerton & Gilliatt 1967a,b, Anderson et al 1970). The essential histological features of the lesions were the greater vulnerability of large myelinated fibres, axonal thinning, segmental demyelination, some Wallerian degeneration and evidence of regeneration. There was a passing reference to shrunken and collagenous fascicles in a median nerve that was electrically inexcitable.

2. The changes observed in nerves subjected to severe tourniquet cuff compression at the knee in the baboon (Ochoa et al 1972). From these it was concluded that the damage to the nerve fibres was a direct result of the applied pressure and not a consequence of secondary ischaemia. Features of these experimental lesions were:

   a. In general, they were restricted to fibres with an axon diameter greater than 5 μm, fine myelinated and non-myelinated fibres being spared. This is consistent with the long established finding that large fibres are more susceptible to compression as well as ischaemia.

   b. Of particular significance was a distortion of the nodes with the formation of paranodal bulbous swellings associated with slippage, folding and rupture of the paranodal myelin lamellae with retraction of the myelin along the internode. The overall effect was to produce a distinctive displacement of the node of Ranvier, one paranode being invaginated by its neighbour to outline a nodal intussusception.

   c. The nodal intussusceptions were maximal under the margins of the cuff and became less conspicuous towards the centre of the compressed segment where they were absent.

   d. The direction of the nodal displacement was always away from the cuff towards uncompressed tissue.

   e. The nodal lesions were regarded as the precursors of the segmental demyelination and axonal thinning that followed, and ultimately the more advanced pathology culminating in axon and myelin degeneration.

3. The changes in a guinea pig model of chronic median nerve entrapment at the wrist were attributed to the physical deformation of nerve fibres from chronic compression (Ochoa & Marotte 1973, Marotte 1974, Ochoa 1980a,b). Though

nodal intussusception was not found in this material, the structural changes again showed a distinctive pattern characterised by:

a. the vulnerability of well-myelinated nerve fibres;

b. gross deformation of the myelin internodes with paranodal slippage of myelin lamellae and the exposure of axons;

c. the myelin segments formed pear or tear drop shaped bulbous swellings. These showed a consistent polarity in which the swellings were formed at the ends of the internodes further from the centre of the lesion with myelin tapering towards it. The arrangement was interpreted as evidence of pressure deformation.

4. Changes identical with those described in the guinea pig by Ochoa and Marotte were reported by Neary et al (1975) in autopsy specimens of the median and ulnar nerve at the wrist and elbow, respectively. In the absence of evidence of nerve dysfunction in the donor individuals during life, these lesions were labelled subclinical entrapment neuropathy.

More recent experimental studies, using a variety of techniques to compress a nerve segment, have supported the earlier conviction that the physical deformation of nerve fibres is responsible for the chronic compression nerve lesion (Horiuchi 1983, Nemoto 1983, Mackinnon et al 1984, 1985, Mackinnon & Dellon 1986).

Comment

There are reasonable grounds for questioning the validity of the claim that the physical deformation of nerve fibres is the primary cause of the lesion in chronic nerve compression.

1. The compression forces in the tourniquet cuff compression experiments were of considerable magnitude (500 and 1000 mmHg), were abruptly applied, and were maintained for 1–3 hours. These pressures were greatly in excess of any that would ever be generated in entrapment situations in the limbs where nerves are exposed to the risk of compression injury. Furthermore, the immediate relief that often follows, for example, decompression of the median nerve in the carpal tunnel syndrome, is inconsistent with such advanced structural changes that would require some time to resolve.

Clearly we are dealing here with lesions that are in the acute compression category and not chronic compression in the sense in which that term is customarily used. On this point there is no dispute. However, these acute lesions are the forerunner of the claims advocating physical deformation of nerve fibres as the primary pathology in chronic compression lesions.

2. The chronic compression lesion attributed to physical deformation is one of well established structural changes. It is difficult to reconcile the immediate relief that at times follows decompression with pathology that would require some time for its resolution.

3. The reports refer to shrunken fascicles and increased amounts of collagen which could be evidence of a vascular lesion. According to Marotte (1974) 'It is possible that it (a proteinaceous exudate) derives from vessels damaged by the compression. However, the structure of blood vessels was not studied.' Gilliatt (1975) regards these as late effects and concedes that 'Ischaemia may well be one of the factors responsible.'

4. It is interesting that Ochoa (1980a,b) attributes these changes to 'minor trauma, or perhaps repeated stretching or friction against flexor tendons.' Note the omission of a reference to compression, the lesion being referred to as chronic entrapment neuropathy.

5. Neither the blood vessels in the compressed segment nor the blood flow through it were studied, despite the possibility that a vascular factor could have contributed to the production of the lesion.

6. A study of the relationship of symptoms to pathology was not possible in the experiments.

7. The chronic lesions described by these

investigators represent well established pathology to which friction has probably contributed. There is no proof that these changes were not preceded by vascular complications that could have initially contributed to their development.

8. If the physical deformation of nerve fibres were the primary pathology in the chronic compression nerve lesion, as has been claimed, then such lesions might be expected to be accompanied by some motor weakness and a sensory deficit because:

   a. well myelinated nerve fibres are selectively damaged;
   b. about 90% of the median nerve fibres at the wrist are sensory fibres;
   c. at the wrist the motor fibres occupy a superfical, exposed and vulnerable position.

However, it is well authenticated clinically that patients with a carpal tunnel syndrome often present with intermittent episodes of pain and paraesthesiae and no objective evidence of sensory or motor involvement. This has been recently confirmed by Szabo and Gelberman (1987), who found that more than 60% of these patients had symptoms of numbness, paraesthesiae and pain with no sensory abnormalities detectable by standard clinical testing.

A more likely explanation for these clinical findings is that the lesion responsible is one based on some vascular mechanism.

Conclusion. Sufficient has been said to cast doubt on the validity of the claim that the physical deformation of nerve fibres is the primary factor in the genesis of the chronic compression nerve lesion in an entrapment situation. It is also a justification for continuing the search for the essential element in the production of these lesions. Such a search has revealed that the missing link is likely to be a vascular factor introduced by compression that impairs the blood supply to normal nerve fibres (Sunderland 1976, 1978).

The vascular factor in the genesis of chronic compression nerve injury

Any nerve that passes through a compartment, opening or tunnel with unyielding walls may be selected as a model to illustrate the manner in which a vascular mechanism could produce the initial lesion when a nerve in such a situation is slowly compressed (Fig. 17.4). The following discussion would also apply if the nerve were gradually compressed against a firm surface.

Median nerve involvement in the carpal tunnel syndrome has been selected to examine the pathogenesis of chronic compression nerve injury because it:

1. illustrates the role and significance of regional anatomical features in the genesis of these lesions;
2. refutes a popular misconception that the lesion is invariably a consequence of the physical deformation of nerve fibres caused by nerve compression;
3. introduces a new pathogenic factor in the genesis of the chronic compression lesion, namely one based on ischaemia of normal nerve fibres.

Two features of the median nerve in the carpal tunnel that have special relevance to the following discussion are: (1) The microstructure of the nerve; (2) The blood flow and intraneural pressures in the compressed segment of a nerve.

The microstructure of the median nerve in the carpal tunnel

1. The nerve is composed of 6–40 fasciculi with an average of 24.
2. The cross-sectional area of the nerve devoted to epineurial connective tissue varies from 70 to 30 per cent with an average of 42 per cent. This epineurial packing protects the fasciculi and their contained nerve fibres from compression, particularly when it is present in large amounts.
3. Sensory outnumber motor fibres by about 9 to 1. Among the former, non-myelinated C fibres of less than 2μm in diameter and A delta nerve fibres of from 2 to 7μm in diameter outnumber the thicker more heavily myelinated fibres by about 4 to 1. Thus the fine fibre group, which includes the nociceptor elements, predominates in the median nerve at the wrist.

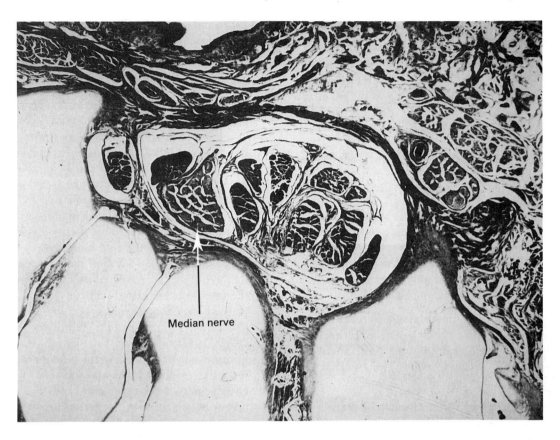

Fig. 17.4 Prepared transverse section at the wrist of a near full-term foetus illustrating the contents of the carpal tunnel. Note the position of the median nerve which has been moulded by neighbouring tendons.

4. Small and large sensory fibres are evenly distributed through the nerve, neither group being isolated or sharply localised.
5. Motor nerve fibres are confined to their own fascicular group, which is located anteriorly.
6. The arrangement of the nutrient vessels to and in the nerve in the carpal tunnel provides the clue to a vascular factor in the genesis of the nerve lesion in the carpal tunnel syndrome.

   a. Peripheral nerves have a profuse local blood supply that is essential for the survival and efficient functioning of nerve fibres.
   b. In the carpal tunnel the only named artery is the median artery. This nutrient artery is itself fine and often absent.
   c. The blood supply to this segment of the nerve is derived from nutrient arteries that enter the nerve above and below the transverse carpal ligament and descend and ascend, respectively, to accompany the nerve into the carpal tunnel where an anastomotic watershed is established between the descending and ascending intraneural systems.
   d. With very few exceptions the largest vessels inside the fasciculi are capillaries. These capillaries are fed by arterioles and drain to venules and veins, all of which are located in the epineurium; venous vessels outnumber arterial. Nutrient vessels pass obliquely through the perineurium, an arrangement that would result in their closure with any swelling of the fasciculus.

The blood flow and intraneural pressures in a compressed nerve segment

What we are concerned with in the aetiology of chronic compression nerve injury is the reaction to pressures that are too low to deform nerves directly but which are sufficient to impair the blood supply to and within the compressed segment of the nerve.

Features of special relevance when considering the modifications to the intraneural blood flow brought about by compression are:

1. The pressure in the veins is lower than in arteries so that veins succumb to external pressure before arteries.
2. There is a normal intrafascicular pressure.
3. The diffusion barrier properties of the perineurium are well documented.

In recent years the microvascular circulation and intraneural pressure systems in an experimentally compressed nerve segment have been intensively investigated by many workers. These studies have established that:

1. The tissue pressure in the carpal tunnel is raised from 2.5 mmHg to 30 mmHg in patients with a carpal tunnel syndrome (Gelberman et al 1981, Werner et al 1983). Bearing in mind the well protected fasciculi in the median nerve in the carpal tunnel, it is most unlikely that pressures of the order of 35 mmHg could physically deform nerve fibres. And yet pressures of this order are sufficient:

   a. to produce symptoms;
   b. to disturb the intraneural microvascular circulation in the compressed nerve segment, and
   c. to interfere with and block all three axon transport systems, fast and slow, anterograde and retrograde (Rydevik et al 1980, Dahlin et al 1982, 1984, 1986, Dahlin & McLean 1986).

2. Nerve fibres may be damaged by a sustained increase in the intrafascicular endoneurial fluid pressure (Myers & Powell 1981).
3. Even a moderate external pressure of 20–30 mmHg on a nerve segment slows the venular blood flow in the epineurium (Rydevik et al 1981) while pressures of 60–80 mmHg completely arrest the blood flow in the compressed nerve segment. Confirmatory data are on record by Bentley & Schlapp (1943), Matsumoto (1983), and Ogata & Naito (1986). According to Szabo & Gelberman (1987), a critical threshold pressure exists between 40 and 50 mmHg at which nerve fibres are jeopardised.

4. Such ischaemic episodes are followed by the occurrence of intraneural oedema when the blood flow is restored. This occurs if the ischaemia is restricted to 6 hours but ischaemia of longer duration than 8 hours is followed by a 'no reflow phenomenon' in the fascicles. Associated with this is a marked intrafascicular oedema and irreversible loss of function (Lundborg 1970, 1975).

5. Compression at 50 mmHg for 2 hours results in epineurial oedema, the endothelium of the epineurial capillaries failing before those in the endoneurium. The latter fail at pressures of 200 mmHg maintained for 4–6 hours (Rydevik et al 1981).

6. The vascular lesions are most prominent at the edges of the compression cuff.

7. Because of the diffusion barrier properties of the perineurium the intrafascicular oedema results in an increase in the intrafascicular pressure.

8. After compression at 80 mmHg for 4 hours there is a fourfold increase in the intrafascicular pressure (Lundborg et al 1983). The raised intrafascicular pressure could still be recorded 24 hours later and in Powell and Myer's (1986) experiments evidence of an intrafascicular oedema was still present 28 days later. This is consistent with the diffusion barrier properties of the perineurium.

9. Even a small increase in the intrafascicular pressure interferes with the blood flow in the endoneurial capillaries (Myers et al 1979, 1982, 1986, Powell and Myers 1983, Myers and Powell 1984).

10. In volunteers subjected to carpal tunnel compression experiments, mild symptoms began to appear at a tissue pressure in the carpal tunnel of 30 mmHg. Increasing this pressure to 50–60 mmHg completely blocked conduction in the nerve. Recovery was prompt and complete following release from pressure (Lundborg et al 1982, Gelberman et al 1983a,b). Of particular interest was the finding that a pressure of 50 mmHg which blocked conduction represented a critical level at which the intraneural circulation was arrested.

The genesis of the chronic compression nerve lesion

There are at least five interrelated pressure systems in the carpal tunnel (Fig. 17.5). For simplification the nerve has been illustrated as if all the nerve fibres were contained in a single fasciculus.

1. The pressure in the nutrient arteries in the epineurium P^A.
2. The capillary pressure inside the fasciculus P^C.
3. The intrafascicular pressure P^F.
4. The pressure in the veins in the epineurium draining the fasciculi P^V.
5. The pressure within the tunnel P^T.

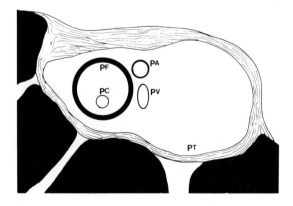

Fig 17.5 Diagrammatic representation of a transverse section across the carpal tunnel illustrating only one of the many fasciculi of the median nerve at that level. P^A and P^V represent pressures in the nutrient arteries and veins in the epineurium. P^C, P^F and P^T represent pressures in the intrafascicular capillaries, inside the fasciculus and in the tunnel, respectively.

In order to maintain an adequate intraneural circulation for the nutrition of nerve fibres, the pressure gradient across this system must be:

$$P^A > P^C > P^F > P^V > P^T$$

These various pressure systems are in delicate balance in a confined space that offers little margin for safety in the event of any local increase in pressure in the tunnel.

If, for any reason, the pressure P^T in the tunnel should slowly increase, then it is logical to conclude that the compression forces falling on the nerve would first be dispersed through and absorbed by the epineurial connective tissue. In this way the fasciculi and their contained nerve fibres would escape injury. The first of the constituents of the nerve to suffer would be the veins in the epineurium.

Obstruction to the venous return from the nerve originating in this way would lead to hyperaemia, venous congestion and circulatory slowing, first in the epineurial and later in the intrafascicular tissues. One of the first signs of impending trouble is the appearance of epineurial oedema. This is because the endothelium of the epineurial capillaries suffers earlier than that of the endoneurial capillaries.

These circulatory disturbances worsen with increasing pressure and ultimately lead, both directly and indirectly, to pathological changes, the most damaging of which take place inside the fasciculi. These pathological changes pass through a series of stages, each of which represents a lesion of increasing severity.

From this it is not to be inferred that the chronic lesion develops in a uniform manner throughout the compressed segment of the nerve so that every fasciculus and every nerve fibre is, at any point in time, affected in the same way and to the same degree. On the contrary, these lesions develop in an irregular manner so that all three of the stages to be described may be present at any given time in different parts of the compressed segment of the nerve. The general trend, however, is one of a changing lesion of increasing severity developing irregularly in space and time as the deforming force persists and increases.

Ischaemia caused by obstruction of the venous return from the fasciculi as the result of pressure on the nerve, followed by intrafascicular oedema and a consequential increase in intrafascicular pressure, imperil and finally destroy nerve fibres by impairing their nutrition and by compression. This sequence of events could account for those structural changes in nerve fibres observed in chronic compression lesions, namely segmental demyelination, axon thinning and, finally, the destruction of the axon with Wallerian degeneration. Furthermore, the paranodal bulbous swellings that have been accepted as a direct effect of mechanical trauma to the nerve fibre could just as easily be caused by another pressure mechanism, namely one in the form of an increasing intrafascicular pressure developing initially as a consequence of obstruction to the venous return from the fasciculi.

However, regardless of whether the damage is caused by direct pressure or has a vascular basis, the fate of the nerve fibres is the same. There is always the possibility, of course, that in some cases the chronic compression lesion represents the combined destructive effects of both factors.

Associated para- and intraneural scarring. The fibrosis and scarred tissue to which fibroblast activity gives rise are a later development in the pathology of the lesion. They first involve the epineurium in the second stage only becoming a feature of the endoneurium in the third phase.

Epineurial fibrosis terminates in a condition often seen at operation in which scar tissue attaches the nerve to neighbouring structures by adhesions, encircles the nerve and encases individual fasciculi. Collagenisation of the endoneurium represents the terminal stage of the lesion. Like epineurial fibrosis it is an irreversible development, but is far more damaging to nerve fibres.

Treatment is an effective decompression of the carpal tunnel immediately objective motor and sensory signs appear. Neurolysis to relieve endangered nerve fibres in the carpal tunnel syndrome should be based on the principles described in Chapter 38.

Stages in the development of the lesion

With increasing compression the lesion passes progressively through a series of stages finally culminating in the destruction of nerve fibres.

Stage 1

Obstruction to the venous outflow from a fasciculus leads, in turn, to a slowing of the intrafascicular capillary circulation, to capillary congestion and an increase in the intrafascicular capillary pressure and then, because of the physical properties of the perineurium, to an increase in the intrafascicular pressure. The intrafascicular circulation is further embarrassed and a vicious circle established. As the capillary circulation continues to slow and the intrafascicular pressure continues to rise, the incarcerated nerve fibres are compressed and their nutrition impaired to a point where they become hyperexcitable and commence to discharge spontaneously. In this respect large myelinated fibres are known to be more susceptible and to suffer earlier than thin finely myelinated and nonmyelinated fibres.

At this stage in the development of the lesion, not all fasciculi or all fibres would be affected to the same degree. Furthermore, whatever changes have occurred are fully and rapidly reversible should the pressure on the nerve be relieved.

This is the stage when subjective sensory symptoms appear in the form of intermittent attacks of pain and paraesthesiae, particularly in the early hours of the morning when they disturb the patient, and a feeling of numbness in the fingers and aching associated with prolonged use of the hand. These symptoms may extend over the entire median field or be restricted to part of it. There is no overt sensory loss at this stage, which is significant when it is remembered that about 90 per cent of the fibres in the median nerve in the carpal tunnel are sensory. The subjective evidence of dysfunction is usually accompanied by a slowing of the conduction velocity.

Stage 2

The capillary circulation has now slowed and congestion developed to a point where the resulting ischaemia damages the capillary endothelium. This leads to the leakage of a proteinaceous exudate into the surrounding tissues which become oedematous. The capillaries of the epineurium are affected earlier than those inside the fasciculi but the accumulation of fluid is concealed within the loosely arranged epineurial tissue where it is free to spread widely. The consequences are more serious when the endothelial lining of the intrafascicular capillaries commences to leak. As protein steadily escapes through the capillary wall it accumulates in the endoneurial tissue because it cannot escape across the perineurial diffusion barrier. As the endoneurial tissue becomes increasingly oedematous there is a consequential increase in the intrafascicular pressure. This and the related ischaemia combine to threaten the survival of the incarcerated nerve fibres by:

1. interfering with their nutrition,
2. deforming them, and
3. promoting the proliferation and increased activity of fibroblasts, culminating in the formation of constrictive endoneurial fibrosis.

As the pressure inside a fasciculus continues to increase some swelling occurs, but this is usually held in check by the relatively unyielding perineurium and the external pressure applied to the nerve. Compression deformation is now reaching levels where the compressed segment may become constricted or flattened against a firm surface.

The nerve becomes swollen and hyperaemic for a variable distance above and below such a compressed segment, owing to the obstruction to the vascular flow in the longitudinal intraneural vessels, the damming back of endoneurial fluid and a further increase in epineurial oedema. In addition; pressure gradients favour the movement of epineurial and endoneurial fluid away from the compressed segment.

This contributes to the enlargement that develops immediately above the upper margin of the compressed segment and it may also result in a smaller swelling just below the lower margin.

Inside a fasciculus, thinned nerve fibres become thinner and undergo segmental demyelination. Finally, some axons are interrupted within their endoneurial sheaths and these nerve fibres then degenerate. At this point the lesion is of a mixed variety. More resistant fibres may still be conducting normally but in most of the surviving thinned

fibres conduction velocity is reduced, a third group has sustained a first degree or conduction block injury, and for still a fourth group the deformation and ischaemia will have damaged fibres to a degree that will be followed by Wallerian degeneration.

This is the stage when the pain and paraesthesiae worsen and objective evidence of nerve involvement appears in the form of a weakness and clumsiness of thenar movements with some muscle wasting but no paralysis, a deepening feeling of numbness with a generalised widespread or patchy defective response to pinprick and light touch.

At this stage, providing whatever is responsible for the compression subsides or the nerve is decompressed, the circulation through the compressed segment recovers, the oedema gradually resolves and the intrafascicular pressure falls. Motor and sensory recovery is delayed depending on whether individual nerve fibres have sustained first or second degree damage and the extent to which irreversible changes have developed. However, if unrelieved, the sensory and motor deficit continues to deepen as more and more fibres are affected. These are unfavourable signs heralding the appearance of irreversible intrafascicular pathology. This is an indication for immediate decompression. Conservative treatment may bring temporary relief, but immediately this is terminated symptoms usually return and further deterioration can be expected.

Stage 3

If long-standing pressure on the nerve is unrelieved, the lesion takes on a more permanent state, a stage being reached when the arterial supply to the nerve is affected in addition to its venous return. Fibroblasts proliferate in the intrafascicular protein exudate and promote the development of an irreversible fibrosis that results in the constriction of increasing numbers of nerve fibres. The final stage is reached when nutrient vessels are obliterated and the affected segment of the nerve becomes converted into a fibrous cord in which only a few fine nerve fibres survive inside fibrosed fasciculi that are encased in a now dense, relatively avascular epineurium. Attempts at axon regeneration through this tissue are rarely successful because of its extent and density. Most regenerating axons terminate at the proximal margin of the compressed segment and add to the swelling of the nerve at that site.

In this advanced stage the median field is usually anaesthetic, though protective sensation may still be present in some patchy areas; the abductor pollicis brevis, and other intrinsic thenar muscles innervated by the median nerve, are now paralysed and wasting is obvious. These signs and symptoms reflect irreversible pathology from which little, if any, improvement can be expected following decompression with or without neurolysis. If some aspects of the lesion are reversible at this late stage there may be some slow improvement when the nerve is decompressed.

Further evidence supporting a vascular based mechanism

Evidence supporting the hypothesis that the chronic compressive lesion has a vascular basis comes from a number of sources:

1. It has been shown experimentally that nerve fibres become hyperexcitable and begin to discharge spontaneously when they become anoxic and their nutrition is impaired, with large fibres suffering earlier than fine fibres (Porter & Wharton 1949).
2. Richards (1951) has also noted that, when a nerve is acutely and abruptly deprived of its blood supply, pain is not a prominent feature of the lesion. If, however, the blood supply is reduced gradually, or intermittently, by a series of episodes, none of which is sufficiently severe to cause necrosis, then the characteristic pains of ischaemic neuritis will appear.
3. A common feature of the pain in this compression lesion is the nocturnal nature of the attacks and the measures taken to obtain relief. The patient is awakened in the early hours by the pain and, to obtain relief, vigorously exercises the limb. It would appear that muscular inactivity during sleep results in venous congestion at the periphery that is sufficient to still further compromise the intrafascicular circulation in the manner previously described. Nerve fibres, already in jeopardy, now respond at a lower threshold to ischaemia and pain results. Vigorously exercising the limb promotes venous return, reverses the cycle, the ischaemic burden on nerve fibres is corrected and pain relieved.

Wilson-MacDonald and Caughey (1984) have demonstrated a significant slowing of nerve conduction at night.

4. Pain in the distribution of the median nerve can be produced by applying cuff compression above the elbow at pressures exceeding the venous pressure but below arterial pressure. This manoeuvre results in peripheral venous congestion with the same consequences as those outlined in the preceding section. Pain is relieved on releasing the pressure.
5. The immediate relief following surgical decompression indicates a lesion that is rapidly and fully reversible and one consistent with a vascular basis. If, however, the primary pathology was based on the physical deformation of nerve fibres as described by its advocates, then it is highly unlikely that this pathology would be immediately corrected by decompression.
6. If relief is not immediate following decompression then the diagnosis is in question, decompression is incomplete or the intraneural pathology has developed to an advanced and irreversible stage.
7. Improvement in the blood flow through the nerve during and following decompression is evidenced by visible changes in the nutrient arteries and the colour of the nerve.

Conclusion

In the final analysis the lesion in chronic compression nerve injury is the result of the combined destructive effects of both physical trauma and ischaemia, each with a time sequence determined by the cause of the compression, with the initial pathology being vascular based.

REFERENCES

Anderson M H, Fullerton P M, Gilliatt R W, Hern J E C 1970 Changes in the forearm associated with median nerve compression at the wrist in the guinea pig. Journal of Neurology, Neurosurgery and Psychiatry 33: 70

Bentley F H, Schlapp W 1943 The effects of pressure on conduction in peripheral nerve. Journal of Physiology 102: 72

Dahlin L B, McLean W G 1986 Effects of graded experimental compression on slow and fast axonal transport in rabbit vagus nerve. Journal of Neurological Sciences 72: 19

Dahlin L B, Danielsen N, McLean W G, Rydevik B, Sjöstrand J 1982 Critical pressure level for impairment of fast axonal transport during experimental compression of rabbit vagus nerve (abstract). Journal of Physiology 325: 84P

Dahlin L B, Rydevik B, McLean W G, Sjöstrand J 1984 Changes in fast axonal transport during experimental nerve compression at low pressures. Experimental Neurology 84: 29

Dahlin L B, Sjöstrand J, McLean W G, 1986. Graded inhibition of retrograde axonal transport by compression of rabbit vagus nerve. Journal of Neurological Sciences 76: 221

Fullerton P M, Gilliatt R W 1967a Pressure neuropathy in the hind foot of the guinea pig. Journal of Neurology, Neurosurgery and Psychiatry 30: 18

Fullerton P M, Gilliatt R W 1967b, Median and ulnar neuropathy in the guinea pig. Journal of Neurology, Neurosurgery and Psychiatry 30: 393

Gelberman R H, Hergenroeder P, Hargens A, Lundborg G, Akeson W 1981 The carpal tunnel syndrome. A study of carpal tunnel pressures. Journal of Bone and Joint Surgery 63A: 380

Gelberman R H, Szabo R, Williamson R, et al. 1983a Tissue pressure threshold for peripheral nerve viability. Clinical Orthopaedics and Related Research 178: 285

Gelberman R H, Szabo R, Williamson R, Dimick M P 1983b, Sensibility testing in peripheral nerve compression syndromes. An experimental study in humans. Journal of Bone and Joint Surgery 65A: 632

Gilliatt R W 1975 Peripheral nerve compression and entrapment: The Oliver Sharpey Lecture. In: Lant A F (ed) Eleventh Symposium on Advanced Medicine. The Royal College of Physicians. Pitman Medical, London, p 144

Horiuchi Y 1983 An experimental study on peripheral nerve lesion — compression neuropathy. Journal of the Japanese Orthopaedic Association 57: 789

Lundborg G 1970 Ischemic nerve injury. Experimental studies on intraneural microvascular pathophysiology and nerve function in a limb subjected to temporary circulatory arrest. Scandinavian Journal of Plastic and Reconstructive Surgery Supplement: 1

Lundborg G 1975 Structure and function of the intraneural microvessels as related to trauma, edema formation and nerve function. Journal of Bone and Joint Surgery 57A: 938

Lundborg G, Gelberman R H, Minteer-Convery M, et al 1982 Median nerve compression in the carpal tunnel — functional response to experimentally induced control pressure. Journal of Hand Surgery 7: 252

Lundborg G, Myers R, Powell H 1983 Nerve compression injury and increase in endoneurial fluid pressure: A 'miniature compartment syndrome'. Journal of Neurology, Neurosurgery and Psychiatry 46: 1119

Mackinnon S E, Dellon A L 1986 An experimental study of treatment methods for chronic nerve compression. Journal of Hand Surgery 11A: 759

Mackinnon S E, Dellon A L, Hudson A, Hunter D A 1984 Chronic nerve compression: an experimental model in the rat. Annals of Plastic Surgery 13: 112

Mackinnon S E, Dellon A L, Hudson A, Hunter D A 1985 A primate model for chronic nerve compression. Journal of Reconstructive Microsurgery 1: 185

Marotte L R 1974 An electron microscope study of chronic median nerve compression in the guinea pig. Acta Neuropathologica Berlin 27: 69

Matsumoto N 1983 An experimental study on compression neuropathy — measurement of blood flow with the hydrogen wash-out technique. Journal of Japanese Orthopaedic Association 57: 805

Myers R R, Powell H C 1981 Endoneurial fluid pressure in peripheral neuropathies. In: Hargens A (ed) Tissue fluid pressure and composition. Williams and Wilkins, Baltimore, p 193

Myers R R, Powell H C 1984 Galactose neuropathy: impact of chronic endoneurial edema on nerve blood flow. Annals of Neurology 16: 587

Myers R R, Costello M L, Powell H C 1979 Increased endoneurial fluid pressure in galactose neuropathy. Muscle and Nerve 2: 299

Myers R R, Mizisin A P, Powell H C, Lampert P W 1982 Reduced nerve blood flow in hexachlorophene neuropathy. Relationship to elevated endoneurial fluid pressure. Journal of Neuropathology and Experimental Neurology 41: 391

Myers R R, Murakami H, Powell H C 1986 Reduced nerve blood flow in edematous neuropathies — a biochemical mechanism. Microvascular Research 32: 145

Neary D, Ochoa J, Gilliatt R W 1975 Sub-clinical entrapment neuropathy in man. Journal of Neurological Sciences 24: 283

Nemoto K 1983 An experimental study on the vulnerability of the peripheral nerve. Journal of the Japanese Orthopaedic Association 57: 1773

Ochoa J 1980a Histopathology of common mononeuropathies. In: Jewett D L, McCarroll H R (eds) Nerve repair and regeneration — its clinical and experimental basis. Mosby, St Louis, p 36

Ochoa J 1980b Nerve fiber pathology in acute and chronic compression. In: Omer G E, Spinner M (eds) Management of peripheral nerve problems. Saunders, Philadelphia, p 487

Ochoa J, Marotte L 1973 The nature of the nerve lesion caused by chronic entrapment in the guinea pig. Journal of Neurological Sciences 19: 491

Ochoa J, Fowler T J, Gilliatt R W 1972 Anatomical changes in peripheral nerves compressed by a pneumatic tourniquet. Journal of Anatomy 113: 433

Ogata K, Naito M 1986 Blood flow of peripheral nerve. Effects of dissection, stretching and compression. Journal of Hand Surgery 11B: 10

Porter E L, Wharton P S 1949 Irritability of mammalian nerve following ischaemia. Journal of Neurophysiology 12: 109

Powell H C, Myers R R 1983 Schwann cell changes and demyelination in chronic galactose neuropathy. Muscle and Nerve 6: 218

Powell H C, Myers R R 1986 Pathology of experimental nerve compression. Laboratory Investigation 55: 91

Richards R L 1951 Ischaemic lesions of peripheral nerves: a review. Journal of Neurology, Neurosurgery and Psychiatry 14: 76

Rydevik B, McLean W G, Sjöstrand J, Lundborg G 1980 Blockage of axonal transport induced by acute graded compression of the rabbit vagus nerve. Journal of Neurology, Neurosurgery and Psychiatry 43: 690

Rydevik B, Lundborg G, Bagge W 1981 Effects of graded compression on intraneural blood flow. Journal of Hand Surgery 6: 3

Sunderland S 1976 The nerve lesion in the carpal tunnel syndrome. Journal of Neurology, Neurosurgery and Psychiatry 39: 615

Sunderland S 1978 Nerves and nerve injuries, 2nd edn Churchill Livingstone, Edinburgh, pp 145, 711

Szabo R H, Gelberman R H 1987 The pathophysiology of nerve entrapment syndromes. Journal of Hand Surgery 12A Supplement: 880

Werner C O, Elmquist D, Ohlin T 1983 Pressure and nerve lesions in the carpal tunnel. Acta Orthopaedica Scandinavica 54: 312

Wilson-MacDonald J, Caughey M A 1984 Diurnal variations in nerve conduction, hand volume and grip strength in the carpal tunnel syndrome. British Medical Journal 289: 1042

18. Traction nerve injury

Two major categories of traction nerve injury are:

1. The acute injury caused by the abrupt application of a force of considerable magnitude, resulting in destructive structural changes and the immediate loss of function.
2. The chronic injury, in which the nerve is stretched so slowly that considerable deformation of its components occurs before signs and symptoms appear. The condition then slowly deteriorates as stretching continues.

CAUSES OF TRACTION NERVE INJURY

1. An injury to the limb that is sufficiently severe to displace parts in such a way as to stretch nerves passing between them. Traction injuries of the brachial plexus are caused when the arm and shoulder girdle are forcibly displaced in relation to the trunk.
2. Damage to a nerve may be caused by transient but severe traction introduced when the dislocated bony parts of a joint or the ends of a fractured bone are violently separated.
3. The passage of a high velocity missile through the limb may create explosive forces along its path and in its wake. Though a nerve in the vicinity may escape direct injury, because it is not in the path of the missile or because its mobility allows it to slip aside, the nerve is unable to withstand the shock waves generated in this way. Injury to the nerve ranges in severity from transient first degree damage to gross laceration and loss of continuity.

Importantly, nerves left in continuity may appear on superficial examination to be uninjured, despite which they harbour widespread intrafascicular third degree damage.

4. Traction on the nerve ends required to bring them together during nerve repair may produce traction lesions at other levels.
5. Premature and forcible postoperative extension of a limb immobilised in flexion to permit tension-free union of the nerve ends introduces traction forces that result in:

   a. suture line failure where healing is incomplete;
   b. damage elsewhere in the system when the suture line holds.

   The suture line is as strong as the nerve elsewhere once healing is completed, while the denervated distal section of the nerve has the same tensile strength as the nerve above the repair.

6. Nerve fibres are stretched and compressed where the nerve is in direct contact with a slowly enlarging aneurysm, cyst, ganglion or tumour. Such deformation usually occurs so gradually that the stretched nerve fibres are able to tolerate considerable distortion without any disturbance of function. Ultimately, however, they become so grossly deformed that they cease to conduct.

PATHOGENESIS OF THE TRACTION NERVE INJURY

The sequence of changes occurring in a nerve as it is stretched is shown in Fig. 18.1. When

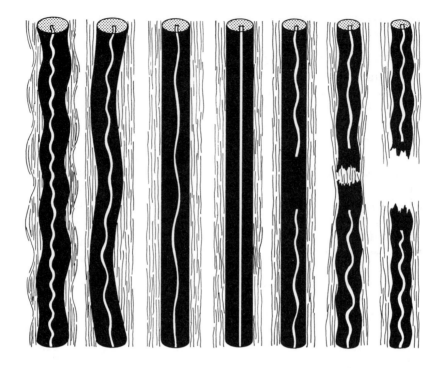

Fig. 18.1 Diagram illustrating the changes occurring in a nerve as it is gradually stretched to mechanical failure. For simplification only one fasciculus and one nerve fibre are shown.

stretched, a nerve first elongates rapidly and easily as the slack in the nerve trunk and its fasciculi is taken up and the undulations eliminated. Though the epineurial tissue assists in maintaining the undulations in the nerve trunk, and gives some elasticity to the nerve by virtue of the lattice type arrangement of its collagen bundles, the component principally responsible for the tensile strength and elasticity of the nerve is fascicular tissue and, in particular, the perineurium.

As stretching continues, the undulations in the nerve trunk and fasciculi are removed and when this is completed further stretching is then resisted by the perineurium. Up to this point the nerve fibres have remained tension free because the deforming force has been expended taking up the slack provided by the undulating arrangement of the nerve fibres inside the fasciculi. However, with increasing elongation, the nerve fibres are ultimately fully straightened and become taut and are then stretched along with the perineurium.

As the fasciculi are stretched, their cross-sectional area is reduced which raises the intrafascicular pressure, thereby leading to compression deformation of the contents of the fasciculus. Tension and compression, as well as directly deforming the nerve fibres, compromise their blood supply, the total effect being one in which nerve fibres suffer from tension, compression and ischaemia.

As elongation approaches the elastic limit, nerve fibres begin to rupture inside the fasciculi. Somewhat later, breaks appear in the perineurium, and the contents of the fasciculi, which are now under great pressure, are extruded through the openings. Finally, fasciculi are torn apart. These lesions often occur at widely spaced intervals along considerable lengths of the nerve. Ultimately, fascicular breakdown involves a sufficient number of fasciculi to cause structural failure of the entire nerve trunk. Tearing of vessels precedes rupture of the fasciculi. The vascular changes vary from hyperaemia to haemorrhages in the epineurium, perineurium and within the fasciculi.

Features of severe traction injuries that make them so serious and difficult to treat are:

1. The intrafascicular rupture of nerve fibres occurs over considerable lengths of the nerve before breaks appear in the perineurium. This, though giving lesions in continuity with preservation of the fascicular pattern, is nevertheless associated with extensive intrafascicular damage and fibrosis which constitute a formidable barrier to regenerating axons.

2. A further difficulty is that these third degree lesions, concealed as they are inside the fasciculi, may be difficult to detect by inspection, while they are not always sufficiently indurated to be felt.

3. The rupture of nerve fibres and fasciculi at different levels over a considerable length of the nerve further complicates regenerative processes.

4. The rupture of blood vessels leads to extensive haemorrhage, particularly inside the fasciculi, which adds to the reaction leading to post-traumatic scarring.

5. As the cross-sectional area of the fasciculi is reduced during elongation, the circulation through them is slowed and finally arrested. Ischaemia of the capillary endothelium results in capillary leakage and the accumulation of a protein exudate in the endoneurial spaces. This not only contributes to the rising intrafascicular pressure but also promotes the formation of collagen which adds to an increasing intrafascicular fibrosis.

6. Rapid stretching of a nerve trunk by as little as 6 per cent may result in severe and extensive damage (Nauck 1931, Sunderland 1978). Orf (1978) gives values of 5–8 per cent with nerve fibres breaking at elongations as low as 2–4 per cent.

7. Traction injuries are associated with severe and lasting retrograde neuronal effects. This has been demonstrated experimentally by Orf (1978).

THE SEVERITY OF TRACTION NERVE INJURIES

The five degrees of nerve injury described in Chapter 25 are represented in the sequence of events and the pattern of failure as a nerve is stretched to its elastic limit and then beyond to the point of mechanical failure.

Initially a point is reached where conduction is blocked before any significant morphological changes can be detected in the nerve. With increasing tension, axons fracture within their endoneurial tubes and a second degree lesion makes its appearance. With the rupture of the endoneurial sheath as well as the axon, there occurs a general disorganisation of the contents of the fasciculi. The damage is, however, confined to the fasciculi which are still taking load, so that the nerve continues to behave as an elastic material. This is a third degree injury. With increasing tension, rupture of the fasciculi marks the onset of a fourth degree injury; this finally proceeds to loss of continuity of the entire nerve trunk, which represents a fifth degree injury. A feature of these lesions is the often extensive longitudinal distribution of the damage.

These changes do not occur evenly either across or along the nerve. Thus lesions are rarely uniform in nature but instead vary in onset, severity, distribution, rate of development and in the manner in which the overall situation deteriorates to a point at which nerve trunk continuity is finally destroyed. This explains why mixed lesions are common in traction injuries.

FACTORS INFLUENCING THE EXTENT AND SEVERITY OF THE TRACTION LESION

The extent and severity of the damage are determined by such factors as the magnitude of the deforming force and the rate of deformation.

The magnitude of the deforming force

This can be arbitrarily assigned to one of three grades of severity — mild, intermediate and violent. Mild traction produces first and second degree injuries, the intermediate causes structural changes representing third degree injury, and violent traction causes widespread tearing of the nerve and finally loss of continuity.

The rate of deformation

When nerves are slowly stretched, with a time scale extending over months or years, they can be stretched well beyond their normal limits and deformed to a remarkable degree without the appearance of signs and symptoms of nerve dysfunction. On the other hand, the same nerve may be stretched so rapidly and violently by a force acting in milliseconds or seconds that conduction and structural failure are instantaneous.

Studies in which human nerves were stretched at rates of elongation of 7.5 cm/minute have shown that, while there are individual variations in the tensile strength of nerves, the greatest elongation at the elastic limit was of the order of 20 per cent, with complete structural failure occurring at maximal elongations of approximately 30 per cent (see Chapter 12). However, for some nerves these values will be as low as 6 per cent. With violent traction structural failure can be expected earlier and at much lower ranges of elongation.

ANATOMICAL FEATURES THAT INCREASE THE VULNERABILITY OF A NERVE TO TRACTION INJURY

The microstructure of nerves and nerve roots

Nerve fibres are at greater risk where the nerve is composed of a single or a few large fasciculi with little supporting epineurial tissue. This is because:

1. The deforming force falls maximally on the major component of the nerve which is fascicular tissue and nerve fibres.
2. Cables of the same size are stronger and more flexible if composed of many strands.
3. Under these conditions all nerve fibres, being concentrated in a single fasciculus, are threatened by the increased intrafascicular pressure that occurs as the nerve is stretched, and which is also responsible for depriving nerve fibres of their blood supply.
4. Rupture of the perineurium results in the involvement of larger numbers of fibres.

5. Regeneration following a third degree injury is seriously complicated in that, with all fibres concentrated in a single fasciculus, the chances of more axons being blocked by intrafascicular fibrosis and of being misdirected into foreign endoneurial tubes are greatly increased.
6. Because the perineurium is absent in nerve roots, they lack the tensile strength of peripheral nerves and so are more vulnerable to traction injury.

Regional features

1. When a considerable length of a nerve is free-running, traction forces are fully spent taking up the slack in the nerve and its fasciculi and the nerve fibres escape injury.

   On the other hand, when only a short free-running length of nerve is available, and particularly when this is fixed at one or both ends, the forces remain concentrated within that length, in which case the elastic limit of the nerve is rapidly exceeded and structural damage occurs. This is seen, for example, in the suprascapular nerve, which is short and relatively fixed where it leaves the upper trunk of the brachial plexus, passes through the suprascapular foramen and its branches enter muscles. Severe traction injuries involving the upper part of the plexus may rupture the suprascapular nerve at its origin, at the foramen, or anywhere between, while its branches may be avulsed from muscle.
2. When a nerve crosses the extensor aspect of a joint it is already under tension during full flexion. Examples are the ulnar nerve at the elbow and the sciatic nerve at the hip joint.
3. Proximity to a joint predisposes to traction damage when that joint is dislocated. Nerves at risk in this respect are the axillary nerve with dislocation of the shoulder joint, the median and ulnar nerves at the elbow joint and the common peroneal (lateral popliteal) at the knee joint.

The relevance of these anatomical features is illustrated by reference to traction injuries of the sciatic nerve in the gluteal region and thigh. In these injuries the lateral popliteal division is more frequently involved and, when both divisions are injured, more often suffers to a greater degree than does the medial popliteal division (Sunderland 1953, 1978).

The fascicular anatomy of the sciatic nerve provides a clue to the greater vulnerability of the lateral popliteal division. This is because, in most individuals, the lateral division is composed of fewer and larger fasciculi and less protective epineurial tissue packing than is the medial division (Fig. 12.4, p. 69).

Additionally, the medial division descends more directly from the sciatic notch and continues into the leg without being firmly fixed other than by the entry of branches into the calf muscles at the knee. Consequently when this division is subjected to violent deformation from the 'near miss' passage of a high velocity missile or by a fracture of the femur, the deforming force is dissipated and spent over a considerable length of the nerve and the nerve fibres escape injury.

On the other hand, the lateral division descends obliquely in the thigh, being angulated and relatively securely fixed at both the sciatic notch and the neck of the fibula. When this nerve undergoes the same violent displacement, the sudden stretch to which it is subjected involves a length of nerve that is strung between two relatively fixed points. There is consequently less slack to take up the displacement and the nerve is subjected to greater stretch. This, in turn, means a more severe injury.

FACTORS REDUCING THE ELASTICITY AND MOBILITY OF NERVES

Adhesions which fix or reduce the mobility of a nerve in its bed, changes in the collagenous tissue of the nerve that reduce its elasticity, deformities that impose a longer course on the nerve, and end-to-end suture under tension all jeopardise nerve fibres by lowering the threshold at which traction begins to produce structural and physiological effects.

TRACTION INJURIES OF THE BRACHIAL PLEXUS

This section on traction injuries of the brachial plexus is included with the object of examining the pathogenesis of these injuries in a clinical setting. In doing so, attention is focussed in particular on:

1. Terminology
2. Structural features of the plexus of particular relevance to traction injuries.
3. The production, distribution and severity of these lesions.

Terminology

Some of the terms used in discussions and reports on brachial plexus injuries introduce an element of ambiguity that could be responsible for confusion and misunderstanding when analysing conflicting claims regarding management policy.

Spinal nerve root. In current anatomical nomenclature the term spinal nerve root is applied to the paired anterior and posterior nerve roots in the spinal canal. However, the spinal nerves formed by the union of paired nerve roots are also referred to as the roots of the brachial plexus which combine to form the trunks of the plexus. Thus the term nerve root could apply to either the nerve roots in the spinal canal or to the spinal nerve in and just beyond the intervertebral foramen. In any consideration of traction injuries of the brachial plexus it is important to distinguish between the two.

The term nerve root should be reserved for the paired anterior and posterior nerve roots in the spinal canal. That part of the plexus extending from the union of nerve roots to the formation of a trunk should be referred to as a spinal nerve.

Avulsion and rupture. These terms should not be used synonymously. Avulsion is the tearing of nerve rootlets from the surface of the cord. It may be partial or complete depending on whether all or only some of the rootlets contributing to a spinal nerve are involved. Nerve root rupture occurs when there is a break in continuity of a nerve root along its course. This is an uncommon lesion. Spinal nerve rupture means a break in continuity of a spinal nerve between its formation in the intervertebral foramen and the trunks of the brachial plexus. The rupture may be partial or complete. There is no such lesion as a spinal nerve avulsion.

Fracture of the spinal nerve at the transverse process is a rupture and not an avulsion.

Preganglionic and postganglionic. These terms are sometimes used to describe the site of the lesion with reference to the posterior root ganglion, a preganglionic lesion being one central to the ganglion and a postganglionic one distal or peripheral to it. These terms, however, could lead to confusion in that, looked at functionally, a preganglionic fibre could be regarded as one conducting to the ganglion and the postganglionic fibre as one conducting away from it. In order to avoid confusion it would be preferable to replace the terms preganglionic and postganglionic with the terms supra- and infraganglionic.

Structural features of the plexus

When the brachial plexus is subjected to a deforming force, the distribution and nature of any damage to the plexus are greatly influenced by structural features of the plexus, some of which protect it from stretch and compression while others render it more susceptible to damage.

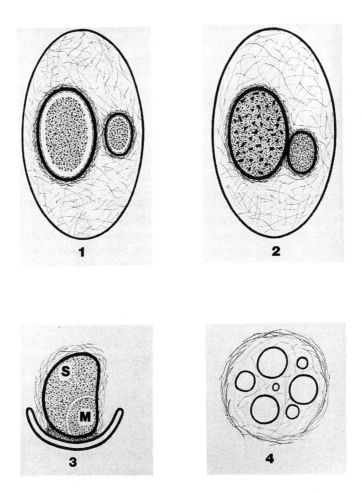

Fig. 18.2   Transerve sections across the nerve root–spinal nerve complex at and just beyond an intervertebral foramen, illustrating the transition from nerve roots to the formation of the single fasciculus of a spinal nerve and its division into several fasciculi (not to scale). The only attachment of the nerve complex to bone is in the cervical region where the spinal nerve is attached to the gutter of the transverse process which it occupies. *S* and *M* sensory and motor components, respectively.

Histological considerations

The structure of nerve roots. Nerve root fibres are loosely held together by endoneurial tissue, which is also specialised about each fibre to form an endoneurial sheath. The collagen fibres of this tissue are finer than the corresponding fibres in peripheral nerve trunks. The endoneurium imparts some tensile strength and elasticity to the nerve root. However, because there is no epineurium, no perineurium, no fascicular structure and no fascicular plexiform arrangement, nerve roots are less tolerant to stretch and compression than are peripheral nerves.

The structure of spinal nerves. The spinal nerve, formed by the union of anterior and posterior nerve roots, is composed of a single fasciculus for a few millimetres after its formation. This fasciculus then divides, the daughter fasciculi participating in plexus formations that result in variations in the size and number of the fasciculi as the nerve continues outwards (Fig. 18.2).

Anatomical considerations

Features in and about the intervertebral foramina of the lower cervical vertebrae

1. As the corresponding anterior and posterior nerve roots enter their corresponding intervertebral foramen they outline a cone of dura at the entrance to the foramen and carry a sleeve of dura laterally which forms a definitive sheath for the nerve root–spinal nerve complex (Fig. 18.3).
2. The nerve root-spinal nerve complex with its dural sheath:
   a. occupies less than 50 per cent of the cross-sectional area of the foramen;
   b. is free to move in and out of the foramen during limb and neck movements because there is no secure attachment of the system to the margins of the foramen which are also smooth.
3. Nerve roots are normally protected from lateral traction on spinal nerves by:
   i. their inherent elasticity
   ii. the wedging of the apex of the dural

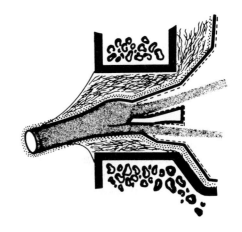

Fig. 18.3 Diagram illustrating the meningeal–neural relations in an intervertebral foramen (not to scale), ——— dura becoming the perineurium; ------ arachnoid; . . . . relative condensation of epidural connective tissue which is continuous laterally with the epineurium of the spinal nerve.

cone into the intervertebral foramen as the cone is drawn outwards along with the nerve root–spinal nerve complex.

During the wide range of movements occurring at the cervical spine, shoulder girdle and shoulder joint, additional stresses are generated that fall maximally on the upper spinal nerves forming the plexus. If these were transmitted directly to the corresponding cervical nerve roots, the latter could suffer traction injury. However, in the case of the fourth, fifth and sixth cervical spinal nerves each, on leaving its foramen, is immediately lodged in the gutter of the transverse process to which it is attached by its epineurial sheath, by reflections of the prevertebral fascia, by slips from the musculotendinous attachments to the transverse processes and by fibrous slips that descend from the transverse process above to blend with the epineurium of the nerve below. The nerve is also held against the bony bar of each transverse process by the vertebral artery whose adventitial coat blends with the sheath of the nerve (Fig. 18.4). The transverse process of the seventh cervical vertebra differs from the others in

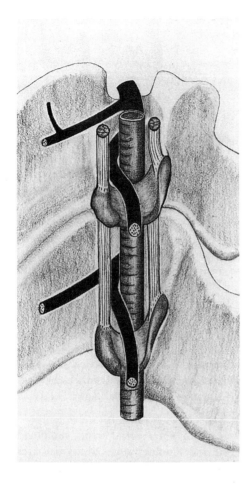

Fig. 18.4 Diagram illustrating the manner in which cervical spinal nerves are forced against the posterior bony bar of each transverse process by the vertebral artery.

that it is more massive and extends further laterally while the gutter characteristic of the transverse processes above is absent.

The eighth cervical and first thoracic spinal nerves lack these attachments as they leave their respective intervertebral foramina.

4. In the lower cervical region it is common for the nerve roots to descend intradurally to a level which may be as much as 8 mm below the foramen that they are to enter. They then perforate the dura in the usual way but must ascend acutely, enclosed in their dural sleeves, in order to reach the foramen over

the lower margin of which they are again angulated as they pass outwards (Fig. 18.5).

Features of the extravertebral part of the plexus

1. The plexiform arrangement of the spinal nerves, trunks and divisions of the plexus contributes to the tensile strength of the system.
2. The undulating course pursued by a nerve trunk in its bed, by the fasciculi in the nerve trunk and by nerve fibres inside the fasciculi protect nerve fibres from traction deformation when the plexus is stretched during movement.
3. The extravertebral part of the brachial plexus may be divided into three parts.

   a. *The upper plexus.* This consists of the fifth and sixth cervical spinal nerves and their extensions laterally (trunks and divisions). This system is securely attached both medially at the cervical transverse processes and laterally by the entry of branches into muscles, e.g. the suprascapular, musculocutaneous, pectoral and axillary nerves and the superior branches of the radial nerve.

   The fifth, sixth and seventh cervical spinal nerves and the upper and middle trunks of the brachial plexus are more obliquely aligned on their way to the limb than are the corresponding elements of the eighth cervical and first thoracic nerves.

   These upper elements are also normally taut owing to the weight of the shoulder girdle and arm, relief being provided by the tone in the elevators of the shoulder girdle. Loss of tone or paralysis of the elevators exposes the upper plexus to chronic stretch and renders them even more vulnerable to traction injury.

   b. *The lower plexus.* This consists of the eighth cervical and first thoracic spinal nerves and their extensions laterally. The lower plexus lacks the attachments to the vertebral transverse processes present in

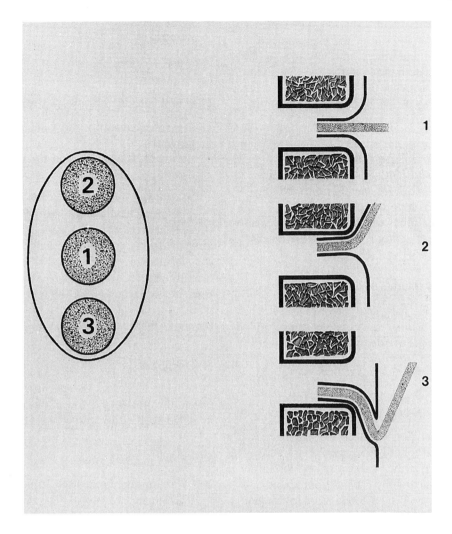

Fig. 18.5 Diagram illustrating variations in the course and position of the nerve root–spinal nerve complex as it approaches and enters the intervertebral foramen. The complex has been represented as a single bundle.

the upper plexus. This means that traction forces directed on this system are freely transmitted medially to the nerve roots and distally down the nerves to the arm.

Regions where the lower trunk of the plexus is in jeopardy are where it crosses:

   i. the firm posterior edge of Sibson's fascia;
  ii. behind the posterior tendinous insertion of scalenus anterior;
 iii. over the first rib.

c. *The middle plexus.* The seventh cervical spinal nerve and its extensions laterally constitute the middle plexus. This system occupies an intermediate position between the upper and the lower plexus. It rarely suffers alone, being more commonly involved with either the upper or the lower plexus.

The distribution and severity of traction lesions of the plexus

The distribution, pathology and severity of the

damage in plexus traction injuries are influenced by such factors as the nature and magnitude of the deforming force and where and how it is applied to the plexus. The basic lesion is one that follows the failure in sequence of nerve fibres, fasciculi and nerve trunks as has been previously outlined for a peripheral nerve. Importantly:

1. Not all fasciculi are affected at the same level, in the same way or to the same degree. Accordingly these lesions have a widespread and irregular distribution through and along the plexus.
2. Severe nerve fibre damage may be concealed within an apparently normal looking plexus.

Distribution of traction lesions

In any injury, the parts may be displaced in such a complicated manner that one, or more, or all parts of the plexus are damaged.

Upper plexus

The upper plexus is at greatest risk when:

1. the angle between the neck and shoulder is abruptly and forcibly increased;
2. the shoulder girdle is abruptly and forcibly depressed such as by a blow from above onto the supraclavicular region or by traction downwards on the arm;
3. the trunk is abruptly and forcibly displaced cranially on the fixed forelimb.

Stresses generated in these ways may:

a. rupture the fifth and sixth spinal nerves at the site of their attachment to the cervical transverse processes where they are composed of a single fasciculus. At this site the spinal nerve may also be forcibly angulated over the costo-transverse bar or around the anterior or posterior tubercles of the cervical transverse processes;
b. tear the attachments of the spinal nerves to the cervical transverse processes before avulsing the nerve roots;
c. avulse branches from muscles;
d. produce lesser degrees of damage along the

nerve between the fixed points referred to previously.

Lower plexus

The lower plexus is at greatest risk when:

a. the arm is abruptly and violently pulled upwards;
b. the trunk is abruptly and forcibly displaced downwards on the fixed forelimb.

Because the lower plexus, unlike the upper, is free of attachments both centrally and distally, stresses generated in the system by traction are dissipated over considerable lengths of the plexus and its median, ulnar and other branches. If sufficiently severe, traction may lead to localised or widespread lesions along the system, even to the point of avulsing nerve roots from the surface of the cord which is the weakest point in the system.

Middle plexus

Occupying as it does an intermediate position between the upper and lower plexuses, it may be involved with either one or the other or both.

Nerve root avulsion injury

Nerve roots may be avulsed from the spinal cord by traction in two ways (Figs 18.6 & 18.7). The first is the end result of traction injuries of the plexus in which tensile stresses are transmitted centrally to stretch and finally avulse nerve roots. In the case of the fifth, sixth and seventh cervical nerve roots, avulsion is preceded by the destruction of two protective mechanisms:

1. Rupture of the protective attachments of the spinal nerve sheath to the transverse processes or fracture of the latter; and
2. Fracturing of the dural cone where it is forcibly drawn into the intervertebral foramen by lateral traction on the spinal nerve.

The eighth cervical and first thoracic nerve roots are more prone to avulsion by this mechanism because they lack protective attachments to the transverse processes, the dural cone alone protect-

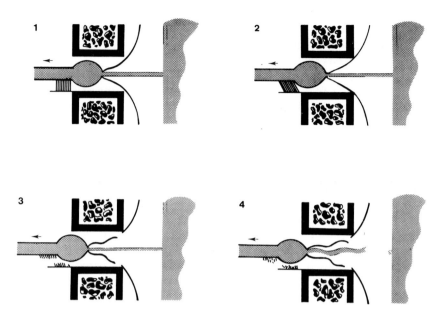

Fig. 18.6 The changes leading to the avulsion of nerve roots caused by lateral traction on spinal nerves. For simplification only one dorsal rootlet is shown.

ing the nerve roots from being overstretched to the point of mechanical failure. In this respect it is worth noting the higher incidence of avulsion injuries of C8 and T1 compared with C5, C6 and C7, whereas the latter sustain a higher incidence of spinal nerve rupture at the transverse processes.

The second mechanism is introduced by those injuries to the cervical spine which deform relationships in such a way that the forces generated by the displacement of the spinal cord act directly on the nerve roots between their attachment to the cord and their entry into the intervertebral foramen. Mechanical failure occurs at the weakest point, which is the site of attachment to the cord, and root avulsion follows while the dural cone is unaffected (Fig. 18.7).

The severity of traction lesions of the brachial plexus

From an examination of the histological features of a nerve trunk in relation to the sequence of changes occurring in a nerve stretched to the point of mechanical failure, there emerges a pattern for these lesions that permits the identification of five types or degrees of injury. These are, in order of increasing severity, impairment or loss of conduction in the affected axons, followed by loss of continuity of axons and then, successively, loss of continuity of nerve fibres, fasciculi and finally the entire nerve trunk. Mixed lesions occur when the damage is not uniform across or along the several parts of the plexus while partial lesions occur when some parts of the plexus escape damage.

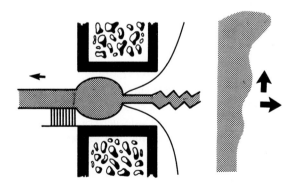

Fig. 18.7 Nerve root avulsion caused by violent displacement of the spinal cord. The dura is undamaged.

Details relating to this grading are provided in Chapter 25. Key features of the grading in relation to traction injuries of the brachial plexus are:

1. With first degree damage:

   a. inspection reveals a normal looking plexus;
   b. recovery occurs spontaneously and is complete;
   c. the appearance of recovery may be delayed for 3–4 months with a time scale that is based on the severity and not the level of the injury.
   d. There are occasions when a conduction block persists and the onset of recovery is suspended until the injured area is freed of offending scar tissue.

2. Second degree damage is characterised by:

   a. a normal looking plexus;
   b. axon degeneration below the injury;
   c. recovery occurs spontaneously and proceeds to completion;
   d. the onset of recovery is delayed because it depends on axon regeneration, structures recovering in the order in which they are reinnervated. Muscles in the proximal part of the limb will therefore recover well before those in the distal part of the limb.

3. Third degree lesions are:

   a. intrafascicular lesions in which fascicular continuity is preserved. They are, therefore, concealed lesions;
   b. axon degeneration is followed by axon regeneration which is complicated by:

      i. intrafascicular scarring which obstructs the passage of regenerating axons;
      ii. the entry of regenerating axons into foreign endoneurial tubes which lead them to functionally unrelated end organs.

   c. axon regeneration is slowed;
   d. the onset of recovery is delayed;
   e. the order of reinnervation and recovery is irregular;

f. recovery is incomplete and imperfect.

4. With fourth degree damage:

   a. fascicular continuity is lost;
   b. the disorganised segment of the plexus is replaced by a mass of matted tissue, scattered through which there may be neuromatous nodules;
   c. axon regeneration is fruitless.

5. Fifth degree damage. This is the lesion in which the affected segment of the plexus has been cleanly severed, ruptured or avulsed.

Nerve root injury

In the case of nerve roots, the absence of perineurial and epineurial tissue means that:

1. The five degrees of injury described for the extravertebral part of the plexus are reduced to three. A first degree injury remains as a physiological conduction block lesion. A second degree injury has the same characteristics as for the extravertebral part of the plexus. A third degree injury involves the rupture of the endoneurial sheath of nerve fibres which means complete loss of continuity of the nerve root. With these lesions the point of avulsion failure is at the attachment of the nerve root to the cord.

   Mixed and partial lesions occur as in the case of the extravertebral part of the plexus.

2. Nerve roots are less tolerant to stretch and compression than are peripheral nerve trunks, so that more serious lesions are produced more readily.

REFERENCES

Nauck E T 1931 Bemerkungen über den mechanisch-funktionellen Bau der Nerven. Anatomische Anzeiger 72: 260
Orf G 1978 Critical resection length and gap distance in peripheral nerves. Acta Neurochirurgica Supplementum 26. Springer-Verlag, Wien
Sunderland S 1953 The relative susceptibility to injury of the medial and lateral popliteal divisions of the sciatic nerve. British Journal of Surgery 41: 300
Sunderland S 1978 Nerves and nerve injuries, 2nd edn. Churchill Livingstone, Edinburgh

19. Friction trauma and nerve entrapment lesions

The literal meaning of entrapment is entanglement or to be caught as in a trap. Nerve entrapment, therefore, implies that the nerve has become attached and fixed in some confined situation by the development of adhesions. This is in contradistinction to compartment compression, where the nerve is free to move within a compartment or tunnel but under conditions where an increasing pressure developing in the compartment would affect the nerve. On this basis the carpal and tarsal tunnel syndromes are based not on entrapment but on compartment compression. Though a distinction should be drawn between compartment compression and entrapment, convention has it that the two should be combined. Entrapment nerve lesions are the most common of the chronic mechanically produced group. They cover a variety of lesions that develop in a nerve where it is running through a confined space, through a constricted opening, or over or around a fibrous band where it is especially vulnerable to mechanical irritation.

The lesions fall into two main categories: (1) The chronic compartment compression entrapment lesion, and (2) The lesion caused by mechanical irritation leading to the involvement of the nerve in the ensuing inflammatory reaction and subsequent fibrosis.

COMPARTMENT COMPRESSION ENTRAPMENT

In this category, a nerve is contained for some part of its course in a compartment with unyielding walls where it is associated with other structures that are subject to space occupying pathology. The nerve is normally free to move in this situation until it becomes attached to neighbouring structures by adhesions. Notable examples in this group are the median nerve in the carpal tunnel and the plantar nerves in the tarsal tunnel.

This type of entrapment lesion is discussed in Chapter 17 on compression nerve injury.

ENTRAPMENT LESIONS CAUSED BY MECHANICAL IRRITATION LEADING TO FRICTION DAMAGE AND THE INVOLVEMENT OF THE NERVE IN THE ENSUING INFLAMMATORY REACTION AND SUBSEQUENT FIBROSIS

The key to the pathogenesis of the entrapment nerve lesion is the local inflammatory reaction that occurs in response to repeated mechanical irritation during limb movements. This reaction culminates in the development of a constrictive fibrosis and the formation of adhesions that attach the damaged nerve at the entrapment site. It is the fixation of the nerve in this way that justifies the use of the term entrapment. The pathogenesis of neural fibrosis is discussed in Chapter 24.

Sometimes unrelieved friction frays and thins the nerve and finally leads to its rupture. This is occasionally the fate of the ulnar nerve behind the medial humeral epicondyle in tardy ulnar palsy when marked osteoarthritic changes and malalignment complicate old supracondylar and condylar fractures of the humerus.

Chronic friction not only damages the protective epineurial tissues but may also involve nerve fibres in superficially located fasciculi. This is particularly likely to occur where the nerve is composed of a single fasciculus or few fasciculi with little supporting epineurial tissue. Nerve fibres damaged in this way regenerate to provide fine regenerating axons that ramify through and end blindly in the fibrosed matrix of the injured segment.

This renders it acutely sensitive to pressure and from traction on the adhesions that attach the nerve at that site.

The fibrous tissue reaction is initially confined to the superficial epineurial tissue but with continuing friction, the reaction ultimately becomes more widespread. In this way the outlines of nerve fibres are finally lost, the nerve at the entrapment site becoming converted into a firm fibrous nodule.

Friction fibrosis from whatever the cause imperils nerve fibres by:

1. constricting them;
2. impairing their blood supply, and
3. forming adhesions that fix the nerve at the injury site.

Traction on the nerve caused during limb movements now deforms a hypersensitive nocigenic focus and results in pain. However, there are those occasions when function deteriorates slowly and painlessly.

Symptoms of nerve entrapment lesions. The cardinal symptom is pain or dull aching after prolonged muscular effort, particularly the overuse of those muscles whose contractions are known to contribute directly to nerve entrapment. Pressure over the entrapment site, providing it is accessible, elicits a painful response. Objective evidence of sensory involvement only appears in the late stages.

Whether or not there is motor disability depends on the motor component of the nerve, the symptoms being muscle weakness progressing to paralysis and wasting.

Treatment. This is conservative in the initial stages and is based on rest. When the condition fails to respond to conservative measures, the nerve should be explored and freed by neurolysis. What form the neurolysis should take depends on the circumstances (Chapter 38).

COMMON POTENTIAL ENTRAPMENT SITES

In general, entrapment sites are located in the vicinity of joints where limb movements make their greatest contribution to mechanical irritation. Such sites are found where:

1. a nerve continually rubs against a rough object such as occurs when it crosses over or under, or is angulated around or over, a rigid fibrous or ligamentous band, the tendinous edge of a muscle, a bony surface, an irregular mass of callus or the irregular bony overgrowths of an arthritic joint;
2. a nerve passes through a fibrous, osseofibrous or osseous foramen or canal through which it moves during movement. The risks of friction injury are greatly increased where the foramen or canal is narrowed or is roughened, or the nerve is, for any reason, inflamed and enlarged;
3. a nerve passes between two closely applied muscles, or through or between the two heads of a muscle against the fibrotendinous edge of one of which it rubs during excessive movements and overuse;
4. any cutaneous nerve is at risk where it passes through deep fascia to become cutaneous. Any chronic inflammatory reaction at this site from trauma will implicate the nerve which becomes fixed at that site;
5. a nerve is subject to chronic irritation and becomes fixed and adherent to neighbouring structures;
6. a nerve becomes enclosed in post-traumatic scarring and adhesions that attach it to its bed and limit its mobility, e.g. entrapment of the ilioinguinal and iliohypogastric nerves in abdominal scars.

Nerves susceptible to friction injury and pathological nerve entrapment

These include the following, details of some of which are provided in a number of texts (Spinner 1978; Sunderland 1978; Mackinnon & Dellon 1989).

1. The spinal nerve in an intervertebral foramen (p. 167).
2. The lower trunk of the brachial plexus at several sites at the thoracic outlet (p. 162).

3. The suprascapular nerve where it passes through the suprascapular foramen. The nerve is relatively fixed at this site, which is a constantly moving point because of the excursions of the scapula during movements of the arm. For this reason the nerve is subject to friction at this site and this could lead to inflammatory swelling and constriction of the nerve. Entrapment lesions of the nerve at this site have been described. Patients present with a dull aching pain in the shoulder region. This pain is aggravated by movements of the shoulder girdle and, when severe, spreads into the neck and down the arm. If the lesion responsible for the pain is not recognised and corrected, weakness and wasting of the spinati appear with, finally, paralysis of these muscles. The motor disability is one in which movements of abduction and external rotation at the shoulder joint are impaired. The entrapped nerve should be decompressed by dividing the transverse scapula ligament.

   The suprascapular foramen is not only a potential entrapment site but the nerve is also relatively fixed at that site so that it could be stretched with displacement of the shoulder. This tension could also be transmitted to the upper trunk of the plexus itself. Chronic irritation and stretching originating in this way could lead to spasm of the spinati and could also cause deep-seated pain in the shoulder region which would be aggravated by movement. This could be the basis of some unexplained lesions of the shoulder region which are characterised by pain and limitation of movement.

4. The axillary nerve and the quadrangular space syndrome. Here the axillary nerve and the posterior humeral circumflex vessels are entrapped in the quadrangular space outlined above by the tendons of the subscapularis and teres minor and the capsule of the shoulder joint, medially by the tendon of the long head of triceps, laterally by the surgical neck of the humerus and below by the tendon of teres major.

5. The radial nerve where it rubs against callus from a fractured humerus.

6. The posterior interosseous nerve where it:

   a. crosses the deep tendinous surface of the extensor carpi radialis brevis muscle;
   b. passes under the tendinous upper border of the superficial head of the supinator muscle (arcade of Frohse);
   c. courses between the two heads of the supinator muscle;
   d. crosses an osteoarthritic humero — radio-ulnar joint.

7. The superficial radial nerve where it crosses deep to the brachioradialis tendon before piercing the deep fascia to become cutaneous.

8. The musculocutaneous nerve where it passes through the coracobrachialis muscle.

9. The median nerve where it passes:

   a. through a supracondylar osseo-fibrous foramen;
   b. under the lacertus fibrosus (bicipital aponeurosis);
   c. between the two heads of the pronator teres;
   d. under the musculotendinous arcade of the flexor digitorum superficialis (sublimis);
   e. around the tendinous radial margin of the flexor digitorum superficialis muscle to become superficial between it and the tendon of the flexor carpi radialis muscle;
   f. through the carpal tunnel.

10. The anterior interosseous nerve where it emerges from between the two heads of the pronator teres muscle.

11. The ulnar nerve where:

   a. it crosses the fibrotendinous edge of the medial intermuscular septum of the upper arm;
   b. it passes behind the medial humeral epicondyle when osteoarthritic changes and malignment have complicated old supracondylar and condylar fractures of the humerus;
   c. it passes under the musculotendinous arcade, formed by the humeral and

ulnar heads of the flexor carpi ulnaris,
to enter the cubital tunnel;

d. it runs in Guyon's canal at the wrist;

e. where its dorsal cutaneous branch turns
round the distal ulna beneath the tendon
of flexor carpi ulnaris.

12. Anterior cutaneous nerves of the abdominal
wall where they pierce the rectus abdominis
muscle.

13. Any cutaneous nerve where it passes
through the deep fascia to become
cutaneous.

14. The sciatic nerve where it passes through
the piriformis muscle.

15. The common peroneal division of the sciatic
nerve where it:

a. passes over the piriformis which brings
it into direct contact with the bone of
the greater sciatic notch against which it
rubs;

b. where it passes between the two
tendinous heads of attachment of the
peroneus longus muscle (fibular tunnel)
at the site where the nerve enters the
peroneus longus. At this site,

   i. it is flattened and its constituent
   fasciculi are separated so that the
   nutrient vessels are exposed and left
   unprotected between them;

   ii. the nerve is attached to bone and
   muscle by deep fascia;

   iii. it is angulated where it turns
   abruptly in its course;

   iv. there is slight sliding movement of
   the nerve during limb movements.

16. The lateral femoral cutaneous nerve where:

a. it is subjected to low grade repetitive
chronic irritation at the site where the
nerve leaves the pelvis and is wedged in
the angle between the inguinal ligament,
the anterior superior iliac spine and
attachment of the sartorius muscle, or
passes through the ligament or the
muscle and finally emerges through deep
fascia to become subcutaneous;

b. it becomes involved in postoperative
scarring in the inguinal region;

17. Sural and superficial peroneal
(musculocutaneous) nerves where they:

a. pass through deep fascia;

b. may be involved in a constrictive fibrosis
following previous trauma to the leg or
foot;

18. A digital nerve subjected to chronic
irritation reacts by forming a tender
enlargement composed mostly of connective
tissue but with fine nerve terminals that
render it acutely sensitive to pressure.
Examples are:

a. Bowler's thumb. The medial digital
nerve of the thumb is involved where
the edge of the hole of the bowling ball
impinges on it when the ball is firmly
gripped.

b. Morton's metatarsalgia. This occurs
where a plantar digital nerve is
compressed where it courses superficial
to the deep transverse metatarsal
ligament between the heads of adjacent
metatarsal bones. The nerve between the
third and fourth metatarsals is the one
most liable to injury.

19. Where any nerve is involved in
post-traumatic scarring and adhesions that
attach and fix it to its bed thereby
introducing an entrapment situation, e.g.
entrapment of the ilioinguinal and
iliohypogastric nerve in abdominal scars,
and the genitofemoral nerve in inguinal
scarring.

Nerve entrapment at the thoracic outlet

In considering the thoracic outlet entrapment
lesion and syndrome it is important to remember
that, in this region, neurovascular structures may
be deformed in many different ways and that it is
necessary to distinguish carefully between them
because operative treatment will only succeed
when the cause has been accurately determined
and effectively corrected.

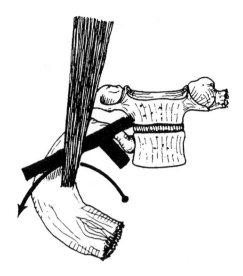

Fig. 19.1 The course taken by the lower trunk of the brachial plexus and the subclavian artery results in both structures being angulated behind the scalenus anterior and over the first rib.

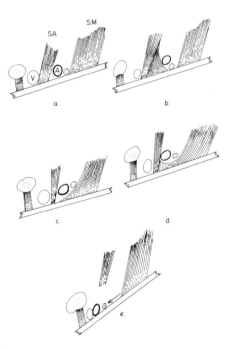

Fig. 19.2 Diagrams of the scalene interval to illustrate: (a) the relations of the subclavian artery and vein, and the lower trunk of the brachial plexus where they cross the first rib; b, c & d variations in the attachments of the scalenus anterior and scalenus medius to the first rib and their effect on the lower trunk of the plexus and the subclavian artery; (e) the effect on the artery and nerve of dividing the attachment of the scalenus anterior to the first rib.

Another feature of the thoracic outlet is the marked slope of the first rib. The head of the rib articulates with the body of the first thoracic vertebra just below its upper margin, while the costosternal junction is at the level of the disc between the second and third thoracic vertebrae.

The lower trunk of the brachial plexus may be injured in the following situations:

1. Where it rubs against a sharp tendinous posterior border of the scalenus anterior (Figs 19.1 & 19.2).

The failure to differentiate between those cases in which the scalenus anterior was at fault and those in which some other mechanism was responsible meant that scalenotomy inevitably became associated with more failures than successes, the operation often aggravating rather than relieving the condition. The explanation of these failures is probably the fact that anterior scalenotomy was either incomplete or that it eliminated one pressure point but left or created others.

In the case of the subclavian artery, dividing the anterior scalene tendon removes the pressure at the site where the artery crosses the rib and is hooked behind the tendon, thereby allowing the artery to slide downwards and forwards to a lower and more anterior position on the rib. This movement, however, brings the artery and the vein more directly into the angle between the clavicle and the rib where they may be compressed.

Following scalenotomy, the lower trunk of the plexus also slides downwards and forwards, following the slope of the rib which may even be increased as a result of the division of the scalene. The nerve then becomes hooked round the firm free posterior edge of Sibson's fascia which becomes the new site of compression and friction (Figs 19.2 & 19.3).

2. Where it is compressed between the clavicle and a normal or abnormal rib. Whether the subclavian artery and lower trunk of the plexus can be compressed between a 'normal' clavicle and first rib in a manner and to a degree sufficient to produce symptoms has been questioned.

There are, however, other reasons why costoclavicular compression in the absence of rib anomalies is an unlikely aetiological factor in all but the exceptional case. Such compression would

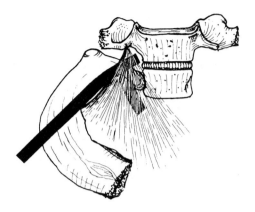

Fig. 19.3 The relationship of the eighth cervical and first thoracic spinal nerves, and the lower trunk of the brachial plexus to the free posterior border of Sibson's fascia.

be intermittent, occurring only when the shoulders are braced back or the arm hyperabducted and these unusual postures maintained or repeated at frequent intervals.

Also, the observation that resection of 'the greater part of the rib' leads to relief is not proof that the mechanism responsible for the symptoms is costoclavicular compression because such an extensive surgical procedure could relieve the plexus from pressure from other causes. For these reasons it will always be difficult to evaluate the role of costoclavicular compression as an aetiological factor in the production of the thoracic outlet syndrome where there is no abnormal rib.

Furthermore, when the space between the clavicle and the rib is reduced, the first structure to suffer should be the subclavian vessels but, though vascular symptoms have been described among the clinical features of costoclavicular compression, they are by no means a characteristic feature of all cases.

While it is conceded that there will be occasions when compression of the neurovascular bundle between a normal first rib and the clavicle is the factor responsible, care should be exercised in making this diagnosis.

Conditions are very different when the costoclavicular space is reduced by an incomplete abnormal rib or callus about a healed fracture of the clavicle. The artery and the lower trunk may then be compressed between the clavicle and the abnormal process, the scalenus anterior intervening but often being displaced posteriorly to indent the artery.

Costoclavicular compression seems to have come into favour as the offending mechanism in the thoracic outlet syndrome largely owing to the failure of scalenotomy, the existence of symptoms in the absence of a rib anomaly and the claim that first rib resection to enlarge the costoclavicular space enjoys a higher success score than other methods in effecting a cure. However, it should be remembered that the resection removes not only the first rib but also any cervical rib associated with it and the attachments of the scalenus anterior as well. Rib resection is therefore an all embracing procedure for an all embracing syndrome and we are left to speculate on the mechanism actually responsible for the neurological complaint.

3. Where it crosses behind the firm free posterior border of Sibson's fascia (Fig. 19.3). The lower trunk of the plexus is normally held posteriorly by the attachment of the firm free posterior edge of Sibson's fascia to the rib. When the scalenus anterior is divided, the lower trunk of the plexus slides downwards and forwards which means that it becomes angulated round the posterior edge of Sibson's fascia against which it rubs during movement. This becomes the site of chronic mechanical irritation that may damage the nerve. The fascial edge may, of course, have been the original source of the trouble in which case the effect of scalenotomy is to aggravate the condition. This fascial edge should be dealt with surgically if permanent relief is to be obtained, but to date its role in mechanically irritating the lower trunk has not been fully appreciated.

Sometimes the lower trunk of the plexus, as it runs laterally, rides across a tendinous scalenus minimus, the nerve occupying the tendinous angle between this muscle and the scalenus medius (Fig. 19.4).

4. Where it crosses the crescentic tendinous fibres of the scalenus medius (Fig. 19.2), there is often a tendinous extension from the antero-medial aspect of the scalenus medius that arches forwards to attach to the first rib where the lower trunk of the brachial plexus normally crosses it. Another anomalous aponeurotic band passes from

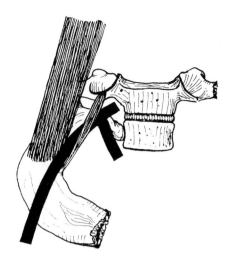

Fig. 19.4 The scalenus minimus attachment is continuous with that of the anterior fibres of the scalenus medius and the lower trunk of the plexus is wedged between the two.

the seventh cervical transverse process behind the lower trunk and in front of the scalenus medius to the upper surface of the first rib. The relations of the band, with the lower trunk emerging anterior to it, exclude it from being a tendinous scalenus minimus or the thickened posterior border of Sibson's fascia. Irritative lesions of the lower trunk may be caused where it rubs across these bands, the lower trunk being particularly liable to damage because it is held posteriorly by the attachments of the posterior free border of Sibson's fascia and so remains in contact with these bands as it runs outwards and downwards.

These bands do not usually extend sufficiently far forwards to involve the subclavian artery because the latter is running from before backwards while the lower trunk is coursing from behind forwards. There are, therefore, usually no circulatory

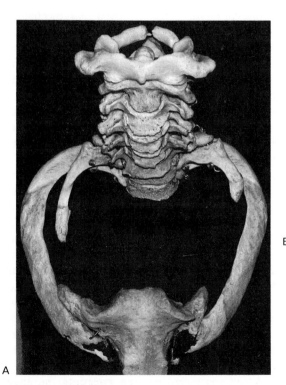

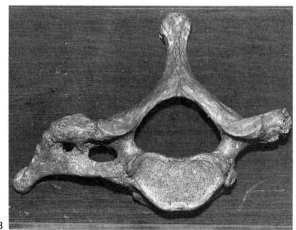

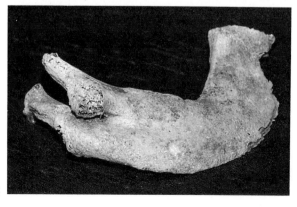

Fig. 19.5 Bony anomalies at the thoracic outlet, illustrating: **a** Bilateral, incomplete, asymmetrical ribs. The spur of bone on each side of the manubrium sterni is the sternal end of each rib. In life each rib was completed by ligamentous tissue. **b** A specimen in which an anomalous first rib is fused with the first thoracic vertebra. **c** A specimen in which a cervical rib is fused with the first thoracic rib to form a double-headed rib.

complications when the scalene band is the offending agent.

5. Where it is compressed in the intermuscular cleft between the scalenus medius and scalenus anterior (Fig. 19.2).

6. Where it is wedged in the narrow tendinous angle between (i) the scalenus medius and scalenus minimus, and/or (ii) the scalenus medius and scalenus anterior.

7. Where it crosses an abnormal rib or the ligamentous extensions associated with such an anomaly (Fig. 19.5).

8. Where it rubs across a boss of bone on the first rib or one formed at the site where an incomplete cervical rib articulates with the upper surface of the first rib.

9. Where it is compressed by an aneurysm of the subclavian artery.

10. Hyperabduction of the arm. Neurovascular symptoms may be produced by hyperabduction of the arm, the position adopted being one in which the arms are elevated above the head with the elbows flexed. This extreme position is adopted by some individuals when sleeping and by others while carrying out occupational tasks that involve working with the arms overhead.

The mechanisms claimed to be responsible for the symptoms are costoclavicular compression and bowing of the axillary artery and the cords of the plexus under the coracoid process and the tendon of pectoralis minor or across the head of the humerus.

SURGERY AND THE THORACIC OUTLET ENTRAPMENT SYNDROME

In the absence of any rib anomaly confirmed by X-rays, it is rarely possible from a clinical examination alone to identify the site and cause of the deformation. Nevertheless, these patients should be thoroughly investigated to establish the mechanism responsible for the symptoms. In doing so steps should be taken to exclude entrapment lesions elsewhere, such as cervical spondylosis and entrapment of the median nerve in the carpal tunnel or beneath a supracondylar ligament, and of the ulnar nerve at the elbow and wrist.

The final diagnosis often depends on an exploratory operation to permit a thorough examination of the various anatomical arrangements that could be at fault, always remembering that more than one factor may be operating. Finding one cause is no reason, therefore, for discontinuing the search for others that might be contributing to the deformation.

Definitive surgery is only undertaken when a careful search has revealed the true cause of the trouble. This is then corrected by appropriate surgical procedures and the neurovascular structures provided with a new bed where they are protected from any further compression, tension or friction.

The past decade has seen many changes in the approach to the surgical treatment of these entrapment lesions. The scalenus anterior has fallen from grace to be replaced by costoclavicular compression as the principal offending mechanism. Again, whereas surgery in the past was directed to correcting or eliminating the particular mechanism that investigation had shown was responsible for the lesion and symptoms, a review of current literature reveals a unified approach in which all lesions are pooled under a common heading, the thoracic outlet syndrome, for the treatment of which one surgical procedure is recommended—first rib resection. Today costoclavicular compression is regarded as the main cause of the thoracic outlet lesion and the symptoms associated with it. The first rib, and not the scalenus anterior or a cervical rib, is regarded as the major offending agent to which surgery should be directed. First rib resection, and not claviculectomy, is the preferred method of decompressing the plexus. However, even the rib resectors are not agreed on the best approach for the removal of this supposedly damaging component. Those advocated include the transaxillary, supraclavicular, subclavicular posterior thoracoplasty type, etc.

It should not be overlooked that with first rib resection the scalene attachment is detached and any cervical rib excised at the same time. Thus rib resection represents a clean sweep of the entire thoracic outlet. And at times it has been found necessary at a later date to resect the mid-third of the second rib.

Finally, one continues to read only too often of patients who have been through many hands and who have already been subjected to multiple

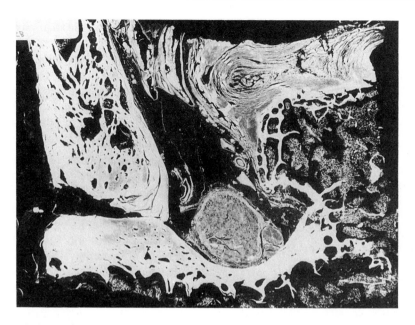

Fig. 19.6   A lumbar spinal nerve in the intervertebral foramen illustrating a posterior sensory component that is much larger than its companion anterior motor component.

procedures without success. Surgical treatment is only as effective as the diagnostic and surgical skill of the surgeon.

THE ENTRAPMENT NERVE LESION IN AN INTERVERTEBRAL FORAMEN

The painful involvement of spinal nerves by pathology developing in and about intervertebral foramina is usually attributed to compression deformation of the nerve in an entrapment situation. However, all is not what it seems to be and, again, anatomical considerations are crucial to an understanding of the genesis of these lesions. Accordingly, the proposition that nerve compression is the responsible aetiological factor needs to be examined in relation to the following regional anatomical features.

1. The walls of an intervertebral foramen or canal are normally smooth.
2. The spinal nerve-nerve root complex with its dural sheath is not firmly attached to the foramen and so moves freely in and out of the foramen with every movement of the vertebral column and limbs (Fig. 18.3, p. 153).

3. The nerve complex occupies less than 50 per cent of the cross-sectional area of the foramen.
4. The posterior sensory component of a spinal nerve is much larger than the anterior motor component (Fig. 19.6).
5. The spinal nerve in the foramen is composed of a single fasciculus that does not divide into multiple fasciculi until it has emerged from the foramen (See Fig. 18.2 p. 152).
6. Included in the foramen and intimately related to the nerve complex and its dural sheath are the spinal artery and veins and the recurrent meningeal or sinu vertebral nerve.
7. The dorsal (posterior) primary ramus.

Cervical foramina

In the case of the cervical region the intervertebral foramen between the fifth and sixth cervical vertebrae can be selected to examine the genesis of the entrapment lesion at this site (Fig. 19.7). Here additional anatomical features of importance are:

1. The zygapophyseal joint is located postero-superiorly;

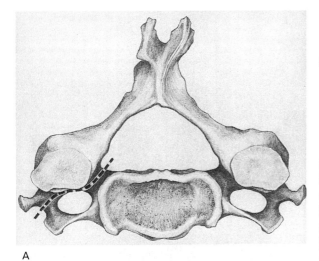

A

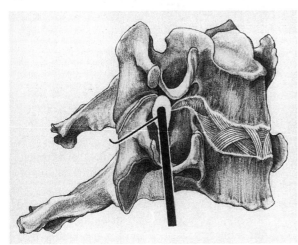

B

Fig. 19.7 Diagrams illustrating the boundaries of a cervical intervertebral foramen (C5–C6) and the gutter of the cervical transverse process lodging the spinal nerve. The apophyseal joint is above and behind the nerve. Any reduction in the intervertebral distance would not significantly alter the vertical diameter of the foramen but would result in tilting that would stretch the apophyseal joint capsule.

2. The neurocentral joint is located antero-superiorly;
3. Both joints form an insignificant amount of the foraminal boundary;
4. The disc takes little part in the formation of the foramen;
5. The boundaries of the foramen are such that any reduction in height of the intervertebral

disc would have little, if any, effect on the dimensions of the foramen or on the alignment of the zygapophyseal joints;
6. As the dorsal primary ramus runs posteriorly it occupies the transverse groove on the lateral surface of the articular pillar. This is bridged by tissue to outline a canal in which there is ample room for the nerve.

Turning now to the pathology responsible for the entrapment nerve lesion in the foramen, this is provided by cervical spondylosis, secondary to disc injury or disease, in which rough irregularities in the form of nodules and osteophytes develop at the vertebral rim and about the zygapophyseal joint. It is generally believed that those appropriately placed encroach upon the foramen as they enlarge and, in doing so, gradually compress the spinal nerve. However, nerve compression is rarely painful (p. 336) and in these cases the deformation occurs so slowly that it is probably of little significance in the production of a painful nerve lesion.

What is important, however, is that the walls of the foramen are no longer smooth but have become rough and irregular. As the spinal nerve moves in and out of the foramen, it is now repeatedly drawn across rough irregularities and traumatised.

Such repeated trauma to the spinal nerve and its sheath:

1. damages spinal nerve fibres. These are particulary vulnerable to injury because they are confined to a single fasciculus with little protective epineurial tissue. Damaged axons regenerate but the axon sprouts end blindly in the traumatised region. In this way a hypersensitive focus is created;
2. promotes an inflammatory response and a reactionary friction fibrosis;
3. compromises the blood supply to nerve fibres because of the deepening fibrosis;
4. finally leads to the formation of adhesions that fix the injured segment of the nerve to its bed so that its mobility in the foramen is lost.

Because the nerve complex is now fixed in the foramen, traction forces, generated in the nerve during limb and neck movements, pull on the traumatised adherent segment of the nerve where hypersensitive axon terminals, whose blood supply has already been impaired, are activated. The resulting impulse activity is registered as pain.

The entrapment nerve lesion in cervical spondylosis is not a compression nerve injury. On the contrary, it is the culmination of a series of complex pathological changes involving traction deformation of a damaged segment of a spinal nerve already subjected to friction trauma, a reactionary fibrosis, and an impaired blood supply due to the fibrosis and fixation by adhesions that destroy its mobility.

Lumbar intervertebral foramina

A lumbar intervertebral foramen, say that between the fourth and fifth lumbar vertebrae, differs in the following significant respects from those of its cervical counterparts (Fig. 19.8).

1. The thick intervertebral disc now forms most of the anterior wall of the foramen. However, the spinal nerve is located superiorly in the foramen and is not in contact with this disc until it has emerged from the foramen. It is the contributing dorsal and ventral nerve roots of this nerve that are intimately related to a disc and it is to the disc above (Fig. 19.9).
2. The zygapophyseal joint forms most of the posterior wall of the foramen.
3. The zygapophyseal joint facets are directed medially and laterally whereas those in the cervical region are directed anteriorly and posteriorly.
4. The medial division of the dorsal primary ramus of the spinal nerve and its accompanying vessels enter a groove between the mammillary and accessory processes which is converted into a tunnel by dense bridging tissue (Figs 19.8 & 19.10). Concealed in this way, the nerve continues medially to curve beneath the zygapophyseal joint where it is incorporated within the capsule of the joint. It is in this section of its course that the nerve is in an entrapment situation. While beneath the joint the nerve

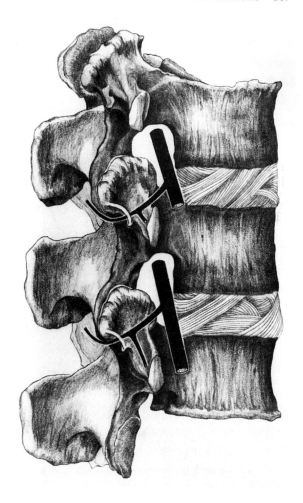

Fig. 19.8 Diagram illustrating the passage of the lumbar nerve through the upper part of the intervertebral foramen where it is behind the vertebral body and immediately below its pedicle. The dorsal ramus is shown crossing the lateral surface of the articular process along with the passage of the medial branch of the ramus through a tunnel beneath the ligamentous tissue joining the mammillary and accessory processes — only the lateral fibres of this ligamentous arch are shown.

gives articular branches to it as well as to the zygapophyseal joint below.

As a consequence of these anatomical features, any reduction in the intervertebral distance from disc prolapse or disease would lead to a number of secondary effects:

1. The vertical diameter of the foramen would

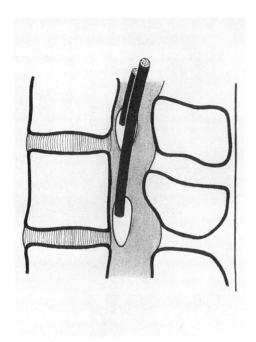

Fig. 19.9 Diagram illustrating the relationship of nerve roots to the intervertebral discs as they descend in the spinal canal to reach their respective foramina. The nerve leaves the foramen proximal to the disc forming its lower anterior boundary but is directly related to the disc above.

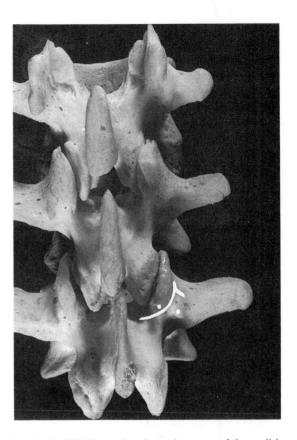

Fig. 19.10 This illustration shows the course of the medial branch of the dorsal primary ramus of the spinal nerve as it curves medially between the mammillary and accessory processes in intimate relationship with the capsule of the zygapophyseal joint.

be significantly reduced as the fourth lumbar body descends caudally on the fifth.

2. The articular facet of the fourth lumbar vertebra would be displaced caudally. This would stretch the capsule of the zygapophyseal joint and promote a reactionary inflammatory swelling.
3. Bulging of the annulus fibrosis and ligamentum flavum, and swelling of the zygapophyseal joint would combine, in varying measure, to reduce the horizontal dimensions of the foramen.
4. Co-existing pathological effects take the form of nodules and osteophytes as described for the cervical region.

Though the spinal nerve is not in contact with the disc until it has left the foramen, these pathological changes could combine to compromise the nerve in its passage to and through

the foramen. Moreover, there is good evidence that the nerve can be compressed and grossly deformed in this way. At the same time, however, the evidence also indicates that such deformation can be symptom free.

It would appear that the offending mechanism is, once again, not solely nerve compression but multifactorial, involving friction trauma, an inflammatory reaction, reactionary fibrosis, ischaemia of nerve fibres and the fixation of the damaged nerve segment with the consequent loss of mobility and increasing vulnerability to traction deformation.

A final word concerns the fate of the medial division of the dorsal primary ramus following distortion of the joint, stretching of its capsule, and an inflammatory reaction with joint swelling and arthritic changes. From the intimate relationship of nerve to joint it is clear that the former could not possibly escape damage under these conditions.

DOUBLE CRUSH SYNDROME. DOUBLE COMPRESSION SYNDROME. DOUBLE ENTRAPMENT SYNDROME

It is a matter of common clinical experience that:

1. It is not unusual to have an overt carpal tunnel lesion of the median nerve masking a second coexisting entrapment lesion of the same nerve fibres at the thoracic outlet.
2. The syndrome attributed to median nerve compression in the carpal tunnel does not always respond to carpal tunnel decompression but is relieved when therapeutic attention is transferred to the thoracic outlet.
3. For years the thoracic outlet was believed to be the source of nerve entrapment but corrective surgery proved ineffective because the unsuspected offending lesion was located in the median nerve in the carpal tunnel.

Even as recently as 1982 Carroll & Hurst reconfirmed that many entrapment lesions erroneously localised to the thoracic outlet were due to compression lesions of the median nerve in the carpal tunnel that were relieved by decompression.

In 1973 Upton and McComas introduced the term, 'double crush syndrome' to describe this phenomenon, which they attributed to disturbances of axoplasmic transport imposed by a proximal lesion that reduced the metabolic safety margin of axons to a second compression at distal levels. Since that time many others, as recently as the 1980s, have reported on this condition (Massey et al 1980, Hurst et al 1985, Pfeffer & Osterman 1986).

The 'double crush' syndrome, more appropriately called double compression or double entrapment syndrome, implies that one insult may be insufficient to impair the function of a nerve whereas two widely separated insults have a cumulative effect that impairs nerve conduction. It is further postulated that the syndrome is based on disturbances of axon transport systems.

Since that time this concept has received considerable experimental attention (Rydevik et al 1980, Nemoto 1983, Seiler et al 1983, Mackinnon et al 1984, Dahlin et al 1984, 1986, Nemoto et al 1987).

There are three known transport systems in axons: fast and slow anterograde, and slow retrograde. It is believed that the survival and functional integrity of axons are largely dependent on materials passing along them in both directions by efficient transport systems. It is believed that nerve compression interferes with these systems, but whether this is a direct or a secondary effect from impairment of the blood supply is not known.

It has now been established that even mild compression at proximal levels impairs axon transport mechanisms to a degree that renders them more susceptible to further compression at a distal level.

In other words one insult is insufficient to impair the function of the fibre whereas two widely spaced insults have a cumulative effect on axon transport mechanisms that add up to functional impairment of the system and a reduction in conduction velocity. This has been confirmed experimentally (Nemoto 1983, Seiler et al 1983, Mackinnon et al 1984, Nemoto et al 1987).

The lesson to be learnt from this information is that with any entrapment syndrome all potential sites along the course of the involved nerve fibres should be carefully examined from the intervertebral foramina to the hand. For example, the eighth cervical and first thoracic nerve fibres could be compromised at the intervertebral foramen, at one or more of several entrapment sites at the thoracic outlet and at the elbow and wrist for both median and ulnar nerves.

REFERENCES

Carroll R E, Hurst L C 1982 The relationship of thoracic outlet syndrome and carpal tunnel syndrome. Clinical Orthopaedics 164: 14

Dahlin L B, Rydevik B, McLean W G, Sjöstrand J 1984 Changes in fast axonal transport during experimental nerve compression at low pressures. Experimental Neurology 84: 29

Dahlin L B, Sjöstrand J, McLean W G 1986 Graded inhibition of retrograde axonal transport by compression of rabbit vagus nerve. Journal of Neurological Sciences 76: 221

Hurst L C, Weissberg D, Carroll R E 1985 The relationship of the double crush to carpal tunnel syndrome. Journal of Hand Surgery 10B: 202

Mackinnon S E, Dellon A L 1988 Surgery of the Peripheral Nerve. Thieme New York

Mackinnon S E, Dellon A L, Hudson A, Hunter D A 1984 Chronic nerve compression: an experimental model in the rat. Annals of Plastic Surgery 13: 112

Massey E W, Riley T L, Pleet A B 1981 Coexistent carpal tunnel syndrome and cervical radiculopathy (double crush syndrome). Southern Medical Journal 74: 957

Nemoto K 1983 An experimental study on the vulnerability of the peripheral nerve. Journal of Japanese Orthopaedic Association 57: 1773

Nemoto K, Masumoto N, Tazaki K et al 1987 An experimental study of the 'double crush' hypothesis. Journal of Hand Surgery 12A: 552

Pfeffer G, Osterman A L 1986 Double crush syndrome: cervical radiculopathy and carpal tunnel syndrome. Journal of Hand Surgery 11A: 766

Rydevik B, McLean W G, Sjöstrand J, Lundborg G 1980 Blockage of axonal transport induced by acute graded compression of the rat vagus nerve. Journal of Neurology, Neurosurgery and Psychiatry 43: 690

Seiler W A, Schlegel R, Mackinnon S, Dellon L 1983 Double crush syndrome: experimental model in the rat. Surgical Forum 34: 596

Spinner M 1978 Injuries to the major branches of peripheral nerves of the forearm, 2nd edn. Saunders, Philadelphia

Sunderland S 1978 Nerves and nerve injuries, 2nd edn. Churchill Livingstone, Edinburgh

Upton A R M, McComas A J 1973 The double crush in nerve entrapment syndromes. Lancet ii: 359

20. Ischaemic nerve lesions due to trauma

Key points in any consideration of ischaemic nerve lesions are:

1. An adequate local blood supply is an essential prerequisite for maintaining the structural and functional integrity of nerve fibres.
2. Should a nerve be deprived of its blood supply, it may continue to receive sufficient oxygen by diffusion from adjacent vascularised tissues to enable it to continue to conduct for some time. However, this alternative source of oxygen applies only to small nerve trunks of small experimental animals.
3. When the blood supply to a nerve is impaired, nerve conduction is lost before the nerve suffers any structural damage. With increasing ischaemia a point is ultimately reached where the blood supply is inadequate to meet the metabolic needs of nerve fibres, though it is still sufficient to satisfy the less demanding needs of the connective tissue elements. At this stage Wallerian degeneration occurs and is later followed by changes that finally convert the nerve into a fibrous cord in which all outlines of nerve fibres are lost.

ANATOMICAL CONSIDERATIONS

The blood supply of peripheral nerves is discussed in Chapter 10. The considerable overlap in the distribution of regional nutrient arteries together with the free and extensive anastomoses between these branches, both on the surface of and within the nerve, means that, though individual regional vessels have specific areas of distribution, collateral circulatory mechanisms are available that ensure an uninterrupted circulation through the nerve in the event of one or even several nutrient arteries being interrupted.

Though the loss of a single regional nutrient artery is unlikely to have any pronounced or permanent effect on the nutrition of the nerve it supplies, the conditions become quite different if extensive occlusion, for example thrombosis, involves the intraneural ramifications of the vessel. This would restrict or prevent the establishment of effective collateral circulations and the flow of blood through the affected segment would then be impaired or arrested. Prolonged local ischaemia produced in this way could damage nerve tissue.

Normally, the anatomical features of the vasa nervorum, their intraneural distribution, and the collateral circulatory systems that they form, provide a considerable margin of safety for the blood supply of a nerve.

PATHOPHYSIOLOGICAL CONSIDERATIONS

Ischaemic nerve lesions constitute a group of great complexity. In some cases ischaemia is the only aetiological factor at work, while in others the ischaemia is a consequence of nerve compression, the two then combining to threaten the survival of nerve fibres.

While it is true that pressure on a nerve results in partial or total ischaemia, and may produce its effects in this way, there is evidence that reversible nerve conduction block due to pressure does differ in certain respects from that produced by ischaemia. Furthermore, in cuff compression of a limb, the pathological changes appear earlier and the effects persist longer in the compressed nerve segment than in the nerve temporarily rendered ischaemic below the compression.

However, in most nerve compression lesions localised ischaemia at the site of deformation will be an inevitable complication, while severe and prolonged compression may so damage blood vessels in the affected segment of the nerve that, even when the pressure is relieved, the circulation may not be restored to the now injured section, which undergoes further pathological change. In this way both compression and ischaemia combine as aetiological agents in first disturbing and then blocking conduction in the affected nerve fibres. Furthermore, since the associated clinical features are determined by the nature and extent of the lesion, and not by the agent or agents responsible for producing it, there is little point in attempting to draw too sharp a line of separation between what is due to compression and what to ischaemia.

Finally, the critical point at which a first degree ischaemic nerve lesion is converted into one of second degree, is somewhere between 4 and 8 hours. This critical time corresponds to the appearance of an endoneurial oedema that reflects damage to capillaries and a more severe involvement of nerve fibres, all of which delays recovery. Ochs (1975) found that cuff compression of 300 mmHg applied to a limb blocked fast axon transport. Complete recovery followed the release of the cuff after 4 hours but 6 hours compression caused an irreversible block of axon transport.

CLASSIFICATION

Nerve lesions due to ischaemia may be classified in the following way:

1. Non-traumatic in origin.

   a. Ischaemic nerve lesions due to arterial embolism.
   b. Ischaemic nerve lesions due to narrowing and occlusion of the arteriae nervorum.
   c. Arterial spasm and pathology from the injection of harmful substances.
   This group will not be discussed.

2. Traumatic in origin.

   a. Ischaemic nerve lesions due indirectly to interference with the blood supply to the nerve trunk by compression and stretch.
   b. Ischaemic nerve lesions due to damage to the arteriae nervorum.
   c. Ischaemic nerve lesions due to damage to the main artery to the limb or to one of its major branches.
   d. The ischaemic factor in combined neurovascular injury.

TRAUMATIC ISCHAEMIC NERVE LESIONS

Following trauma to a limb, disturbances of motor and sensory function may be due to an impaired blood supply to non-neural tissues consequent on damage to the main limb artery, to direct damage to peripheral nerves, to the secondary involvement of nerve trunks as the result of ischaemia or to a combination of these causes. In such cases exclusion, or confirmation, of suspected arterial damage and an accurate assessment of the precise nature and extent of the motor and sensory changes with reference to the distribution of individual nerves will greatly assist in determining the role of ischaemia as a possible aetiological factor in the production of neurological complications.

ISCHAEMIC NERVE LESIONS DUE TO COMPRESSION AND STRETCH

It is often difficult, because of the arrangement of the arteriae nervorum and the manner in which they supply the capillary bed of the nerve, to distinguish those structural and functional changes that are attributable to circulatory disturbances from those that are due to compression.

Furthermore, the reduction in the cross-sectional area of fasciculi produced by nerve stretching raises the intrafascicular pressure which, in turn, results in the compression of both nerve fibres and intrafascicular capillaries. Increasing pressure directly applied to the nerve or introduced indirectly by stretching, slows and finally arrests the circulation. The adverse effects of compression and stretching on the intraneural vessels and the microvascular circulation have been discussed in Chapters 17 and 18.

ISCHAEMIC NERVE LESIONS DUE TO DAMAGE TO THE ARTERIAE NERVORUM

Arteriae nervorum may be involved at the time of injury or later during the extensive mobilisation of an injured nerve preparatory to transposition, nerve repair or both. Ischaemia may also follow destruction of the vessels or arteriolar spasm.

Damage to the arteriae nervorum at the time of the injury

Damage to a major nutrient artery, or system of nutrient arteries, may lead to severe and extensive ischaemic nerve lesions. These lesions more commonly affect the median nerve in the forearm and the sciatic nerve. This is because of peculiarities in the arrangement of the arteriae nervorum that sometimes leave long sections of these nerves so dependent on a single major nutrient artery that injury to this vessel seriously interferes with the blood supply to the nerve.

The neurological manifestations of nerve trunk involvement due solely to ischaemia are confined to the distribution of the affected nerve. Thus the accidental injection of bismuth into the inferior gluteal artery has resulted in severe damage to the sciatic nerve, presumably because of the embolic blocking of its major nutrient supply in this region, the arteria comitans nervi ischiadici. A similar situation has arisen when the hypogastric artery has been therapeutically embolised to control pelvic haemorrhage (Chapter 10).

In the case of the median artery, injuries that directly involve this nutrient vessel are usually associated with such extensive damage to structures at and in the vicinity of the elbow that they lead to severe ischaemic complications that collectively constitute the syndrome of Volkmann's ischaemic contracture. In these cases direct damage to the nutrient artery may no longer be solely responsible for the ischaemia, additional factors now operating in the form of damage to the main artery of the limb, and compression of the nerve and its nutrient artery as the result of swelling beneath the

relatively unyielding fascia of the elbow and upper forearm.

Damage to the arteriae nervorum during mobilisation of the nerve

The complete and extensive separation of a nerve from neighbouring structures is frequently required in order to permit its transposition to a new site or to facilitate end-to-end nerve repair after the loss of a segment. This procedure may require the sacrifice of many large nutrient vessels, and the question naturally arises as to whether or not this will adversely affect the nutrition of the nerve.

The nature of the anastomoses between regional nutrient arteries supplying the nerve indicates that the arrangement is one that provides for the development of effective collateral circulations after one or several regional arteries have been ligated. Clinical and experimental observation relating to the effects of excluding the regional sources of supply confirm the physiological efficiency of such collateral circulations. These are established and maintained by the large longitudinal anastomosing channels on the surface of the nerve and by finer anastomotic chains placed more deeply between the fasciculi. Damage to the former throws an additional burden on the latter which may, at times, be inadequate for the needs of the nerve.

Regional peculiarities in the blood supply that leave long sections of a nerve solely dependent on a single major nutrient artery represent a potential weakness, though there is good evidence that, even under these apparently unfavourable conditions, the anastomoses at the peripheral limits of the solitary channel are such that there is only a remote possibility of segmental ischaemia resulting from the loss of such a single nutrient vessel. On the other hand, damage to the longitudinal arterial anastomotic systems on the surface of the nerve during mobilisation could jeopardise its blood supply. In order to avoid this complication it is essential to preserve these superficial longitudinal systems by dividing the parent nutrient arteries some distance from the nerve before they branch into their primary ascending and descending branches that are to constitute the major longitudinal anastomotic systems on the surface of the nerve (Fig. 38.1 Chapter 38).

It should also be noted that nerve stretching introduced when traction is applied to the proximal and distal nerve stumps, in order to effect end-to-end repair, compromises the intraneural circulation.

ISCHAEMIC NERVE LESIONS DUE TO DAMAGE TO THE MAIN ARTERY TO A LIMB OR TO ONE OF ITS MAJOR BRANCHES. ISCHAEMIC PARALYSIS

In this category the main artery to a limb (e.g. subclavian, axillary, brachial, femoral, popliteal or one of their major branches) is lacerated or severed and subsequently ligated, or the vessel is suddenly occluded by post-traumatic spasm, embolism or thrombosis. The nerves, however, escape direct injury at the time of wounding but suffer with the other tissues that are rendered ischaemic by the arterial lesion.

The consequences of interrupting the main arterial supply to a limb depend on the rate at which a collateral circulation becomes effective in preserving affected tissues. The factors which control the development of a functionally effective collateral circulation are not fully understood but they include:

1. the availability of collateral channels through which the circulation could be restored;
2. the functional efficiency, as opposed to the anatomical existence, of such collateral channels;
3. the state of the vessel wall in terms of its elastic properties;
4. the presence of arterial disease resulting in pathological narrowing of the vessel lumen;
5. a pressure in the system sufficient to maintain an adequate circulation through the collateral channels and through the limb.

Clearly there is room here for individual variations which go some way to explaining why, following apparently identical degrees of arterial damage, some patients are more prone to ischaemic complications than others.

Interruption of the main artery to a limb may terminate in one of three ways:

1. Failure to establish an effective collateral circulation culminating in tissue necrosis that necessitates the amputation of the part.
2. Collateral channels commence to function so rapidly that the blood supply to the affected tissues is restored before degenerative changes have time to develop. Under these conditions the ischaemic effects are limited to muscle weakness and disturbances of sensation that are minimal and transient so that within a few weeks there may be no detectable abnormality.
3. Between the two extremes of loss of the limb on the one hand and full recovery on the other, there are degrees of circulatory impairment in which tissues suffer varying degrees of ischaemic damage depending on factors that control the amount of blood reaching them by alternative channels. Nerves suffer with the other soft tissues of the limb, and to a degree that depends on the severity and duration of the ischaemia to which they are subjected. It is this third group which provides examples of the syndrome of ischaemic paralysis.

The syndrome of ischaemic paralysis

The syndrome of ischaemic paralysis refers to the disability that follows the traumatic interruption of a main limb artery without direct damage to peripheral nerves at the site of wounding.

Under these conditions it is often difficult to decide how much of the disability is attributable to nerve trunk ischaemia and how much to irreversible ischaemic changes affecting non-neural tissues. This is because unrelieved ischaemia contributes to the residual disability in two ways:

1. A constrictive fibrosis hinders regeneration in those nerve fibres that have undergone Wallerian degeneration and impairs nerve conduction in others.
2. Ischaemic changes involving muscles, tendons and tendon sheaths, articular and

periarticular structures, fascia and connective tissues, adversely affect physiological systems and mechanisms at the periphery and so create obstacles to functional recovery.

The diagnosis of nerve ischaemia secondary to arterial injury, and an estimate of the disability attributable to this factor, ultimately rests on an assessment of the total clinical picture embracing the precise nature and distribution of the motor and sensory disturbances, the condition of the muscle and the nutritional state of the limb. In the final analysis only the passage of time may disclose the true position.

Features of ischaemic paralysis originating in this way are:

1. It is most commonly seen in the upper limb but may follow wounds of the femoral and popliteal arteries.
2. Usually it is the main artery to the limb that is affected but damage to smaller vessels, such as the radial and ulnar arteries, may result in a similar but less extensive disability.
3. The distribution of the neurological disturbances depends on the size of the damaged vessel, the level at which it is interrupted, and factors controlling the development of an efficient collateral circulation.
4. The effects may be confined to, and are always maximal in, the hand and foot, though they may extend to the elbow and knee.
5. The more proximal the level of the vascular lesion, the greater the chances of ischaemic paralysis.
6. The clinical manifestations of the syndrome include partial paralysis of muscles, the degeneration and fibrous tissue replacement of muscle tissue, disturbances of sensation and colour changes affecting the skin.
7. *Motor function.* Muscle involvement is maximal at the periphery of the limb, where it is generalised and unrelated to the regional distribution of individual nerves. Such a generalised motor disability must be attributed to ischaemia, since direct nerve damage could only be responsible for these same effects if all three major nerves innervating the hand and forearm were injured at the site where the artery is damaged. This, though possible, is highly unlikely. Furthermore, in the case of the lower limb, coincidental damage to both nerve and artery is for anatomical reasons limited to the popliteal artery and medial popliteal nerve, anterior tibial artery and nerve, and femoral artery and nerve. In no case would direct damage to one of these nerves account for the wide distribution of the motor defect in the lower limb. While it is possible for one nerve to suffer more than others in ischaemia, direct damage to the nerve at the site of wounding should be suspected if the distribution of the motor loss points strongly to one particular nerve.

The affected muscles are first swollen and then become firm, indurated, fibrosed and shortened in contractures. Passive movements which stretch these muscles are not free and are often painful. In uncomplicated nerve injury, on the other hand, the paralysed muscles are softer in consistency, they atrophy more rapidly and passive movements are freer and fuller in range; under certain circumstances, however, such denervated muscles may undergo fibrosis, and periarticular changes may restrict joint movements.

8. *Sensation.* The area of defective sensation follows a more 'glove and stocking' pattern as opposed to the regional anatomical distribution of one or more individual nerves.

Paraesthesiae and pain are common after ischaemic lesions. The incidence of pain is, however, much higher when the vascular damage is associated with a nerve injury. Within the affected area there may be a delayed but extremely unpleasant response to deep pin prick and pressure. This is attributed to the greater resistance of fine myelinated fibres to ischaemia.

9. *Nutrition.* There is a high incidence of nutritional disturbances which vary in

severity from mild oedema, breaking of the nails and ulceration of the digits, to more marked changes in the form of superficial necrosis of the tips of the digits. Both the pain and the trophic changes may be sufficiently severe to cause the patient considerable concern.

10. *Evolution*

1. Immediate or acute phase. This occupies the first few weeks. The changes are most marked in the hand or foot and involve the oedematous infiltration of ischaemic regions. The hand is swollen and cold and the skin cyanotic or claret coloured with bluish or red mottling. The swelling involves both subcutaneous tissues and muscle, giving them a 'doughy' consistency. The skin becomes indurated, thickened and dry. The affected parts can be moved both actively and passively, but movements are difficult to perform owing to stiffness and the pain caused by stretching ischaemic muscles.

The patient frequently experiences paraesthesiae that are intensified by touch, deep pressure and cold and are relieved by warmth so that the patient carefully protects the affected parts. Cutaneous sensation is diminished or lost over a distribution of the glove and stocking type. All forms of sensation are affected, stimuli being incompletely perceived, poorly localised and imperfectly differentiated; pin prick and pressure give rise to a delayed, unpleasant and diffuse response. Deep sensation is also impaired but not to the same degree.

2. Delayed or chronic phase. This is the stage of degeneration and fibrosis of muscles and the conversion of protein exudate into fibrous tissue. Fibrosis and muscle contracture, together with the joint deformities to which they give rise, limit the motor function of the affected parts, particularly those movements involving the hand and digits. Joints become fixed in abnormal positions and the range and freedom of movements is still further restricted. The development of adhesions involving subcutaneous tissues, tendon sheaths and fasciae limits the free play of one structure over another.

The skin becomes smooth, shiny and thin while the discolouring of the immediate phase is intensified. Spindling of the digits occurs, the nails become talon-like and the digits the site of trophic ulceration.

The pathogenesis of ischaemic nerve lesions

The nature, severity and consequences of nerve trunk ischaemia depend on the duration of the ischaemia and whether or not an adequate collateral circulation is available. Affected nerves present a wide variety of pathological changes ranging from those characteristic of conduction block, to Wallerian degeneration, disorganisation of the nerve trunk and necrosis. Generally speaking, they correspond to the first four degrees of nerve injury described in Chapter 25. Mixed lesions are common because the pathological changes are not usually uniform throughout the involved section of the nerve.

Where the injury results in both ischaemia and severance of the nerve, the ischaemic changes are always more severe in the distal segment because the interruption of the longitudinal arterial channels imposes a greater burden on those mechanisms operating to produce an effective collateral circulation. For this reason, the distal segment of a severed nerve should be handled with particular care during mobilisation in order to preserve those regional nutrient arteries that have survived the injury and upon which the nutrition of an already jeopardised nerve depends.

First and second degree ischaemic lesions

Acute ischaemia leads to a first or second degree injury, depending on how quickly an effective collateral circulation develops or arteriolar spasm is relieved. The circulation may be restored so rapidly that the changes are restricted to those that represent first degree involvement (Chapter 25) in which the axon survives in continuity and there is no Wallerian degeneration. Minor changes in the axon and myelin are quickly and fully reversible so that signs of recovery appear early and function is rapidly and completely restored.

If the restoration of an adequate circulation is somewhat delayed, the ischaemia reaches a point where it leads to the breakdown of the axon and the sequence of changes that constitute Wallerian degeneration. If the local circulation is restored before more advanced structural changes develop, the endoneurial tubes, whose outlines have been preserved, transmit regenerating axons to the periphery in such a way that function is fully restored, though both the onset and progress of recovery are delayed in comparison with a first degree ischaemic lesion. (Chapter 25).

Third degree ischaemic lesions

Chronic or prolonged ischaemia is followed by the more severe and permanent destruction of nerve tissue. In the well-established lesion, a considerable length of the nerve is affected; this is thinned, greyish in colour, fibrotic and firm to palpation. Histologically, the epineurium and perineurium show little change other than an increase in fibroblasts; the fascicular pattern is retained, though individual fasciculi are atrophied. The changes are maximal and severe inside the fasciculi and take the characteristic form of a gross thickening and collagenisation of the endoneurium. The endoneurial tubes, from which the myelin and axon have been removed as the result of Wallerian degeneration, are reduced in diameter both by shrinkage and endoneurial thickening until they are finally obliterated and transformed into strands of dense collagenous tissue. Isolated collections of myelin may be left trapped and plugging some endoneurial tubes, owing to the absence of an adequate circulation and the phagocytic response which are responsible for removing the debris of degeneration. Degeneration of Schwann cells proceeds until finally the intrafascicular tissue is transformed into dense, relatively acellular collagenous sheets and strands. Involvement of the intraneural vessels, which is maximal inside the fasciculi, includes such changes as intimal proliferation and thrombosis. Later there is an increase in the number of small vessels about which aggregations of polymorphs and lymphocytes may be seen.

These vessels are evidence of an improving collateral circulation based on new vessels. Larger occluded nutrient vessels may be recanalised but this usually comes too late to be of any value for, by this time, the destruction and collagenisation of endoneurial tubes is irreversible, though the improved blood supply does arrest further deterioration.

These various changes involve long stretches of the nerve and create conditions that are unfavourable for regeneration, since new axons are faced with a dense barrier of tissue of considerable length through which they must force their way. Though regenerating axons are seen, they are small and regeneration is incomplete. This represents the final stages of a third degree injury. Some regeneration and recovery are possible if collagenisation is not too advanced and the restoration of an adequate local circulation is not unduly delayed.

Fourth degree ischaemic lesions

The nerve is converted into a relatively avascular, grossly shrunken, fibrotic strand which may lose its identity in the scar tissue of an associated soft tissue injury. Collagenisation is complete inside the fasciculi where all traces of the endoneurial tubes have vanished; the overall appearance is one of dense acellular collagenous bands with patchy hyaline changes. A fibroblastic proliferation in the perineurium is replaced by a progressive fibrosis. This sheath finally loses its identity and merges with the adjacent tissue. In this way the distinctive outlines of the fasciculi are obliterated and the internal structural features of the nerve trunk are lost; the epineurium is less severely affected but does show fibrosis. Collectively, these advanced changes represent the transformation of an organised peripheral nerve trunk into a disorganised strand of fibrous tissue.

COMBINED NEUROVASCULAR INJURIES

In this type of ischaemic lesion both the artery and the nerve or nerves with which it is intimately associated are injured simultaneously by the same wounding mechanism.

The close relationship between blood vessels and nerves in certain regions predisposes to combined neurovascular injuries from penetrating wounds. Such combined injuries occur more frequently with wounding above the elbow than with wounding in the leg and elsewhere in the arm. This finding is readily explained by the closer relationship in the upper arm between large nerves and important vessels.

As we have seen in the previous sections, arterial damage alone may result in serious disturbances of motor and sensory functions. The effects of an injury in which both nerve and artery are damaged at the same site will, therefore, be twofold: (1) those due to denervation following any one of the five degrees of nerve injury described in Chapter 25, and (2) those due to an impoverished blood supply to the tissues that adversely affects their survival and their functional capacity when the injured limb survives.

The arterial lesion may be one of laceration, severance, spasm, thrombosis, ligation, or arterial and arteriovenous aneurysms. When the limb is left with a barely adequate blood supply, peripheral circulatory deficiencies may indirectly disturb nerve function in two ways:

1. Persistent ischaemia of peripheral tissues, and the changes to which it gives rise, reduce the effectiveness of reinnervation.
2. Persistent ischaemia of the nerve trunk, and the resulting fibrosis, interfere with regenerative processes and with the function of nerve fibres that have regenerated and reinnervated the periphery.

In addition, when an aneurysm is present, it may compress and deform the nerve trunk and, since injured nerve fibres are more susceptible to compression ischaemia, this adds to the neurological disturbance.

For these reasons such combined injuries produce complex effects which depend, inter alia, on the relative extent and severity of the damage to artery and nerve or nerves. Usually, however, collateral circulations are established so rapidly that the arterial lesion is not an embarrassment to nerve regeneration.

Traumatic aneurysms and nerve lesions

Nerve lesions associated with traumatic aneurysms may result from:

1. Direct trauma to the nerve at the time of injury,

2. Ischaemia introduced by the arterial injury or developing subsequent to the surgical treatment of the aneurysm,
3. Pressure from the aneurysm itself. Here evidence of a nerve lesion is not present immediately following the injury but appears as the aneurysm enlarges and the nerve becomes intimately related to the wall of the aneurysmal sac. These are usually cases of first and second degree involvement of the nerve, though the division of nerve fibres has been attributed to pressure erosion by a pulsating aneurysm.

The nature and distribution of the motor and sensory defects are determined by the nerve or nerves affected and the nature and severity of the nerve injury. Pain and paraesthesiae present the following features:

1. Pain is more common in these cases than in uncomplicated nerve injuries.
2. They usually date from the time of the injury, which suggests that they are more intimately related to the arterial lesion than to the aneurysmal swelling.
3. In general, they are diffuse, maximal in the hand or foot, and are unrelated to the regional distribution of any one nerve or nerves.
4. Pain varies in quality and intensity. It is usually burning in quality and paroxysmal in intensity.
5. Pain developing or increasing in intensity indicates an extension of the aneurysm.
6. Slight to moderate pain tends to fade gradually.
7. An aneurysm should be suspected in those patients in whom severe pain persists and is not related to the regional distribution of a peripheral nerve.

THE EFFECT OF CONCOMITANT VASCULAR INJURY ON NERVE REGENERATION

Ligation of a damaged main artery to a limb leads to widespread effects in non-neural tissues, recovery from which depends on the establishment and efficiency of collateral circulations. This factor complicates attempts to evaluate the influence of arterial damage on the processes of regeneration in man. An additional difficulty is that this factor cannot be isolated from the many other variables that operate simultaneously to adversely affect the course of recovery.

As a generalisation, it may be accepted that the course of spontaneous regeneration is much the same regardless of whether or not there is an associated vascular injury while a satisfactory end-result after nerve repair is not necessarily excluded by a vascular complication.

At the same time there is now good evidence that the outcome of nerve repair is better when a severed nerve and vessel are repaired at the same operation (p. 58). Nor should the importance of the peripheral blood supply to a nerve ever be underestimated.

REFERENCES

Ochs S 1975 Axoplasmic transport — a basis for neural pathology. In: Dyck P J, Thomas P K, Lambert E H (eds) Peripheral neuropathy. Saunders, Philadelphia, Ch 12, Vol 1, p 243

21. Nerve injury caused by the injection of therapeutic agents. Cryogenic lesions. Ionising radiation.

NERVE INJURY CAUSED BY THE INJECTION OF THERAPEUTIC AGENTS

These nerve injuries are caused when a therapeutic agent is inadvertently injected directly into the nerve or into the tissues immediately surrounding it (Sunderland 1978, Hudson et al 1978, Gentili et al 1979, 1980a–c). Substances proved harmful to nerve fibres and nerve trunks cover a wide variety of agents; the vehicle for the agent may be equally as damaging. A separate and special category in this group are those nerve lesions deliberately produced to block conduction, either temporarily or permanently, for therapeutic purposes.

The nerve may be damaged by:

1. the needle as it passes into or through the nerve in such a way as to penetrate fasciculi. Trauma from the needle is more likely to occur when the nerve is composed of large fasciculi as opposed to a number of small, widely separated fasciculi between which the needle may more easily pass;
2. the destructive, sclerosing or toxic action of the agent;
3. the injection of the material into a fasciculus which damages some nerve fibres and compresses others. In more severe lesions delayed complications in the form of a constrictive intrafascicular fibrosis complete the destruction of nerve fibres. Under these circumstances regenerating axons are unable to find their way through the scarred tissue and useful regeneration cannot be expected;
4. the injection of the material into the interfascicular epineurial tissue. The fibrosis which follows constricts fasciculi and impairs their blood supply;
5. the injection of the material into the surrounding tissues, with destructive effects which could spread to involve the nerve either directly or subsequently in constrictive scar tissue;
6. pressure from a haematoma;
7. involvement of nutrient vessels causing spasm or thrombosis, followed by ischaemic necrosis of nerve tissue;
8. direct injection into a major nutrient vessel such as the inferior gluteal artery and its branch to the sciatic nerve.

Injection injuries may be localised to a few fasciculi or have more widespread effects depending on the way in which the lesion is produced. Intraneural injections are more damaging than extraneural and the consequences are far more serious when the agent is injected under pressure into a fasciculus. Permanent constrictive scarring, in and about the nerve, may be sufficient to prevent recovery in the affected fibres.

The most important factors determining the severity of the nerve injury are the nature and amount of the injected material and its location in relation to the nerve.

Pathological changes include an intense inflammatory and early fibrotic reaction about the nerve, which may appear swollen and hyperaemic in the early stages. Late findings include a thickened or shrunken nerve with an irregular contour which may show a lateral neuroma, of firm or soft consistency, reflecting needle trauma localised to one bundle or part of the nerve, paraneural scarring with dense adhesions firmly binding the nerve to the surrounding tissues, and intraneural fibrosis, confirmed by internal neurolysis, which gives the nerve an indurated feeling. The lesions are usually localised to the site of the injection but on occasion the damaging material may track for long distances up and down the nerve to cause more extensive lesions. In particularly severe cases the nerve may be necrotic over long distances.

The buttock and the outer aspect of the upper arm enjoy a traditional acceptance as sites for deep injections. Consequently, the sciatic and the radial nerves are the two most frequently at risk.

In the buttock, the sciatic nerve is composed of numerous small fasciculi which are separated by a large amount of connective tissue. This arrangement provides some protection from injections that inadvertently involve it in that the needle is more likely to pass between fasciculi.

The peroneal division is more vulnerable than the tibial division of the sciatic nerve probably because: (1) it is composed of less epineurial tissue and fewer and larger fasciculi that allow more direct access to nerve fibres by the injurious agent, and (2) it slightly overlaps the tibial division and so is more superficially placed.

Care should be taken when using the gluteal region for an intramuscular injection to select a site which keeps both the needle and the injected material well clear of the sciatic nerve. In order to ensure this, the surface anatomy of the nerve must be kept constantly in mind. The nerve lies along a curved line joining (1) the junction of the upper and mid-thirds of a line from the posterior superior iliac spine to the outer border of the ischial tuberosity; and (2) a point mid-way between the ischial tuberosity and the upper border of the greater trochanter of the femur.

These surface markings place the nerve in the inferomedial quadrant of the gluteal region. The injections should therefore be into the superolateral quadrant.

In the case of the radial nerve, the injection site is into the outer aspect of the upper arm where the nerve is often composed of one or two major fasciculi with little protective connective tissue. This is an arrangement that predisposes to more severe damage should the nerve be penetrated. Intramuscular injections should be into the deltoid (1) above the lower point of its insertion where the nerve is turning forwards through the intermuscular septum after leaving the spiral groove, and (2) below

the deltoid branch of the axillary nerve which is coursing horizontally forwards on the deep surface of the muscle at the level of the surgical neck of the humerus.

With deep injections it is important to keep in mind the regional anatomy of nerve trunks in order to ensure that the site selected is well clear of any major nerve.

Clinical features of injection nerve injury

In most cases the onset is immediate or follows within a few minutes of the injection. This reflects the rapidity with which nerve tissue is damaged. A delayed onset suggests a more slowly acting agent and/or its location in the surrounding tissues with slow spread to involve the nerve trunk. There is intense pain at the time which persists in about half the cases. Severe pain may become the most disturbing feature of the lesion, taking on the characteristics of causalgia and finally requiring a sympathetic block or sympathectomy to relieve it. There is an associated motor and sensory loss which may be complete or incomplete. Motor fibres are more susceptible than sensory fibres and suffer to a greater degree when both are affected.

Decision making in the treatment of injection injury

The first step is to attempt some estimate of the severity of the nerve damage. This varies from the rapidly reversible changes causing only transient loss of function, to destructive lesions with permanent constrictive scarring in and about the nerve which is sufficient to prevent recovery in the affected fibres. There is, of course, no way of knowing precisely where the material is located within, or in relationship to, the nerve. Some indication of the extent and severity of the damage may be obtained from a knowledge of the destructive action on nerve tissue of the agent used, the amount injected, the rapidity with which the signs and symptoms of nerve involvement appeared, whether function is totally or incompletely lost and whether the condition remains stationary or improves. Deterioration would suggest developing fibrosis.

For practical purposes the severity of the lesion can be expressed in three grades:

1. *Lesions of maximal severity.* These are caused by very toxic and destructive agents which cause extensive necrosis and replacement fibrosis of the nerve. Spontaneous recovery is unlikely and the lesion will later require surgical excision and repair. With particularly destructive agents in large amounts exposure of the nerve with lavage to dilute and remove the agent as quickly as possible is worth considering. Unfortunately, the damaging effects of the agent are immediate, particularly when the injection is into the substance of the nerve. The results of such treatment have not been encouraging.

2. *Lesions of moderate severity.* These are caused by the direct action of the agent on axons, resulting in Wallerian degeneration, and by the reactive fibrosis which constricts nerve fibres, fasciculi and the nerve trunk. Spontaneous recovery is possible but it is delayed for long periods and will, most likely, be incomplete. These are the cases where recovery may be aided by neurolysis.

3. *Mild transient lesions.* Here the direct action of the agent on axons is confined to producing a reversible conduction block lesion. Recovery is rapid in these cases.

As regards the prospects for spontaneous recovery of an acceptable quality following injection injury of the sciatic nerve the possibilities are:

a. Early and complete recovery. If signs of recovery appear within a few hours or days then the prospects of complete recovery are good. These patients represent a very small minority, though the number could be greater than the records suggest because such a transient complaint may not be recorded.

b. Delayed recovery of 6 weeks to 18 months.

c. Incomplete recovery. The majority are left with some permanent defect.

d. No recovery. Every series has its quota of patients with no recovery.

In the face of this generally unsatisfactory outcome the next question to ask is what has surgical exploration to offer, when should it be undertaken and what is to be done with the exposed nerve?

The nerve should be explored when: (i) the injected agent is known to be particularly destructive; (2) there is severe persistent pain; and (3) after an acceptable delay to allow signs of regeneration to appear, the lesion is still complete or any residual function is of no practical value.

Objections to early exploration are:

1. Some patients will, if left alone, recover either completely or to a useful degree.
2. The onset of recovery proceeding to a useful end-result is often delayed for periods as long as 12 months.
3. Unnecessary operative manipulation may add to the damage to the nerve.
4. Exploration does not always remove the difficulty of deciding, in the doubtful case, whether or not to excise the damaged segment and repair the nerve.

Exploration shortly after the injury is premature. Unless the agent used is known to be particularly destructive, exploration should not be contemplated within the first 6 weeks of the injury so that any spontaneous recovery from a reversible conduction block lesion can be given a reasonable opportunity to reveal itself.

Exploration at or shortly after 6 weeks is justified on the following grounds:

1. In skilled hands the operation presents no problems.
2. It is desirable to confirm, at the earliest possible opportunity, the state of the nerve by inspection, palpation and nerve conduction studies.
3. It is essential to identify, with the least possible delay, severe damage in the form of extensive necrosis requiring some form of surgical repair. However, because the results of high sciatic repairs, either by end-to-end suture or by grafting, are generally poor, doubtful lesions should be subjected to no more than neurolysis and then left until it is clear that there is going to be no spontaneous recovery. The time limit for this is 6 months in the case of the radial nerve and 12 months for the sciatic. The shorter delay for the former is because of the shorter distances to be covered by

regenerating axons to reach their end organs. The position is thus one of trial neurolysis followed later, if necessary, by resection and suture or grafting.

4. Constrictive scar tissue should be removed by external and internal neurolysis as soon as possible in order to provide damaged nerve fibres with the best available environment in which to regenerate. If exploration is too long delayed, continued scarring and fibrosis in and around the nerve add to the difficulties of neurolysis and reduce the prospects of getting useful spontaneous recovery.

5. Even if neurolysis anticipates the onset of spontaneous recovery, nothing is lost and much gained by improving the local terrain for the continuation of useful regeneration. Spontaneous recovery does not always proceed to completion in the undisturbed nerve, and there is always the chance that neurolysis performed at this time could improve the overall quality of the recovery.

6. Internal neurolysis must be carried out with special care, for there is the grave risk of severing fine fasciculi containing fibres that would recover spontaneously if left undisturbed (Chapter 38).

7. The results following neurolysis are often disappointing. This is to be expected because of the concealed intrafascicular pathology in so many lesions that cannot be adequately dealt with by this procedure.

NERVE INJURY CAUSED BY COOLING AND FREEZING

The information provided by studies on the effect of cooling human nerves relates to the disturbances of function and speculation on the likely nature of the nerve lesion produced by cooling (Weber 1847, Waller 1861, Bickford 1939, Sinclair & Hinshaw 1951, Glasgow & Sinclair 1962). Bickford reported function failing in the order: cold, motor, vasomotor, 'first' pain, touch, 'second' pain and warmth. However, Sinclair and Glasgow were unable to detect any consistent difference between the times of failure of cold and warm sensibility.

Even as early as 1922, Bielchowsky and Valentin

reported that the most effective way of achieving temporary interruption of conduction for therapeutic purposes was to freeze the nerve with ethyl chloride, 5 minutes freezing being sufficient for the thickest nerve. The method, however, proved unreliable.

In earlier experimental studies cooling the nerve did not go below $-4°C$, with significant structural and functional changes being found only at temperatures below 10°C (Trendelenberg 1917, 1918, Denny Brown et al 1945, Torrance & Whitteridge 1948, Whitteridge 1948, Lundberg 1952, Dodt 1953, Widdicombe 1954, Douglas & Malcolm 1955, Paintal 1965a,b, 1967, Buck et al 1966, Schaumburg et al 1967, Franz & Iggo 1968, Kawano & Matsumura 1968, Pribor & Novak 1969).

The following account of the damaging effects of cold on peripheral nerve is based on the comprehensive studies of Denny Brown et al (1945).

Cooling between 10° and 0°C for 30 minutes to 2 hours caused changes in nerve fibres that constitute a continuous series ranging from a mild reversible conduction block with or without oedema, to axon swelling and a cellular reaction culminating in Wallerian degeneration in more severe lesions. The more resistant connective tissue and, in particular, the perineurium and epineurium, survive so that the general architecture of the nerve is preserved. While an associated vascular stasis and ischaemia could be responsible for some of the nerve fibre damage, the direct effect of cold on myelin and on enzyme systems sustaining the nerve fibre appear to have special significance. Regeneration occurs with these lesions and is completed by the third month.

When the nerve was frozen solid by a spray of carbon dioxide (Denny Brown et al 1945), disorganisation and necrosis of the fascicular contents were conspicuous within 2 or 3 days. These changes involved swelling and fragmentation of the axons and endoneurium, and degeneration of myelin, and endoneurial and Schwann cells. Associated with these changes was a marked inflammatory reaction in the epineurium and perineurium, which were infiltrated with polymorphonuclear leucocytes, lymphocytes, plasma cells and proliferating fibroblasts. However, the perineurium and the epineurium survived. The vessels were hyperaemic with occasionally some extravasation of red blood cells. Within 10–14 days phagocytic activity was well advanced, being more marked at the site of injury where myelin dissolution was almost complete, than distally along fibres still undergoing Wallerian degeneration. At the proximal end of the affected region endoneurial and Schwann cell activity was marked and regenerating axons were already entering the affected segment.

By the end of 3 months the degenerated tissue had been almost completely removed from the affected segment which remained excessively cellular owing to the increased number of endoneurial and Schwann cells. The regenerated fibres were thinner than the original fibres and regeneration, although apparently complete, was still complicated by those factors combining to disorganise the pattern of innervation.

More recent studies have used the cryoprobe to take temperatures well below 0°C. Gaster et al (1971) cooled 3 mm segments of nerves to 0 to −60°C for 60 seconds with a cryoprobe placed on the surface of the nerve. They reported no changes until temperatures of −10°C were reached when the first disturbances in function were observed. The neurological disability deteriorated progressively as the temperature was lowered to −20°C, when there was complete loss of function. The findings suggest that, if the exposure time is shortened to 60 seconds, then nerve fibres can tolerate temperatures down to −5°C.

In a similar series of experiments others froze nerves by cryoprobe at temperatures from −60°C to −100°C for periods ranging from 1 to 4 minutes (Carter et al 1972, Beazley et al 1974). They found:

1. that all lesions were of the second degree type and recovered completely;
2. a linear relationship between the duration of the exposure and the delay in the onset of recovery;
3. no relationship between the temperature and the duration of loss of function.

Mira (1971, 1972a,b, 1979, 1981) used a liquid nitrogen cyroprobe to freeze the sciatic nerve of the rat, the point of the probe being directly applied to the nerve which was rapidly frozen at −180°C for a duration that did not exceed 30–40 seconds. This method resulted in local necrosis of axons and disorganisation of their myelin sheaths. There was no disruption of the connective tissue components of the nerves, the microvessels or the basal lamina surrounding each nerve fibre. Thus these were pure second degree lesions with full anatomical and physiological recovery. The maintenance of continuity of the several connective tissue sheaths of the nerve, particularly the basal laminae, is a fundamental factor in axon regeneration and Mira regarded this model as the best for the study of uncomplicated axon regeneration.

Additional features of cryogenic nerve lesions revealed by these several investigations include:

1. Nerves are resistant to cooling down to temperatures of 10°C, below which the degree of the neurological disability is proportional to the intensity of cooling.
2. Cold can seriously disturb function at temperatures short of freezing.
3. Motor function succumbs before, and suffers to a greater degree than sensory function. Motor loss becomes evident at about 10°C and a mild sensory loss at 7°C. The loss of both functions becomes total between 5°C and 0°C. However, there is some evidence that nerves can tolerate temperatures down to −5°C for 60 seconds.
4. The various sensory modalities do not fail simultaneously, nor does failure occur progressively and in a regular and consistent manner.
5. Function is rapidly restored as recovery from cooling takes place, sensory functions recovering before motor and the various sensory modalities returning in the reverse order from that in which they were lost.
6. Differences in the susceptibility of the various modalities of sensation to cooling cannot be satisfactorily related to fibre size.
7. Non-myelinated fibres are more resistant to cold block than myelinated fibres.
8. Conflicting views persist regarding the relationship between fibre size and susceptibility to cooling. Some claim that the largest fibres are the most susceptible (Denny Brown et al 1945, Whitteridge 1948, Torrance & Whitteridge 1948,

Widdicombe 1954). According to others the finer fibres are blocked by cooling before the larger (Dodt 1953, Douglas & Malcolm 1955, Byck et al 1966) and there is the third view that there is no relationship between fibre size and susceptibility to cold, fibres of all sizes suffering concurrently during cooling (Paintal 1965, Schaumburg et al 1967, Kawano & Matsumura 1968).

9. There are species, and conceivably individual, differences in the resistance of nerves to cold.

10. The axons and myelin of mammalian nerve fibres are selectively damaged by exposure to cold. The pathological changes fall into a continuous series from simple oedema without damage to nerve fibres on the one hand, to necrosis of all axons and Schwann cells at the other extreme. The structure and continuity of the epineurium, perineurium and basal lamina of individual nerve fibres are preserved. Regeneration is rapid and complete. Lesions, expressed in terms of nerve trunk damage, are of first or second degree severity, with the contents of some fasciculi suffering third degree damage.

NERVE INJURY CAUSED BY IONISING RADIATION

Reports in both the experimental and clinical literature regarding effect of radiation on nerves, regenerating axons and the quality of recovery after nerve repair express conflicting views. The subject has been reviewed by Sunderland (1978). Some have been unable to detect any adverse effects in their experiments using dosages of 4000–6000+ rads (Janzen and Warren 1942, Hicks and Montgomery 1952, Clemedson and Nelson 1960, McGuirt and McCabe 1977). Contrary views have been expressed by others. Linder (1959) found that exposing the rat sciatic nerve to smaller doses of ionising radiation but over a longer period produced delayed effects in the form of localised degenerative changes and fibrosis. The findings suggested that these changes were primarily vascular in origin. Despite these structural changes, electrophysiological studies revealed no disturbances in conduction. On the other hand, Arnold et

al (1961) reported depressed conduction in the saphenous nerve.

In Bergström's (1962) studies the changes ranged through hyperaemia and nerve swelling, an inflammatory infiltration and fibroblastic proliferation in the epineurial connective tissue, fragmentation of myelin sheaths leading to the degeneration of nerve fibres, and Schwann cell proliferation. Focal areas of necrosis with thickening of vessel walls were also observed.

Cavanagh (1968) found that, following a crush injury of the sciatic nerve, exposure to 1000–2000 rads resulted in failure of Schwann cells to proliferate, with individual Schwann cells still showing evidence of radiation damage 9 months later.

From their experimental studies of the effect of radiation on grafted facial nerves Yamamoto and Fisch (1982) concluded that radiation has an inhibitory influence on axon regeneration.

The most detailed study, however, is one by Spiess (1972), who irradiated the sciatic nerve in rats with doses between 3000 and 8000 rads. With lower dosages the conduction velocity was still within normal limits 3 months later. However with doses of 5000 rads, early structural changes signifying radiation damage were observed at 2 months. With doses of more than 6000 rads severe changes were still present 6 months later.

Primary radiation damage to neural structures involved alterations in the contour and structure of the axons with changes in the neurofilaments, the destruction of some axons, evidence of commencing demyelination, the complete disintegration of some nerve fibres, and the appearance of an angiomesenchymal reaction that was regarded as the forerunner of secondary radiation effects in the form of fibrosis and ischaemia.

Thus the early changes in nerves following exposure to ionising radiation are the direct effect of radiation on axons whereas the late effects are the results of an angiomesenchymal reaction culminating in intense fibrosis that constricts and finally replaces nerve fibres, and causes the obliteration of vessels and further ischaemic damage.

Clinical considerations

Knowledge of the effects of ionising radiation on

human nerves is largely the outcome of studies on radiation-induced nerve involvement during the treatment of malignant lesions of the breast and parotid gland.

Cutaneous nerves are the most resistant of the subcutaneous tissue components to acute radiation but when they are involved the lesions are distributed irregularly and vary in severity across and along the nerve. The changes appear to be delayed effects in the form of conspicuous intra and paraneural fibrosis secondary to changes in the vessels and connective tissue that are more susceptible to radiation damage.

Postoperative radiation therapy directed to the supraclavicular and axillary regions following surgery for carcinoma of the breast introduces the risk of radiation damage to the brachial plexus which represents the most common, and clinically the most significant of the peripheral nerve lesions due to ionising radiation. The incidence appears to be related to the dosage. On balance, higher dosages produce symptoms earlier than lower dosages. In Stoll and Andrew's (1966) studies, the incidence was approximately five times higher with higher dosages.

A conspicuous feature of these lesions is the long delay between irradiation and the appearance of symptoms and signs of brachial plexus damage.

The initial symptoms are usually sensory in nature with pain, paraesthesiae, hypoaesthesia and weakness affecting the hand and fingers. However, the distribution of the motor and sensory disturbances naturally depends on the particular parts of the plexus affected. Severe pain is often the predominant symptom in the well-established lesion and spontaneous remissions or improvement of this pain are unusual. The pain is apparently the result of an impaired blood supply to nerves that are also threatened by an increasing fibrosis. The clinical course of the condition is one of steady deterioration of neurological function.

There is always the difficulty of distinguishing clinically between damage to the plexus from radiation therapy and that due to metastatic infiltration. The two present many features in common and uncertainty can only be resolved by exploration, inspection and the examination of biopsy material.

Points favouring metastatic involvement of the plexus are: (1) exploration of the plexus and the examination of biopsy material confirms the presence of metastatic infiltration; (2) the symptoms of plexus involvement antedated the use of radiation; (3) the existence of widespread metastatic complications elsewhere in the body.

The absence of such evidence would confirm radiation as the offending agent. Of course both radiation damage and metastatic invasion could co-exist.

The histological examination of biopsy material, and that obtained at autopsy, has confirmed the extensive, though patchy, fibrosis in, through and around the plexus which at times makes identification of the neural structures extremely difficult. Within the scarred region fibrosis constricts and obliterates the fasciculi and their contained nerve fibres. Many axons and myelin sheaths have disintegrated, or are in the process of disintegrating, the perineurium and endoneurium are thickened and blood vessels obliterated. A conspicuous feature of advanced lesions is the considerable amount of scar tissue present. It is as if radiation had been responsible for bringing about a delayed change in the behaviour of fibroblasts, leading to their unrestrained proliferation and the continued deposition of collagen. Thus the changes in the plexus do not appear to be due to direct radiation damage but are secondary effects in which the nerve fibres suffer as the result of the ischaemia and a constrictive fibrosis that follows the reaction of connective tissue and the destruction and obliteration of blood vessels. In severe damage all traces of the nerve may finally be lost in a mass of scar tissue. The fibrosis introduces a further complication by compromising lymph flow and drainage not only from the arm but also from the supraclavicular region. The resulting oedema leads to more fibrosis, scarring and ischaemia, all of which hasten the destruction of nerve fibres.

Treatment of this distressing complication of radiation therapy has not to date been encouraging. The problem is to arrest and reverse the remorseless deterioration that is a feature of these lesions.

Neurolysis to free imperilled nerve fibres introduces the risk of destroying an already depleted blood supply and of still further impoverishing nerve fibres. The results of neurolysis have not been encouraging except perhaps in the early stages. Omentoplasty designed to revascularise the plexus and improve the blood supply to nerve fibres, and to dampen the activity of fibroblasts has met with mixed success (Uhlschmid & Clodius 1978, Brunelli 1980, Narakas 1984).

The surgical treatment of malignant tumours of the parotid gland often requires sacrificing parts of the facial nerve and repairing the defect by grafting. Regarding the influence of postoperative radiation therapy on the outcome of facial nerve grafting, there are conflicting views. Some have concluded on experimental grounds and clinical experience that postoperative radiotherapy, at clinically acceptable dosage levels, has either no,

or a negligible effect, on the outcome of facial nerve grafting (Conley 1961, Miehlke et al 1972, McGuirt 1976, 1980, McGuirt and McCabe 1977). On the other hand, others are equally as convinced that this practice has a markedly detrimental effect on the return of facial function after grafting (Lathrop 1963, Pillsbury and Fisch 1982, Stearns 1982, Yamamoto and Fisch 1982).

These studies are complicated by the many other co-existing variables that affect the course and quality of the recovery after nerve grafting. However, on balance, the evidence suggests that postoperative radiotherapy in these cases does increase the risk of adversely affecting the outcome after nerve grafting.

REFERENCES

Injection nerve injury

Gentili F, Hudson A R, Kline D, Hunter D 1979 Peripheral nerve injection injury: An experimental study. Neurosurgery 4: 244

Gentili F, Hudson A R, Kline D, Hunter D 1980a Early changes following injection injury of peripheral nerves. Canadian Journal of Surgery 23: 177

Gentili F, Hudson A R, Hunter D, Kline D 1980b Nerve injection injury with local anesthetic agents: a light and electronmicroscopic, fluorescent microscopic and horseradish peroxidase study. Neurosurgery 6: 263

Gentili F, Hudson A R, Hunter D 1980c Clinical and experimental aspects of injection injuries of peripheral nerves. Le Journal Canadien des Sciences Neurologiques. May: 143

Hudson A R, Kline D, Gentili F 1978 Peripheral nerve injection injury. In: Omer G E, Spinner M (eds) Management of peripheral nerve problems, Saunders, Philadelphia, p 639

Sunderland S 1978 Nerves and nerve injuries, 2nd edn. Churchill Livingstone, Edinburgh, p 173

Nerve injury caused by cooling and freezing

Beazley R M, Bagley D H, Ketcham A S 1974 The effect of cryosurgery on peripheral nerves. Journal of Surgical Research 16: 231

Bickford R G 1939 The fibre dissociation produced by cooling human nerves. Clinical Science 4: 159

Bielschowsky M, Valetin B 1922 Die histologischen Veränderungen in durchfrorenen Nervenstrecken Journal für Psychologie und Neurologie. Leipzig, 29: 133

Byck R, Goldfarb J, Schaumburg H, Sharpless S K 1966 Reversible differential block of saphenous nerve by cold. Proceedings of International Congress of Biophysics, Vienna, September 1966. No. 436

Carter D C, Lee P W R, Gill W, Johnston R J 1972 The

effect of cryosurgery on peripheral nerve function. Journal of the Royal College of Surgeons of Edinburgh 17: 25

Denny-Brown D, Adams R D, Brenner C, Doherty M M 1945 The pathology of injury to nerve induced by cold. Journal of Neuropathology and Experimental Neurology 4: 305

Dodt E 1953 Differential thermosensitivity of mammalian A-fibres. Acta Physiologica Scandinavica 29: 91

Douglas W W, Malcolm J L 1955 The effect of localized cooling on conduction in cat nerves. Journal of Physiology, London 130: 63

Franz D N, Iggo A 1968 Conduction failure in myelinated and nonmyelinated axons at low temperatures. Journal of Physiology, London 199: 319

Gaster R N, Davidson T M, Rand R W, Fonkalsrud E W 1971 Comparison of nerve regeneration rates following controlled freezing or crushing. Archives of Surgery, Chicago 103: 378

Glasgow E F, Sinclair D C 1962 Dissociation of cold and warm sensibility in experimental blocks of the ulnar nerve Brain 85: 67

Kawano M, Matsumura H 1968 An electron microscopic study of pathological changes of the great occipital nerve following local cooling. Acta Medica, Nagasaki 12: 353

Lundberg A 1952 Potassium and the differential thermal sensitivity of the membrane potential spike, and negative after potential in mammalian A and C fibres. Acta Physiologica Scandinavica 15: (Supplementum 15) 1.

Mira J C 1971 Maintien de la continuité de la lame basale des fibres nerveuses myélinisées après une congélation localisée. Comptes Rendus des Séances de l'Académie des Sciences Série D 273: 1836

Mira J C 1972a Variations du nombre et du calibre des fibres nerveuses myélinisées après une 'section' des axones par congélation localisée. Comptes Rendus des Séances de l'Académie des Sciences Série D275: 979

Mira J C 1972b Effets d'une congélation localisée sur la structure des fibres nerveuses myélinisées et leur régéneration. Journal de Microscopie 14: 155

Mira J C 1979 Quantitative studies of the regeneration of rat myelinated nerve fibres: variations in the number and size of regenerating fibres after repeated localised freezings. Journal of Anatomy 129: 77

Mira J C 1981 Degeneration and regeneration of peripheral nerves: Ultrastructural and electrophysiological observations, quantitative aspects and muscle changes during reinnervation. International Journal of Microsurgery 3: 102

Paintal A S 1965a Block of conduction in mammalian myelinated nerve fibres by low temperatures. Journal of Physiology, London 180: 1

Paintal A S 1965b Effects of temperature on conduction in single vagal and saphenous myelinated nerve fibres of the cat. Journal of Physiology, London 180: 20

Paintal A S 1967 A comparison of the nerve impulses of mammalian non-medullated nerve fibres with those of the smallest diameter medullated fibres. Journal of Physiology, London 193: 523

Pribor D B, Novak R 1969 The relation of the cryoprotective action of dimethyl sulfoxide to salt damage to frog sciatic nerves. Cryobiology 6: 126

Schaumburg H, Byck R, Herman R, Rosengart C 1967 Peripheral nerve damage by cold. Archives of Neurology, Chicago 16: 103

Sinclair D C, Hinshaw J R 1951 Sensory changes in nerve blocks induced by cooling. Brain 74: 318

Torrance R W, Whitteridge D 1948 Technical aids in the study of respiratory reflexes. Journal of Physiology, London 107: 6P

Trendelburg W 1917 Langdauernde Nervenausschaltung mit sichere Regenerationsfähigkeit. Zeitschrift für die gesamte Experimentelle Medizin 5: 371

Trendelburg W 1918 Über langdauernde Nervenausschaltung mit sichere Regenerationsfähigkeit. Zeitschrift für die gesamte Experimentelle Medizin 7: 251

Waller A 1961 On the sensory, motory and vaso-motory symptoms resulting from refrigeration of the ulnar nerve. Proceedings of the Royal Society 11: 436

Weber E M 1847 Über den Einfluss der Erwärmung und Erkältung der Nerven auf ihr Leitungsvermögen. Archives d'Anatomie, d'Histologie et d'Embryologie (Strasbourg) 342

Whitteridge D 1948 Afferent nerve fibres from the heart and lungs in the cervical vagus. Journal of Physiology, London 107: 496

Widdicombe J G 1954 Receptors in the trachea and bronchi of the cat. Journal of Physiology, London 123: 71

Nerve injury caused by ionising radiation

Arnold M C, Harrison F, Bonte F J 1961 The effect of radiation on mammalian nerve. Radiology 77: 264

Bergström R 1962 Changes in peripheral nerve tissue after irradiation with high-energy protons. Acta Radiologica 58: 301

Brunelli G 1980 Neurolysis and free microvascular omentum transfer in the treatment of postactinic palsies of the brachial plexus. International Surgery 65: 515

Cavanagh J B 1968 Prior X-irradiation and the cellular response to nerve crush: duration of effect. Experimental Neurology 22: 253

Clemedson C J, Nelson A 1960 In: Errera M, Forssberg A (eds) Mechanisms in radiobiology, Vol. 2. Academic Press, New York, p 144

Conley J J 1961 Facial nerve grafting. Archives of Otolaryngology 73: 322

Hicks S P, Montgomery P O'B 1952 Effects of acute radiation on the adult mammalian central nervous system. Proceedings of the Society of Experimental Biological Medicine 80: 15

Janzen A H, Warren S 1942 Effects of roentgen-rays on the peripheral nerve of the rat. Radiology 38: 333

Lathrop F D 1963 Management of the facial nerve during operations on the parotid gland. Annals of Otolaryngology Rhinology and Laryngology 72: 780

Linder E 1959 Über das funktionelle und morphologische Verhalten peripherer nerven längere Zeit nach Bestrahlung. Fortschritte auf dem Gebiete der Röntgenstrahlen und der Nuklearmedizin 90: 618

McGuirt W F 1976 Effect of radiation therapy on facial nerve cable autografts Transactions. Ophthalmology and Otology 82: 486

McGuirt W F 1980 Cable grafting and irradiation. Archives of Otolaryngology 106: 445

McGuirt W F, McCabe B F 1977 Effect of radiation therapy on facial nerve cable autografts. Laryngoscope 87: 415

Miehlke A, Stennert E, Schuster R 1972 Über die Regeneration peripherer Nerven nach Einwirkung ionisierender Strahlen. ORL 34: 88

Narakas A O 1984 Operative treatment for radiation-induced and metastatic brachial plexopathy in 45 cases, 15 having an omentoplasty. Bulletin of the Hospital for Joint Diseases Orthopaedic Institute 44: 354

Pillsbury H C, Fisch U 1982 Extratemporal facial nerve grafting and radiotherapy. In: Graham M D House W F (eds) Disorders of the facial nerve. Raven Press, New York, p 463

Spiess H 1972 Schädigungen am peripheren Nervensystem durch ionisierende Strahlen. Springer-Verlag, Berlin

Stearns M P 1982 The effect of irradiation on nerve grafts. Clinical Otolaryngology 7: 161

Stoll B A, Andrews J T 1966 Radiation-induced peripheral neuropathy British Medical Journal 1: 834

Sunderland S 1978 Nerves and nerve injuries, 2nd edn. Churchill Livingstone, Edinburgh, p 177

Uhlschmid G, Clodius L 1978 A new use for the freely transplanted omentum. Management of a late radiation injury of the brachial plexus using freely transplanted omentum and neurolysis. Chirurgie 49: 714

Yamamoto E, Fisch U 1982 Effects of electron irradiation on results of facial nerve grafting In: Graham M C, House W F (eds) Disorders of the facial nerve. Raven Press, New York, p 179

22. Miscellaneous causes of nerve injury

NERVE INJURY CAUSED BY HIGH VELOCITY AND OTHER MISSILE WOUNDING

Missiles, travelling at high velocity, frequently cause wounds that are unexpectedly severe and out of all proportion to the size of the missile. These widespread, and often severe, effects are due to the violent motion set up in the tissues through which the missile passes.

Forces generated when a high velocity missile strikes and passes through tissues take the form of shock wave pressures on impact, high pressure regions in front of and lateral to the moving body, and pressures associated with the formation of a temporary explosive cavity in the track of the missile which changes shape in successive pulsations. As a result, structures adjacent to, and often considerable distances from this cavity are abruptly compressed, stretched, and deformed. This leads to further tissue damage. Thus not only is tissue directly in the path of the missile destroyed, but neighbouring structures are also damaged.

Missiles travelling at high velocities through limbs can produce a great variety of nerve injuries. Nerves directly in the path of the missiles are severed and large segments of them may be destroyed. Nerves which are off, but adjacent to, the track of the missile may be sufficiently elastic and mobile to withstand the stresses and strains generated about and in the wake of the missile. On the other hand, the forces created may be so severe that even nerves some distance away from the path of the missile are affected. These may suffer all degrees of damage, ranging from the transient paralyses of function seen in first degree injuries to the gross tears and loss of continuity that are irreparable and leave a permanent disability. It is important to note that, though nerves may be in continuity and appear on examination to be intact, they may harbour widespread microscopic lesions that are prejudicial to spontaneous recovery. Severe stretch injuries of peripheral nerves are often caused by high velocity missile wounding.

Shotgun wounding involving peripheral nerves also presents some special features.

1. The close range (contact to 14 feet) shotgun wound may contain not only sterile shot but also organic wadding.
2. The number of shot concentrated in a given area depends on the range, being progressively reduced with distance owing to scattering.
3. At close range the energy is concentrated in a small area so that there is always gross destruction of soft tissue. Peripheral nerves are more commonly injured than arteries. The extent of the nerve injury varies from lesions in continuity to transection or large segmental defects.
4. Shotgun wounding involves impact and blast effects. The damage caused by a close range shotgun blast is similar to that just described in some high velocity missile wounds, though the blast effect is greater in the latter and the direct injury effect greater in the former.
5. As the range increases the shot pattern scatters and the energy is dispersed over a wider area. Extensive segmental destruction is then less likely, while the chances of multiple wounding at widely separated sites are increased.

NERVE INJURIES ASSOCIATED WITH CLOSED FRACTURES AND DISLOCATIONS

Serious nerve injury complicating closed fractures and dislocations is uncommon. Spontaneous recovery is the rule in those cases where severe traction can be excluded and routine exploration is not justified.

The nerve may be damaged at the time of the accident or it may escape at that time only to be involved during the treatment of the fracture or dislocation, or at a later date by changes that develop as the result of the original injury. Though it may at times be difficult to determine the precise chronological sequence of events at and following the accident, nerve lesions complicating bone and joint injuries may be classified as primary, early secondary and late secondary, remembering that these distinctions are not always clear.

Immediate involvement. Primary lesion

In these cases the nerve is damaged at the moment of fracture or dislocation by:

1. the same force that fractures the bone or dislocates the joint. Thus a violent blow on the outer aspect of the upper arm may not only fracture the humerus but also simultaneously crush the radial nerve against the bone;

2. Some secondary mechanism that is introduced indirectly by the fracture or dislocation at the time of the accident, e.g. direct impact from a bony fragment, stretch following separation of the bone ends, pressure from a displaced bone shaft, fragment or articular surface, or trauma between the bone ends. The radial nerve may escape direct injury at the time of the accident but be impaled on a spike of bone or suddenly and violently stretched as the bone ends of the fractured humerus separate.

These lesions are characterised by the abrupt and total loss of function over the distribution of the injured nerve dating from the time of the accident. Sometimes they escape immediate notice because of the preoccupation with the bone or joint injury which dominates the clinical picture, so that nerve involvement is only detected some time later.

Early involvement. Early secondary lesion

This type of lesion is characterised by:

1. the abrupt loss of function caused when the nerve is damaged during clumsy and unskilful manipulations or operative procedures undertaken to reduce the fracture or dislocation. Though the open reduction and fixation of fractures is usually safe in capable and experienced hands, it carries with it the decided risk of damage to neighbouring nerves;

2. a delayed gradual onset in which function is at first impaired and then gradually deteriorates until it fails completely. The nerve lesion in these cases may be due to:

a. Involvement of the nerve in scar tissue or callus.

b. The development of a friction neuritis secondary to repeated trauma inflicted on the nerve where:

  i it is stretched by an unreduced or incompletely reduced dislocation or bony fragment around which it rides during movement;

  ii it rubs across a sharp projecting bony fragment or irregular bony surface;

  iii it is adherent to bone.

In these cases the clinical manifestations of nerve involvement appear 1–2 months after the accident. It is, of course, possible for a lesion which is of the primary type initially to develop into a secondary lesion;

3. deteriorating neurological function in the distribution of a nerve which is compressed by an incorrectly applied and ill-fitting plaster cast or splint. The loss of function in these cases may be painless.

Late involvement. Delayed secondary lesion

These are the 'tardy' lesions of delayed onset in which some years elapse before signs and symptoms of nerve involvement appear and become fully established. The onset is insidious and the deterioration of function gradual and progressive but irregular. These delayed effects are due to the development of complications, consequential on the fracture or dislocation, that result in slow compression, stretch or friction of the affected nerve. Characteristic of this group is the tardy ulnar palsy that follows injuries about the elbow joint.

The nature and severity of the nerve injury

The nerve may be damaged by compression, stretch and/or friction. The lesion may be circumscribed or extensive, nor is it necessarily uniform in severity or distribution either across the nerve or along the length affected. Nerve damage associated with bone and joint injuries varies from first to fifth degree involvement (Chapter 25), from simple rapidly reversible conduction block at one end of the scale to severance by a bony spike or rupture from violent traction at the other.

Of particular significance are the traction or stretch injuries, which may be serious but fortunately are not common. Here the forces act along the nerve and, if the violence is severe, this damage may extend for considerable distances proximal and distal to the fracture site; the nerve may be ruptured or anatomical continuity preserved despite the severity of the damage.

Dislocations may cause nerve injuries varying in severity from transient paralysis, such as occurs following involvement of the axillary (circumflex humeral) nerve in dislocation of the shoulder joint, to the severe and extensive tears that may involve the lateral popliteal (common peroneal) nerve in injuries that rupture ligamentous structures and dislocate the knee joint.

Signs of nerve involvement associated with a closed fracture usually indicate a lesion in continuity that will recover spontaneously. This, however, is not invariably the case, particularly in stretch or traction injuries which may result in extensive damage along the nerve trunk or even in rupture of the nerve. An offending bony spike in proximity to the nerve should suggest the possibility of more severe damage while a palpable swelling on the nerve is evidence that at least some of the nerve fibres have sustained a third degree injury. Though the chances of achieving a satisfactory functional result under these conditions are considerably reduced, there are occasions when good recovery may still occur spontaneously.

OBSTETRICAL, BIRTH AND NEONATAL NERVE INJURIES

Nerve injury in the mother may result from pressure on the roots of the sciatic nerve in the pelvis by the foetal head or from trauma caused by the blades of obstetrical forceps during a difficult delivery. The lumbosacral cord is particularly vulnerable to injury where it crosses the ala of the sacrum and the effects of the lesion are maximal in the fibres for the lateral popliteal division of the sciatic nerve. A combination predisposing to nerve compression by the foetal head is small women and large babies. Lesions of the lateral popliteal and saphenous nerves may follow pressure inadvertently applied in the region of the knee during delivery. Recovery is usually well advanced by the 2nd to the 3rd month but may be delayed for a year.

In the newborn the facial nerve, the brachial plexus and the radial and posterior interosseous nerves are most prone to injury. Nerve involvement is rare in the lower limb but has been described for the sciatic, lateral popliteal and obturator nerves. In sciatic nerve injuries the lateral popliteal fibres usually suffer most because of their greater vulnerability to pressure and stretch (p. 68). It is possible that the nerves of the lower limb are involved more frequently than is recorded, nerve damage passing unrecognised because recovery occurs so rapidly.

Aetiology

Nerve injuries in the newborn may be due to:

1. Pressure on the nerve during uterine development from constriction of a limb by the umbilical cord or amniotic bands.
2. Pressure on the nerve during difficult parturition from:

   a. compression against the sacral promontory, symphysis pubis, or the bony prominence of a normal or deformed pelvis, and compression due to uterine pathology;

   b. a rigid cervix or uterine contraction rings;
   c. the use of forceps to aid delivery;
   d. fractures.

3. Stretch as the result of:

   a. abnormal tension on the nerve caused when a limb is maintained in an abnormal position in utero for a long period. Thus acute flexion of the extended leg at the hip in breech presentation may stretch the sciatic nerve over the dorsal aspect of the hip joint and the obturator nerve under the superior ramus of the os pubis;

   b. traction on the limb or forcible intra-uterine manipulations to assist delivery. By far the most common peripheral nerve injuries in the birth palsy group are those involving the brachial plexus.

4. Ischaemic lesions of the sciatic nerve resulting from injections into the umbilical cord. Several cases of neonatal sciatic palsy have been described in which the aetiology has remained obscure. The findings, however, have suggested that the nerve lesion was caused by the accidental injection of an analeptic drug into an artery instead of a vein in the umbilical cord. The drug is believed to pass by way of the umbilical artery to the hypogastric artery where it results in arterial spasm or thrombosis which involves the blood supply not only to the sciatic nerve but also to other tissues.

5. Intramuscular injections. Nerve injury due to therapeutic injections in the newborn.

6. Involvement in regions of subcutaneous fat necrosis. The cause of subcutaneous fat necrosis in the newborn is not known though it is usually attributed to obstetrical trauma. In these cases the nerve lesion could be due to direct trauma or could originate secondarily from involvement in the fibrosis which replaces the necrosing tissue. Lesions affecting the outer aspect of the arm above the elbow may be responsible for damage to the radial nerve.

Pathology

Most lesions are examples of first degree injury which recover rapidly and completely. Severe pressure or stretch may cause second and third degree damage, while ischaemia may lead to extensive lesions which carry a high incidence of incomplete recovery.

NERVE INJURIES CAUSED DURING ANAESTHESIA, COMA, DRUG NARCOSIS AND THE UNDISTURBED SLEEP OF THE FATIGUED AND WASTED INDIVIDUAL

These constitute a special group of compression, stretch and ischaemic nerve lesions.

Nerve damage observed postoperatively has been the subject of many reports. When relaxed under anaesthesia the patient is more susceptible to the effects of abnormal positioning of the limbs and may be subjected to postural insults against which he is unable to protest. Under these conditions nerves may be damaged and the injury not detected until the patient has recovered from the anaesthetic. Illustrative examples are pressure on the radial, median or ulnar nerves against the edge of the operating table, the involvement of the brachial plexus from abnormal positioning on the table, and pressure on the lateral popliteal and saphenous nerves by the straps of the stirrups used for the lithotomy position.

Some post-anaesthetic lesions of the brachial plexus are due to compression but most are stretch injuries. In the case of the other nerves compression is the offending agent. Tourniquet paralysis, which may be produced during the course of an operation, is discussed under compression injuries.

Patients should be examined preoperatively as a routine procedure, to detect or exclude any signs and symptoms referable to nerve damage. Should, for any reason, a pre-existing established nerve lesion pass unnoticed, help in differentiating this from damage of immediate origin may be provided from an electromyographic examination of the affected muscles. Electromyographic evidence typical of nerve involvement does not appear in limb muscles until 16–21 days after denervation.

Peripheral nerves may be damaged when they are subjected to unrelieved compression against an unyielding surface for periods of hours or even days. This occurs in the stuporous alcoholic in the classical 'Saturday night' paralysis, in prolonged coma due to drugs, injury or metabolic disturbances and in the deep undisturbed sleep of the very fatigued individual when warning sensations are no longer perceived. Under these conditions nerves are more vulnerable where:

1. the nerve contains little epineurial connective tissue packing;
2. the individual is extremely wasted so that the protective padding of softer tissue is greatly reduced or absent;
3. there is underlying nerve pathology in the form of a latent neuropathy, based on a metabolic disorder, obliterative disease of the nutrient arteries or some other cause.

The duration and intensity of the deformation determine the severity of the nerve damage which varies from a conduction block first degree injury to one of third degree and even, in unusual circumstances, to necrosis of the nerve.

IATROGENIC NERVE INJURIES

Iatrogenic nerve injuries are those inflicted during clinical management by misadventure based on ignorance or unavoidable circumstances. In avoiding iatrogenic damage there is no substitute for a sound knowledge of regional anatomy.

The literature relating to iatrogenic nerve lesions up to 1977 is reviewed in Sunderland's *Nerves and Nerve Injuries* (1978). Only more recent and relevant references are included here. A reference that should be consulted is one by Bonney (1986).

Injection injuries

1. Therapeutic injections. When administering any form of intramuscular injection it is necessary to keep in mind the regional anatomy of nerve trunks in order to ensure that the site selected for the injection is well clear of any nerve. The radial and sciatic nerves are the principal victims but any nerve is at risk in the hands of the careless and ignorant. This subject is also discussed in Chapter 21.
2. Needle trauma to a nerve during nerve block anaesthesia. Selander et al (1977) have shown that a 45° bevelled needle is less likely to damage fasciculi.

3. Intrafascicular needle recording. The effects of microneurography electrode penetration of the rat sciatic nerve have been studied by Fried, Frisen and Mozart (1989). Such penetrations always produced lesions resulting in the degeneration of myelinated and nonmyelinated axons, followed by regeneration which was not complete 9 and even 16 weeks later.
4. The median nerve may be damaged:

   a. during axillary arteriography or catheterisation, or subsequently by compression from a haematoma;
   b. during brachial arteriovenous fistula construction for maintenance haemodialysis;
   c. from misplaced intravenous injections in the cubital fossa (Berry & Wallis 1977);
   d. directly or by compression from a haematoma following puncture of the lower brachial artery for arterial gas sampling (Luce et al 1976, Pape et al 1978);
   e. during exposure of the brachial artery in the cubital fossa for cardiac catheterisation (Schneck 1960).
5. The brachial plexus may be damaged during subclavian vein catheterisation and following axillary arteriotomy-angiography (O'Keefe 1980, Joyce & Stewart-Wynne 1983).
6. Sciatic nerve paresis following internal iliac artery embolisation to control pelvic haemorrhage. It is assumed that the procedure leads to a blocking of the inferior gluteal artery and its major branch to the sciatic nerve (p. 58).

Nerve injuries caused by the tight application of a bandage, plaster cast or tourniquet

1. Compression injury of the common peroneal nerve at the neck of the fibula caused by the misapplication of a cast.
2. Tourniquet paralysis.

The 1980s have seen a remarkable increase in interest in tourniquet physiology and pathology, particular attention being given to an evaluation of the inflatable tourniquet, the fate of the tissues both under and below the tourniquet, the complications of excessive tourniquet pressures and how to avoid them, and the duration of tourniquet applications and all directed to making the procedure safe and reliable (Bolton & McFarlane 1978, Klenerman & Hulands 1979, Saunders et al 1979, Klenerman 1980, 1982, 1983, Klenerman et al 1980, 1982, Hurst et al 1981, Yates et al 1981, Lundborg & Rydevik 1982, Shaw & Murray 1982, Aho et al 1983, Sapega et al 1985, Newman & Muirhead 1986, Nitz et al 1986, Lundborg 1988).

Characteristic features of tourniquet paralysis.

1. They are more common in the upper limb than in the lower because of the exposed position of the major nerves above the elbow as compared with the protected course pursued by the sciatic nerve in the thigh.
2. The radial nerve is the most commonly and seriously affected but the sciatic nerve, particularly the common peroneal division, is not immune. The greater vulnerability of the radial nerve is explained by its direct relationship to the humerus where it is usually composed of a single fasciculus, or two or three major fasciculi, with little protective epineurial tissue. The same applies to the common peroneal nerve in the distal part of the thigh.
3. Motor nerve fibres are the most susceptible.
4. The nerve lesion varies from first to third degree damage.
5. Spontaneous recovery is usually complete or well advanced by the third month but may be delayed for six.
6. The following points relate to safety margins for the application of the tourniquet:

   a. The conventional inflatable wide cuff should be used.
   b. The pressure should be not much greater than that required to achieve a bloodless field.
   c. The duration of application should not exceed 2 hours and this should be reduced if there is evidence of peripheral vascular disease.

Sapega et al (1985) recommend limiting the ini-

tial application to 1–1.5 hours with a release period of 5 minutes, followed by an additional 1–1.15 hours of compression.

Nerves at risk during the open or closed reduction of a fracture or dislocation

While the open reduction and fixation of fractures is usually safe in capable and experienced hands, it carries with it the risk of damaging neighbouring nerves.

1. Axillary nerve and the shoulder joint.
2. Radial nerve and fractures of the humerus.
3. Interosseous nerve and fracture dislocations about the humeral-radioulnar joint.
4. Median and ulnar nerves in fractures about the elbow joint.
5. The sciatic nerve at the hip joint when reducing a dislocation or during hip replacement.
6. The sciatic nerve and fractures of the femur.

Nerve injuries caused when the patient is deeply anaesthetised

When relaxed under anaesthesia the unprotesting patient is more susceptible to the abnormal positioning of the limbs and may be subjected to postural insults against which he is unable to complain. Under these conditions nerves may suffer compression and stretch damage, for example the radial, median and ulnar nerves against the edge of the operating table, involvement of the brachial plexus from abnormal positioning on the table and pressure on the common peroneal and saphenous nerves by the straps of the stirrups in the lithotomy position.

There is also the risk of nerve compression injury from the use of a tourniquet during the course of an operation.

Inadvertent transection of a nerve and nerve injury occurring during a surgical procedure

1. The palmar cutaneous branch and the thenar motor branch of the median nerve during carpal tunnel surgery.
2. The infrapatellar cutaneous branch of the

saphenous nerve in incisions about the knee joint.

3. Transection of the accessory nerve or greater auricular nerve at the posterior border of the sternocleidomastoid muscle during the biopsy removal of a cervical lymph node.

4. Transection of the ilioinguinal, iliohypogastric, genitofemoral and even the femoral nerves with incisions in the inguinal region.

5. Surgical procedures at the wrist where the median nerve is mistakenly used instead of the palmaris longus tendon for a tendon graft.

6. The median and ulnar nerves may be inadvertently included in a ligature or clamp applied to the brachial or ulnar artery, respectively, to control haemorrhage.

7. The long thoracic nerve may be inadvertently severed during surgical procedures on the axilla.

8. Traction injury of the brachial plexus during cardiac surgery involving standard median sternotomy with wide retraction of the sternum (Seyfer et al 1985).

REFERENCES

Aho K, Saino K, Chianta M, Varpanen E 1983 Pneumatic tourniquet paralysis. Journal of Bone and Joint Surgery 65B: 441

Berry P R, Wallis W E 1977 Venepuncture. Lancet, i: 1236

Bolton C, McFarlane R 1978 Human pneumatic tourniquet paralysis. Neurology 28: 787

Bonney G 1986 Iatrogenic injuries of nerves. Journal of Bone and Joint Surgery 68B: 9

Fried K, Frisen J, Mozart M 1989 De- and regeneration of axons after minor lesions in the rat sciatic nerve. Effects of micro-neurography electrode penetrations. Pain 36: 93

Hurst L N, Weiglein O, Brown W F, Campbell G J 1981 The pneumatic tourniquet: a biomechanical and electrophysiological study. Plastic and Reconstructive Surgery 67: 648

Joyce D A, Stewart-Wynne E G 1983 Brachial plexopathy complicating central venous catheter insertion. The Medical Journal of Australia p 82

Klenerman L 1980 Tourniquet time — how long? Hand 12: 231

Klenerman L 1982 The tourniquet in operations on the knee: a review. Journal of Royal Society of Medicine 75: 31

Klenerman L 1983 Tourniquet paralysis. Journal of Bone and Joint Surgery 65B: 374

Klenerman L, Hulands G H 1979 Tourniquet pressure for the lower limb. Journal of Bone and Joint Surgery 61B: 124

Klenerman L, Menakshi B, Hulands G H, Rhodes A M 1980 Systemic and local effects of the application of a tourniquet. Journal of Bone and Joint Surgery 62B: 385

Klenerman L, Crawley J, Lowe A 1982 Hyperemia and swelling of a limb upon release of a tourniquet. Acta Orthopaedica Scandinavica 53: 209.

Luce E A, Futrell J W, Wilgis E F S, Hooper J E 1976 Compression neuropathy following brachial arterial puncture in anti-coagulated patients. Journal Trauma 16: 717

Lundborg G 1988 Nerve injury and repair. Churchill Livingstone, Edinburgh, p 80

Lundborg G, Rydevik B 1982 The bloodless field in hand and arm surgery: theoretical and practical aspects. Läkartodmomgem, Stockholm 79: 4035

Newman R J, Muirhead A 1986 A prospective evaluation of a safe and effective low pressure tourniquet system. Journal of Bone and Joint Surgery 68B: 625

Nitz A J, Bodner J J, Matulionis D H 1986 Pneumatic tourniquet application and nerve integrity: motor function and electrophysiology. Experimental Neurology 94: 264

O'Keefe D M 1980 Brachial plexus injury following axillary arteriotomy — angiography. Journal of Neurosurgery 53: 583

Pape K E, Armstrong D L, Fitzhardinge P M 1978 Peripheral median nerve damage secondary to brachial arterial blood gas sampling. The Journal of Pediatrics 93: 852

Sapega A A, Heppenstall R B, Chance B, et al 1985 Optimizing tourniquet application; release times in extremity surgery. Journal of Bone and Joint Surgery 67A: 303

Saunders K, Louis D, Weingarden S, Waylonis W 1979 Effects of tourniquet time on postoperative quadriceps function. Clinical Orthopaedics and Related Research 143: 194

Schneck S A 1960 Peripheral and cranial nerve injuries resulting from general surgical procedures. Archives of Surgery, Chicago 5: 53

Selander D, Dhuner K-G, Lundborg G 1977 Peripheral nerve injury due to injection needles used for regional anesthesia. Acta Anaesthesiologica Scandinavica 21: 182

Seyfer A E 1985 Upper extremity neuropathies after cardiac surgery. Journal of Hand Surgery 10A: 16

Shaw J A, Murray D G 1982 The relationship between tourniquet pressure and underlying soft-tissue pressure in the thighs. Journal of Bone and Joint Surgery 64A: 1148

Sunderland S 1978 Nerves and nerve injuries, 2nd edn. Churchill Livingstone, Edinburgh

Yates S K, Hurst L, Brown W F 1981 The pathogenesis of pneumatic tourniquet paralysis in men. Journal of Neurology, Neurosurgery and Psychiatry 44: 759

23. Neuromas

TERMINOLOGY

Reference to the meaning attached to the term neuroma in the literature reveals differences that necessitate stating specifically what is meant by the term in this text on nerve injury. Here neuroma is used to describe a post-traumatic phenomenon in the form of a non-neoplastic disorganised bulbous enlargement that develops at the ends of a severed peripheral nerve or at the site of injury to a nerve in continuity.

Since this book is devoted exclusively to the subject of nerve injury and nerve repair, and having established the post-traumatic basis of the *neuroma*, it will be convenient henceforth to delete the prefix post-traumatic from the term.

Proximal and distal neuromas. These are the bulbous enlargements found at the cut ends of a severed nerve. Both are associated with a peripheral nerve, hence the term neuroma, but the proximal differs significantly from the distal neuroma in that the former contains regenerating neural elements and the latter does not.

Spindle neuroma. A localised swelling of a nerve in continuity caused by the proliferation of the connective tissue elements of the nerve in response to trauma. With some injuries in continuity the swelling also contains regenerating axons and proliferating Schwann cells.

THE PATHOGENESIS OF NEUROMA FORMATION

An important function of the Schwann cells and endoneurial sheath is to insulate axons from the surrounding tissues. After second degree injuries this insulating function of the endoneurium confines regenerating axons to endoneurial tubes, thereby inevitably guiding them back to the end organs they originally innervated. If this limiting barrier is destroyed, regenerating axons escape into, and branch freely within, a disorganised mass of fibroblasts and Schwann cells to form a swelling that is usually referred to as a neuroma. However the simple term, bulb, is probably more appropriate. The connective tissue absorbs, distorts and limits this disorderly axonal growth and spread so that ultimately the neuroma ceases to enlarge. Thus the presence of a swelling on a nerve is evidence that the endoneurium has been breached and that an injury of at least third degree severity has been sustained. Conversely, lesions that do not break the endoneurium are not associated with neuroma formation.

The development, structure and size of a neuroma depend on:

1. the numbers of axon sprouts that emerge from ruptured endoneurial tubes and escape into the surrounding connective tissue;
2. the extent to which their further growth in this new environment is distorted and disorganised;
3. related changes in the connective tissue characterised by the proliferation of Schwann cells and fibroblasts in response to trauma and the presence of regenerating axons.

The following is an arbitrary and simple classification of neuromas based on considerations of convenience.

1. Neuromas on nerves in continuity.

2. The formation of bulbs at the ends of severed nerves.
3. Suture line neuromas.
4. Amputation stump neuromas.
5. Painful neuromas.

NEUROMAS ON NERVES IN CONTINUITY

Localised swellings on nerves in continuity are of two main types, those in which the perineurial sheath of fasciculi is not broken and those in which it is (Fig. 23.1).

Lesions in which the perineurium is not broken. Pseudo-neuromas

1. Spindle-shaped swellings may develop on nerves where they are subjected to repeated

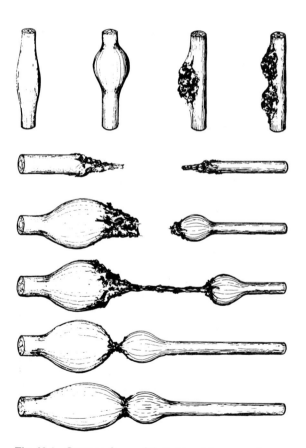

Fig. 23.1 Common forms of 'bulbs' involving nerves in continuity and the ends of a severed nerve.

friction or irritation. Initially the enlargement is due to an increase in the connective tissues of the nerve, nerve fibres escaping direct injury. However, there are further developments if physical trauma persists and the reactionary fibrosis continues to increase.

Nerve fibres ultimately suffer both from direct injury and indirectly from the deepening fibrosis that constricts nerve fibres and impairs their blood supply.

Symptoms of this involvement include paraesthesiae, a deepening numbness of the area served by the affected nerve, and severe pain when the swelling is compressed or the nerve stretched. Examples of this type of neuroma are the interdigital neuroma in Morton's metatarsalgia, and the nodule found on the lateral femoral cutaneous nerve in meralgia paraesthetica where the nerve passes beneath or through the inguinal ligament. In bowler's thumb neuroma the medial digital nerve of the thumb is repeatedly compressed and traumatised as the thumb is firmly held against the edge of the hole in the bowling ball.

The terminal stage in the development of these neuromas is marked by their conversion into a collagenised and relatively avascular mass in which nerve fibres have been constricted by fibrosis. Wallerian degeneration occurs below the lesion and attempts at spontaneous regeneration through the neuroma are unsuccessful, though regenerating axons will grow into and terminate in the enlargement to increase its sensitivity to deformation. Needless to say, the destruction of nerve fibres is not always complete, for circumstances may be such that some survive.

2. The enlargement may be a sequel to a third degree injury resulting in the degeneration and regeneration of axons. The normal undamaged perineurium is resistant to penetration by regenerating axons so that in this type of injury the reaction is confined within the damaged fasciculi. When axons commence regenerating, axon tips are obstructed in their growth by the intrafascicular fibrosis. Confronted with this obstacle the axons continue to sprout, become swollen, and twist and turn in their efforts to continue their advance. All this leads to the formation of a spindle-shaped enlargement of the nerve trunk

that is usually small and firm or hard. Since the swelling is confined to fasciculi, its size and form depend on the size and number of the fasciculi affected. The largest spindle neuromas are found at levels where a nerve is composed of a single large fasciculus or a few large fasciculi. Intrafascicular haemorrhage, which usually occurs with third degree injuries, and the associated cellular reaction contribute to the swelling. In more severe third degree injury these vascular and cellular complications also involve the interfascicular tissue, thereby adding to the size of the neuroma.

It is worthy of note that extensive intrafascicular damage may involve considerable lengths of a nerve without the formation of a swelling. Under these circumstances the changes are evenly distributed and ultimately convert the fasciculus into a fibrous cord.

Neuroma formation when the perineurium is ruptured by the injury

When some fasciculi are breached or severed, regenerating axons escape into the interfascicular epineurial tissue where they continue to grow, branch and ramify widely in a disorganised way. This occurs in association with proliferating fibroblasts, Schwann cells, macrophages and capillaries to form a mass in which the proportion of cells to collagen fibres varies as does its vascularity. With time, progressive fibrosis converts a soft swelling into a firm hard nodule. This is the genesis of the largest swellings observed on injured nerves in continuity. The multiple scattered nodules seen in tears of the brachial plexus are also formed in this way, the plexiform arrangement preventing the separation of nerve ends which remain linked by a neuromatous mass.

Depending on the location of the damaged fasciculi in the nerve these pathological developments may cause a general enlargement at the site of the injury or, if the lesion is partial and more superficially placed, the neuroma projects from the surface of the nerve. Such a partial nerve injury may be one in which the damaged fasciculi are: (1) breached but not severed; (2) severed though the ends have been prevented from retracting because of the nature of the fascicular plexuses; or

(3) severed with retraction and separation of the ends of the fasciculi.

Though these various grades of injury may, and usually do, occur in combination it is convenient to consider neuroma formation in each case.

Lateral neuroma formation associated with breaks in the perineurium

When the protective perineurial sheath is breached, the subjacent contents of the fasciculus are herniated through the opening under the influence of the intrafascicular pressure. This mass of extruded tissue, which forms a swelling on the surface of the fasciculus, consists of injured nerve fibres, Schwann cells, fibroblasts and vessels into which regenerating axons may subsequently grow. This extrusion varies from a small lateral swelling to more extensive irregular involvement of the nerve trunk depending on the number of fasciculi affected, their size and the site where they are ruptured.

Lateral neuroma formation associated with fascicular severance and minimal retraction of the fasciculi

There is little, if any, neuroma formation where only a few superficial fasciculi are severed without retraction of the fascicular ends. This is because the region between the severed fasciculi is soon occupied by blood clot, fibroblasts and Schwann cells which rapidly restore fascicular continuity. Though all axons in the affected fasciculi are severed, the close proximity of the fascicular ends and the bridging tissue of Schwann cells and fibroblasts mean that when regenerating axons reach this region few go astray. The end result is an irregularity of the surface of the nerve at the site of injury or a small lateral swelling. Though usually small, the consistency and dimensions of these lateral neuromas depend on such factors as the size of the affected fasciculi, the distance between the severed fascicular ends, the nature and extent of the local cellular reaction and the number of axons obstructed and deflected by the bridging tissue.

Lateral neuroma formation associated with fascicular severance and wide separation of the ends of the fasciculi

When the ends of the severed fasciculi are well separated, swellings form on their proximal and distal ends as described for severed nerve trunks. These lateral swellings may become continuous to form an irregular lateral enlargement or may fail to meet and remain separated by a notch. Under these conditions more regenerating axons go astray or are obstructed in their growth. Thus large lateral neuromas, and particularly those that are notched, are evidence of greater damage to the nerve.

THE FORMATION AND MICROSTRUCTURE OF BULBS ON SEVERED NERVES

The distance separating the ends of a severed nerve trunk varies depending on the length of nerve destroyed and the extent to which the nerve ends retract. Because of the greater elasticity of the fasciculi, their ends retract still further within the loose epineurial framework. The region between the nerve ends is occupied by blood clot, the damaged tissue of the nerve bed and neighbouring structures and sometimes foreign material.

The changes occurring at the proximal nerve end result in the formation of a 'bulb' that differs in certain significant respects from that which develops at the distal nerve end. (Fig. 23.1).

The proximal bulb or neuroma

The changes result in the early appearance of three zones in the proximal stump:

1. A proximal zone of normal nerve with the exception of those axons that are disintegrating because of retrograde neuronal degeneration. This action passes without any sharp line of demarcation into:
2. An intermediate zone where the nerve fibres are undergoing Wallerian degeneration and are becoming converted into endoneurial tubes occupied by Schwann cells. The remaining architectural features of the nerve trunk are preserved. Injuries that sever the

nerve usually result in some retrograde nerve fibre degeneration that may extend centrally for distances of 3–4 centimetres.

3. A distal or terminal zone. This includes the severed ends of the fasciculi and the epineurial tissue through which they have retracted. It is a disorganised region of blood clot, tissue fluid and a cellular reaction involving fibroblasts and Schwann cells that have emerged from the ends of the severed fasciculi. The escape of tissue fluid and cells from the cut end of the fasciculi is aided by the intrafascicular pressure from above. The terminal zone of loose vascular cellular tissue formed in this way varies in amount according to the magnitude of the reaction, but the overall effect is to form a club-shaped swelling at the end of the proximal stump.

With the onset of regeneration axon sprouts descend along the endoneurial tubes and finally escape into the disorganised matrix of the terminal zone, where they branch and rebranch irregularly to contribute to the general disorganised structure of the bulb.

The intermediate and terminal zones now present additional features that give the fully developed neuroma its characteristic form and structure (Figs 23.2 & 23.3).

1. The proximal zone of normal nerve is essentially unchanged;
2. The intermediate zone shows fasciculi occupied by fine regenerating axons descending along endoneurial tubes in intimate relationship with Schwann cells. Later these fibres become myelinated and their complex sheath reconstituted, but their dimensions and structure are never fully restored;
3. The distal or terminal zone is now composed of organising blood clot and a tangled, disorganised mass of fibroblasts, Schwann cells, vessels and fine branching regenerating axons.

The axons enter this distal zone singly, or in small collections or bundles that range in diameter from 10 to 50 μm. Since they are no longer con-

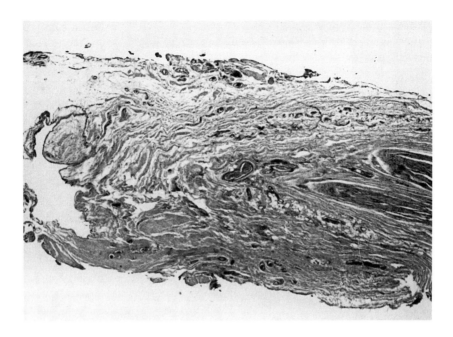

Fig. 23.2   Longitudinal section through the distal or terminal zone of disorganised tissue of a proximal neuroma.

fined within fasciculi the axons fan out, and the complexity and irregularity of their growth in this new situation are influenced by the density and arrangement of the fibroblast–Schwann cell matrix. This is usually such that the axons are obstructed, deflected and distorted as they grow and branch. As a result, axons or bundles of axons cross and zig-zag through the tissue and interlace in patternless confusion. Individual axons end blindly in club-shaped swellings or discs, or are deflected into whorls or convolutions, some of which return along the regenerating fibre. Axonal growth, though grossly disorganised, is profuse, with axons branching and rebranching as they wind irregularly through the tissue. Though most regenerating axons end blindly in the terminal zone, some succeed in passing through it to continue on towards the distal stump or into the tissues forming the nerve bed. Associated with this axonal growth is a further proliferation of Schwann cells and fibroblasts, all of which adds to the bulk of the neuroma.

The sum total of these changes is the formation of a pronounced swelling that varies in size and consistency depending on its vascularity and the amount and density of each of its major components: axons, Schwann cells, fibroblasts and collagen fibres.

Enlargement ceases only when axon growth is finally spent in the Schwann cell–fibroblast framework of this mass.

It takes about 3 weeks for a neuroma to reach a size that can be detected by palpation.

Since axon growth tends to be more active the closer the lesion is to the parent neurons, bulbs forming at proximal levels are usually larger than those developing when the nerve is severed at the periphery.

With the passage of time the loose vascular cellular tissue of the early stages is usually replaced by a denser sclerotic connective tissue matrix that finally gives the bulb a firm to hard and nodular consistency, and a greyish white colour.

Infection and the presence of foreign bodies are additional complications that promote fibrosis and, in this way, contribute to the final form, size and consistency of the bulb.

The bulb may be circumscribed and well-encapsulated in a fibrous sheath or it may be less well-defined and firmly attached to surrounding tissues by adhesions. These often contain regenerating axons that have escaped from the

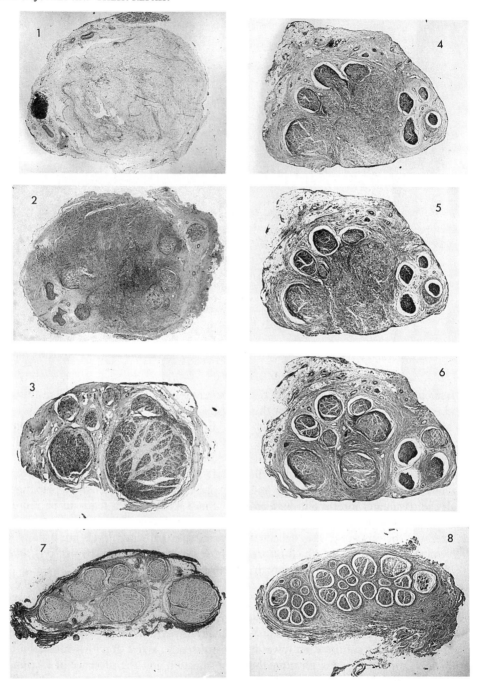

Fig. 23.3 Transverse sections through neuromas to illustrate variations in histological structure at different levels.
1. The featureless poorly staining distal extremity of the neuroma.
2. Traces of fasciculi are appearing in the section.
3. Intraneural fibrosis is present both inside and external to the fasciculi.
4, 5 and 6 illustrate the gradually improving structure of the nerve stump as sectioning is carried proximally. Some fasciculi have been involved over greater distances than others.
7 and 8. Sections from the same nerve to illustrate the reduction in the density and amount of the interfascicular connective tissue. Both sections would be regarded as favourable for repair though conditions in 7 would be more favourable than those in 8.

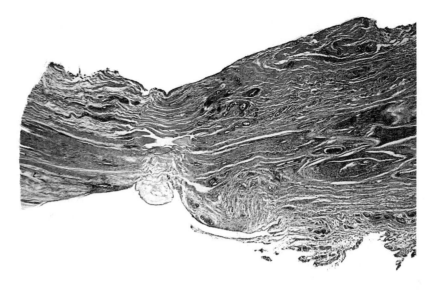

Fig. 23.4 Histological preparation, illustrating a band of tissue linking the proximal neuroma to smaller swelling on the distal nerve end.

bulb and extended further afield. This latter arrangement is commonly seen in extensive injuries involving adjacent tissues and the early development of adhesions that foster the wider dispersal of regenerating axons.

The proximal bulb may be widely separated from any distal swelling with strands radiating irregularly from each to anchor it to neighbouring tissues. On the other hand, proximal and distal bulbs may be linked by a band of tissue carrying regenerated axons or they may be fused with, or without, a junctional neck of varying thickness (Fig. 23.4).

When the nerve stumps are involved in scar tissue, the bulbs are found at the margin of the scar and, though adherent to this tissue they are rarely buried in it. The arrangement is one that suggests that the scar tissue is forming an impenetrable barrier against which growing axons and proliferating Schwann cells accumulate to form a relatively circumscribed mass.

THE CLINICAL SIGNIFICANCE OF THE PRESENCE OR ABSENCE OF A NEUROMA

It is important to note that a bulb does not always form at the end of the proximal stump of a severed nerve. Sometimes regenerating axons and proliferating Schwann cells and fibroblasts wander freely to become dispersed in damaged tissue planes, fascia and muscle, thereby attaching the nerve end to its bed. Pressure and traction on these areas may be painful.

In these cases it is not uncommon on exploring a nerve to find either one or both nerve stumps gradually merging into a mass of fibrous tissue in which all traces of continuity of the nerve trunk are lost.

In an experimental study by the author on neuroma formation, using an Australian marsupial (*Trichosurus vulpecula*), a segment of both median and ulnar nerves was removed between the axilla and the elbow. The duration of the experiments ranged from 9 to 485 days. The relevant findings of this study were:

1. Distal bulbs were absent in all 32 specimens examined.
2. A prominent proximal bulb was present in 13 specimens of each nerve.
3. A slight proximal swelling was present in 8 median and 7 ulnar specimens.
4. There was no trace of a proximal bulb in 11 median and 12 ulnar specimens.

These several observations have particular relevance to the diagnostic significance of a neuroma at the proximal end of a severed nerve. While it is correct to interpret the presence of a proximal neuroma as proof of a persisting potential for axon regeneration, it cannot be assumed from the absence of such a neuroma that the proximal stump is no longer a viable source for regenerating axons. This is because axon regeneration at the proximal nerve end does not always result in the formation of a neuroma.

Finally, lesions in continuity that are clinically complete, but show a bulb at the site of injury, may recover spontaneously. Thus a palpable bulb on an injured nerve in which there is complete interruption of conduction does not necessarily exclude the possibility of some spontaneous recovery, while the absence of a neuroma under the same conditions is no proof that the nerve has not been severed.

THE DISTAL BULB OR NEUROMA

Severed fasciculi retract within the epineurium so that the free end of the nerve is composed solely of epineurial tissue. The nerve fibres undergo Wallerian degeneration whilst proliferating Schwann cells escape from the ends of the fasciculi and intermingle with the fibroblasts derived from the damaged endoneurium, perineurium and epineurium. This cellular response, and the organising blood clot and oedema associated with the injury, may lead to the formation of a club-shaped swelling at the end of the distal stump that may also become attached by adhesions to the nerve bed. In most cases the Schwann cell–fibroblastic reaction is insufficient, or not sufficiently circumscribed, to form a significant enlargement at this site. That there is now no intrafascicular pressure to promote the escape of Schwann cells from the ends of the fasciculi may partly explain why the Schwann cell outgrowth from the distal stump is never as great as from the proximal. This feature, together with the absence of regenerating axons that contribute directly to the swelling, and indirectly to it by stimulating Schwann cell activity, explains why the distal bulb remains smaller and of simpler structure than the proximal. Any swelling that does form is usually reduced when its connective tissue framework contracts. Should regenerating axons reach and end blindly in the Schwann cell–fibroblast mass at the end of the distal stump they will cause a further enlargement of the distal bulb which, however, always remains the smaller of the two.

SUTURE LINE NEUROMAS

There is a high incidence of neuroma formation at the site of a nerve repair.

Where there are marked dissimilarities in the fascicular patterns at the nerve ends, and the fasciculi are small and widely separated by a large amount of interfascicular epineurial tissue, the cut ends of some fasciculi in the proximal stump will become opposed to interfascicular tissues in the distal during the repair. Consequently, when axon regeneration commences, large numbers of growing axon tips inevitably enter interfascicular epineurial tissue where they branch and rebranch in disarray and finally end blindly, combining with proliferating Schwann cells and fibroblasts to form a postoperative neuroma that may be even larger than that present prior to operation.

A large tender suture line neuroma developing in this way, though an indication of the vital regenerative capacity of axons, is a forerunner of failed repair, of the development of a potentially troublesome suture line problem, and poor recovery.

Where, on the other hand, the fasciculi are large and closely packed, this aberrant axon growth is less likely to occur and lead to marked bulb formation.

AMPUTATION STUMP NEUROMAS

Following the amputation of a limb, neuromas form at the ends of divided nerves. These neuromas present all of the characteristic features of bulbs forming on the proximal stump of a severed nerve. In amputation stumps, however, they assume particular importance because they often occupy an unprotected position at the new extremity of the limb where they are subject to repeated blows, pressure and irritation. These traumatic effects are more serious when the bulbs are located in a weight-bearing area. Such chronic irritation causes further structural changes in the bulb that lead to an increase in its size and sensitivity. Under these unfavourable conditions the customary tenderness of the bulb may be replaced by an acute hypersensitivity so that the slightest pressure or traction on the bulb becomes extremely painful.

Neuromas resulting from the amputation of a limb are also of interest because of their possible influence on the appearance and persistence of phantom sensations, and also because of their possible role in the causation of stump and phantom limb pain.

Neuroma formation following nerve section performed during amputation presents the following special features.

1. The only bulb to form develops at the end of the sectioned nerve. There is no distal segment to receive the axon outgrowths, which now wander freely in the surrounding tissues.

2. Every nerve trunk, large and small, cutaneous and deep, is severed at the level of the amputation. Each develops a neuroma that, inter alia, depends on the size of the parent nerve trunk. Thus the stump becomes the site of multiple neuromas that vary in size and tenderness and the degree to which they are exposed to pressure. Even the smallest of these may be a source of trouble.

3. Healing of the nerve ends occurs in a traumatised region where non-neural tissues are healing simultaneously. For this reason:

   a. It is unusual for neuromas to develop and lie freely in the surrounding tissues. They tend, on the contrary, to become adherent to one another and to other tissues such as skin, fascia, muscle, tendon, bone or deep scar tissue. As it forms, a neuroma may become embedded in a mass of scar tissue that is often extensive, especially after prolonged infection and delayed healing; in the extreme case this mass may be of almost cartilaginous consistency. Attachments to skin and other tissues leads to traction on the neuroma during movement.

   b. Regenerating axons grow irregularly from the nerve ends into the surrounding connective tissue. From the interaction between these two tissues either a circumscribed bulb appears at the nerve end, or axons continue to wander diffusely through the healing connective tissue framework of the stump so that, ultimately, the nerve ends gradually merge into scar tissue; variations range between these two extremes. The bulbs in amputation stumps tend to be larger than those observed after the severance of a single nerve in an intact limb. This is probably because in the amputation stump axon growth proceeds more freely in the greater mass of healing tissue surrounding the nerve.

   Even when a well-defined bulb is formed, regenerating axons continue to escape into the disorganised matrix of healing tissue, where the irregular arrangement of the connective tissue scaffolding results in further modifications to their growth. Firstly, they may travel considerable distances from their source; for example, axon tips from a sciatic bulb may migrate to the front of the thigh by first reaching and then ascending along the popliteal artery. Secondly, they meet repeated obstacles which force them to twist, spiral and divide in an irregular manner. This free and repeated axon branching has, in turn, two important implications.

   In the first place the different tissues in the stump become reinnervated in a disorderly manner which greatly complicates the pattern of sensory impulses flowing centrally from the stump. Secondly, axon branching means that each regenerating axon now gives rise to many sprouts. This leads to a considerable increase in the number of free terminals and an increase in the density and complexity of the innervation of the stump. The new axons remain immature and the manner in which they innervate the tissues may make the stump hypersensitive and convert it into a potential source of nociceptor impulses.

c. Contraction of the scar tissue of the stump, especially after infection and delayed healing, impairs the blood supply and constricts axons, neuromas and their parent nerves.

4. Some neuromas of a weight-bearing stump are exposed to constant pressure, friction and irritation.

5. Stump neuromas vary in shape, size composition and consistency, tenderness and in their relationship to other tissues. Repeated irritation and deformation in a pressure bearing area induces additional changes that lead to a further increase in size. The presence of a foreign body also causes a neuroma to be larger than would otherwise be the case.

The composition and consistency of neuromas are determined by two features:

a. the relative amounts of nerve and fibrous tissue and the degree of scarring. In long-standing neuromas the nerve fibres appear to be of larger calibre and more numerous than in the case of recent bulbs;

b. the vascularity of the bulb. Though the degree of vascularity varies, neuromas usually have a rich arterial supply and are enmeshed in a basket-like arrangement of veins that drains to larger vessels. A vascular factor in pain causation is also likely.

6. Tenderness depends on the density of innervation by hypersensitive sensory terminals.

7. The extent to which the neuroma is involved in scar tissue and adhesions varies, as does the particular tissue to which it may be attached, e.g. bone, tendon, muscle, skin.

8. Neuromas command attention because they are the most obvious evidence of disorderly axon growth. Of equal importance, however, is the diffuse, disorderly reinnervation of the stump tissues by immature axon terminals, particularly those from cutaneous nerves,

that convert the stump into a potential source of abnormal sensory impulses.

NEUROMAS AS A SOURCE OF NOCICEPTOR ACTIVITY

As previously outlined, a neuroma consists of a matrix of connective tissue, enlarged by the activity of proliferating fibroblasts, in which is embedded a tangled mass of regenerating and regenerated axons, and Schwann cells. Axon growth, though grossly disorganised, is profuse with axons branching and rebranching as they wind through the tissue in patternless confusion. The sum total of these changes is the formation of a pronounced swelling which varies in size and consistency depending on its vascularity and the amount and density of each of its major components: axons, Schwann cells, fibroblasts and collagen fibres.

The following additional histological features are of particular significance because they are responsible for increasing the sensitivity of a neuroma to pressure and traction. This is the underlying basis for the tender, painful neuroma.

1. Most regenerating axons end freely in the neuroma, remain of fine calibre, are inadequately sheathed and are nonmyelinated.

2. The second feature concerns the relationship established between Schwann cells and nonmyelinated axons. In a normal nerve it is common for a Schwann cell to envelop several nonmyelinated axons, each axon being separated from its neighbours by a fold of Schwann cell cytoplasm. In the neuroma, however, Schwann cells often continue to envelop several nonmyelinated nerve fibres but these are now arranged in direct contact and in a manner suggesting an ephaptic relationship. (Fig. 23.5).

When a neuroma is attached by adhesions to surrounding parts, it will be disturbed by any movement or displacement of these parts. Deformation caused by traction forces generated in this way is a common source of nociceptor activity.

Not all neuromas are abnormally sensitive or painful to physical deformation. Why some

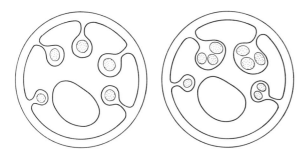

Fig. 23.5 The relation of multiple axons to a single Schwann cell. Normally each axon is separated from its neighbours by a fold of Schwann cell cytoplasm. In neuromas several axons are often in direct contact without any intervening folds of cytoplasm.

neuromas should be exquisitely sensitive and painful while others are insensitive, even in the same individual, remains obscure.

It is possible that the susceptibility of a neuroma to physical deformation could be influenced by the extent to which axons in the neuroma mature and acquire protective insulating sheaths.

In the author's experience, it is usually the small hard nodule that is insensitive, presumably because the aborted axons are few in number and well protected from physical deformation by the overgrowth of fibrous tissue which forms the major component of the neuroma.

On the other hand, large soft neuromas appear to be the principle offenders. Here there has been a prolific growth and branching of regenerating axons so that the bulk of the neuroma is composed of inadequately sheathed fine fibres and highly sensitive bare axons and axon terminals.

The treatment of painful neuromas is discussed in Chapter 38.

Neuromas as abnormal impulse generating systems

The presence of free axon terminals, bare axons and fine, immature inadequately sheathed nerve fibres in large numbers provides the basis for the generation of nociceptor discharges in response to pressure and stretch. In addition, abnormal changes in the impulse generating properties of fine free nerve terminals may be initiated by circulating or locally produced algesic substances.

However, this notion fails to explain why some neuromas are painful and others are not.

The neuroma as a spontaneous discharging focus of abnormal activity in C and A delta afferent fibres, which is mechanosensitive, chemosensitive and sensitive to hypoxia, is now well documented (Wall & Gutnick 1974a,b, Howe, Loeser & Calvin 1977, Govrin-Lippmann & Devor 1978, Wall & Devor 1978, 1983, Devor & Janig 1981, Korenman & Devor 1981, Nystrom & Hagbarth 1981, Scadding 1981, Desantis & Duckworth 1982, Devor & Bernstein 1982, Blumberg & Janig 1984, Burchiel 1984a,b, Burchiel and Russell 1985, Burchiel, Wyler & Heavner 1986).

Pathologically altered regions of an injured nerve may not only provide foci of spontaneous activity but they may also introduce two additional possibilities in the generation of abnormal activity: (1) the spread of the electrical activity generated in one fibre to interfere with conduction in adjacent fibres, and (2) the formation of artificial synapses between bare axons.

Fibre interactions occurring in these ways, particularly those involving sensory fibres, are relevant to any consideration of causalgia and other disordered sensory phenomena associated with nerve injury (Chapter 34).

Fibre interaction and the formation of artificial or ephaptic synapses

The axons of nerve fibres bound together in a fasciculus are separated from each other by complex myelin–Schwann cell–endoneurial sheaths, though the myelin component is absent in nonmyelinated fibres and at the nodes of myelinated fibres. This complex sheath functions as an insulator that normally prevents action currents associated with the passage of nerve impulses along one fibre from interfering with the electrical activity, and therefore impulse conduction, in neighbouring fibres.

There is now much experimental evidence confirming that action currents associated with the passage of impulses along one or a group of fibres may spread to excite quiescent neighbouring fibres or to modify their activity. Such mutual interactions have, as might be expected, also been recorded after injury to nerve fibres.

Any injury, however, that leads to failure of the insulating properties of the nerve sheath, whether it be nerve section, crushing by ligature or even moderate compression, introduces another type of fibre interaction at the site of injury in the form of an artificial synapse created where denuded axons are in contact. In this way the electrical activity in, for example, motor fibres is relayed to sensory fibres, thereby generating abnormal activity in them.

Studies of such artificial synapses have shown that:

1. sensory fibres have a lower threshold and far less accommodation than motor fibres;
2. sensory fibres have less capacity to resist

stimulation in this way. This is particularly so in the case of nociceptor fibres of the C group which are readily excited by fibre interaction;
3. artificial synapses show the same susceptibility to anaesthetics and anoxia as other synapses;
4. transmission across the artificial synapse is facilitated by cooling and depressed by warming;
5. the lower accommodation of sensory nerves offers an explanation for the directional properties of the artificial synapse which favour transmission from motor to sensory fibres.

REFERENCES

Blumberg H, Janig W 1984 Discharge pattern of afferent fibres from a neuroma. Pain 20: 335
Burchiel K J 1984a Effects of electrical and mechanical stimulation on two foci of spontaneous activity which develop in primary afferent neuromas after peripheral axotomy. Pain 18: 249
Burchiel K J 1984b Spontaneous impulse generation in normal and denervated dorsal root ganglia: sensitivity to alpha-adrenergic stimulation and hypoxia. Experimental Neurology 85: 257
Burchiel K J, Russell L C 1985 Spontaneous activity of ventral root axons following peripheral nerve injury. Journal of Neurosurgery 62: 408
Burchiel K J, Wyler A, Heavner J E 1986 Peripheral and central nervous system. Methods of Animal Experimentation 7: Part B 217. Academic Press, New York
DeSantis M, Duckworth J W 1982 Properties of primary afferent neurons from muscle which are spontaneously active after a lesion of their peripheral processes. Experimental Neurology 75: 261
Devor M, Bernstein J J 1982 Abnormal impulse generation in neuromas: electrophysiology and ultrastructure. In: Culp W J, Ochoa J (eds) Abnormal nerves, and muscles as impulse generators: Oxford University Press, New York, p 363
Devor M, Janig W 1981 Activation of myelinated afferent ending in a neuroma by stimulation of the sympathetic supply in the rat. Neuroscience Letters 24: 43

Govrin-Lippmann R, Devor M 1978 Ongoing activity in severed nerves: source and variation with time. Brain Research 159: 406
Howe J F, Loeser J D, Calvin W H 1977 Mechanosensitivity of dorsal root ganglia and chronically injured axons: a physiological basis for the radicular pain of nerve root compression. Pain 3: 25
Korenman E M D, Devor M 1981 Ectopic adrenergic sensitivity in damaged peripheral nerve axons in the rat. Experimental Neurology 72: 63
Nystrom B, Hagbarth E 1981 Microelectrode recordings from transected nerves in amputees with phantom limb pain. Neuroscience Letters 27: 211
Scadding J W 1981 The development of ongoing activity, mechanosensitivity, and adrenaline sensitivity in severed peripheral nerve axons. Experimental Neurology 73: 345
Wall P D, Devor M 1978 Physiology of sensation after peripheral nerve injury, regeneration, and neuroma formation. In: Waxman S G (ed) Physiology and pathobiology of axona. Raven Press, New York, p 377
Wall P D, Devor M 1983 Sensory afferent impulses originate from dorsal root ganglia as well as from the periphery in normal and nerve injured rats. Pain 17: 321
Wall P D, Gutnick M 1974a Properties of afferent nerve impulses originating from a neuroma. Nature 248: 740
Wall P D, Gutnick M 1974b Ongoing activity in peripheral nerves: the physiology and pharmacology of impulses originating from a neuroma. Experimental Neurology 43: 580

24. Neural fibrosis

Neural fibrosis is a serious complication of nerve injury, threatening as it does the structural and functional integrity of nerve fibres that are left in continuity, creating a barrier to the passage of regenerating axons when nerve fibres have been severed, and compromising the blood supply to nerve fibres, regenerating and otherwise, at the site of the injury.

Neural fibrosis can occur as a consequence of: (1) trauma to a nerve; (2) interference with the circulation through a nerve; (3) interruption of the blood supply to a nerve; (4) wound infection; or (5) the destructive action of certain therapeutic agents injected into the nerve.

An understanding of the pathogenesis of this complication is essential for the rational application of neurolysis to relieve imperilled nerve fibres. The role of neurolysis in the treatment of nerve injuries is discussed in Chapter 38.

NEURAL FIBROSIS SECONDARY TO TRAUMA

Trauma takes the form of a crush or traction injury, chronic friction, or as an iatrogenic event following an ill-advised and carelessly performed neurolysis.

Neural fibrosis occurs in the following situations:

1. when the nerve and surrounding tissues are damaged but the nerve itself is left in continuity;
2. when the nerve is cleanly transected with minimal damage to surrounding tissues and nerve repair is followed by suture line healing. The subject of suture line scarring is deferred until suture line problems are discussed in later chapters;
3. when a length of the nerve trunk is lost with considerable co-existing damage to the structures constituting the nerve bed.

Neural fibrosis is a common aftermath of trauma that damages a nerve and the surrounding tissue, with a distribution that is determined by the severity of the injury. Trauma of increasing severity affects in turn the tissues and structures forming the bed of the nerve, the superficial epineurium surrounding the nerve, the interfascicular epineurial connective tissue and finally the perineurium and endoneurial tissue.

The reaction to the injury

The injury not only damages the connective tissues of the nerve but also severs or ruptures fine blood vessels and lymphatics with haemorrhage occurring into the damaged area. This sets up a diffuse chronic inflammatory reaction that is characterised by an increase in the number of fibroblasts either from mitosis or by invasion. These cells and the collagen they form are the principal elements responsible for the pathogenesis of neural fibrosis.

Fibroblasts have an oval smooth contoured nucleus and a cytoplasm with long processes that are rich in endoplasmic reticulum and mitochondria but contain few fibrils. The collagen fibrils that they produce on demand are formed outside the cell but from tropo-collagen molecules secreted by the fibroblast.

Following an injury, fibroblasts rapidly increase in number in the damaged tissues as part of an inflammatory reaction in response to the injury.

The collagen fibres elaborated in response to fibroblast activity are first fine and randomly arranged but with time they increase in number and become coarser and arranged in bundles. These bundles are irregularly arranged but will become oriented along lines of mechanical stress, though the lattice arrangement characteristic of normal epineurial tissue is not restored.

Collagen fibres can shorten (Wright 1958) so that when damaged connective tissue heals it contracts and constricts structures that it envelops. As healing nears completion the contracting scar tissue gradually becomes less cellular and the surviving cells pyknotic and compressed between collagen bundles.

The now scarred area is relatively avascular, most of the vessels disappearing as local metabolic needs decline or as the result of constriction by collagen fibres. In any event, the end result is an area of dense fibrosis with few blood vessels. Additional features of this fibrosis worth noting are:

1. It is uneven in its distribution and the effects may be localised or diffuse depending on the nature, distribution and severity of the damage to the nerve.
2. In general, the more severe the injury the more extensive, dense and permanent the eventual scarring.
3. The reaction is always more severe when blood vessels are severed or ruptured, with haemorrhage occurring into the damaged connective tissue.
4. The considerable individual and racial variations in the extent and density of scarring is a matter of common observation.
5. The collagen fibres elaborated by epineurial fibroblasts are thicker and more numerous than those formed by endoneurial fibroblasts. Should perineurium be breached and epineurial fibroblasts gain access to the interior of a fasciculus, then the deposition of thick collagen fibres in that situation would have far more serious consequences for the nerve fibres.

The role of myofibroblasts

The possible role of myofibroblasts in the pathogenesis of neural fibrosis calls for comment.

Myofibroblasts are an important component of granulation and healing tissues (Gabbiani et al 1971, 1972, Majno et al 1971, 1972, Montandon et al 1973, Ryan et al 1973, 1974, Majno 1979). These cells are derived from active fibroblasts by a process of metaplasia in which the fibroblast undergoes three characteristic changes.

1. Bundles of parallel fibrils appear in the cytoplasm with a high content of actomyosin.
2. The nuclear surface changes from a smooth to a folded contour.
3. Very fine extensions develop from the surface of the cell that connect cells to one another and to the stroma.

Myofibroblasts have contractile properties, and structurally and functionally they are similar to smooth muscle cells. Myofibroblast contraction and shortening in response to endogenous agents are transmitted to the tissue as a whole and in this way is responsible for post-inflammatory contractures.

The pathogenesis of contractures in neural fibrosis is due to collagen shortening and the contracture of myofibroblasts. These two elements combine to play an important role in the formation of restrictive and constrictive scar tissue that at the same time gives mechanical strength to the scar. However, they are processes that have potentially harmful consequences for those structures enveloped by the constrictive scar tissue as well as for the mobility and elasticity of the nerve trunk.

The distribution and consequences of neural fibrosis

1. Fibrosis affecting the tissues constituting the bed of the nerve and the superficial epineurium. Adhesions formed in this way secure the nerve to its bed and, at the same time, encircle it with a ring or band of scar tissue (Fig. 24.1). This complication may convert a minor nerve injury into something more serious as the scar tissue:

a. increases in density and contracts;
b. buries the nerve over a variable but often considerable distance in dense scar tissue;
c. constricts the nerve;
d. compresses major nutrient vessels passing to

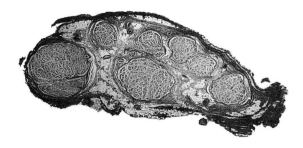

Fig. 24.1 Fibrosis of the superficial epineurium with severed adhesions at the right of the section.

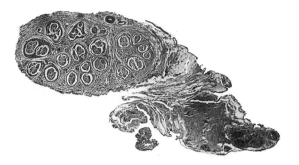

Fig. 24.3 Extensive external and intraneural epineurial fibrosis with adhesions.

and within the nerve, thereby impairing its blood supply;

e. impairs the passage of nutrients from capillaries to nerve fibres;

f. firmly attaches the nerve to neighbouring structures.

A nerve bound down by adhesions ceases to be a mobile structure. With its mobility reduced in this way the nerve is repeatedly disturbed with every limb movement and local muscle contraction. Deformation occurring in this way adversely affects function and is also a common source of pain.

2. Fibrosis affecting the interfascicular epineurial connective tissue and perineurium. This varies in amount and consistency and may be generalised, localised or irregularly distributed in transverse and longitudinal directions (Figs 24.2 & 24.3). The consequences and complications of scarring in this situation are: (1) the constriction of fasciculi (2) a reduction in the elasticity of the nerve and its capacity to adjust to traction; (3) involvement of the intraneural nutrient vessels and vascular networks. This compromises the blood supply to nerve fibres and leads to a failure to meet their metabolic needs.

3. Intrafascicular fibrosis following trauma. Here the fibrosis is the outcome of third degree or intrafascicular damage, usually caused by traction; in which capillaries are ruptured along with nerve fibres. Intrafascicular fibrosis also occurs as a terminal complication of chronic nerve compression. The intrafascicular damage is not usually localised but has a widespread, somewhat irregular, distribution along the affected fasciculi (Chapter 18) (Figs 24.4 & 24.5). This reaction is confined within the fasciculi and the scarring that follows

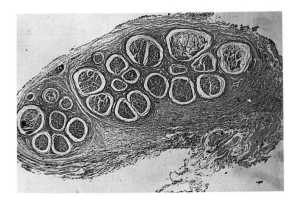

Fig. 24.2 Generalised fibrosis of the epineurial tissue.

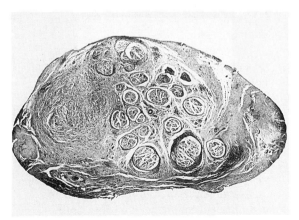

Fig. 24.4 Generalised fibrosis of the epineurium with involvement of the perineurium of some fasciculi and the fibrous tissue replacement of others.

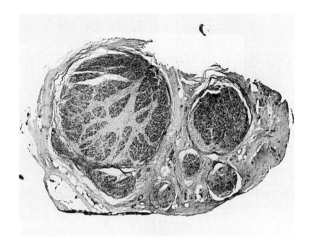

Fig. 24.5 Fibrosis involving the intrafascicular endoneurium and epineurium.

has a corresponding distribution and is responsible for:

a. the loss of elasticity of the involved fasciculi;
b. creating an impenetrable barrier to the advance of regenerating axons.
c. impairing the blood supply to those nerve fibres surviving in continuity. The blood flow through the capillary bed of the fasciculi is decisive in maintaining the nutrition of nerve fibres, and particularly the axons, and in ensuring their survival.

Nutrient materials conveyed in the capillaries for nerve fibres must be transported across the capillary endothelium, the complex sheath of the axon and the interval between these two.

Transcapillary transport and exchange depend, inter alia, on such factors as blood flow velocity and the condition of the capillary endothelium. Diffusion across the endoneurial tissue interval is influenced by its composition and the distance separating capillaries and nerve fibres, that is, the density of the capillary network. In the case of the endoneurial sheath, basal lamina and Schwann cell layer, the transfer is more complicated, involving as it does both diffusion and the active transport of materials that require attachment to and release from mobile and fixed carriers in the system. Any thickening of the capillary wall, fibrosis of the endoneurium, or thickening of the complex sheath of the nerve fibre would impede the transfer of nutrients from vessel to nerve fibre and its constituents (Fig. 24.6).

NEURAL FIBROSIS SECONDARY TO INTERRUPTION OF THE BLOOD SUPPLY TO THE NERVE. THE ISCHAEMIC LESION

Ischaemic nerve lesions are discussed in Chapter 20. Only the related neural fibrosis is discussed in this section.

Ischaemia is due to a variety of causes: arterial embolism, obliterating arterial disease, occlusion or traumatic destruction of the arteriae nervorum and the occlusion of a single major nutrient vessel such as the arteria medianes in Volkmann's ischaemic contracture.

The nature, severity and consequences of nerve trunk ischaemia depend on the duration of the ischaemia and the availability of an adequate collateral circulation. Affected nerves, therefore, present a wide variety of pathological changes. However, because the connective tissue is the most resistant of the components of a nerve to the abrupt loss of its blood supply, the reaction finally culminates in the degeneration and fibrous tissue replacement of all other elements.

In the well-established lesion, a considerable length of the nerve is thinned, greyish in colour, fibrotic and firm to palpation. The epineurium and perineurium show little change other than a proliferation of the perineurial fibroblasts; the fascicular pattern is retained though the fasciculi are atrophied. Inside fasciculi the changes are maximal and severe and take the characteristic form of a gross thickening and collagenisation of the endoneurium. The endoneurial tubes, from which the myelin and axon have been removed as the result of Wallerian degeneration, are reduced in diameter both by shrinkage and endoneurial thickening until they are finally obliterated and transformed into strands of dense collagenous tissue. Isolated collections of myelin may be left trapped and plugging endoneurial tubes, owing to the absence of an adequate circulation and the phagocytic response, both of which are responsible for removing the debris of degeneration.

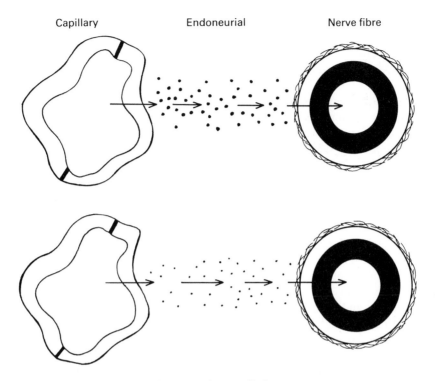

Capillary   Endoneurial   Nerve fibre

Fig. 24.6 Endoneurial fibrosis impairs the passage of nutrients from capillaries to axons.

Degeneration of Schwann cells proceeds until finally the intrafascicular tissue is transformed into dense, relatively acellular collagenous sheets and strands. Involvement of the intraneural vessels, which is maximal inside the fasciculi, includes such changes as intimal proliferation and thrombosis.

These various changes involve long stretches of the nerve and create conditions that are unfavourable for regeneration, since the new axons are faced with a dense barrier of tissue of considerable length through which they must force their way.

The nerve is finally converted into a relatively avascular, grossly shrunken, fibrotic strand which may lose its identity in the scar tissue of an associated soft tissue injury. Collagenisation is complete inside the fasciculi where all traces of the endoneurial tubes have vanished; the overall appearance is one of dense acellular collagenous bands with patchy hyaline changes. The proliferation of perineurial fibroblasts is replaced by a progressive fibrosis until the perineurium finally loses its identity and merges with the adjacent tissue. In this way the distinctive outlines of the fasciculi are obliterated and the internal structural features of the nerve trunk are lost. These advanced changes represent the transformation of an organised peripheral nerve trunk into a disorganised strand of fibrous tissue.

NEURAL FIBROSIS SECONDARY TO INTERFERENCE WITH THE CIRCULATION THROUGH THE NERVE

The development and distribution of the neural fibrosis that occurs when the circulation through the nerve is compromised is best illustrated by reference to the events that follow the steadily increasing compression of a nerve where it is passing through a compartment with unyielding walls. The genesis of the nerve lesion created in this way is discussed elsewhere (see Chapter 17). In this section we are concerned only with the neural fibrosis that becomes a significant feature of the lesion.

Here it is sufficient to say that if, for any reason, the pressure in the compartment rises and continues to do so, the circulation to, through and from the nerve is compromised in the following way.

The epineurial nutrient veins are the first structures to suffer. This compromises the venous drainage from the epineurium and later from the fasciculi, the overall effect of which is to slow the blood flow through the capillary network in the epineurial and endoneurial tissues. The resultant capillary congestion and stasis are later followed by the failure of the capillary endothelium which becomes permeable to plasma proteins so that a protein-rich exudate escapes into the surrounding tissues. This exudate provides a nidus for the proliferation of fibroblasts and the deposition of collagen fibres as a consequence of which the epineurial and endoneurial tissues become the site of a deepening fibrosis.

In the case of the epineurium the exudate spreads freely and the resulting adhesions attach the superficial epineurium to neighbouring structures and the fasciculi to one another.

The consequences are more serious in the case of the intrafascicular endoneurium because:

1. individual nerve fibres become surrounded by increasing amounts of collagen;
2. the exudate is prevented from leaving the fasciculi because the perineurium forms an impermeable barrier to the passage of large molecules;
3. osmotic pressure gradients are now such that fluid is drawn into the fasciculi.

The overall effect of these developments is to increase the intrafascicular pressure. The steadily increasing intrafascicular pressure and deepening fibrosis threaten the survival of nerve fibres and finally lead to their destruction: (a) from direct compression and constriction, and (b) by compressing and constricting capillary networks which deprives nerve fibres of their blood supply and essential nutrients; (c) by increasing the collagen deposited between capillaries and nerve fibres, thereby impairing the transfer of nutrients from the former to the latter.

The final outcome of unrelieved compression is the gradual fibrous tissue replacement of the contents of the fasciculi, the outlines of nerve fibres being lost as the affected nerve segment is converted into a cord of fibrous tissue in which fascicular outlines can still be identified.

NEURAL FIBROSIS AND INFECTION

When a wound is infected, the inflammatory element in the reaction to trauma is greatly increased. However, as long as the perineurium is undamaged the inflammatory reaction is confined to the epineurial connective tissue which offers little resistance to the spread of infection to and along the nerve and between the fasciculi.

The perineurium on the other hand provides an effective barrier to the spread of local inflammatory processes. Normal fasciculi are frequently found surrounded by advanced infection and fibrosis, the histological picture indicating that the undamaged perineurium is particularly resistant to even severe and prolonged infection. Immediately the perineurium is broken, however, infection enters the damaged fasciculus which becomes involved in a rapidly spreading inflammatory reaction that extends proximally and distally inside the fasciculus.

Infection excites an acute inflammatory reaction characterised by the invasion of the damaged tissues by large numbers of leucocytes and macrophages, an increase in the number of newly formed vessels, and capillary permeability that results in the appearance of an exudate. These changes represent a defence phase. When this has been successfully completed, and the debris phagocytosed and removed, a reparative phase takes over in which fibroblasts proliferate and increase in activity with the deposition of excessive amounts of collagen. In this process, inflammation and repair are a continuum that culminates in the formation of dense scar tissue.

NEURAL FIBROSIS CAUSED BY THE DESTRUCTIVE OR TOXIC ACTION OF CHEMICAL AGENTS

Here the nerve is injured when a therapeutic agent is inadvertently injected directly into the nerve or into the tissues immediately surrounding it. Apart from the direct damage to tissues by the needle, substances harmful to nerves cover a wide variety of therapeutic and prophylactic agents, the vehicle for the agent in some cases proving equally as damaging.

Material may be injected into a fasciculus, into the interfascicular epineurial tissue, or into the tissues immediately surrounding the nerve.

Material admitted directly into a fasciculus causes an inflammatory reaction resulting in a destructive fibrous tissue response that is confined within the fasciculus. Under these circumstances regenerating axons are unable to find their way through the scarred tissue and useful regeneration within the affected fasciculus cannot be expected.

Material injected into the interfascicular tissues is free to spread and track widely through and along the nerve depending upon the pressure used to inject it. The reaction that follows leads to scar-ring that constricts the fasciculi, impairs the blood supply to their contents and gives the nerve an indurated consistency. The effect on the contained nerve fibres depends on the degree to which the resulting fibrosis deforms fasciculi and impoverishes their blood supply.

Material injected into the tissues surrounding the nerve is also free to spread widely through these tissues and into the nerve itself. The resulting pathological changes include an immediate acute inflammatory reaction about the nerve, which may appear swollen and hyperaemic in the early stages. This is followed by the usual fibroblastic response that ultimately encases the nerve in dense scar tissue with adhesions firmly binding the nerve to the surrounding tissues, all of which can be confirmed subsequently during neurolysis.

REFERENCES

Gabbiani G, Ryan G B, Majno G 1971 Presence of modified fibroblasts in granulation tissue and their possible role in wound contraction. Experientia 27: 549

Gabbiani G, Hirscheil B J Ryan G B et al 1972 Granulation tissue as a contractile organ. A study of structure and function. Journal of Experimental Medicine 135: 719

Majno G 1979 The story of the myofibroblasts. American Journal of Surgical Pathology 3: 535

Majno G, Gabbiani G, Hirschel B J et al 1971 Contraction of granulation tissue in vitro: similarity to smooth muscle. Science 173: 548

Majno G, Ryan G B, Gabbiani G et al 1972 Contractile events in inflammation and repair. In: Lepow I H, Ward P A (eds) Inflammation: mechanisms and control. Academic Press, New York, p 13

Montandon D, Gabbiani G, Ryan G B, Majno G 1973 The contractile fibroblast: Its relevance in plastic surgery. Plastic and Reconstructive Surgery 52: 286

Ryan G B, Cliff W J, Gabbiani G et al 1973 Myofibroblasts in an avascular fibrous tissue. Laboratory Investigation 29: 197

Ryan G B, Cliff W G, Gabbiani G et al 1974 Myofibroblasts in human granulation tissue. Human Pathology 5: 55

Wright G P 1958 An introduction to pathology, 3rd edn. Longmans, London, p 231

25. A classification of nerve injury

'Except ye utter by the tongue words easy to be understood, how shall it be known what is spoken'.
Corinthians Chap. 14, ix.

Prior to 1940 nerve lesions were categorised on the basis of such general and vague terms as contusion, concussion, stretch, compression, laceration and division. However, the deficiencies and inadequacies of such a classification were not fully appreciated until the early years of World War II when nerve injuries from battle casualties, which had increased rapidly in numbers, became the subject of special study and created a demand for a meaningful classification of nerve injury. This produced two new classifications, both based on nerve fibre and nerve trunk pathology. Seddon (1943, 1975) introduced a classification based on three types of nerve injury, neurapraxia, axonotmesis and neurotmesis and Sunderland (1951, 1978) classified nerve damage into five degrees. The latter's classification will be presented here, since it includes the three types described by Seddon and, in addition, has certain advantages that will emerge as the discussion proceeds.

To be convincing and clinically acceptable any classification of nerve injury should satisfy the following criteria:

1. have a sound pathological basis;
2. be all-inclusive, i.e. it should cover all types and degrees of nerve injury;
3. relate to the clinical events associated with a lesion;
4. have diagnostic, prognostic and therapeutic significance;
5. involve a terminology that is readily understood;
6. have the added attractiveness of simplicity.

If a classification is too complicated nobody will use it.

Sunderland's classification, which is based on histological features of the nerve trunk, recognises five degrees or types of nerve damage increasing in severity from loss of conduction followed successively by loss of continuity of axons, then of nerve fibres followed by the fasciculi and, finally, the entire nerve trunk (Fig. 25.1). Each of these types presents special features that call for separate consideration.

The proposed classification relates solely to lesions producing loss of function. Those which result in perversions of function, as opposed to paralysis and loss of sensibility, also constitute a separate category. In addition, injuries may not be of uniform severity, either across or along the nerve trunk, in which case some axons, nerve fibres and fasciculi are more severely affected than others. Partial and mixed lesions are produced in this way.

The classification about to be described is based on the histopathology of the lesion and not on the cause which is represented by a great variety of agents — mechanical, thermal, chemical and ischaemia. The same agent may produce any one of the first four degrees, depending on its intensity and the time for which it operates, while mechanical trauma may be responsible for all five. Finally, the lesion may be sharply localised to a short segment of the nerve or it may involve a considerable length of the nerve. The latter is particularly likely to occur with traction injuries.

The pathological and clinical features of each of the five degrees of damage will now be examined to, inter alia, test the validity of the classification

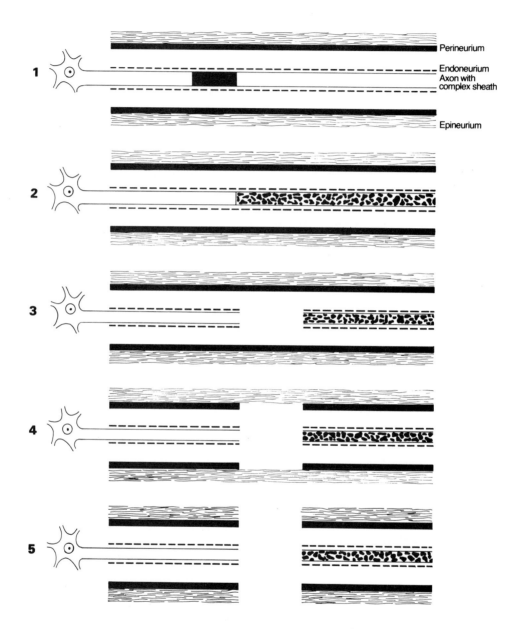

Fig. 25.1 Diagram illustrating the five degrees of nerve injury. *1*. Conduction block. *2*. The lesion confined to the axon within an intact endoneurial sheath and resulting in Wallerian degeneration. *3*. Loss of nerve fibre continuity (axon and endoneurial sheath) inside an intact perineurium. *4*. Loss of fascicular continuity with nerve trunk continuity depending solely on epineurial tissue. *5*. Loss of continuity of the entire nerve trunk.

from which it will be seen that it satisfies the above-mentioned criteria in every respect.

FIRST DEGREE INJURY

The basis of a first degree injury, which corresponds to neurapraxia in Seddon's classification, is interruption of conduction at the site of injury.

Pathology

This has been described in Chapter 13. The essential pathological features of this injury are:

1. Continuity of the axon is preserved.
2. There is no Wallerian degeneration.
3. Local changes are of a minor nature and are fully reversible so that the structural features and physiological properties of the affected nerve fibres are fully restored.
4. Thick nerve fibres are more susceptible than fine and motor fibres are more susceptible and suffer to a greater degree than sensory fibres.
5. Motor nerve fibres, those serving the various sensory modalities and sympathetic fibres fail sequentially in the following order: motor; proprioceptor; touch; temperature; pain and sympathetic. Recovery occurs sequentially in the reverse order.
6. The principal causal agents are mild compression and ischaemia.

Clinical features

The essential clinical feature is that after a quiescent period of variable but short duration, the affected axons again conduct across the injured segment and function is rapidly and completely restored.

The motor defect

1. Motor function is lost in the field of the injured nerve.
2. The onset of paralysis in uncomplicated first degree compression injury may be gradual or sudden and is always painless. The condition may be arrested on the verge of paralysis so

that only a paresis results. Paresis could be due to the maximal involvement of a small number of the motor fibres to a muscle, or to the partial involvement of all or a large number of them. The co-existence in any given case of normal, paresed and paralysed muscles is due to variations in susceptibility among motor fibres and to the fact that some occupy more protected positions in the nerve than others.

3. The affected muscles do not fibrillate.
4. There is no reaction of degeneration in the paralysed muscles.
5. Conduction across the injured segment of the nerve is either slowed or lost. In the case of the latter the nerve conducts above and below the block but not across it.
6. Recovery may commence so early and advance so rapidly that there is no time for wasting to appear. Muscles atrophy when the onset and progress of recovery are delayed. This delay in first degree injuries is rarely long enough for wasting to become as marked as that observed after axon degeneration. Lest atrophy be attributed to disuse of the affected limb, it should be pointed out that it is maximal in the involved muscles even if it is not confined to them. Furthermore, wasting improves only with the onset of recovery, and its disappearance closely parallels the return of power in the affected muscles.

The sensory defect

1. In a fully developed first degree injury all forms of sensation are lost in the autonomous area innervated by the injured nerve.
2. Loss of proprioception is frequently the only sensory defect present because cutaneous sensory defects are often so transitory that they escape detection unless the patient is examined immediately following, or soon after, the injury.
3. Even when clinical testing fails to detect any sensory deficit, patients may show electrophysiological evidence of sensory nerve involvement.

4. Where all cutaneous sensory modalities are affected, touch is usually affected to a greater degree than nociception.
5. Within even a few days of the injury, the only residual sensory disturbance, other than the proprioceptor defect, may be one of paraesthesiae that rapidly subside. This explains the dissociated loss that is so commonly observed clinically.
6. A prolonged sensory loss indicates a more severe injury with an even greater delay in the return of motor function.

Sympathetic nerve fibres are the most resistant to this form of injury.

Onset and course of recovery

After a quiescent period of variable but short duration the nerve fibres suddenly reawaken to activity.

Motor recovery

The pattern of motor recovery presents the following features:

1. The onset of recovery in the paralysed muscles is delayed for periods ranging from a few days to several months, though most cases will show some signs of recovery within 6 weeks.
2. There is no serial order of reinnervation of muscles determined by the site of origin and length of their branches.
3. The affected muscles recover simultaneously, or in a somewhat irregular and random manner in which case they recover in rapid succession within a few days of each other, so that all muscles are contracting shortly after the first appearance of motor recovery.
4. The pattern of recovery cannot be explained on the basis of Wallerian degeneration followed by axon regeneration.
5. Variations in the severity of the conduction block sustained by individual nerve fibres in the nerve trunk account for variations in the duration of the paralysis for individual muscles and in the time required for the full restoration of function.
6. The early reappearance of muscle contractions in response to voluntary effort does not necessarily mean a speedy return to normal function.
7. Concerning the recovery of motor function, it is necessary to draw a distinction between the onset of recovery and its progress to the point where it meets the clinical and electrophysiological criteria for normality. The first muscles to show signs of reinnervation are not necessarily the first to recover completely.
8. The onset of recovery may be consistently delayed in some muscles in comparison with others. This is usually due to the fibres innervating them occupying a more exposed position in the nerve trunk at the injury site.
9. A cutaneous sensory defect that does not recover rapidly indicates a severe injury and justifies the prognosis that the onset of motor recovery and the restoration of full motor function will be considerably delayed.
10. In general there is a relation between the duration of the compression and the severity of the resulting lesion, longer compression times being associated with delayed recoveries. The length of the nerve damaged is also a factor affecting recovery.
11. Complete recovery inevitably follows this type of injury, since axonal continuity is preserved and the changes responsible for the interruption of conduction are fully reversible. Full restoration of function may, however, be delayed for 3–4 months after the injury and, in more severe cases, this period may be extended. A residual defect indicates a loss of axons and a disturbance of the pattern of innervation, and is evidence of a more severe injury.

Sensory recovery

Cutaneous sensory loss is usually transient, sensation recovering well in advance of motor and proprioceptor functions, and returning so rapidly that it is not usually possible to study the precise manner in which it does so. Touch, which is affected to a greater degree than pain, recovers more slowly. Paraesthesiae indicative of disturbed conduction may persist for several days.

Sympathetic nerve fibres

Among the various fibre types these, along with nociceptor fibres, are the first to recover.

Explanation of the dissociated functional loss in first degree injury

It has been repeatedly confirmed that motor and proprioceptor fibres are more susceptible to compression than those which serve sympathetic functions and sensations of pain and touch. The preservation of normal cutaneous sensation in the presence of well-established paralysis, is often a striking feature in many of these patients. Possible explanations are:

1. A relationship between fibre size and susceptibility in which fibres succumb to compression-ischaemia in order of their size.
2. The location of sensory fibres in the nerve trunk, together with their inherent resistance to pressure and ischaemia, may be such that they are able to resist pressures just sufficient to block motor conduction. Compression, however, may reach levels at which these protective mechanisms fail and the sensory fibres then suffer the same fate as neighbouring motor fibres. If this is so, the motor fibres, which have already succumbed at lower pressures, should become progressively more severely affected as the pressure increases to a level at which conduction in sensory fibres fails. Such an interpretation receives support from the clinical finding that paralysis is prolonged when it is associated with a sensory defect.

   On the other hand, the location of the sensory fibres may be such that their inherent resistance is ineffective at quite low thresholds, in which case sensory defects make their appearance concurrently with impairment of motor function. The motor fibres would not now be involved to the same degree and should, therefore, recover

more rapidly. This interpretation is supported by the course of recovery observed in some patients.

3. These views on the basis of the dissociated effects characteristic of first degree injury must be regarded as provisional only. They obviously leave unexplained the fundamental problem of the inherent and differential susceptibility of nerve fibres to pressure and ischaemia.

   In the face of continuing uncertainty on this issue, we are left with the conclusion that the greater resistance of cutaneous sensory fibres in these injuries is due to some as yet unrecognised property which renders them less susceptible to pressure and ischaemia. The evidence rather suggests that the dissociation depends, not on a single factor but on a combination of them.

Variant forms of first degree injury

Delayed conduction block

In the classical first degree injury recovery occurs spontaneously. There is, however, a subdivision of this group that is worthy of note but about which little is known. This is the type of lesion in which, after a long delay without recovery, exploration and simple neurolysis are followed by the early onset of recovery, which then progresses in a manner that is identical in every respect with that observed after a classical first degree injury.

This phenomenon can usually be explained by the surgical procedure fortuitously coinciding with the onset of spontaneous recovery. Though this explanation accounts for some cases, it is common experience that there remain those odd injuries associated with prolonged loss of function in which fibrous constriction of the nerve or some obscure local pathology is apparently responsible for maintaining a conduction block that persists until the nerve is released, following which there is a burst of recovery. How long conduction can be blocked in this way without threatening axonal continuity, and precipitating a severe type of lesion, remains unknown but it can certainly be for many months.

Conduction block superimposed on a recovered second degree injury

Axon regeneration from a classical second degree injury (see below) may proceed to completion without the anticipated onset of motor and sensory recovery. The lesion now takes on the features of the prolonged conduction block injury described above, the onset of recovery being delayed until the damaged segment of the nerve is freed by neurolysis.

It is important not to confuse this situation with that in which premature neurolysis coincides with the onset of recovery in a normally regenerating nerve that has suffered second degree damage.

SECOND DEGREE INJURY

Second degree injury corresponds to axonotmesis in Seddon's classification.

Pathology

The pathology of second degree injury has been described in Chapters 14 and 15. Recapitulating, the essential pathological changes are:

1. The axon is severed or axonal mechanisms are so disorganised that the nerve fibre undergoes Wallerian degeneration below the injury.
2. Continuity of the endoneurial sheath of the nerve fibre and the basal lamina of the Schwann layer are preserved.
3. Axonal continuity with the periphery is restored by axon regeneration.
4. Each regenerating axon as it advances is confined within the endoneurial tube that originally contained it. This ensures that the axon is inevitably directed back to the end organ that it originally innervated.
5. This ensures that the restored pattern of innervation is identical in every respect with the original pattern of innervation.
6. Complete functional recovery is the inevitable end result.

Clinical features

The peripheral defect

1. There is complete loss of motor, sensory and sympathetic functions in the autonomous distribution of the nerve.
2. With the disintegration of the axon, nerve conduction below the lesion is lost 24–72 hours after the injury.
3. Fibrillations and other electrical signs of denervation are present in denervated muscles.
4. The denervated muscles atrophy.

Onset and course of recovery

1. The interval between injury and the onset of recovery is influenced not only by the severity of the injury but also by the level of the injury because regenerating axons have greater distances to travel after high as opposed to low level lesions.
2. Since recovery depends on the regeneration of severed axons, the paralysed muscles are now reinnervated in the order in which they were originally supplied by the nerve, so that the onset of recovery in individual muscles proceeds in serial order from above downwards, proximal muscles recovering before those innervated at more distal levels.
3. The onset of sensory recovery is in strict conformity with the distance that must be grown by the regenerating sensory processes.
4. The advance of regenerating sensory axon tips can often be followed down the nerve by tracing the progress of the point at which Hoffmann–Tinel's sign can be elicited. In second degree injuries this procedure is of some prognostic significance because the regenerating sensory processes are confined to their original tubes. This means that the pattern of sensory innervation is ultimately fully reconstituted.
5. All functions are completely restored, since the restored pattern of innervation is identical with that obtaining before the injury. In the exceptional case there may be traces of a residual defect that can only be due to a retrograde neuronal degeneration

that has reduced the number of the surviving axons. This, however, rarely occurs with an injury that leaves all but the axons of the nerve intact.
6. Owing to the increased delay before the onset of recovery, and the additional time required to reinnervate the entire peripheral field by axon growth, the delay before function is fully restored exceeds that observed after first degree injuries and is to be measured in months as opposed to weeks.

THIRD DEGREE INJURY

Pathology

The pathology of third degree damage has been described in Chapters 14, 15 and 18. Summarising, the essential features of these injuries are:

1. They are intrafascicular injuries that may be localised to a segment of the nerve or widely distributed along considerable lengths of the nerve.
2. They involve:
   a. the disintegration of axons and Wallerian degeneration;
   b. the disorganisation of the internal structure of fasciculi;
   c. the loss of endoneurial tube continuity;
   d. the fasciculi are left in continuity and their general arrangement in the nerve trunk is preserved;
   e. the retrograde effects are severe, particularly when the nerve is injured at proximal levels. Some affected neurons degenerate which reduces the number of axons available for regeneration.
3. The intrafascicular damage may also include haemorrhage, oedema, vascular stasis and ischaemia. The intrafascicular fibrosis that follows then constitutes a serious obstacle to regeneration.
4. The interfascicular epineural tissue is often damaged as well with the formation of scar tissue in which the injured fasciculi, though in continuity, become embedded.

5. Common causes of this type of nerve injury are:
   a. Traction that is sufficient to rupture nerve fibres without disrupting the fasciculi (Chapter 18).
   b. Compression that either directly, or indirectly through ischaemia, results in the destruction of nerve fibres and their fibrous tissue replacement so that fasciculi are finally converted into fibrous cords at the site of the injury. This is the lesion that follows chronic progressive compression in a compartment with unyielding walls (Chapter 17).
6. Regeneration is hampered by the following adverse developments.
   a. The numbers of neurons and axons that survive to regenerate are reduced.
   b. The onset of axon growth may be considerably delayed because of the additional time required for cell bodies to recover and this recovery may be incomplete.
   c. Intrafascicular fibrosis blocks some axons, delays others in their growth, diverts others from their proper course and later, by constricting those that are successful in negotiating the scar tissue between the nerve fibre ends, adversely affect their subsequent growth, development and function. This disorderly axon growth may be so pronounced that the affected fasciculi develop a fusiform swelling at this site.
   d. Loss of continuity of the nerve fibres means that regenerating axons, though still confined within the fasciculi, are no longer confined to the endoneurial tubes that originally contained them. Since there is no known mechanism directing axons into their original or functionally related endoneurial tubes many fail to do so and instead are misdirected into foreign ones.

Because of these complications, the outcome of regeneration following a third degree injury is one in which the restored pattern of innervation is left both incomplete and imperfect compared with the original and function suffers accordingly.

7. The outcome of the erroneous cross-shunting of axons depends on the fibre composition of the affected fasciculi. The consequences are minimal when the fibres of a fasciculus are from the same, or from different but functionally related sources. However, where the fasciculi are composed of fibres from functionally unrelated structures, and particularly when motor and sensory fibres are intermingled in the same fasciculus, many axons find their way into foreign tubes. This represents wasteful regeneration.

At proximal levels, the fibres from the most distal structures are intermingled and widely distributed over the fasciculi, whereas those from branches of high origin are more discretely localised. It follows, therefore, that in high lesions the consequences of an injury that ruptures the endoneurial tubes are more serious for distally innervated than the proximally innervated structures. In this way the level of the lesion becomes a factor influencing the extent and quality of the recovery.

Details of the fibre composition of the fasciculi at various levels for the different peripheral nerves are available elsewhere (Sunderland 1978). Such information provides the clue to the profound peripheral disability and poor results that sometimes follow lesions in continuity, in which both inspection and palpation of the nerve at the site of injury suggest only minimal damage.

Clinical features

Motor, sensory and sympathetic functions are lost in the autonomous field of the injured nerve.

Onset of recovery

This is delayed for longer periods than is the case with second degree injury because of:

1. the more severe retrograde disturbances from which recovery takes place more slowly;

2. the additional time taken by regenerating axon tips to traverse scar tissue that obstructs and slows them, and

3. the extended denervation of peripheral tissues consequent on (1) and (2). This in turn, increases the time required, following reinnervation, for the denervated tissues to undergo those further changes required for functional recovery to occur.

While structures may recover in the order in which they were originally innervated, this may be modified because some regenerating axons, faced with fewer obstacles, make faster progress than others. Recovery in individual structures is slower and is usually incomplete, a paresis and/or sensory defect persisting as an expression of imperfections in reinnervation. Muscles that do recover often take longer to do so for the following reasons:

i. They have been denervated for longer periods and additional time is required to reverse the changes that have developed in the denervated tissues;

ii. It may be possible to compensate for imperfections in the restored pattern of innervation by re-educational measures but this requires additional time and delays the completion of recovery.

iii. Some muscle fibres may, for one reason or another, remain denervated. This loss may be offset by the 'use' hypertrophy of those muscle fibres that have fully recovered. This also delays the completion of recovery.

Hoffmann–Tinel's sign in third degree injury. Once the endoneurial tubes have been ruptured, Hoffmann–Tinel's sign ceases to be a reliable guide to prognosis and the quality of the recovery. Though confirming the presence and the advance of regenerating sensory processes, the sign is of limited prognostic value because sensory 'axons' could now be in and descending down motor endoneurial tubes.

The end result. In third degree damage there is a residual defect that varies in degree depending on the loss of axons, the extent and severity of intrafascicular fibrosis, and the extent of the erroneous cross-shunting of regenerating axons occurring at the site of injury. Severe stretch injuries lead to the intrafascicular rupture of nerve fibres over considerable lengths of the nerve, while additional intrafascicular complications are introduced by compression ischaemia and vascular damage, all of which aggravate intrafascicular scarring. Under such adverse conditions, and particularly at levels where the nerve fibres of different branches are intermingled and widely represented in many if not all injured fasciculi, little if any recovery is to be expected. An important point is that the nerves so affected may, to external observation and examination, show surprisingly little evidence of the severe disorganisation that has taken place inside the fasciculi.

FOURTH DEGREE INJURY

Pathology

In fourth degree injuries the fasciculi are ruptured or so disorganised that they are no longer sharply demarcated from the epineurium in which they are embedded and which shares in the reaction. Continuity of the nerve trunk is preserved, though the involved segment is ultimately converted into a tangled mass of ruptured fasciculi, scar tissue, Schwann cells, and regenerating axons that may be enlarged to form a neuroma. Wallerian degeneration follows the usual pattern.

As in third degree injuries, factors are present that retard and complicate regeneration, but in the case of fascicular disorganisation they are far more serious. The retrograde neuronal effects are more severe following these injuries and there is also a high incidence of neuronal degeneration and a correspondingly greater reduction in the number of surviving axons. Furthermore, regenerating axons, now no longer confined to ruptured fasciculi, are free to enter the interfascicular tissue where many become lost and terminate blindly, while the chances of others entering foreign tubes are greatly increased. Scarring is more severe and extensive and is responsible for large numbers of growing axons being blocked and others going astray. As a result few axons reach the periphery and make useful connections.

Clinical features

There is complete loss of motor, sensory and sym-

pathetic functions in the field served by the nerve. Though some spontaneous recovery may occur it rarely proceeds to a useful degree. This is the type of injury that requires excision of the damaged segment and surgical repair of the nerve.

FIFTH DEGREE INJURY

A fifth degree injury is one in which there is loss of continuity of the nerve trunk. The distance separating the nerve ends varies, while local pathology depends on when the injured region is examined, because both the reaction at the site of the injury and the subsequent regeneration modify the picture. The nerve ends may remain separated, or they may become joined by an attenuated strand of tissue composed of a fibroblastic and Schwann cell framework transmitting regenerating axons. The latter arrangement is seen only after sufficient time has elapsed to enable the neural, Schwann cell and fibroblastic activity to bridge the gap. The amount of scar tissue that is formed between the nerve ends varies from a small connecting strand to an extensive mass of tissue in which the nerve ends are completely buried. This scar tissue, as well as the separation of the nerve ends, constitutes a formidable barrier to the advance of regenerating axons. Bulb formation may occur on the proximal stump, the distal stump, or on both. The proximal neuroma and the distal bulb may be joined to form an irregular bulb, linked to form a dumbell-shaped structure, or be buried in a common mass of scar tissue.

Wallerian degeneration occurs in the distal segment. Though some regenerating axons may reach and descend along the distal stump to reinnervate the periphery, such spontaneous recovery is usually of little value because the axons are few in number, and the chances of restoring functionally useful end organ connections are slender indeed. Some regenerating sensory processes may give a Hoffmann–Tinel's sign that, under these conditions, is an unreliable guide both to the nature of the injury and the quality of the end result.

Motor, sensory and sympathetic functions are lost in the autonomous distribution of the severed nerve.

Recovery after an untreated fifth degree injury is negligible for the following reasons:

1. The retrograde neuronal reaction is particularly severe and large numbers of neurons fail to survive.
2. The majority of regenerating axons fail to reach fasciculi and the endoneurial tubes of the fasciculi at the distal stump owing to:

   a. the separation of the nerve ends. Even when the ends are close together, large numbers of regenerating axons escape into the intervening tissue as they emerge from the open end of the proximal stump. This wasteful regeneration increases with the distance between the nerve ends;
   b. dissimilarities in the cross-sectional areas of the nerve ends consequent on denervation shrinkage of the distal stump;
   c. dissimilarities in the fascicular patterns of the nerve ends; the fascicular patterns of the nerve ends only correspond in every respect after clean severance;
   d. the scarring between the nerve ends which obstructs some axons and misdirects others, either away from endoneurial tubes or into functionally unrelated ones.

The chances of restoring useful connections are, of course, greatly aided by suturing the nerve ends, but despite this there still occurs a significant loss of axons and distortion of the fibre pattern. Factors influencing the extent and quality of the recovery after nerve suture are discussed in Chapter 39.

PARTIAL NERVE INJURY

Partial nerve injuries are those in which some nerve fibres escape injury while others sustain a variable degree of damage. Though the term is usually applied to partial severance or partial fourth degree involvement of the nerve trunk, it also includes first, second, and third degree injuries.

The nature of the peripheral defect, the course of recovery and the end result depend on the fibre composition of the damaged fasciculi, the particular sector of the nerve injured and the particular type of injury sustained by each fibre.

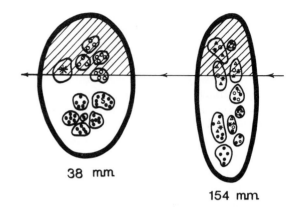

Fig. 25.2 Transverse sections from a specimen of the radial nerve taken 38 and 154 mm above the lateral humeral epicondyle. The partial injury at 38 mm involves all fibres destined for the superficial radial branch and the branches to the radial wrist extensors. The partial injury involving the same sector at 154 mm involves only some of the fibres destined for the superficial radial branch and the branches to the brachioradialis, brachialis and radial wrist extensor muscles.
The code for the different branch fibres is:
o, Superficial radial; ●, Posterior interosseous; S, Supinator; ★, Combined radial wrist extensors; △, Brachioradialis; ▲, Brachialis.

1. If the damaged fasciculi contain a proportion of the fibres from each of several branches, there will result a widely distributed paresis and/or sensory impairment. On the other hand, if they contain all the fibres destined for a particular muscle or muscles, or cutaneous area, the result will be a sharply localised paralysis and/or discrete area of sensory loss (Fig. 25.2).
2. The fascicular pattern of the nerve at that level. The nerve which is composed of numerous, small and widely separated fasciculi possesses an advantage when it is subjected to mechanical trauma falling unevenly across the nerve (Fig. 25.3). In partial injuries the intraneural damage will be confined to the small fasciculi lying in the path of destruction, so that such lesions tend to be self-limiting. The consequences of a partial lesion of corresponding extent and severity are more serious where the fasciculi are large and few in number; this is particularly so where all the nerve fibres are concentrated in a single fasciculus. Under

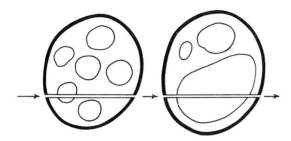

Fig. 25.3

these conditions rupture of the perineurium leads to more widespread changes throughout the fasciculus. Most of the nerve fibres comprising the nerve are then involved either directly, or indirectly as the result of:

a. the associated vascular damage,
b. the herniation of the fascicular tissue through the break in the perineurium, and
c. scar tissue formation. Such damage to the nerve usually requires total resection and suture, whereas damage limited to a few small fasciculi may only require local excision of the involved sector and partial repair.

3. The particular sector of the nerve injured and the branch fibre composition of the affected fasciculi which is influenced by the level of the injury.

   The manner in which variations in the fibre composition of fasciculi are produced by fascicular intercommunications has been described in Chapter 7. For some distance above its origin, each branch is represented in the nerve by a fasciculus, or group of fasciculi, which is sharply localised and superficially situated. These fasciculi subsequently intercommunicate at higher levels with adjacent bundles composed of fibres from different branches, which results in an intermingling of the fibres of originally separate systems. Further scattering and mixing of the fibres of individual branches gradually continue as the intercommunications are repeated at

successive levels. Finally, the various branch systems come to be widely represented over the fasciculi in varying combinations and proportions, though each bundle does not necessarily contain fibres from every branch.

The longer the nerve, and the more distal the origin of a branch, the greater the diffusion and intermingling of its fibres at proximal levels. When, however, the fasciculi of a branch with a high origin commence to fuse with others they do so with fasciculi that have already acquired fibres from most, if not all, of the distal branches. As a result, the fibres of such proximal branches are rapidly mixed with those from several sources but, since their intraneural course is too short to permit extensive scattering, they remain relatively discretely localised though in combination.

Thus, at any level, some fasciculi are composed solely or predominantly of fibres for a branch or branches that are soon to leave the nerve, while the remainder are composed of fibres, in varying combinations and proportions for more distal branches.

Partial lesions will, therefore, produce variable peripheral effects depending on the fibre composition of the damaged fasciculi which is determined, in turn, by the level of the injury (Fig. 25.2). When the damaged fasciculi contain a few of the fibres of some, or all, of the branches, the resultant loss of function is minimal and widespread, and might even escape detection clinically. On the other hand, where a partial injury damages fasciculi that contain all or the majority of the fibres representing a particular branch, the peripheral effect would be sharply localised and clinically demonstrable.

Thus a partial nerve injury at one level may either escape detection or give a widely distributed paresis, while a corresponding lesion at another level may produce a sharply localised paralysis or sensory loss.

MIXED NERVE INJURY

Mixed nerve injuries are those in which all nerve fibres are affected but to a varying degree. These are common injuries.

In injuries sufficiently severe to cause partial severance or partial fourth degree involvement, it is unlikely that the remaining fibres in the nerve will have escaped some injury. These lesions would be more properly classed as mixed lesions in which all fibres were affected but to a varying degree.

Finally, within fasciculi surviving in continuity it is possible to meet with every grade of intrafascicular damage ranging from a first degree injury to one in which intrafascicular disorganisation follows the destruction of endoneurial tubes. Nerve lesions in continuity commonly present such a spectrum of damage.

Such mixed lesions result in the complete loss of motor, sensory and sympathetic functions in the autonomous distribution of the injured nerve. Since the damage falls unevenly across the nerve so that some parts and some fibres are more severely affected than others, the duration of the loss of function, the order and onset of recovery in the reinnervated parts, and the end result will show irregularities depending on the distribution of each type of injury, and the extent to which individual fibres are damaged.

IRRITATIVE LESIONS

There are neurological conditions in which the clinical picture is characterised by abnormal motor and sensory phenomena that include one or a combination of the following:

Motor:	Muscle twitching, fasciculation and spasm.
Sympathetic:	Abnormal sweating and vasomotor disturbances.
Sensory:	Paraesthesia, spontaneous pain, and abnormal responses to touch, heat and cold.

In such conditions it is first necessary to exclude the possibility of a central lesion. This done, there remain those cases in which perverted functions are unquestionably due to localised pathology in the peripheral nerve trunk.

Such abnormal activity and responses may occur under three conditions:

1. They may constitute the sole disability associated with nerve involvement.
2. They may be associated with a progressive lesion of the nerve trunk in which gradual deteriorating function ultimately culminates in complete loss of function. It is during the course of this deterioration that abnormal signs and symptoms indicative of an irritative lesion may appear.
3. They may appear during the early stages of recovery following complete interruption of conduction in the nerve, persisting until the completion of those refinements of the recovery process on which normal function depends.

The pathogenesis of these abnormal irritative phenomena is obscure, but the association with regressing and recovering nerve lesions suggests that they have their origin in changes to the structure, nutrition and physiological properties of nerve fibres that fall short of interruption of conduction but are of such a nature as to give rise to abnormal spontaneous activity in those fibres.

REFERENCES

Seddon H J 1943 Three types of nerve injury. Brain 66: 237
Seddon H J 1975 Surgical disorders of the peripheral nerves, 2nd edn. Churchill Livingstone, Edinburgh, p 32
Sunderland S 1951 A classification of peripheral nerve injuries producing loss of function. Brain 74: 491
Sunderland S 1978 Nerves and nerve injuries, 2nd edn. Churchill Livingstone, Edinburgh, p 133

Changes in denervated structures

26. Changes in denervated bones, joints, periarticular structures and tendons

GENERAL CONSIDERATIONS

A nerve injury may be followed by changes in bones, joints and tendon sheaths of the affected parts. These changes are usually sited at and below the wrist and ankle and are particularly marked following severe injuries of the brachial plexus and sciatic nerve, involving as they do most of the innervation to the limb.

Severance of a peripheral nerve not only deprives bones, joints and periarticular structures of their sensory innervation, and vessels of vasomotor control, but also, and importantly, muscles of their motor innervation.

The role of disuse and inactivity in the production of the changes following denervation

The changes in bones, articular and periarticular structures and in the connective tissues of fascial planes that follow denervation and the paralysis of muscles on the one hand, and those developing during unrelieved immobilisation without denervation on the other, are alike. In each case, the development and nature of the changes are more closely related to disuse and inactivity than to any other factor. This makes it difficult to evaluate the effects directly attributable to denervation of the affected parts.

Disuse and inactivity promote venous and lymphatic stasis and lead to nutritional disturbances in the tissues that accelerate the formation of tissue fluid and its accumulation in tissue spaces. Swelling and oedema may also be increased as the result of a co-existing soft tissue injury, wound infection, and bone fracture, while ligation of the major

artery supplying the limb may introduce an additional complicating factor.

Exudate gravitates to dependent parts, tracking along muscles to their attachments in the vicinity of joints where it collects to result in the softening, relaxation and stretching of joint capsules and ligaments. These changes are eventually followed by fibrosis, the formation of adhesions in tissue planes and about joints, and muscle contractures. Osteoporosis is a further result of the impaired circulation and is a conspicuous feature of some 'irritative' lesions where pain compels immobilisation of the affected parts.

The important factors contributing to the development of bone and joint pathology that may seriously impair joint functions are, therefore, the inactivity of muscles from paralysis or immobilisation, and the complications that follow venous and lymphatic stasis and vasoconstrictor paralysis or irritation. Subsequently, muscle contractures, adhesions and fibrosis develop that result in articular stiffness and rigidity, and in the restricted movement at joints.

The role of vasomotor disturbances in the production of the changes following denervation

The vasodilatation that follows the division of sympathetic pathways contributes to circulatory disturbances and the complications to which they give rise. Vasomotor effects may also follow the pathological involvement, as opposed to the complete division, of sympathetic pathways. Thus scarring at the site of a partial nerve injury, or in the proximal stump of a severed nerve, may create trigger zones of great sensitivity that initiate abnormal vasomotor reflexes that operate over unaffected pathways. Bone and joint changes are more common where cutaneous trophic disturbances are a prominent feature of the nerve lesion, the relationship suggesting a common origin for both. These changes are most marked in the hand and the foot.

The role of the sensory loss in the production of the changes following denervation

Recurrent trauma to an insensitive and unprotected part, such as occurs when a denervated foot is subjected to weight-bearing, adds to the severity of the denervation changes.

ARTICULAR AND PERIARTICULAR STRUCTURES

Anaesthesia renders joints and periarticular structures more susceptible to trauma, firstly because of the loss of protective sensory mechanisms, and secondly because a joint that is insensitive is more likely to be ill-treated. Injury increases the effusion of fluid in and about the joint, thereby predisposing to fibrosis and the formation of adhesions. These changes are less severe in pure motor lesions because unaffected protective sensory mechanisms and pain ensure rest following joint injury.

Because high lesions give maximal peripheral involvement, severe changes are more common after irreparable injuries of the brachial plexus and of the median, ulnar and sciatic nerves in the proximal part of the limb.

The importance of anaesthesia and trauma in the aetiology of joint pathology accompanying denervation should be stressed.

The consequences of denervation on articular and periarticular structures relate to joint weakness and instability, joint stiffness and limitation of movement, deformities and dislocation.

Joint weakness and instability

Joints are particularly susceptible to trauma and dislocation when an insensitive joint is subjected to repeated trauma, is rendered insecure by the paralysis of supporting muscles and is weakened by the softening, relaxation and stretching of the joint capsule and its supporting ligaments. In general, joint pathology is most destructive in weight-bearing joints. Particularly vulnerable in this respect are the joints of the foot in lesions of the sciatic nerve when weight-bearing has been permitted without adequate protection and support.

Joint stiffness and limitation of movement.

These complications are due to fibrosis and adhesions that involve the capsule and ligaments of the joint and in this way restrict or prevent free movement.

Deformity

The paralysis of some muscles and the unopposed action of contracting antagonists results in the development of deformities. In the early stages these are reducible, either passively or by the contraction of unaffected muscles, but in time they will, if neglected, become fixed and irreducible. An illustrative example is the griffe deformity of ulnar nerve lesions (Fig. 26.1).

Joint dislocation

Weakening of the joint capsule and supporting structures predisposes to dislocation. Recurrent trauma to an insensitive and insecure joint may finally lead to its total collapse and disintegration. Dislocation of the shoulder joint may occur in this way as a complication of neglected brachial plexus injury.

BONE

The changes observed in bones after nerve injuries depend on the age of the patient at the time of the injury and the duration of denervation. In general the changes become more marked, particularly in the small bones of the hands and feet, as the duration of denervation increases. They also tend to be more prominent with nerve injuries at the root of the limb when the territory denervated or rendered inactive is more extensive.

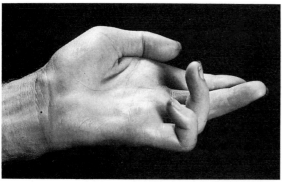

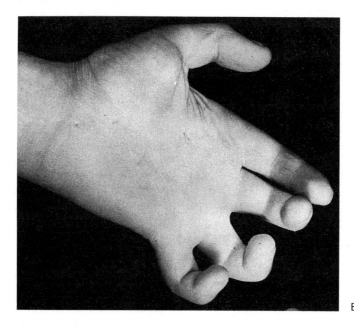

Fig. 26.1   The irreducible ulnar griffe deformity of ulnar nerve lesions

Adult bones

In adult bones, both form and contour are already firmly established though bone remains sensitive throughout life to influences that may modify its structure. Accordingly, though the general form and contour of denervated bones are preserved, the texture is altered. The cortex is reduced in thickness with a corresponding increase in the diameter of the medullary canal. With advanced atrophy the cortex may become converted into a thin shell of bone. The trabeculae of cancellous bone become thinner, some even disappearing, so that the overall effect is one of decalcification and increased porosity (osteoporosis). These changes are greater in the vicinity of joints. Following re-innervation and the restoration of function, the original architecture of the bone is not fully restored. Trabeculae that have disappeared are not reformed though those surviving become thicker, leading to the appearance of a trabecular pattern in which the framework is composed of coarser but more openly arranged strands. This new pattern provides permanent and unmistakable evidence that the bone has suffered a period of disuse osteoporosis.

In the case of the carpal and tarsal bones the osteoporosis is often marked, being usually patchy at first and only later becoming generalised. This radiological picture is not, however, specific for nerve injuries as it is also seen when there is imposed inactivity but no nerve damage. It is also of interest that the changes associated with nerve injury are not confined to the bones in the region innervated by the injured nerve.

Failure to support and protect the denervated foot in sciatic nerve lesions predisposes to stress fracturing of the weakened metatarsals.

Growing bones

Young bones in which growth is continuing actively are more vulnerable to abnormal influences introduced by nerve injury.

Nerve injuries sustained during this period, in addition to modifying the texture of the bone, may also affect bone growth. The nature of the changes induced in this way naturally depends on the duration and distribution of the denervation and the extent to which the affected limb is immobilised as a result of the injury. Furthermore, disturbances of bone growth originating in this way may modify joint surfaces, thereby predisposing to dislocation.

Where there is muscle paralysis, the forces responsible for moulding bone structure are absent with the result that bony prominences, markings and other features that are produced by muscle growth and pull are poorly developed.

The changes in bone consequent on denervation could be due directly to the loss of some neurotrophic influence or indirectly to vascular changes and/or disuse resulting from the nerve injury.

Neurotrophic factor

There is no evidence of a specific neurotrophic factor affecting the growth and structure of bone.

The sympathetic nervous system and vascular changes

Osteoporosis is common in those lesions in which trophic changes become a prominent feature of the lesion. These 'trophic' effects are believed to be an expression of disturbed vasomotor function and it could be that the accompanying bone changes have a similar origin.

The role of the sympathetic nervous system in bone growth and the maintenance of bone structure is by no means clear. Some maintain that sympathectomy of the limb is without effect on bone. Others are equally convinced, from both experimental and clinical evidence, that sympathectomy results in an acceleration of bone growth and a slight increase in the length of the sympathectomised limb, both of which are attributed to the increased blood supply that follows sympathectomy.

Sensory innervation

Selective nerve section has shown that sensory innervation is without effect on the growth and structure of bone.

Motor innervation

There is much clinical and experimental evidence indicating that muscle activity influences the growth and form of bone and the maintenance of bone structure. For this reason:

1. Nerve injuries do not provide suitable material for a separate evaluation of neural and muscular influences on bone because muscle activity is dependent on nerve supply and any interference with the latter inevitably results in changes in the former.
2. The changes in bone following nerve section on the one hand and immobilisation without denervation on the other are alike, the rate of onset and extent of the changes being, in each case, more closely related to the degree of disuse of the part than to any other factor.

Conclusion

The bone changes associated with a nerve injury are due principally to the disuse arising from muscle paralysis, though there is some evidence that vascular changes may also contribute to the final condition.

Bone repair

Nerve injuries do not, per se, retard or in any other way disadvantage the union and consolidation of fractures.

27. Changes in denervated muscle

DENERVATION ATROPHY

For information on the changes produced in muscles by denervation we are forced to rely largely on experimental studies, supplemented, where possible, by the histological examination of biopsy material taken from human muscles prior to or during an operation (Sunderland 1978).

Though clinical observation and the examination of biopsy tissue fail to provide the range and wealth of material that can be obtained experimentally, they nevertheless are consistent with the account that is to follow, which is based on an experimental study by Sunderland and Ray (1950).

Muscle tissue may survive denervation for at least 2 years. Over this period its general form is preserved and, though distinctly paler than normal, it retains a colour and a texture that identifies it as muscle tissue. Fibrillation and the shortening of the muscle on removal indicate that contractile tissue survives denervation for this long period.

Experimentally, there is a rapid initial loss of weight, the muscle sustaining a 30 per cent loss by the end of the 1st month. This increases to 50 to 60 per cent by the 2nd month beyond which the process then slows, a relatively stable state being reached somewhere about the 4th month. From this time onwards the weight loss varies between 60 and 80 per cent.

Attention is directed to the marked loss of weight that occurs within the first 2 months of denervation.

THE HISTOLOGY OF DENERVATION MUSCLE ATROPHY

In the absence of secondary complications, such as those due to vascular and lymphatic stasis and direct injury, muscle fibres become grossly atrophied but retain those histological characteristics upon which their identification depends (Fig. 27.1).

While the entire muscle is affected, the changes do not affect all muscle fibres uniformly so that the microstructure of the muscle tissue varies throughout the muscle.

The extrafusal muscle fibre

The earliest and most characteristic change in the structure of a denervated muscle fibre involves a loss of sarcoplasm and a reduction in its calibre. This change is generalised and proceeds at about the same rate throughout the muscle. The fibres atrophy rapidly in the initial stages so that by the 2nd month the average cross-sectional area of the fibre is reduced by 70 per cent. The process then slows appreciably until by the 4th month the atrophy advances only a further 10 per cent. From this time onwards the atrophy varies between 80 and 90 per cent.

The fibres suffer more severely than the loss in weight of the muscle indicates so that the calibre of the fibres provides a more accurate measure of the effects of denervation than does the weight of the muscle. The difference between weight loss and reduction in fibre calibre is accounted for by a relative increase in the amount of connective tissue that compensates in some measure for the greater atrophy of the fibres.

While it is true that some muscle fibres degenerate and are lost, this is not the fate of the majority. The question of muscle fibre degeneration is discussed later.

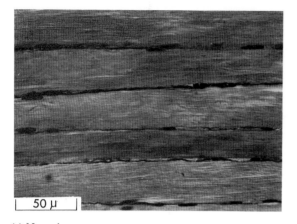

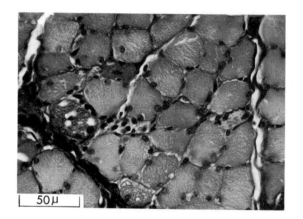

(a) Normal

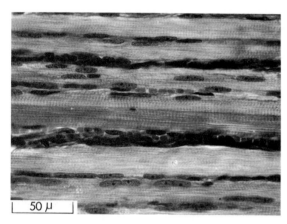

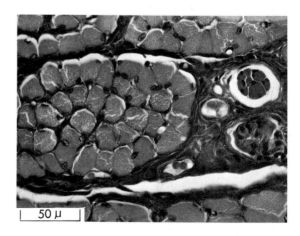

(b) *PT: D* 49; *M* 55; *F* 67

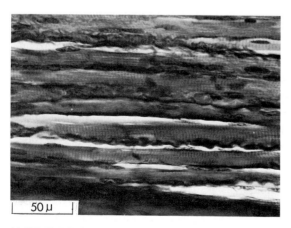

(c) *PT: D* 112; *M* 72; *F* 82

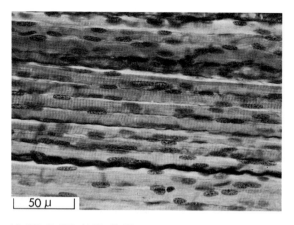

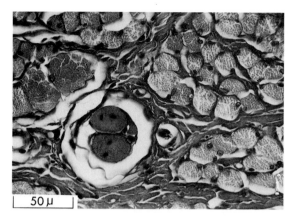

(d) *PT: D 229; M 74; F 87*

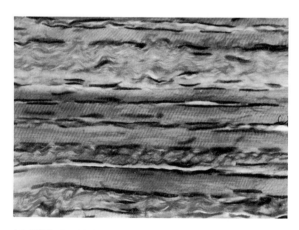

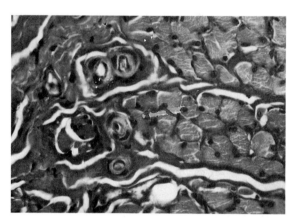

(e) *FCU: D 485; M 69; F 91*

Fig. 27.1   Longitudinal and transverse sections of a normal pronator teres muscle and muscles denervated for 49, 112, 229 and 485 days. *D* = duration of denervation in days; *PT* = pronator teres; *FCU* = flexor carpi ulnaris; *M* = % muscle atrophy; *F* = % muscle fibre atrophy (Australian marsupial; *Trichosurus vulpecula*).

Motor end plates

Surviving fibres still carried an end plate regardless of the period of denervation though it is not possible to decide whether they suffer any reduction in number. End plates, however, become more difficult to detect as the atrophy of the fibres reaches maximal values, since they then extend across the full width of the fibre so that great care is required to distinguish their nuclei from other nuclear aggregations within the fibre. The end plate nuclei do not undergo the enlargement observed in the case of the subsarcolemmal nuclei but remain unchanged. End plates have been identified in human material after a year's denervation; thereafter fibre atrophy makes their identification difficult.

The neuromuscular spindle

Atrophic changes involve the intrafusal as well as the extrafusal fibres but not to the same degree.

The periaxial space remains patent and well defined, is not encroached on by connective tissue and there is little, if any, thickening of the capsule which does not lose its identity by blending with the surrounding connective tissue. As a result, spindles have been readily identified in experimental material 16 months after denervation.

Connective tissue

The entire muscle is surrounded by a layer of condensed areolar connective tissue, the epimysium, from which a large number of septa pass into the substance of the muscle. These fine septa divide and fuse in an irregular manner so that the muscle fibres are collected into a number of bundles or fasciculi that vary in size and shape, and which are enclosed in a thin but well defined layer of connective tissue, the perimysium. Within each bundle individual muscle fibres are closely packed together. Each fibre is invested in, and separated from its neighbours by, a delicate sheath of connective tissue, the endomysium, which, at the periphery of the bundle, is continuous with the perimysium. The normal histological picture is such that any increase in connective tissue can be easily recognised.

During the 1st month of denervation the essential reaction is one of atrophy of muscle fibres; obvious changes are not detected in either the amount or the features of the connective tissue. Proliferation of connective tissue appears first in the perimysium and later the endomysium, while the deposition of new collagen in both regions is always preceded by a marked increase in the number of fibroblasts. This great increase in fibroblasts is, together with muscle fibre atrophy, the most characteristic feature of the histological picture of denervation. Cellular proliferation in the endomysium, which precedes any thickening of this interstitial layer, produces large numbers of nuclei that are sandwiched between still tightly packed muscle fibres.

The proliferation of fibroblasts that is first evident in the perimysium at the end of the 1st month peaks at the 3rd month, by which time there is also a considerable increase in the cellularity of the endomysium. Between the 1st and 3rd months this increasing cellularity is followed by a progressive thickening of the perimysium followed by the endomysium, both becoming composed of coarser and more tightly packed fibres that stain more deeply. By the 3rd month, the endomysial thickening has progressed to such a degree that individual atrophied muscle fibres are now separated from one another instead of being packed tightly together. From this time onwards there is little further thickening of the endomysium and perimysium. This increase in connective tissue is relative rather than absolute, there being in fact an overall reduction in the amount of connective tissue as the muscle atrophies.

The connective tissue increase does not result in any disorganisation of the overall internal architecture of the muscle. The final picture is one in which the septa outlining the bundles and the spaces between the atrophied fibres are occupied by thickened connective tissue. At no stage are atrophying muscle fibres replaced by fibrous tissue; this only occurs in those scattered small foci where muscle fibres have degenerated.

The survival of muscle fibres following denervation should not be surprising in view of evidence that muscle may develop its characteristic features in the total absence of a nerve supply. Furthermore, good and in some cases complete restoration of function can occur in reinnervated human muscles following periods of denervation of at least 12 months, provided the quiescent muscle has been maintained in the best possible condition by appropriate physiotherapy (Chapter 29).

MUSCLE DEGENERATION. FIBROSIS. CONTRACTURE

Under certain circumstances grossly atrophied muscle fibres become involved in irreversible changes that lead to the loss of the fibre and its replacement by connective tissue. Such extreme changes are clearly not general and the findings suggest that factors other than denervation, but which are conceivably associated with it, are responsible for the degeneration.

The onset and distribution of the degenerative changes

The degeneration of muscle fibres is a delayed phenomenon when it does occur. It is not usually seen before the 6th month but is clearly evident by the 9th month and is well advanced by the twelfth. Initially the degenerative changes are in the form of scattered foci affecting small numbers of muscle fibres. More fibres are progressively affected until the foci enlarge and merge, thereby involving more extensive areas. The overall picture is consequently one in which the degenerative changes occur irregularly and vary in severity throughout the denervated muscle.

The nature of the degenerative changes

At some stage the ultrastructural changes characteristic of the atrophic process may, for reasons not yet fully understood, terminate in the degeneration of the fibre. This degeneration occurs in three different ways in the same muscle, though each ultimately leads to the disappearance of the muscle fibre.

1. Progressive thinning and obliteration of the muscle fibre. Atrophy continues and the calibre of the muscle fibre is progressively reduced until the shrunken fibre is finally composed of a very fine strand that gradually merges without any clear line of demarcation into the fibrous strands of the endomysium. The affected area is not invaded by phagocytes, the appearance suggesting that the change occurs so gradually that local adjustments do not require the intervention of these elements.

2. Nuclear clumping with the disintegration of the muscle fibre. Here the nuclei of the atrophying fibre collect into clumps which give the fibre an irregular outline in longitudinal section. The fibre then fragments. Though there is some phagocytic activity at the site of the muscle fibre fragments, this is only occasionally to a marked degree and is not a conspicuous feature of the degeneration.

3. Swelling, vacuolation and disintegration. Here local swelling and vacuolation of the fibre occur with rupture of the sarcolemmal membrane and fragmentation of the fibre. Unlike the two previously mentioned forms of degeneration, the affected area is invaded by phagocytes and the histological picture suggests a more acute and rapid form of degeneration.

An increase in connective tissue and the appearance of fat cells accompany the disintegration, obliteration and loss of muscle fibres but there is no evidence that muscle fibres are converted into fibrous tissue or fat, the change being one of replacement rather than conversion.

The terminal stage is one in which all trace of organised muscle fibres is lost, the original structure being now represented by strands of fibrous tissue with columns of fat cells amongst which are scattered clumps and short chains of nuclei that alone represent the original muscle fibre.

FIBROSIS

Widespread interstitial fibrosis involving muscles, tendon sheaths and capsular structures is a familiar picture in cases of longstanding denervation, particularly where the nerve injury has been aggravated by gross infection and ischaemia. These changes are so prejudicial to the restoration of function, if and when reinnervation takes place, that they should be kept to a minimum by appropriate therapy.

Fibrosis in denervated striated muscle is the end result of two changes.

1. The proliferation of fibroblasts that precedes the deposition of fibrillar material leads to an increase in the connective tissue of the muscle. The collagen fibres gradually become coarser and more closely packed until each atrophied muscle fibre is enclosed in, and separated from its neighbours by, a greatly thickened endomysium while each fasciculus is enveloped in a thickened perimysium.

2. Muscle fibre degeneration and its replacement by fibrous tissue. The fibrosis that develops in denervated muscles is due essentially to circulatory disturbances originating within an inactive paralysed muscle. It ultimately results in the formation of contractures in muscles, with adhesions that attach them to surrounding structures

thereby reducing their mobility. These changes fix the muscle in the position in which it has been immobilised or allowed to shorten. In this way joint movement becomes restricted, while a joint may also become fixed in an unnatural position as a result of the unopposed action of normal muscles.

Fibrosis and contractures appear earlier and are more extensive and severe in the ischaemic lesions of vascular injury than is the case in an irreparable nerve injury.

The following three types of histological changes have been described in biopsy specimens of muscles removed from patients with serious damage to the main artery of the limb or to the vessels supplying the affected muscles, and even trivial damage causing slow haemorrhage within fascial-bound spaces: (1) massive necrosis of muscle fibres; (2) dense interstitial fibrosis enclosing fibres that may be normal, atrophied or necrosed; (3) scattered foci of necrosis with patchy interstitial fibrosis, due to the pressure from a tight plaster, crushing of the limb, fractures with arterial contusion, or slow haemorrhage within fascial planes.

CONTRACTURE

Contractures in muscles develop as the result of a variety of causes.

1. In paralysed muscles subjected to prolonged unrelieved immobilisation. The basic lesion is an interstitial fibrosis in the muscle that is shortened or lengthened depending on the position in which it has been immobilised.
2. In the unopposed antagonist of a paralysed muscle. The muscle imbalance introduced by loss of a component of the muscular apparatus acting on the joint involves a redistribution of muscle power and a new equilibrium to which the antagonist adapts by a gradual change in its structure, so that in time it adjusts itself to its new position by

becoming structurally shortened. If unrelieved, this results in an interstitial fibrosis, permanent shortening, capsular changes and finally joint fixation.
3. As the result of ischaemic changes in affected muscles.
4. The spontaneous or therapeutic immobilisation of a part in a position to relieve pain may result in contractures in muscles that have been rendered inactive as a result of the immobilisation.
5. Irritation of a damaged nerve by a foreign body or scar tissue causing spasm of the muscle.
6. Physiopathic reflex contractures characterised by immobilisation of the part accompanied by prominent trophic and vasomotor disturbances.

Contractures of the variety outlined in (4), (5) and (6) are no longer common but were given prominence and attracted considerable attention, in particular by several French and German writers during World War I. They appear to have been the product of prolonged infection, with treatment of the patient and the denervated parts that would be considered inadequate and unsatisfactory by modern standards.

Contractures due to fibrosis are to be distinguished from those due to the increased muscle tone or spasm that develops in certain irritative lesions. Spasm is relieved by nerve block and warming, both of which are without effect on muscle contracture due to fibrosis.

Factors influencing the onset, course and severity of the changes developing in denervated muscles and the measures available to prevent or correct them are discussed in the next chapter.

REFERENCES

Sunderland S 1978 Nerves and nerve injuries, 2nd edn. Churchill Livingstone, Edinburgh, p 229
Sunderland S, Ray L S 1950 Denervation changes in mammalian striated muscle. Journal of Neurology, Neurosurgery and Psychiatry 13: 159

28. Factors influencing the development and severity of the changes in denervated muscle

GENERAL CONSIDERATIONS

Again we are largely dependent on experimental studies for information concerning the factors that influence the development and nature of the changes occurring in denervated muscles. Of significance are factors peculiar to species, to individuals within species, to individual muscles and to different muscle fibres within the same muscle. Mechanical, thermal and electrical influences have also been shown to affect the changes occurring in denervated muscles.

The muscle wasting that is such a characteristic feature of denervation is due mainly to the atrophy of muscle fibres. There is much clinical and experimental evidence to indicate that, in the uncomplicated case, this atrophy does not normally terminate in the dissolution of the fibre. When degeneration occurs it is initially focal in its distribution and only later becomes widespread as the adverse conditions responsible for the disintegration of muscle fibres continue to operate.

Against this background it is of clinical interest to enquire why the degeneration of muscle fibres should be an uncommon event following uncomplicated denervation and, because precise information is lacking on this point, to speculate on the factors that could be responsible for the degeneration when it becomes a prominent feature of the pathology of the muscle.

From a study of denervation phenomena in striated muscle it is clear that the nerve supply to a muscle is essential for maintaining the structure of muscle fibres and muscles, the enzymatic and metabolic activity of muscle fibres, the histo-chemical profile of muscle fibres and the functional integrity of muscle fibres.

Though there is now a reasonably clear picture of the behaviour of muscle fibres following denervation, our knowledge of the processes involved remains incomplete. However, even though the mechanism is not understood, some factors have been identified that influence the onset, development, and severity of the changes in denervated striated muscle (Sunderland 1978).

THE TROPHIC FACTOR

The axonal link between the nerve cell and the muscle fibre provides for complex inter-relationships additional to and independent of those connected with the transmission of nerve impulses. The well-being of muscle fibres could normally be due to some as yet unidentified neurotrophic factor provided by the neuron, the loss of which could be responsible for the atrophy of denervation.

There is now considerable support for the belief that the mechanism by which the motor nerve exerts a trophic influence over the muscle involves axon transport systems, and that denervation changes are due to the loss of a trophic substance that is transported down the axon, released at the nerve endings and taken up by the muscle.

The mechanism by which the hypothetical trophic substance gains entry to the muscle from the nerve terminal remains conjectural. We are, therefore, left with an established trophic influence of nerve on muscle, mediated by an unidentified hypothetical substance or substances, that operate by way of mechanisms that are the subject of considerable speculation.

The concept of such a neurotrophic influence, however, leaves unexplained the atrophy of tenotomy and immobilisation that develops in essentially the same way as that following denervations despite the fact that the pathway between the nerve cell and the muscle is preserved (Sunderland & Lavarack 1959, Sunderland 1978).

THE HISTOLOGICAL FACTOR

In order to enter the muscle fibre, nutrient materials conveyed in the capillaries to the muscles must be transported across the capillary endothelium, the sarcolemma, and the interval between these two membranes. Transcapillary transport and exchange depend, inter alia, on such factors as blood flow velocity and the condition of the capillary endothelium. Diffusion across the interstitial space will be influenced by its composition and the distance separating capillaries and muscle fibres, that is, the density of the capillary network. In the case of the sarcolemmal membrane transfer is more complicated, involving as it does both diffusion and the active transport of materials that require attachment to and release from a mobile or fixed carrier in the membrane.

Whether or not denervation introduces changes that embarrass transport mechanisms and the uptake of substances provided by the capillaries remains to be clarified. Any thickening of the capillary wall, deposition of collagen tissue in the interstitial space or adverse changes in the molecular structure of the sarcolemmal membrane could be expected to have the effect of impeding the transfer of nutrients from vessel to muscle fibre.

THE VASCULAR FACTOR

The blood flow through the capillary bed of the muscle is decisive in maintaining the nutrition of muscle fibres, thereby ensuring their survival. Information relating to the blood flow through denervated muscle is conflicting.

Following a nerve injury the circulation through denervated muscle is altered by: (1) the vasoconstrictor paralysis, and (2) the loss or reduction of muscle activity due to the paralysis of some muscles and the disuse or immobilisation of normally innervated muscles.

The experimental evidence has it that, at the time when muscle tissue is atrophying most rapidly, the blood flow through the muscle, and particularly through its capillary bed, increases to a level that ensures a blood supply to denervated muscle fibres that is sufficient to meet their metabolic and functional requirements. From this it is concluded that muscle atrophy is not the result of an impaired blood supply.

Again, the atrophy following denervation exceeds that due to disuse, as the examination of the distribution and degree of wasting associated with an ulnar nerve paralysis and immobilisation of the hand will reveal. Here, though wasting is generalised, it is obviously greater in the ulnar than in the median field. This would suggest that more than a vascular factor is involved in the genesis of muscle atrophy.

However, there is other evidence to the contrary. Though the vasoconstrictor paralysis leads to an immediate increase in the blood flow through denervated muscles, this effect is temporary owing to the gradual return of some tone in the denervated vessels. Furthermore, the rate of flow is ultimately diminished by the reduced muscular activity to a level that threatens the survival of atrophied muscle fibres.

Muscle contractions during exercise and, to a lesser degree, the passive stretching and shortening that occur during limb movements, have an important effect on the circulation through muscle, the blood flow being low at rest but increased many times during activity.

The adverse effects of inactivity on the flow of blood to and through a muscle has more profound effects than the vasomotor paralysis. Failure of the pumping action of the muscles leads to venous and lymphatic congestion and stasis which are maximal in the most dependent part of the limb, namely the hand and the foot, where gravity imposes a further burden on venous return from the limb. This, in turn, results in the accumulation of metabolites in the muscle, an oxygen deficit and a carbon dioxide excess, all of which contribute to the dilatation of the vascular bed and the venous stasis. The overall effect of these changes is to impair the nutrition of muscle fibres, which consequently atrophy.

Finally, venous and capillary congestion and stasis, and the thrombosis that threatens under these conditions, may so impair the nutrition of the muscle fibres that they degenerate and are replaced by connective tissue.

Accepting prolonged muscle inactivity whatever its cause, and the vascular impairment to which it gives rise, as the essential aetiological factors leading to the degeneration of muscle fibres one would expect degenerative changes to be:

1. focal in their distribution in the initial stages, becoming more generalised as the vascular complications extend;
2. influenced by the degree to which muscle activity is reduced;
3. more common and more severe in peripherally situated muscles where the circulation is likely to be more seriously impaired. Thus the muscles of the hand and foot should be more vulnerable than those of the forearm and leg;
4. all other things being equal, as common in normal muscles subjected to prolonged disuse as in muscles subjected to prolonged denervation;
5. increased in extent and severity as the period of denervation is prolonged.

In general the findings are consistent with these assumptions.

The picture suggests that more widespread involvement results from the enlargement and fusion of smaller scattered foci of degeneration. Thickening of the arteries and narrowing of the lumen have been described in denervated muscles. These changes became accentuated after 1 year's denervation, so that arteries are ultimately obliterated and many capillaries compressed out of existence. Degenerative changes are, however, also seen where there is no such advanced vascular pathology.

Thus the general proposition that loss of muscle activity and the vascular impairment associated with it are the principal offenders responsible for muscle fibre degeneration and replacement fibrosis is consistent with the development, distribution and nature of the changes observed experimentally in denervated muscle.

The significance of venous and lymphatic stasis in the production of degenerative lesions should not be underestimated.

THE METABOLIC FACTOR

This concerns the capacity of a denervated cell to utilise substrates that are made available and which, in turn, raises the further question of whether the nervous system exercises a control over biochemical mechanisms inside the cell. The metabolism of muscle fibres depends, inter alia, on the availability of substrates in sufficient amounts to meet the functional needs of the cells, the passage of these substrates across membranes, and their uptake by the cell. This involves complex membrane transport systems and the utilisation of these substances by cellular activity that is subject to intracellular regulatory mechanisms.

It has been suggested that the metabolism of muscle fibres is regulated, in an as yet unexplained way, by substances elaborated in the motor neuron and transported down the axon into the muscle fibre. Following nerve section, these 'activating' elements could no longer reach the muscle, with the result that the utilisation of substrates and metabolic recovery processes would be impaired and the muscle fibre would atrophy.

That this is not the only factor operating, however, is shown by the advanced wasting that follows disuse from immobilisation and tenotomy, despite the fact that in both these cases the muscle has an intact nerve supply.

THE FATIGUE FACTOR

Could the ceaseless fibrillation that is a characteristic feature of denervation contribute to the atrophy of denervated muscle fibres? Though there is a broad correspondence between the two, there is still insufficient evidence to decide whether fibrillation is the cause of the atrophy or merely an accompanying phenomenon. The following experimental evidence is contrary to a causal relationship.

1. If the final common motor pathway is preserved, but isolated from all impulses impinging on it, atrophy follows essentially the same pattern in the affected muscles as that observed after denervation and yet there is no fibrillation.
2. The atrophy associated with immobilisation and tenotomy occurs in much the same way

as that following denervation; fibrillation is a prominent feature in the latter but is absent in the former.

3. The electrical stimulation of denervated muscle is said to retard the atrophy but has no significant effect on the fibrillation.

4. Denervated muscle commences to atrophy before the onset of fibrillation.

INHERENT FACTORS

Variations as between species. A study of the denervation changes reported for different experimental mammals indicates that, though the overall picture is substantially the same, the weight loss occurs more rapidly in the initial stages in some animals than in others.

Variations as between individuals. Both clinical and experimental observations show that the rate of atrophy of denervated muscles is subject to a wide range of individual variation. Some patients with peripheral nerve injuries show marked wasting within 3 months, while in others wasting occurs more slowly and is spread over a longer period.

Variations as between different muscles. Muscles differ in the manner and rate at which they atrophy following denervation. This cannot be explained on the basis of differences in tension or disuse.

Variations as between different muscle fibres in the same muscle. At any given time the various parts of a denervated muscle show different stages of atrophy, some muscle fibres being more affected than others. After excluding vascular complications, stretch, disuse and other factors contributing to the atrophic process, we are forced to the conclusion that the removal of a trophic influence and/or disturbances of nutrition affect some fibres sooner and to a greater degree than others.

MECHANICAL AND THERMAL FACTORS

In the previous chapter atrophy and the degenerative changes in denervated muscle, together with the fibrosis associated with them, have been related to such variables as disuse, the impaired circulation to which it gives rise, and the nutritional disturbances that follow.

Conditions that increase, extend and prolong disuse, and still further prejudice an already impaired circulation through the denervated muscle, hasten atrophy and encourage muscle fibre degeneration and fibrosis. Such conditions also adversely affect the restoration of function following reinnervation of the muscle. On the other hand, conditions that prevent or minimise disuse and improve the circulation through the denervated muscle retard atrophy and assist muscle fibres to survive. In this way they provide for improved recovery following reinnervation.

Conditions that have been studied in relation to denervation atrophy will now be discussed.

The influence of movement, inactivity and the position of the limb

It is now well established that the condition of denervated muscles and the rate at which they recover following reinnervation are adversely affected by prolonged immobilisation of the affected parts, the position in which they are fixed, and overstretching.

Prolonged inactivity, due either to paralysis or to immobilisation by splints or casts, prejudices venous return and leads to venous stasis. As a result the pressure in the muscle vascular bed is raised and the circulation through it is reduced. The extent to which immobilisation alters the blood flow through the muscle depends on such factors as the time for which it operates and whether it is intermittent or continuous.

Unrelieved immobilisation: (1) increases the rate of wasting; (2) increases the severity of the atrophic changes and encourages degeneration and fibrosis in denervated muscles; (3) delays the onset of functional recovery in reinnervated muscles and slows its subsequent progress.

Atrophy is maximal when muscles are immobilised in both a shortened and overstretched position and is minimal when they are splinted in a neutral or resting position.

Clinically, it has been established that stretching paralysed muscles delays, and may even prevent, functional recovery after they are reinnervated.

An associated bone, joint or soft tissue injury may demand priority of treatment that involves such prolonged and extensive immobilisation that the survival of denervated muscle fibres is threatened. Under such unfavourable conditions degenerative changes are not necessarily confined to the paralysed muscles but may also affect normal muscles rendered inactive by the immobilisation.

On the other hand, in simple uncomplicated nerve injuries, splinting to relax and prevent overstretching of paralysed muscles and the development of deformities from the unopposed action of other factors should never be carried to excess. Splinting should be relieved regularly and the affected parts massaged and manipulated in order to exercise not only the denervated muscles but also those rendered inactive by the immobilisation. Regular movements, active and passive, improve the circulation by reducing venous stasis and assisting venous return, and lead to earlier functional recovery in reinnervated muscles. Splinting designed to permit normal muscles to perform a full range of movement but which finally returns the paralysed muscles to a position of rest has, therefore, a distinct advantage.

Influence of trauma

Denervated muscle fibres are particularly susceptible to trauma in the form of repeated overstretching that accelerates atrophy and favours the development of degenerative changes.

The influence of gravity

When vasomotor tone in the peripheral vessels is lost, and the supporting and pumping action of striated muscles on the venous system fails or is impaired, blood accumulates in the dependent parts causing venous congestion and ultimately a reduction in blood flow through the capillary bed. These conditions are aggravated when the limb is maintained in a dependent position for long periods, the impaired circulation then being maximal in the hand and foot.

Postural venous congestion and oedema are detrimental to the survival and well being of muscle fibres and, where possible, should be prevented by appropriate posturing of the limb, the use of supporting bandages wherever practicable, and by regular exercises designed to utilise the contractions of normal muscles to promote venous return.

The influence of temperature

Exposure to cold makes additional demands on the circulation in the denervated muscle that it is unable to meet. This leads to further impairment of the nutrition of denervated muscle fibres so that recovery will be retarded even if the rate of atrophy is not accelerated. Denervated parts should be kept warm and well protected from exposure.

Conclusions

Conditions aggravating muscle atrophy, contributing to muscle fibre degeneration and retarding recovery following reinnervation are:

1. Vascular and lymphatic stasis.
2. Unrelieved immobilisation.
3. Immobilisation in a stretched position.
4. Cold.

Conditions that maintain atrophied muscle fibres in a healthy state, prevent those changes that threaten their survival, and hasten recovery following reinnervation are warmth, and immobilisation in a position of rest relieved at regular intervals to allow active and passive exercises planned to reduce vascular and lymphatic stasis and to promote the flow of blood through the muscle. Co-existing non-neural injuries that demand temporary but unrelieved immobilisation must naturally take priority.

THE EFFECT OF ELECTRICAL STIMULATION ON THE CHANGES OCCURRING IN DENERVATED MUSCLES

Regarding the effect of electrical stimulation on denervated muscle, the important question to be settled is whether or not this has any special advantage in maintaining denervated muscle fibres in a healthy state, in preventing the development of those changes that threaten their survival, and in hastening recovery following reinnervation.

Data relating to this question are available from both experimental and clinical sources and here there is a mass of conflicting information.

The following beneficial effects have been attributed to electrical stimulation.

1. Though it does not entirely prevent muscle atrophy, it does slow the process, delaying and reducing the wasting so that denervated muscle fibres survive, and await reinnervation, in a less atrophied state than would otherwise be the case.
2. As assessed by electromyography, it reduces the time between the reappearance of motor unit activity and the return of voluntary contractions.
3. It hastens the return of voluntary contractions by accelerating the rate of axon regeneration. Such a role is discussed and excluded in Chapter 15.
4. It improves the quality of motor recovery following reinnervation.
5. It has a psychological advantage in that it demonstrates to a patient that a muscle that is paralysed can be made to contract.
6. Despite any persisting uncertainties surrounding the value of electrical stimulation, it would be wrong to deny the patient a form of therapy that certainly does no harm and might be beneficial.

Conditions under which electrical stimulation is claimed to be effective in retarding experimental denervation atrophy are:

The strength of the stimulus. Treatment to be of any value must induce strong contractions. Stimuli causing feeble contractions are ineffective. Strong contractions have been avoided by some on the grounds that they may damage atrophied muscle fibres, though this view is not supported by the experimental evidence.

Strong stimulation is claimed to be effective at all stages of denervation. Unfortunately stimulation strong enough to be effective is often too uncomfortable to be tolerated by a patient.

Fatigue. In order to avoid the danger of fatiguing atrophied muscle fibres during treatment a rest interval of 1–10 minutes is recommended between each group of stimuli.

The site of the muscle. Treatment is more effective with superficially placed muscles that are readily accessible. It is least effective for deeply placed and inaccessible muscles.

The size of the muscle. Strong, generalised contractions are more easily induced in small than in large muscles.

The nature of the stimulus. Electrotherapy produces its most beneficial effects prior to reinnervation, so that galvanism is the only worthwhile form of stimulation. The form of the stimulating shocks used varies (sinusoidal, exponentially rising currents, rectangular pulses) but this factor is apparently without significance providing strong contractions are elicited.

The frequency of treatment. The effectiveness of electrotherapy is proportional to the frequency of treatment. Thus treatment given twice daily is more effective than when given once a day which, in turn, is more effective than its use on alternate days.

The duration of each treatment. The effect of electrical stimulation is proportional to the duration of each treatment.

The state of the muscle. Though stimulation of the denervated muscle retards atrophy, muscle weight once lost cannot be restored by stimulation during the denervation period.

Muscles should be stimulated under conditions that favour the development of maximum tension by the muscle fibres. Thus the beneficial effects of electrical stimulation are greatest when the muscles are stimulated under conditions that permit maximum isometric contraction, whereas stimulation is ineffective in tenotomy atrophy where isometric tension cannot be developed.

All the conditions required for electrotherapy to produce its most beneficial effects are not present in every patient. Treatment must frequently be modified and adjusted to meet the particular condition and interests of individual patients. However, any departure from the optimal conditions must be expected to reduce the effectiveness of the method.

How the alleged beneficial effects of electrical stimulation are achieved is not clear. It could be by:

1. improving the blood flow through the muscle as a result of the induced muscle contractions. This is assumed on the grounds that, normally, muscle activity increases the circulation and because electrical stimulation is less effective when there is a co-existing injury to a major blood vessel. However, according to the experimental evidence, there appears to be no significant increase in the volume of the capillaries or improvement in blood flow as the result of electrically induced exercise;
2. by improving the venous return from the muscle, thereby preventing the accumulation of damaging metabolites;
3. by some unspecified direct effect on the metabolism of the atrophying muscle fibres. How and in what way this is effected is not known.

The beneficial effects of electrical stimulation claimed by some are denied by others on the following grounds:

1. The clinical value of electrical stimulation is difficult to assess because so many other co-existing variables are combining to influence the onset, course and quality of motor recovery. This makes it difficult to determine any special claim to which electrical stimulation might be entitled.

2. Even among the advocates of electrical stimulation there is disagreement on such questions as the strength of the current to be used, when treatment should be commenced and terminated, the duration and frequency of stimulation and so on.

3. It has been stated that galvanic stimulation accelerates the return of the volume of the muscle to its predenervated state and that stimulation in the later stages of recovery is still effective in improving the quality of muscle function. For this reason continuation of electrical treatment is advised until motor recovery is well advanced. This claim should not be allowed to pass unchallenged.

In the author's experience, which is shared by many others, electrical stimulation has little effect at any stage of denervation and certainly nothing is to be gained by extending electrical treatment beyond the onset of recovery. Following the reappearance of muscle contractions in response to voluntary effort, a programme of voluntary exercises is more effective than contractions induced electrically.

4. Electrical stimulation is uncomfortable, tedious and demanding in terms of both time and effort. More importantly, in order to obtain the advantages claimed by its advocates, treatment necessitates an intensive and prolonged programme based on a demanding and time consuming regimen of electrical stimulation that makes excessive demands on trained personnel to say nothing of the inconvenience caused to patients. Needless to say, the costs of such a programme are considerable. For this reason one is justified in questioning whether the alleged benefits claimed for electrical stimulation are sufficiently significant to justify the greatly increased costs involved.

5. In the early 1940s the author conducted a study at a Base Military Hospital in which some patients received electrical stimulation and others did not. The results in the two groups were essentially the same, from which it was concluded that electrotherapy conferred no special advantages over and above those obtainable by a planned programme of massage, warmth, antigravity measures and a daily routine of active and passive muscle exercise carried through a full range of movements. Admittedly this was an inadequate study, neglecting as it did the full import of current strength, the intensity, frequency and duration of treatment and the necessity for a daily regimen far more demanding than was used at that time. However, the results were clear enough and, though perhaps open to other interpretations, echoed the experience of many others.

In all of these deliberations some critical questions are left unanswered.

1. Does the use of electrical stimulation consistently give better results?

2. Does the use of electrical stimulation significantly improve the quality of the recovery?
3. Does the use of electrical stimulation consistently hasten the onset of recovery?
4. How much worse off are patients who are denied this form of therapy?
5. A cost-effective/benefit study is needed to determine if the improvement conferred by electrical stimulation is so much better as to justify the greatly increased costs and inconvenience involved.

Until satisfactory answers to these questions are available the following conclusions seem to be not unreasonable.

1. Electrical stimulation is not a replacement for other treatment methods such as massage, warmth, antigravity measures and a daily routine of muscle exercises with movements taken actively and passively through a full range.
2. It has yet to be convincingly demonstrated that electrical stimulation of denervated muscle provides a definite bonus to treatment by retarding muscle atrophy, preserving muscle fibres in a more favourable state pending reinnervation, hastening the onset and course of motor recovery and improving the quality of the end result.
3. At the present time the case for electrical stimulation as an adjunct to muscle recovery should be listed as not proven.
4. Clinically, there is no hard evidence to suggest that the addition of electrical stimulation to the therapeutic basket adds consistently or significantly to the recovery of muscle following reinnervation.
5. A cost effective study will finally be necessary to decide whether electrical stimulation is a worthwhile clinical therapeutic undertaking. The information currently available would suggest that the end does not justify the means.
6. Some will undoubtedly continue to use it and others will refrain from doing so and

the overall results will probably be the same in each case.

MEASURES DIRECTED TO IMPROVING THE BLOOD SUPPLY TO DENERVATED MUSCLES

The use of physical methods to improve the blood flow through the muscle will be largely determined by the consultant's view of the role of the vascular factor as an aetiological agent in the production of denervation atrophy and the more serious degenerative changes that may be associated with denervation. To those who maintain that the circulation through the muscle and its capillary bed is increased following denervation, nothing is to be gained by resorting to physical methods designed to increase an already adequate blood supply. On the other hand, those who believe that venous congestion contributes to the denervation changes will do all that is possible to assist venous return by massage, passive movements and warmth induced by hot packs and baths, diathermy and ultrasonic radiation.

The value of warmth as a therapeutic agent has also been challenged on the grounds that by increasing the metabolic rate it could make further demands on an already depleted circulation.

THE EFFECT OF CHEMICAL AND BIOLOGICAL AGENTS

The effects of a wide variety of substances on muscle atrophy have been investigated experimentally. The evidence suggests that they play only a minor role in modifying the course of denervation atrophy.

Attempts to alter the course of atrophy by changing the level of vitamin intake have not been successful; a vitamin intake regarded as normally adequate for the animal is also adequate for optimum recovery following reinnervation. Experiments with a wide range of chemical agents acting on the muscle fibre and at the myoneural junction offer no encouragement for the successful treatment of denervation muscle atrophy by this method.

Studies along these lines have not to date significantly increased our understanding of the mechanisms involved in denervation atrophy nor have they offered any prospects of improvement in the destitute field of corrective therapy.

REFERENCES

Sunderland S 1978 Nerves and nerve injuries, 2nd edn. Churchill Livingstone, Edinburgh, pp 289 & 298
Sunderland S, Lavarack J O 1959 Changes in human muscles after permanent tenotomy. Journal of Neurology, Neurosurgery and Psychiatry 22: 167

29. The capacity of reinnervated human muscles to function efficiently after prolonged denervation

INTRODUCTION

The changes that develop in a muscle that has been deprived of its nerve supply are well known, though some details relating to the processes involved remain obscure. It is now clear that, despite denervation of several years' duration, muscle tissue can, and does, survive in a grossly atrophied but histologically recognisable state. Morphological studies alone do not, however, provide an answer to the question of whether or not the changes produced in a muscle by prolonged denervation become irreversible and incompatible with the restoration of useful function when the muscle is satisfactorily reinnervated.

This chapter is directed to a consideration of four items relating to this question that are of considerable clinical interest and importance.

1. How long can muscle fibres survive denervation in a histologically recognisable state?
2. For how long does a denervated muscle retain the capacity to recover and function efficiently when it is finally reinnervated?
3. Is a persisting paresis in a muscle, reinnervated after prolonged denervation, due to residual changes within the muscle that are directly attributable to the denervation, or does the fault lie in the manner in which the muscle has been reinnervated? To answer this question requires a knowledge of the factors that are responsible for the persisting paresis under these conditions.
4. If the ultimate fate of denervated muscle is degeneration and replacement by fibrous tissue, when does this occur? This essential piece of information determines when all thought of obtaining an acceptable recovery from nerve repair should be abandoned.

Despite their considerable practical importance, little information is available on these points.

THE SURVIVAL OF DENERVATED MUSCLE FIBRES AND THEIR RECOVERY FOLLOWING REINNERVATION AFTER PROLONGED DENERVATION

In man, observations on the motor recovery after delayed nerve repair, and the examination of biopsy material and electromyographical recordings, all offer indisputable evidence that muscle fibres may survive denervation for periods well in excess of 12 months. In the case of the electromyographical evidence, fibrillation potentials have been recorded from muscles denervated for 15 years.

Regarding the quality of the recovery after reinnervation under these conditions, conclusions based on experimental studies are inconclusive and unsatisfactory. What is needed is precise and detailed information on the quality of the motor recovery that is achievable in human muscles when nerve repair has unavoidably been delayed for very long periods. Unfortunately, the clinical records are usually quite inadequate for the purpose of determining at what point in time the prospects of obtaining an acceptable recovery after delayed nerve repair have declined to zero, nerve repair then becoming a fruitless exercise.

One study that has been directed to this question has shown that very good or complete restoration of function may follow the reinnervation of muscles that have been denervated for at least 12 months, providing the quiescent muscle has been maintained in the best possible condition by appropriate therapy (Sunderland 1950, 1978). Data relating to the quality of the recovery in muscles that have remained denervated for more than a year in a patient following delayed repair of the radial nerve are given in Table 29.1.

It remains to account for the residual paresis in muscles that fail to recover completely after long delayed nerve repair, since the possibility remains that the duration of denervation may have been responsible for or at least contributed to the incomplete recovery in these muscles. This introduces for consideration the basis of the residual functional deficit in reinnervated muscles.

THE BASIS OF THE RESIDUAL FUNCTIONAL DEFICIT IN REINNERVATED MUSCLES

The residual paresis of a reinnervated muscle may

Table 29.1 Patient K H McN. Machine gun bullet wound of the right cubital fossa and supracondylar region with destruction of a segment of the radial nerve below the origin of the innervation to brachioradialis. Range and power of movements are expressed as a percentage of those on the contralateral side; the value for the range precedes that for the power. Wasting is expressed as the difference in the circumference of the forearms at corresponding levels. ECRL: Extensor carpi radialis longus; EDC: Extensor digitorum communis; ECU: Extensor carpi ulnaris; APL: Abductor pollicis longus; EPL: Extensor pollicis longus

Interval between injury and nerve suture	313 days
Interval between suture and last examination	330 weeks
Return of voluntary contractions in weeks	ECRL 20. EDC 34. ECU 35. APL 40. EPL 40
Wrist extension	Full/Full
Grip	70
Synergic extension of the wrist	Good
Extension of the fingers	
Simultaneously	Full/75
Independently	
Index	75/4
Middle	Full/35
Little	75/5
Thenar abduction	80/35
Thenar extension	Full/50
Wasting: when maximal	35 mm
at last examination	7 mm

be due to the loss of some functioning units and/or a persisting reduction in the functional efficiency of reinnervated muscle fibres.

Reduction in the number of functioning units

Several factors combine to reduce the number of muscle fibres that survive and are satisfactorily reinnervated.

1. The loss of some muscle fibres from direct injury or muscle fibre degeneration secondary to changes introduced by the nerve injury.
2. The failure of regenerating axons to reach the muscle owing to:

   i. a reduction in the number of surviving neurons as the result of retrograde degeneration, together with the failure of some regenerating axons to enter endoneurial tubes in the distal stump. This means that some muscle fibres are never reinnervated.
   ii. misdirected axon regeneration at the suture line whereby axons enter foreign endoneurial tubes that direct them to functionally unrelated end organs so that the reconstituted axonal pathway is of no functional value.

3. The failure of functionally appropriate axons after entering the muscle to re-establish connections with their old end organs and their inability to form new endings because of local changes, such as fibrosis. The difficulty and slowness in the formation of new motor end plates increases with the period of denervation.

Reduction in the functional efficiency of reinnervated muscle fibres

The functional efficiency of reinnervated muscle fibres may be adversely affected by: (i) persisting changes directly affecting muscle fibres, and (ii) neurogenic factors that reduce the functional effectiveness of axon regeneration.

Intrinsic factors affecting muscle fibres

1. Satisfactorily reinnervated muscle fibres may fail to recover fully owing to the irreversibility of changes that have developed within them as the result of prolonged denervation.
2. Intramuscular changes, such as increasing fibrosis, impair the co-ordinated activity of groups of muscle fibres. Fibrosis is minimal in denervated muscles that have been well cared for but is increased when the parts have been neglected and subjected to prolonged immobilisation.

Neurogenic factors

1. Axons that fail to re-establish connections with their original end organs may form new endings that are less efficient than the original.
2. The erroneous cross-shunting of axons, and the fibre mixing to which it gives rise at the site of repair, may lead to:

   a. the formation of functionally inappropriate connections with a muscle. This may so distort the normal pattern of innervation that the functional efficiency of the system suffers.
   b. the restoration of functionally related connections in which, however:

      i. a particular muscle fibre is now innervated not by its original but by another motor axon and,
      ii. one type of muscle fibre is reinnervated by an axon originally innervating a muscle fibre of another type. The innervation of a 'slow' muscle by axons originally innervating fast muscle does not always convert slow muscle to normal fast muscle but only to some mixed form.

3. Retrograde and trans-synaptic neuronal changes consequent on injury may persist and adversely affect patterns of motor activity.
4. Incomplete sensory reinnervation of muscle and skin could contribute to the motor disability. Thus any residual defect in the restoration of functionally effective proprioceptor mechanisms would interfere with proper motor function.
5. The branching of regenerating axons and collateral axon sprouting within the muscle itself may result in neurons reinnervating a much larger territory than was previously the case. These extra pathways could make additional demands on the parent neuron and overloading occurring in this way could adversely affect motor function. The significance of this factor remains obscure.
6. Though axons may re-establish satisfactory end organ connections, they may fail to mature into pathways that will excite a normal response in the reinnervated muscle fibre. This may be due to one or a combination of persistent defects in the neuron, irreversible changes in the endoneurial tube or irreversible changes in the muscle.

   The incomplete maturation of regenerated axons is probably one factor responsible for the experimental finding that after nerve repair the conducting properties of regenerated axons are never fully restored. Persisting defects in the conduction properties of individual nerve fibres and defects in neuromuscular function could also contribute to the disorganisation of patterns of activity on which normal motor function depends.
7. The full restoration of muscle function after nerve repair requires more than the re-establishment of axonal continuity between neurons and terminal end organs in the muscle. In addition to the factors referred to in the preceding sections, it also depends on the restoration of neuromuscular units in sufficient numbers and in the appropriate functional combinations to provide for those complex patterns of activity that alone determine the strength and precision of motor function.

The loss of some muscle fibres and the reduced efficiency of others may be offset by the hypertrophy of those that have fully recovered, while central adjustments may compensate to some degree for defects arising from the erroneous cross-shunting of regenerating axons at the suture line and the incomplete maturation of those that reach their destination.

THE EXPLANATION FOR THE DETERIORATION IN THE QUALITY OF THE MOTOR RECOVERY WITH INCREASING DELAYS IN THE REPAIR OF THE NERVE

It is a matter of common knowledge that, all other things being equal, the quality of the motor recovery falls off as the delay before repairing the nerve increases. Is this to be explained by changes in the muscle that are directly or indirectly attributable to the denervation, or is it due to some factor of an unrelated nature? This section is devoted to a consideration of this question.

While experimental investigations provide a picture of the complexities of reinnervation processes, and the manner in which the restored pattern becomes progressively more distorted as the period of denervation increases, the extent to which a residual functional defect after delayed reinnervation is attributable to denervation changes developing within the muscle remains uncertain.

In the absence of any suitable test for the recovery of voluntary movements in the experimental animal, the restrictions that are imposed on functional recovery by pathological changes developing in the muscle must remain purely inferential. It is conceivable that abnormal changes detected histologically may still be compatible with recovery of a useful degree. Furthermore, considerable doubt exists as to how much of the residual functional deficit (clinical material) is attributable to changes developing within the muscle as the result of denervation, and how much to a reduction in the number of appropriate axons reaching the muscle and to the failure of restored pathways to mature into functionally efficient units. Though it is certain that several factors are operating, it is important to determine the relative contribution of each. That the duration of denervation is of significance is not denied, but the point at which it becomes critical cannot be decided until it is possible to effect a separate evaluation of the various factors contributing to, and complicating, the recovery.

After nerve repair at high levels, recovery in the hand muscles is less complete than in proximally innervated muscles. This has been attributed by some to the longer period for which the distal muscles have remained denervated. This is an unlikely explanation for the following reasons. After *immediate or early* suture, the distal muscles will have been denervated for a much shorter period than would be the case for the proximal muscles when repair at the same level has been delayed for 12 months. Despite this, the quality of the recovery in the distal muscles after early or immediate suture is still inferior to that recorded for the proximal muscles after a delayed repair. Briefly, conditions are more favourable for recovery in the proximal than in the distal muscles because:

1. the nerve fibres supplying the proximal muscles occupy a greater cross-sectional area of the nerve at the site of suture;
2. they are more sharply localised in the nerve at proximal levels than the fibres destined for structures further distally. Thus, in the competition for endoneurial tubes after high repair, the axons for the distal muscles suffer a distinct disadvantage in comparison with those destined for more proximal branches in that they are fewer in number and are not localised in the nerve;
3. the consequences of loss of axons and disorderly reinnervation are more serious for the distal muscles than for the proximal. The latter often combine as prime movers in executing movements and for this reason the reinnervation of one member of the group by fibres originally supplying another does not seriously disturb the pattern and so assists in the restoration of function. On the other hand, the muscles controlling the digits function as independent but well integrated and co-ordinated systems in every movement, combining to give that delicacy, refinement and precision of action which, in the case of the hand, is the basis of manual dexterity. In these complex and finely

adjusted movement patterns each muscle has a specific role to play. Consequently, any disturbance of the nerve fibre pattern during regeneration seriously impairs the restoration of function.

The complete or satisfactory recovery in some muscles, together with the explanation advanced to account for the poor recovery in muscles innervated in the distal part of the limb, make it unlikely that changes within the muscle resulting from prolonged denervation (within the periods reported) could have been responsible for the residual defect in those muscles that failed to recover completely. We must, therefore, seek elsewhere for the factors responsible for a persisting motor deficit. These are more likely to be based on the failure of axons to reach the muscle in sufficient numbers and from appropriate neurons rather than on irreversible changes developing within the muscle as a result of prolonged denervation. There is much additional evidence supporting the view that the basis of the residual motor deficit after delayed nerve repair is neural rather than muscular in origin.

1. The retrograde neuronal effects are more severe after high nerve section, thereby leading to a higher incidence of degeneration and a greater reduction in the number of surviving axons.
2. Many regenerating axons fail to reach fasciculi and endoneurial tubes in the distal stump owing to:

    i. dissimilarities in the cross-sectional areas of the nerve ends consequent on the progressive shrinkage of the distal stump with increasing periods of denervation;
    ii. dissimilarities in the fascicular patterns at the nerve ends;
    iii. some scarring at the suture line which is inevitable, regardless of how well and expeditiously the nerve is repaired, owing to the fact that healing excites a reaction that obstructs and deflects some axons in their passage across the suture line.

3. The failure of regenerated axons to mature

completely impairs the conduction properties of restored pathways.
4. Nerve suture may have been effected under tension that still further reduces the chances of satisfactory regeneration.

A further point in support of the interpretation that the residual motor disability is due essentially to a reduction in the number of appropriate axons reaching the muscle is that such residual motor defects are common after immediate and early repair despite the fact that there has been insufficient time for the condition of the denervated muscle to deteriorate to a degree that would complicate reinnervation.

In view of the several factors that combine to reduce the number of functionally useful axons that reach a muscle it is surprising that full recovery should be recorded in some muscles. Possible explanations for this are:

1. After high nerve repair complete recovery is never observed in any of the distal muscles but only in the proximal. At proximal levels the fibres innervating proximal muscles are localised in the nerve in a manner that favours the restoration of correct connections during regeneration. This and other factors favouring recovery in the proximal muscles have been mentioned in an earlier section.
2. The compensatory hypertrophy of satisfactorily reinnervated muscle fibres could offset the loss of other fibres.
3. Muscles are often recorded as normal on the basis of limited clinical tests. These, though exacting, may not take into consideration every complex movement pattern in which the muscle participates or the capacity of the muscle to sustain prolonged effort. If muscles are subjected to sufficiently detailed testing, residual defects will often appear that represent the functional expression of an incomplete and imperfect pattern of reinnervation.
4. Central adjustments may compensate for the incomplete reinnervation of a muscle and for any disturbances of innervation due to the misdirected growth of axons.

CONCLUSIONS

1. The full restoration of muscle function after nerve repair requires more than the re-establishment of axonal continuity with the terminal endings in the muscle. Of related importance are:

    i. the restoration of functionally appropriate or related and, therefore, useful connections as opposed to non-functional connections;

    ii. the maturation of the newly restored pathways into functionally mature and efficient nerve fibres;

    iii. the presence of nerve fibres in sufficient numbers, and functioning in the appropriate combinations, to permit the restoration of those patterns of activity on which normal neuromuscular function depends;

    iv. the capacity of the reinnervated muscle fibres to respond in sufficient numbers to give precision and power to motor performance;

    v. the restoration of appropriate proprioceptor mechanisms.

2. Complete or very good recovery may occur in reinnervated human muscles that have been denervated for at least 12 months providing axons can be directed in sufficient numbers to their original or functionally related end organs, and the quiescent muscle has been maintained in an optimal condition by appropriate therapy. From this it is concluded that, within at least the 1st year of denervation, the changes that develop in the denervated muscle do not necessarily assume proportions that render them irreversible.

3. The residual paresis in a reinnervated muscle has a multifactorial neurogenic basis.

4. The most potent factors responsible for the residual deficit in muscle function following reinnervation after prolonged denervation are those that lead to:

    i. a reduction in the number of functionally useful axons reaching the muscle and, therefore, a reduction in the number of satisfactorily reinnervated muscle fibres;

    ii. fibre mixing at the site of nerve repair that distorts the normal pattern of innervation;

    iii. the persistence of retrograde and trans-synaptic neuronal changes that impair patterns of activity at central levels.

5. Additional factors that may operate are:

    i. changes developing in the muscle as a result of the denervation that reduce the chances of restoring useful neuromuscular connections or which prevent muscle fibres that have been satisfactorily reinnervated from functioning normally;

    ii. changes in endoneurial tubes that delay or prevent the conversion of restored axonal pathways into functionally mature and efficient fibres.

The evidence suggests that these two factors are of minor significance within the 1st year of denervation.

REFERENCES

Sunderland S 1950 Capacity of reinnervated muscles to function efficiently after prolonged denervation. Archives of Neurology and Psychiatry (Chicago) 64: 755

Sunderland S 1978 Nerves and nerve injuries, 2nd edn. Churchill Livingstone, Edinburgh, p 312

30. Changes in denervated skin and subcutaneous tissues. Trophic changes

GENERAL CONSIDERATIONS

The skin and the subcutaneous tissues are innervated by sensory and sympathetic nerve fibres that reach their destination by way of the cutaneous branches of peripheral nerves. In this way the blood vessels of the skin and subcutaneous tissues, the sweat glands and the arrectores pilorum receive a motor innervation and the skin its sensory supply. The cutaneous sympathetic fibres of a peripheral nerve are distributed over the same area as that served by its sensory fibres so that, following a nerve injury, the area of sympathetic loss corresponds closely to that deprived of its sensory innervation. The peripheral distribution of both cutaneous sympathetic and sensory fibres also provides for an overlap of adjacent territories served by different nerves.

This chapter is concerned with the changes occurring in the cutaneous and subcutaneous tissues that follow denervation (Sunderland 1978). Disturbances of sensation, other than those that threaten the integrity and survival of these tissues, are considered elsewhere.

In the absence of any evidence supporting the existence of specific trophic nerve fibres, the trophic regulatory control which the nervous system normally exercises over the skin and subcutaneous tissues would appear to be served by way of the sensory and sympathetic pathways whose combined activity provides for and controls the full and complex functional requirements of these tissues.

THE PATHOPHYSIOLOGICAL BASIS OF CHANGES IN THE SKIN

Injury to a peripheral nerve gives rise, in the denervated cutaneous and subcutaneous tissues, to characteristic circulatory and nutritional disturbances that vary from the trivial to the severe. Though the changes produced in this way are conveniently referred to as trophic changes, it is again emphasised that they have their origin in the pathological interference with sensory and sympathetic mechanisms.

The significance of the cutaneous sensory loss is that it renders the area insensitive and, therefore, more susceptible to repeated injury that finally results in blistering and ulceration.

Severance of sympathetic fibres results in two important changes in the denervated insensitive skin and subcutaneous tissues: (1) loss of sweating that results in dryness; and (2) alterations in the blood flow that may deteriorate to a point where the nutrition of the denervated tissues suffers so that they then undergo more obvious and, in some cases, more serious trophic changes.

The impaired circulation, together with the loss of sensation and the dryness of the affected skin, combine to render the skin particularly susceptible to injury and to provide the final touches to the trophic picture in the form of blistering and ulceration.

THE NATURE OF THE CHANGES IN THE SKIN

1. Changes in the blood flow through denervated skin and subcutaneous tissues.
2. Histological changes.
3. Changes in the texture of the skin, nails and hair.
4. Changes in the texture of the skin to immersion in water.

5. Changes in the colour of the skin.
6. Changes in the temperature of the skin.
7. Changes in the amount and consistency of the subcutaneous tissues.
8. Ulceration.

Blood flow through denervated skin and subcutaneous tissues

There are regional differences in the vasomotor responses of different vascular beds, vasomotor reactions of the hands and feet being unique and not at all characteristic of other cutaneous areas or deeper tissues.

The major vascular effects following severance of sympathetic fibres are due initially to the loss of vasoconstrictor tone and subsequently to the introduction of other complications that still further modify the blood flow through the vascular bed of the denervated skin and subcutaneous tissues.

Factors contributing to alterations to the peripheral circulation are:

1. The loss of vasomotor tone and reflexes that are dependent on intact vasoconstrictor pathways. Though the vascular effects produced in this way are influenced by the duration of the denervation, they may be conveniently grouped into an immediate and a delayed category, the transition from one to the other occurring gradually about 3 weeks after injury.

    Immediate effects of denervation. The warm phase. These take the form of an immediate vasodilatation due to the removal of vasoconstrictor tone so that the blood flow is greatly increased and the denervated area becomes flushed and warm. The nutrition of the denervated tissues does not usually suffer, though trivial injuries to the insensitive skin may cause blistering and ulceration.

    Delayed effects of denervation. The cold phase. As the blood flow through the denervated tissues gradually slows, the immediate or warm phase is replaced by a delayed or cold phase in which the affected part, and even the entire hand or foot, becomes abnormally susceptible to cold.

    The end result is one in which the affected tissues are usually colder than normal areas. Although the circulation can increase in response to non-neurogenic factors, the persistent tendency to an impaired circulation is ultimately responsible for the development of marked nutritional changes in the skin and subcutaneous tissues.

2. Tone gradually returns in permanently denervated vessels.

3. The responses of the small cutaneous and subcutaneous vessels to cold have long been recognised. Local cooling produces arteriolar constriction and slows the capillary return.

4. The increased sensitivity of denervated vessels to circulating adrenaline and noradrenaline, to which there is a lowered threshold and prolonged response. This increased sensitivity takes several days to develop.

5. The retrograde changes that are associated with partial and complete nerve injuries could involve sympathetic neurons and the resulting disordered patterns of activity could adversely affect cutaneous vascular mechanisms by way of uninjured pathways.

6. Scarring or other changes developing at the site of partial nerve damage may create trigger zones of abnormal sensitivity that cause pain and sympathetic disturbances that predispose to the development of, or aggravate, established trophic changes.

7. Though the precise role of vasodilator nerve fibres and antidromic vasodilator mechanisms in peripheral vasomotor activity is not known, their involvement in a nerve injury might adversely affect the cutaneous circulation.

8. Blood vessels in the normal tissues adjacent to the denervated area continue to respond to vasomotor activity and this could, in turn, modify the movement of blood from normal to abnormal tissues.

9. Our knowledge of the factors influencing the calibre of veins is incomplete. However, there is evidence that veins have constrictor tone and dilate when their nerve supply is removed and that they are relaxed by blood

containing an excess of carbon dioxide. These changes would predispose to venous stasis and would also embarrass the return of blood from the denervated part.

10. Vessels, denervated as the result of long-standing nerve lesions, do not appear to be subject to pathological changes of an obliterating nature that might contribute to an impairment of the cutaneous circulation.

11. Co-existing vascular pathology, such as the ligation or thrombosis of a major artery to the limb, might be expected to add to the circulatory embarrassment, thereby aggravating trophic disturbances in the denervated area. Though this is sometimes the case, it is not invariably so. Thus trophic changes may fail to appear in combined arterial and nerve lesions and yet be pronounced where there are no such arterial complications.

12. The effect of disuse on the blood supply and nutrition of denervated tissues is considerable. Inactivity imposed by the paralysis of muscle and by prolonged immobilisation enforced by pain, indifference on the part of the patient, or splinting necessitated by treatment for the nerve injury or for a co-existing bone, joint, or extensive soft tissue injury, sometimes result in trophic changes extending to involve normally innervated but inactive areas.

13. The paralysis of some muscles and the immobilisation of others impairs the venous return and leads to venous stasis that is maximal in the most dependent parts of the limb, namely the hand and the foot. Oxygen lack, excess carbon dioxide and the increased blood acidity that are to be expected under these conditions all produce arteriolar dilatation by local action. The accumulation of 'metabolites' produced locally under these unfavourable conditions also affects the calibre of vessels and in this way contributes indirectly to disturbances of the circulation. Histamine constricts arteries but dilates capillaries and yet still produces a marked vasodilatation in denervated tissues. Serotonin has a similar effect.

Histological changes

Changes in the dermal plexus, free nerve terminals and encapsulated sensory receptors

The outlines of the denervated dermal plexuses and finer nerve terminals persist as trains of Schwann cells surrounded by a fine endoneurial sheath. How long they persist in this form is not known, but regenerating 'axons' will utilise them for at least 1 year and there is presumptive evidence that this period could be extended, but again by how much is not clear.

There is some uncertainty regarding the fate of the denervated encapsulated receptors — Pacinian and Meissner's corpuscles and the Merkel cells. It is the author's belief based on clinical experience that they must persist, at least into the 2nd year of denervation.

In high second degree injuries, spontaneously regenerating 'axons' are inevitably directed back to their old endings so that the original pattern of innervation is fully restored. These regenerating 'axons' may take 6–9 months to reach the hand and yet complete sensory recovery is the end result. The return of some sensation in the hand, indicating the presence of reinnervated mechanoreceptors following nerve repair delayed, for one reason or another, for up to 12 months extends the survival period to well into the 2nd year.

Denervated Pacinian corpuscles have been identified 40 weeks after denervation in the macaque (Wong et al 1971, Krishnamurti et al 1973) and 9 months after a brachial plexus injury in man (Lyons and Woodhall 1949) and Carlsted et al (1986) have reported them surviving denervation for 5 and 22 years in humans.

Dellon and his associates (1975, 1976, 1981), in accounts of their comprehensive study of the fate of sensory corpuscles after nerve division, include statements in which degeneration and atrophy are used in a confusing way. For example (Dellon 1981): 'the capsular structure degenerated by 10 months' . . . 'We conclude that the denervated Meissner corpuscle undergoes progressive degeneration, beginning first with its axon terminal, then with enzyme systems within the lamellar cell (e.g. acetylcholinesterase) and then with atrophy of the lamellar cell complex itself.'

'It may be concluded that the Merkel cell–neurite complex also undergoes progressive degeneration post denervation.'

However, it is clear from a complete and careful study of their writings on this subject that degeneration refers only to the fate of the axon terminal and atrophy to the lamellar complex that survives long periods of denervation in a ghost state, but for how long is still not known.

That sensory corpuscles survive in an atrophied state pending the arrival of regenerating axon terminals is confirmed by the studies of Burgess et al (1974) and Jabaley and his associates (1976, 1980).

With the passage of time following nerve repair there are three possibilities.

1. Specialised receptor systems continue to survive in an atrophied state, awaiting the arrival of a functionally appropriate nerve terminal to rejuvenate them.
2. If denervated receptors do degenerate with time, an appropriate 'axon' arriving in the skin must have the capacity to fashion a new receptor from the remnants of the old.
3. The elements of sensation that are restored do not require the elaborate receptor apparatus and mechanisms claimed to be a prerequisite for discriminative sensory recovery. There is some evidence that this could well be the case.

Finally, the falling off in the quality of the sensory recovery after delayed nerve repair calls for an explanation. Is it due to a loss of sensory end organs or to some other factor? An examination of this question suggests that the decline in sensory performance with delayed nerve repair depends more on the nature of the nerve injury than on the fate of denervated sensory end organs.

We have already seen that, after high second degree nerve injuries, sensory recovery is ultimately complete despite the fact that sensory end organs in the hand have been denervated for 6–9 months. This is because the restored pattern of sensory innervation is precisely the same as the original in this type of injury.

After nerve repair conditions are very different. In the first place many regenerating sensory 'axons' fail to reach the skin. Secondly, many that do, fail to develop into fully mature sensory nerve fibres, and thirdly we do not know the consequences of cross-innervation when a sensory 'axon' that originally innervated one receptor now establishes a connection with another of a different type. As a consequence of these misadventures the restored pattern of sensory innervation differs significantly from the original. Under these circumstances a sensory deficit can hardly be attributed solely to the 'degeneration of receptors'.

Changes in sweat glands

What little evidence is available on the survival of sweat glands following denervation indicates that they continue to respond to pharmacological agents 3 months (Sakurai and Montagna 1965) and 10 months (Braeucker 1928) after denervation. What has been written above concerning the outcome as regards sensory recovery after high second degree nerve injuries applies equally to sweat glands. The collective clinical evidence indicates that these structures survive denervation into the 2nd year.

Changes in the texture of the skin, nails and hair

Changes affecting the texture of the skin are usually present in the hand or foot in the established case. They first appear as a mild scaliness of the skin which, in some patients and particularly in those where the limb is immobilised, progresses to the formation of thicker epidermal collections. The dry denervated skin desquamates at a slower rate than does the normal skin, with the result that the epithelium thickens, hardens and adheres to the surface as rough brownish-white bran-like flakes or sheets. This hyperkeratosis characteristically involves the palm and sole. Under conditions of disuse this hyperkeratosis also involves the unaffected regions of the hand or foot, but usually not to the same degree as that observed over the denervated area, so that the latter remains clearly outlined. Beneath this crust the skin is thin, smooth and delicate.

The epithelium becomes thinner in longstanding irreparable injuries as well as in 'irritative' lesions complicated by pain and severe vasomotor disturbances. This epidermal atrophy results in the papillary and skin creases becoming shallower and less distinct, though they are never obliterated. In the well-established and long-standing case the denervated skin finally becomes thin, smooth, shiny and cyanotic. Pin-pricks that fail to mark the normal skin readily penetrate this fragile covering and produce free bleeding.

Though changes in the appearance and growth of the nails are common after nerve injury they develop more slowly and only become a prominent feature of the picture in long-standing cases of ir-reparable or severe injuries. The finger nails are affected more often and to a greater degree than the toenails, while the changes following median nerve damage are more pronounced than those ob-served after ulnar lesions. These changes vary in nature and degree and take about 6 months to develop fully. In general, they present one or a combination of the following abnormalities (Sunderland and Ray 1952). The finger nails develop striations, ridges and other blemishes, be-come dry, and lose their lustre. They also become more brittle and break more easily. Wasting of the digital pads leads to abnormal curving of the nail, both in the transverse and longitudinal planes, so that in the advanced state they present a talon or beaked appearance. This is most frequently ob-served in the index finger. The nails share in the atrophy, often becoming smaller than the cor-responding nail of the normal hand or foot.

1. After uncomplicated nerve injuries nail growth in the denervated digits is retarded in some cases but not in others. When growth is affected the retardation is only slight.
2. When arterial ligation is superimposed on the nerve injury, growth is consistently and markedly retarded in the denervated digits and greatly exceeds the slight slowing recorded after uncomplicated nerve injuries. There are three reasons why this greater slowing should not be attributed solely to the vascular injury:
   a. it outlasts the period of circulatory embarrassment;
   b. the non-denervated digits of the involved hand are not affected;
   c. complete nerve recovery results in an

equality of growth in the involved and corresponding normal digits.

The hair in denervated areas behaves in a vari-able manner. Hypertrichosis is a feature in some patients while in others the hair is less abundant and grows more slowly. In causalgia, however, there is an obvious loss of hair over atrophic, shiny, cyanotic skin.

Changes in the texture of the skin to immersion in water

O'Riain (1973) has reported the interesting obser-vation that the well-known phenomenon of normal wrinkling of the skin that follows the immersion of the hands in warm water for 15–30 minutes does not occur in denervated skin, which retains its smooth appearance.

Changes in the colour of the skin

The colour of the skin is determined by:

1. Its pigmentation.
2. The character of the blood in the subpapillary venous plexus. The extent to which the oxygenated blood is reduced before its passage to this venous plexus largely depends on the rate of blood flow through the cutaneous vessels. Thus the blood in the subpapillary venous plexus will be more arterial in type when the flow is rapid and more venous in character when the rate of flow is slowed.
3. The thickness and texture of the skin and subcutaneous tissues.
4. The prevailing environmental temperature.

White skin may range in colour from pallor through salmon pink to red and finally to a dull claret or cyanotic colour.

Pallor is the result of constricted vessels and a reduced blood flow. Where there is a rapid flow of well oxygenated blood through moderately con-stricted vessels the skin is pink. With dilated vessels the pink deepens to red if the rapid flow is maintained but, should the circulation through the tissues be slowed, the skin then takes on a dull claret or cyanotic colour.

Pink coloured skin is warm, indicating a rapid flow of well oxygenated blood through the tissues, whereas pallor and the deeper red colours are found in cold limbs, the evidence pointing in these cases to a reduction in the circulation.

In nerve injuries the colour of the denervated skin is subject to considerable variation depending not only on the factors enumerated above but also on the nature and persistence of the vasodilation and the extent to which the denervated vessels become hypersensitive to cold, circulating agents and local metabolites. The hand, which is usually more exposed than the foot, is more subject to colour change than the latter which, relatively protected beneath the bed clothes or by protective footwear, is less affected by the external temperature.

Pallor is uncommon but, when present, it is more frequently seen in the foot. The deeper reds predominate in causalgia, particularly when the affected hand or foot is cold and the limb is in a dependent position. Here the colour may be generalised, graded or mottled but it usually deepens as the digits are descended. The colour rapidly improves when the limb is elevated and warmed. Localised pressure applied to the cyanotic area and also to a normal cutaneous area produces a blanching of the skin in each case which, on release of the pressure, persists for a longer time in the former. These findings reflect the loss of tone in the vasoconstrictor system.

Changes in the temperature of the skin

The temperature of the skin is influenced by the rate of blood flow through the cutaneous vessels. Heat exchange at the surface can be so modified by mechanisms controlling this rate of flow that a constant body temperature is maintained despite wide variations in the environmental temperature.

Defective vasomotor mechanisms, and the cutaneous circulatory disturbances to which they give rise, are responsible for changes in the temperature of the denervated skin following nerve injury. Immediately following denervation the skin becomes flushed and warm owing to the vasodilatation that follows the vasoconstrictor paralysis. This warm phase continues for about 3 weeks, during which the affected part remains warm and does not respond by cooling on exposure to cold. This phase may be prolonged in some incomplete irritative lesions of the sciatic and median nerves with causalgia and marked vasomotor disturbances. Under these conditions the affected cutaneous areas may also be moist or even sweat profusely.

The capacity of the denervated skin to resist cold is reduced and its temperature falls as the blood flow through the denervated tissues is gradually reduced by persistent vasodilatation, inactivity and immobilisation. The cyanotic, claret coloured skin of this delayed phase is cold and in striking contrast to the warm pink to red skin of the early phase. This temperature change may be confined to the denervated part or may extend to involve the entire hand or foot.

Skin temperature follows the environmental temperature. In hot weather the part is not cold but when exposed in cold weather it cools more readily, more rapidly and to a greater degree than the corresponding normally innervated tissues. It also remains colder for a longer period and warms only slowly after the external temperature has been raised. These changes may be confined to the denervated region, though usually the entire hand or foot feels and is colder than the opposite normal member. Under these conditions the hand is usually colder than the foot because it is usually more exposed, while the foot is protected by clothes and footwear.

Additional factors affecting the temperature of the denervated part are:

1. the instability of the cutaneous vessels consequent not only on the denervation but also on their increased sensitivity to circulating agents and local influences;
2. the thickness of the subcutaneous tissue and the amount of fat that it contains and,
3. the reduced local heat production due to paralysis of some muscles and the inactivity of others which is further reduced by exposure to cold.

The cold phase persists as long as the denervation. As the circulation improves with reinnervation the normal responses to temperature change are gradually restored, though the affected part remains unduly sensitive to cold for a long time.

Changes in the amount and consistency of the subcutaneous tissues

Reference has previously been made to the manner in which circulatory disturbances and inactivity following muscle paralysis and immobilisation lead to venous and lymphatic congestion and stasis. Oedema may follow, though it is not common in uncomplicated nerve injury in the upper limb. It frequently occurs as a swelling of the foot, and occasionally of the leg, in lesions of the sciatic nerve.

Oedema and the disturbed nutrition of the subcutaneous tissue ultimately reduce its elasticity and lead to fibrosis. These changes give an indurated consistency to the skin and reduce its mobility.

In time the subcutaneous tissues share in the atrophy and, in the case of the terminal pads of the affected digits, this leads to a distinctive tapering or spindling of the fingers. This feature is most evident in the index, which normally shows some tapering in comparison with the other digits (Fig. 30.1). Wasting of the digital pads contributes to the abnormal curving of the nails during their growth and finally results in them taking on a talon-like or beaked appearance.

Although this subcutaneous atrophy is always maximal in the digital pads, the remaining segments of the digits and the subcutaneous tissues of the hand and foot also suffer. The changes in the toes are less obvious than those involving the fingers, mainly because of the shape and smaller size of the former, and the smaller amount of subcutaneous tissue normally present in them. The change is also more noticeable following median nerve injury because of the shape of the index which favours tapering as wasting occurs.

Ulceration

Dryness, atrophy, loss of elasticity and a poorer circulation, together with a loss of cutaneous sensation and the protection that it provides, all combine to render denervated tissue extremely susceptible to cold and injury. Such trophic changes are always more pronounced in the hand and foot, which accounts for the frequency with which ulceration is found in these regions. In addition, they are usually more marked in the foot than in the hand owing to the greater impairment

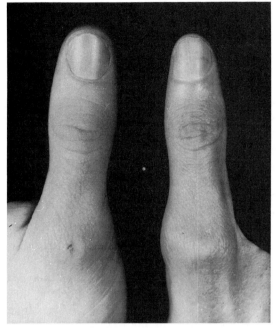

A

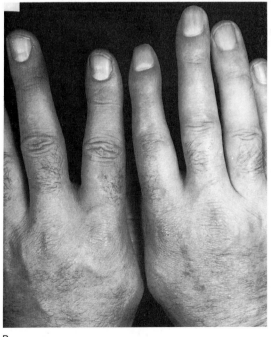

B

Fig. 30.1 Wasting of the thumb and and index finger in patients with median nerve lesions

of the circulation and the greater incidence of oedema in the former after sciatic nerve injury, though the hand, being more exposed than the foot, is more prone to injury.

Trauma to insensitive skin modified by trophic changes is the important factor causing the characteristic trophic ulceration associated with some nerve lesions. Burns, pressure, friction, chemicals and other mild injuries, that are normally avoided by protective reflex or voluntary action or which are too trivial to damage normal healthy skin, will cause ulceration under these abnormal conditions. Whether or not ulceration occurs largely depends on the care and protection given to the affected part.

Though every part of the affected area is unduly susceptible, ulceration more commonly affects those areas that are habitually exposed and are, therefore more liable to injury. These are the inner side of the hand, the radial side of the index finger, the dorsum of the fingers and nail beds, and pressure bearing areas such as the sole, particularly the heel and the metatarsal heads of the big and little toes. Burns from cigarettes, hot water and domestic appliances are a common source of injury to the hand while pressure and friction from ill-fitting socks and footwear, that are tolerated by the normal foot, readily produce blisters and ulceration of the denervated sole. Such damage is more likely to occur under conditions where the vitality of the tissues is still further reduced by, for example, exposure to cold.

Ulcers on the fingers and hand respond rapidly to treatment but those involving the sole and toes are difficult to heal. This is because of the generally poorer condition of the foot and the repeated trauma produced during walking, both of which adversely affect healing. Minor trauma in the form of cuts and burns in the denervated area often take an unduly long time to heal.

THE INCIDENCE, DISTRIBUTION AND SEVERITY OF TROPHIC CHANGES

It is difficult to evaluate and express the severity of the trophic changes other than in such general terms as insignificant, mild and severe.

Whether or not such complications develop, and the severity of those that do, depend on a number of factors chief amongst which are the particular nerve injured, the nature and level of the nerve lesion and the duration of denervation.

Incidence

When they do occur, trophic changes are uncommon, mild and transient in simple nerve lesions in which the denervated parts have been well cared for and protected against cold and trauma, and where recovery occurs spontaneously and rapidly. Trophic effects, however, are common and severe when the nerve has suffered irreparable damage and there is prolonged denervation. They are also a prominent feature in some partial injuries, particularly of the irritative variety, that are complicated by severe pain or causalgia and marked vasomotor disturbances.

Distribution

When trophic changes do develop they are, with few exceptions, confined to the hand or foot, and, in particular, to the digits. These sites are more prone to involvement because they are more exposed to injury and because they are the most dependent parts of the limb and are served by the most peripheral section of the vascular tree.

It is there that the harmful effects of an impaired circulation and venous congestion and stasis will be greatest. In addition, greater vasomotor instability has been claimed for the skin of the hands and feet in comparison with other cutaneous areas.

This explains why trophic changes are more common and severe after injuries involving the brachial plexus, and the median, ulnar, sciatic, medial popliteal and tibial nerves because these nerves provide the major sensory, motor and vasomotor innervation to the hand and foot.

The distribution of trophic changes corresponds closely to the territory served by the injured nerve but sometimes neighbouring normally innervated tissues are affected when they share in the disuse introduced by the injury.

Severity

The severity of the trophic changes depends on the duration of denervation which, in turn, depends on the site and nature of the injury. Trophic changes more commonly develop and are usually of greater severity after high lesions because:

1. the vasomotor paralysis is more extensive;
2. the territory subjected to disuse, either directly or indirectly as the result of the injury, is greater;
3. the tissues are denervated for longer periods owing to the greater distance to be covered by regenerating axons;
4. retrograde neuronal changes are more severe and so are more likely to distort central patterns of activity and to adversely affect regenerative processes and the restoration of function.

The most severe changes are seen when the denervated tissues are neglected and are exposed to cold and injury. This emphasises the need for the constant care and protection of the denervated parts, particularly during the early stages, for the skin has already become unduly susceptible to cold and trauma, and the associated cutaneous sensory loss renders the part more liable to injury. The high incidence of ulceration during the first few weeks after the injury is due to the failure of the patient, and sometimes inexperienced nursing staff, to realise how easy it is to injure skin that is both insensitive and already unduly susceptible to cold and trauma.

ORDER OF APPEARANCE OF TROPHIC CHANGES

The order of appearance of trophic changes, while subject to some individual variation, proceeds very much according to the following pattern:

1. Immediately conduction is lost in a peripheral nerve a well-defined area of skin, corresponding to the cutaneous distribution of the nerve, becomes insensitive, flushed, warm and dry. The subsequent sequence of changes depends on the duration of denervation and the care which the affected tissues receive.
2. An increased susceptibility of the insensitive skin to trauma is present from the outset and persists until reinnervation is completed.
3. An initial warm phase lasts for approximately 3 weeks, during which only minor trophic changes develop in the tissues, with the exception of ulceration due to trauma.
4. Both the colour and the temperature then gradually change as the circulation through the affected part slows. The part becomes colder and the colour increases in depth until, in the well established and long-standing case, the part is cold and cyanotic. Though this transition may commence at the end of the 1st week, it is usually delayed until the 3rd week. The cold phase then persists until it is corrected by reinnervation and the restoration of function.
5. Changes in the texture and consistency of the skin closely follow changes in its colour and temperature. They are mild in the early stages but become progressively more pronounced until they are a prominent feature 3–6 months after the injury, after which the only further significant changes are those due to trauma and ulceration. Thin, atrophic, shiny and cyanotic skin develops much earlier in lesions with severe pain
6. Minor changes in the nails in the form of blemishes and increased brittleness appear early and are usually noticeable by the 2nd month. The characteristic deformed curving is a later development and appears to be related to the rate and degree of atrophy of the digital pad of the terminal phalanx.
7. Marked atrophy of the digital pad and spindling of the index finger become a prominent feature at and after the 6th month. In the absence of any recovery there is little further change after the 6th month, apart from the tissue damage caused by repeated trauma, while the tendency to ulceration remains.
8. Trophic changes are arrested and then regress with reinnervation and the restoration of function. Pronounced digital pad atrophy and nail deformation, which are terminal features of irreparable injuries or those showing little recovery, are, however, permanent.

REFERENCES

Braeucker W 1928 Uber die Innervation der Schweissdrusen und die chirurgische Behandlung der Hyperhidrosis. Klinische Wochenschrift 7: 683

Burgess P R, English K B, Horsch K W, Stensaas L J 1974 Patterning in the regeneration of type 1 cutaneous receptors. Journal of Physiology 236: 57

Carlsted T, Lugnegård H, Andersson M 1986 Pacinian corpuscles after nerve repair in humans. Peripheral Nerve Repair and Regeneration 1: 37

Dellon A L 1976 Reinnervation of denervated Meissner corpuscles. Journal of Hand Surgery 1: 98

Dellon A L 1981 Sensory corpuscles after nerve division. In: Evaluation of sensibility and re-education of sensation in the hand. Williams & Wilkins, Baltimore, p 47

Dellon A L, Witebsky F G, Terrill R E 1975 The denervated Meissner corpuscle: a sequential histological study after nerve division in the rhesus monkey. Plastic and Reconstructive Surgery 56: 182

Jabaley M E, Burns J E, Orcutt B S, Bryant W M 1976 Comparison of histologic and functional recovery after peripheral nerve repair. Journal of Hand Surgery 1: 119

Jabaley M E, Dellon A L 1980 Evaluation of sensibility by microhistological studies. In: Omer G E, Spinner M (eds) Management of peripheral nerve problems. Saunders, Philadelphia, p 954

Krishnamurti A, Kanagasuntheram R, Vy S 1973 Failure of reinnervation of Pacinian corpuscle after nerve crush: an electron microscopic study. Acta Neuropathologica 23: 338

Lyons W R, Woodhall B 1949 Atlas of peripheral nerve injuries. Saunders, Philadelphia

O'Riain S 1973 New and simple test of nerve function in the hand. British Medical Journal 3: 615

Sakurai M, Montagna W 1965 Observation on the eccrine sweat glands of *Lemur Mongoz* after denervation. Journal of Investigative Dermatology 44: 87

Sunderland S 1978 Nerves and nerve injuries, 2nd edn. Churchill Livingstone, Edinburgh, p 472

Sunderland S, Ray L J 1952 The effect of denervation on nail growth. Journal of Neurology, Neurosurgery and Psychiatry 15 : 50

Wong W C, Kanagasuntheram R 1971 Early and late effects of median nerve injury on Meissner's and Pacinian corpuscles of the hand of the macaque (*M. fascicularis*). Journal of Anatomy 109: 135

Diagnosis. Motor sensory and sympathetic functions and their evaluation

31. Diagnosis of nerve injury

The purpose of this chapter is to stress the over-riding importance of accurate diagnosis as the essential prerequisite for planning the treatment of the lesion.

TERMINOLOGY

Symptom. Subjective evidence of dysfunction as described by the patient.

Sign. Objective evidence of dysfunction as revealed by observation and examination of the patient.

Syndrome. A combination of symptoms and signs that consistently occur together to mark a well-defined pathological state.

GENERAL CONSIDERATIONS

When a region traversed by a nerve is involved in an open or closed injury, damage to the nerve should always be suspected until it can be excluded.

The possibility of damage to a nerve at more than one level should be kept in mind where there is multiple wounding of a limb.

Where the careful inspection and gentle examination of a nerve exposed in a wound reveals loss of continuity or a traumatised section of the nerve, the diagnosis is not in doubt and it is then possible to proceed forthwith to plan appropriate treatment. However, a different approach is called for when this type of information is not available. This involves the use of diagnostic procedures to determine: (1) The identification of any nerve injured; (2) The site of the injury; (3) The nature, extent and severity of the injury.

This information is a necessary prerequisite not only for establishing a diagnosis but also for predicting the likely outcome of the injury and for formulating management policy.

Obtaining this information requires:

1. A detailed knowledge of:
   a. the regional anatomy of peripheral nerves;
   b. variations in the course, relations and distribution of individual peripheral nerves;
   c. their branch pattern;
   d. anomalous innervations;
   e. the function of the parts usually innervated by each nerve and the effect on function of anomalous innervations.

2. A searching clinical history directed with particular reference to:
   a. the onset and course of the condition, and
   b. the wounding mechanism including the site and depth of a therapeutic injection, the use of a tourniquet and the ligation of a vessel. These provide useful clues to, inter alia, the nature, extent and severity of the injury. In stab wounds the damage is more likely to be localised and to involve transection of the nerve, whereas the damage will be more extensive in traction and crush injuries to the limb.

3. A systematically conducted clinical examination to reveal the status of motor, sensory and sympathetic functions (Chapters 32, 33, 35).

4. If some time has elapsed since the injury and providing any open wound has healed:
   a. the site of the injury should be palpated to ascertain if a neuroma is present on

the nerve. Neuromas take some time to develop and are usually not obvious before the 3rd month. If present, they indicate damage of third, fourth or fifth degree severity and, if sensitive, the presence of regenerating 'axons';

b. percussion should be carefully applied along the course of the injured nerve from below upwards to ascertain if Hoffmann–Tinel's sign can be elicited. Such a sign indicates the presence of regenerating sensory 'axons', though this is an unreliable guide to the outcome of regeneration;

c. the presence of an aneurysm and its relationship to a neighbouring nerve should be noted.

5. An evaluation of motor function based on:

   a. the distribution and degree of muscle wasting;
   b. the appearance or absence of visible or palpable contractions in individual muscles in response to voluntary effort;
   c. measurements of the range and power of individual movements in response to voluntary effort;
   d. the ability to perform complex coordinated movements involved in manual and digital skills.

   Relevant tests are discussed further in Chapter 32.

6. Sensory testing to determine the distribution and nature of any sensory disturbance, impairment or deficit, cutaneous and deep, with particular reference to the elements of protective sensation, tactile and discriminative sensation, proprioception and the stereognostic sense. Such testing is discussed further in Chapter 33. Concerning paraesthesiae and pain, attention should be directed to the following features:

   a. Time of onset, distribution, quality and severity.
   b. Is the condition continuous or intermittent? The duration of intervals between episodes.

   c. Precipitating, exacerbating and ameliorating factors.
   d. Is the condition increasing or diminishing in severity and distribution?

7. Tests to detect disturbances of sympathetic function are usually confined to the hand or foot and relate to sweating, to the state of the peripheral circulation as this is reflected in the colour and temperature of the affected part, and associated features in the form of trophic changes.

ADDITIONAL DIAGNOSTIC AIDS

There is no substitute for the routine approach to the clinical investigation of a nerve injury outlined above. However, there are times when additional tests are required to confirm or modify a provisional diagnosis.

Radiological examination

This should be directed to a study of the displaced ends of a fractured bone, callus formation, a dislocation, the presence of bony abnormalities and foreign bodies, all with reference to the possibility of their being responsible for a co-existing nerve injury.

Electrodiagnosis

A number of electrodiagnostic methods are available for detecting peripheral nerve injury, for determining the level of the lesion and for evaluating its severity. They include:

1. the muscle response to nerve trunk stimulation;
2. changes in the electrical excitability of the affected muscles;
3. the interpretation of muscle action potentials in electromyograms of the affected muscles;
4. changes in the conduction time and nerve conduction velocity of motor fibres as determined by stimulation electromyography.

Electrodiagnostic methods have their greatest value in handling difficult and perplexing diagnostic problems. In this respect both the application of the techniques and the interpretation of the findings should be left in the hands of experts; they are not the province of the amateur or novice. Special texts on this subject are available and should be consulted for details. A general outline of what the tests have to offer is given in Chapter 32.

MISCELLANEOUS PROCEDURES

Axon reflex testing, myelography, the examination of the cerebrospinal fluid and recording evoked somatosensory cortical potentials are procedures of special relevance only to the investigation of brachial plexus injuries.

NERVE BLOCK

There are occasions when unusual motor and sensory findings confuse the diagnosis and raise the question of whether parts normally served by the injured nerve are receiving an anomalous innervation from another source. This possibility can be settled by blocking the nerve suspected of being the offender and in this way revealing the source of the confusion.

Care should be taken, during the administration of the injected local anaesthetic, to ensure that the injected solution does not spread to involve normal adjacent nerve trunks.

EXPLORATION AS A DIAGNOSTIC AID IN A NERVE INJURY OF UNCERTAIN PATHOLOGY

Exploration of a nerve solely as a diagnostic procedure is only indicated under the following exceptional circumstances:

1. where there are grounds for suspecting nerve severance after injuries known to be associated with a high incidence of loss of continuity or other pathology believed to be inconsistent with spontaneous recovery. Such is likely to be the case:

   a. with penetrating injuries caused by sharp objects;

   b. after severe stretch injuries, particularly of the brachial plexus;
   c. when the position of a spike or sharp fragment of bone suggests direct damage to the nerve.

2. where the site, nature and severity of the causal injury point to severe damage to a nerve at the root of the limb. To await the onset of spontaneous recovery under these circumstances would involve unduly long delays. In the event of nerve repair subsequently becoming necessary such delays would further prolong treatment unnecessarily and could prejudice the end result. A case in point is an injury to the sciatic nerve in the buttock;

3. the danger to be avoided during early exploration is the temptation to interfere with nerves that would recover if left undisturbed. Early exploration will, in many cases, reveal a nerve in continuity which often shows pathological changes that do not constitute a threat to successful spontaneous regeneration.

FACTORS INFLUENCING THE DIAGNOSTIC ROUTINE

Though an all-embracing approach to the diagnosis of nerve injuries has been outlined, it should be understood that there will be occasions when it will be expedient to modify this routine.

Clearly the routine can be dispensed with when a nerve is known to have been severed.

Other relevant factors are:

The age of the patient. The patient may be too young to communicate and cooperate in the examination.

The general condition of the patient. While it is important to establish at the earliest possible opportunity whether a major nerve has been injured, the selection of diagnostic procedures is determined by the condition of the patient; whether he is conscious or unconscious, alert or confused, agitated or composed, comfortable or in severe pain, exhausted or refreshed.

Under unfavourable conditions the clinician

may have to be content with a brief examination confined to the simplest procedures that can be quickly completed in order to disturb a still desperately ill patient as little as possible. More detailed testing can be undertaken as soon as he is well enough to collaborate.

At the other end of the scale is the patient who presents in good general health with a history of a slow but progressive deterioration in motor and sensory function. Such patients are able to co-operate and so no restrictions apply to the tests selected to reveal the nature of the nerve injury.

The nature and extent of co-existing injuries. Sometimes severely injured patients have sustained multiple injuries that necessitate deferring the full investigation of a known or suspected nerve injury. The co-existence of severe and extensive injuries to neighbouring structures such as soft tissue, bone and joints may limit the scope of the clinical examination.

The availability of specialist facilities. If the services of experienced personnel and access to specialised technological aids are not available, the approach would need to be modified accordingly and a detailed investigation delayed until these facilities are available.

THE NEED FOR REPEATED CLINICAL EXAMINATIONS

Though the identity of the nerve injured can be established from a single examination, further examinations at selected intervals are required in order to decide whether the condition is stationary, improving, or deteriorating. This information determines what further action is indicated.

ASSESSING THE NATURE AND SEVERITY OF THE NERVE INJURY

Peripheral nerves may be injured in many different ways, from the acute lesions due to violent trauma at one end of the scale to the slow, but progressive, loss of function resulting from gradual deformation at the other. They may be complete or incomplete and vary in severity from a conduction block to complete severance. An estimate of the nature and severity of the lesion is based on information derived from several sources:

1. the manner in which nerve function was lost or is deteriorating;
2. the wounding mechanism;
3. the condition of the nerve if it is exposed in the wound;
4. the nature and distribution of the peripheral disability.

The manner in which nerve function was lost or is deteriorating

The nature of the onset and the manner in which the disability has progressed reflect the pathology of the lesion.

The acute lesion with abrupt loss of function. This may date from the injury or the nerve may escape at that time only to be damaged during procedures undertaken for the treatment of the injury such as:

1. careless wound debridement or inadvertently clamping or ligating a nerve when controlling haemorrhage;
2. the reduction of a fracture or dislocation;
3. the application of a tourniquet or an ill-fitting plaster;
4. a misplaced therapeutic injection.

In these cases the nerve may or may not have been left in continuity.

The chronic lesion with slow progressive deterioration of function. These are lesions in continuity in which progressively increasing numbers of nerve fibres are affected, individual fibres sustaining increasing degrees of damage as the deforming force continues to operate. Such lesions may develop as the result of:

1. complications introduced by an earlier injury; for example, injuries about the elbow joint as a precursor of tardy ulnar palsy;
2. chronic intermittent deformation from external forces which provides the background to occupational compression lesions;
3. pathology developing in the absence of any external trauma; for example, compression-stretch from an enlarging aneurysm, compression within a confined

space (the entrapment neuropathies), or angulation and/or friction over an abnormal process (cervical rib).

The wounding mechanism

A study of the wounding mechanism often provides a clue to the severity of the lesion. Note should also be taken of the condition of the wound, whether healing was normal or delayed, and the extent and duration of any sepsis.

1. Though the wounding mechanism in acute injuries is usually obvious, there are occasions when it remains obscure, such as when a nerve injury associated with a fracture could be due to the force fracturing the bone, or indirectly to trauma from the bone ends, or to stretch as they are violently displaced.
2. The severity of the nerve injury increases with the severity of the wounding mechanism.
3. Nerve lesions associated with open injuries are likely to be more severe than those occurring in closed injuries. Exceptions of note are severe stretch injuries, unrelieved plaster compression lesions of the common peroneal nerve at the neck of the fibula, and the laceration, or even severance, of a nerve by the sharp spur of bone from a closed fracture.
4. Nerve involvement due to sharp penetrating wounding usually takes the form of partial or complete severance.
5. High velocity missile wounding. The nerve may be severed by direct hit or sustain a lesion in continuity of variable degree from 'near-miss' deformation (p. 193). The risk of severe damage is higher with this type of wounding, particularly when the associated limb bone is fractured. Most, however, are lesions in continuity which recover spontaneously.

The state of the exposed nerve

If the nerve is exposed in the wound it should be delicately examined to determine whether it is normal in appearance, bruised, lacerated or severed.

The nature and distribution of the peripheral disability

The clinical examination distinguishes between complete and partial lesions. The latter fall into four categories.

1. A partial lesion may date from the time of the injury. Here the peripheral defect is determined by the fascicular fibre composition at the level of the injury. If the different branch fibres are widely represented in most fasciculi, a partial lesion causes a widespread paresis and reduction in the quality of sensation. If the injured fasciculi are composed solely of all fibres from only one or two branches, the peripheral defect will be localised to, and maximal in, the field of those branches.
2. A partial lesion may represent a stage in the development of a lesion which is progressing slowly to complete loss of conduction, failure occurring more rapidly in some fibres than in others.
3. The lesion may have been complete originally but has been converted into the incomplete variety by regeneration, which is confined to some fibres only or which is proceeding more rapidly in some fibres than in others.
4. The partial lesion may represent a state of arrested, or permanently incomplete, recovery.

PROGNOSIS

The clinical examination should conclude with a forecast of the likely outcome as based on the estimated nature and severity of the nerve lesion and any associated non-neural damage. These considerations determine the subsequent management of the case.

32. Nerve injury and motor function

Repeated examinations and evaluations of motor functions following nerve injury and nerve repair are required:

1. as part of the diagnostic process to determine the site, nature and extent of any nerve involvement.
2. at the first examination to establish a baseline against which to compare assessments at subsequent examinations and in this way to determine whether the condition is stationary, improving or deteriorating.
3. to monitor the onset and course of recovery and in this way to provide information of prognostic significance, and
4. as part of the final assessment when there is no further improvement and the overall use and performance of the affected parts of the limb and the patient's ability to cope with a wide range of daily activities are under review.

To meet these requirements it is essential that the information on which the evaluation is based should be accurate and reliable. To ensure that this is so, it is necessary to recognise and exclude complicating factors that could lead to errors in the evaluation. Some of these factors operate from the time of the injury while others appear subsequently.

The topics discussed in this chapter include terminology, disturbances of motor function caused by nerve injury, and the evaluation of motor function. The histological changes in denervated muscle and the pattern of motor recovery after nerve repair are discussed separately in Chapters 27 and 44, respectively.

PART 1. GENERAL

TERMINOLOGY

Agonists or prime movers, synergists, antagonists and fixators are terms given to muscles that participate in specific but different ways to give precision and efficiency to complex voluntary movements (see below).

Paresis. The condition when a muscle is partially denervated so that the response to voluntary effort is weakened. This occurs:

1. in partial nerve injury when only some of the fibres of a muscle are denervated;
2. when a previously paralysed muscle has been:

   a. reinnervated by still immature regenerating nerve fibres;
   b. incompletely reinnervated for any one of a number of reasons.

Paralysis. The condition when a muscle has been totally deprived of a nerve supply and so is unable to respond to voluntary effort.

Isometric contraction. Contraction of a muscle against a force sufficient to prevent shortening and movement.

Isotonic contraction. Contraction of a muscle allowed to shorten and to produce movement.

Supplementary, or trick action of muscles. This relates to the ability of a muscle or muscles to produce a movement that they do not normally perform, until the prime mover held to be solely responsible for producing that movement is paralysed.

OF MUSCLES AND MOVEMENTS

1. It is movements and not individual muscles that are under voluntary control.

2. A voluntary movement requires the delicately co-ordinated action of several muscles not necessarily innervated by the same nerve, each of which contributes to producing the movement in a different way, all combining in a co-ordinated manner to give refinement, steadiness and precision to the movement.

The degree of co-ordination demanded between these various muscles is such that the absence or impairment of any one is sufficient to disorganise the action of others and in this way to impair the efficiency of the entire movement.

It is therefore important to know not only what muscles are involved in the production of any particular movement but also the role assigned to each in producing it. The testing of voluntary movements as an expression of motor function is based on this knowledge.

Prime movers or agonists. These are the muscles that produce the desired movement in response to voluntary effort. A prime mover does not act alone.

Antagonists. These muscles act in direct opposition to the prime mover. As the latter contracts, the antagonist resists in a carefully graduated manner to control and regulate the rate, steadiness, strength and range of the movement.

Synergists. When a muscle is capable of producing more than one movement as a prime mover, other muscles, called synergists, are called upon to prevent all but the desired movement. For example, the abductor pollicis longus and extensor pollicis brevis, acting together, radially abduct the thumb but in doing so they also radially abduct the hand. In order to counteract the unwanted movement of the hand, the ulnar abductors of the wrist contract to prevent the undesired action of the prime movers.

Fixators. These are muscles that are called into action to immobilise and stabilise the site from which the prime mover is acting, thereby enabling it to function in the most effective manner.

3. A muscle may have a different role in the performance of different movements. Individual muscles are, therefore, involved in many more voluntary movements than those customarily ascribed to them when only their function as a prime mover is considered.

4. A prime mover will not do its work if gravity will do it instead.

5. Proprioceptor mechanisms play a key role in the performance of voluntary movements. When proprioceptor mechanisms are impaired motor function inevitably suffers. Visual guidance can compensate for some of this loss. However, the motor deficit is revealed when attempts are made to perform purposeful movements in the dark or in the absence of visual guidance.

6. The importance of the hand in these matters is self evident. No part of the body possesses a greater range of purposeful movements than the hand and the finely and delicately coordinated digital movements involved in daily tasks. Manual dexterity and manipulative skills are particularly dependent on innervation patterns, both motor and proprioceptor, that regulate and control the coordinated activity of prime movers, antagonists, synergists and fixators.

7. The co-ordination between prime movers, antagonists, synergists and fixators is such that the absence of one is sufficient to impair or disorganise the action of the others. In this way the movement becomes clumsy, ill-directed and less efficient. It is, therefore, important to know not only what muscles are normally involved in any particular movement, but also the role assigned to each in that movement. A movement that the patient is unable to perform is often attributed solely and directly to the paralysed muscle or muscles, the possibility being overlooked that the function of uninvolved muscles might also be impaired by the elimination of the paralysed members. Consequently, when a muscle is paralysed not only must the loss of its action as a prime mover be considered but also the effect of that loss on the function of unaffected muscles. An example is provided by the weakening of the grip that follows paralysis of the extensors of the wrist. This is because the long digital flexors, which also flex the wrist, operate effectively only when wrist flexion is prevented by the synergic contraction of the wrist extensors.

In arriving at any conclusion regarding the actions of muscles on the basis of the disturbance of movement, consideration should always be given to the interdependence of muscles in executing a particular movement, for muscles function as well-integrated and co-ordinated groups, combining to give delicacy, refinement and precision to the movement.

8. Though an individual muscle may by virtue of its attachments, the direction of its fibres, and the design of the joint surfaces over which it passes, perform a variety of actions as a prime mover, the effect of its contraction is finally determined by the function of other muscles in the movement pattern. If any of these components are paresed or paralysed, then the manner in which the movement is impaired will often indicate the basis of the disability. For example, when all three carpal extensors contract pure extension at the wrist results, the ulnar adductor action of the ulnar extensor being prevented by the radial abducting action of the radial extensors. If the extensor carpi ulnaris is paralysed, voluntary extension at the wrist is accompanied by radial deviation of the hand since the radial abductors are now unopposed. This radial deviation on extension diminishes as the extensor carpi ulnaris recovers.

9. Volition directed to simple movements, such as isolated flexion of the terminal phalanx of the thumb, flexion and extension of the wrist and so on, is the cornerstone of the clinical testing of motor function. This, however, is an artificial and oversimplified approach to the evaluation of useful motor function because it neglects the more important role of a muscle in the execution of complex, highly integrated and co-ordinated movements.

PART 2. DISTURBANCES OF MOTOR FUNCTION CAUSED BY NERVE INJURY

Prerequisites for efficient motor function are:

1. muscles that are normally innervated and vascularised,
2. tendons that move freely in their sheaths and across other structures;
3. joints and periarticular structures that permit a free and unrestricted range of movement, and

4. a normal sensory innervation to these parts.

Defects in any of these will adversely affect motor function.

Disturbances of motor function caused by nerve injury include:

1. the loss of tone and reflexes in denervated muscles;
2. muscle wasting;
3. the development of deformities;
4. the absence of voluntary contractions in denervated muscles;
5. the impairment and loss of voluntary movements;
6. changes in the excitability of denervated muscles revealed by electrodiagnostic procedures.

Loss of tone and reflexes

Division of a peripheral nerve results in the loss of tone and tendon reflexes, e.g triceps, biceps and Achilles tendon reflexes.

Muscle wasting

The muscle wasting is due to a combination of denervation and disuse. Denervation atrophy is confined to the muscles innervated by the injured nerve. Disuse atrophy involves normally innervated muscles that have been rendered inactive by the lesion or by immobilisation; in individual cases it is not as marked as that due to denervation. A characteristic feature of disuse atrophy is the absence of fibrillation.

Development of deformities

The paralysis of some muscles and the unopposed action of others involve the redistribution of forces acting on joints. The unopposed antagonists adjust to a new position by becoming structurally shortened and this may lead to the development of deformities. These may be present at rest or only become evident during movements performed by unaffected muscles. Such deformities can give valuable information concerning the paresis or paralysis of muscles.

The absence of voluntary contractions

The absence of visible and palpable contractions of a muscle in response to voluntary effort is presumptive evidence of denervation. In this respect, it is important to remember that: (1) the test applies only to muscles that are superficial and accessible to inspection and palpation, and (2) it is common for the contractions from a normally innervated muscle to so displace a paralysed muscle, with which it is in contact, as to create the impression that the latter is contracting.

The impairment and loss of movements and the evaluation of motor function

The involvement of motor nerve fibres shows up as weakness or paralysis of muscles which, in turn, is reflected in the impairment or loss of movements.

PART 3. THE EVALUATION OF MOTOR FUNCTION

Methods for evaluating the status of motor function are directed to: (1) the wasting of the affected muscles; (2) changes in the excitability of muscles to electrical stimulation as revealed by electrodiagnostic procedures; and (3) The condition of muscles and movements.

THE EVALUATION OF WASTING

There is no method for measuring wasting that satisfies the rigorous standards demanded for a comparative study. Categories of mild, moderate and severe, subjective though they may be, are useful even if they are of little value for this purpose.

Wasting may be expressed as the difference between the circumference of the limbs, measured at regular intervals, at fixed levels with reference to an easily identifiable bony landmark such as the medial humeral epicondyle and the apex of the head of the fibula. This is the preferred method for clinical use.

However, any metrical study of wasting based on this method is complicated by:

1. the difficulty of ensuring that the measurement is always taken at precisely the same level. This can be avoided by marking the level permanently with some sort of indelible point on the skin;
2. soft tissue injury and the destruction of tissue;
3. swelling or oedema which obscures the wasting;
4. the amount of subcutaneous tissue, particularly fat;
5. immobilisation of the limb in a cast;
6. the development of a 'use hypertrophy' in the uninvolved limb that may obscure the true amount of residual wasting.

The displacement method of evaluating wasting requires two identical cylinders filled to the same level with water into which, say, the hands are immersed to a given level. The difference in the amounts of water displaced is taken as a measure of the wasting. The method is suitable for the forearm and hand, and the leg and foot but is still too cumbersome for clinical use, bearing in mind the limited value of this information in the totality of evaluating motor function.

ELECTRODIAGNOSTIC TESTING

This is used for the recognition of nerve injury, for detecting the onset of recovery and for following its progress.

Nerve trunk stimulation

The simplest form of electrodiagnosis is stimulation of the nerve trunk both above and below the site of the suspected lesion. The nerve trunk may be stimulated by means of superficial or skin electrodes, by needle electrodes introduced in the vicinity of the nerve trunk, or by direct stimulation during surgical exposure of the nerve.

Nerve trunk stimulation above the lesion will indicate whether conduction is normal, completely or incompletely interrupted, or impaired.

Two points should be kept in mind in interpreting the results of nerve trunk stimulation: (1) the anomalous and supplementary innervation of muscles, and (2) a nerve undergoing Wallerian degeneration will continue to respond to electrical stimulation below the lesion for 3–4 days after the injury.

Stimulating the nerve trunk below the lesion should be delayed for 1 week, when it becomes of value in identifying a first degree injury. This is because the nerve trunk below a lesion undergoing Wallerian degeneration will have become un-responsive to electrical stimulation by this time whereas the first degree lesion is one in which the damaged nerve conducts above and below the lesion but not across it. This simple test gives in-formation relating to the site of the nerve lesion in first degree injuries.

Changes in the response of a muscle to electrical stimulation

A muscle may be stimulated electrically either directly through the skin or indirectly by way of the motor nerve which innervates it. The stimulus may be of the galvanic variety or take the form of electrical pulses of varying shapes and frequencies. The nerve trunk may be stimulated by means of superficial or skin electrodes, by needle electrodes introduced in the vicinity of the nerve trunk, or by direct stimulation during surgical exposure of the nerve.

A muscle is a complex of tissues consisting, inter alia, of two excitable elements, nerve fibres and muscle fibres. Nerve fibres are more readily ex-citable than muscle fibres, so that in normally innervated muscle the nature of the response to electrical stimulation is imparted by the nerve fibre component.

Following denervation the nerve fibres retain their excitability for about 3–4 days when frag-mentation of the axons reaches a degree where continuity with the muscle is lost. Denervated muscle fibres are then left as the sole remaining excitable element and impart their own charac-teristic response to direct electrical stimulation. This excitability persists as long as contractile tissue survives.

These changes are the basis of a number of well-established electrodiagnostic tests for the recog-nition of nerve injury, for the detection of the onset of recovery and for following its progress.

Of the several electrodiagnostic methods based on the measurement of the excitability of a muscle to electrical stimulation, the strength duration method is the most useful and has largely replaced other methods. The strength duration curve shows whether a muscle is normally innervated or com-pletely denervated. If the curve shows features characteristic of both denervation and normal in-nervation, then the muscle is partially denervated. The precise form of the curve then provides some information of the ratio of normal to denervated muscle fibres in the muscle (Fig. 32.1).

The strength duration curve of normal muscle

Because nerve fibres respond to currents of much shorter duration than muscle fibres, the response of normal muscle to stimulation is characteristic of the nerve fibres alone, and the strength duration curve has the short time constant characteristic of nerve fibres. The current strength required to elicit minimal contraction of the intact muscle remains the same over a wide range of pulse dur-ations until the short pulse durations are reached when the current strength has to be increased. This gives a continuous, almost flat curve with an upward trend in voltage at the extreme left of the curve when short duration stimuli are used. The current intensity necessary for excitation rises steeply with pulses between 0.1 and 0.01 milli-seconds (Fig. 32.1a).

The strength duration curve during nerve fibre degeneration

As the nerve fibres degenerate, the rapid nerve fibre response declines and the slower muscle fibre response emerges and eventually predominates. This is reflected in the form of discontinuities or kinks that usually appear in the curve between the 3 and 10 milliseconds pulse durations. These kinks divide the curve into two parts, one a rapid com-ponent with a short time constant characteristic of the declining nerve fibre response, and the other with a long time constant or slow curve charac-teristic of the growing muscle fibre response which is now unmasked by commencing nerve fibre degeneration. The former is rapidly replaced by

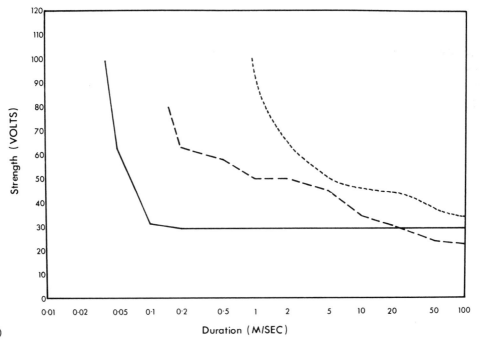

Fig. 32.1(a)

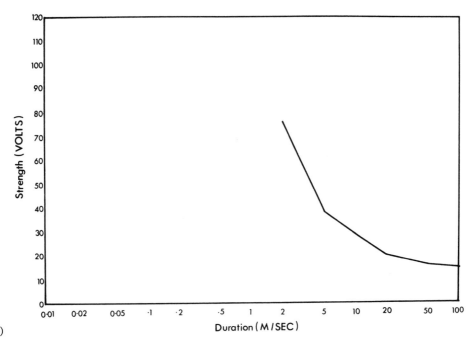

Fig. 32.1(b)

Fig. 32.1 Strength duration curve profiles of normal, denervated, and incompletely innervated muscles. **a.** S/D curves from a left lateral popliteal nerve lesion. ———— Normal peroneus longus. – – – – Peroneus longus undergoing denervation atrophy. . . . . . The denervated peroneus longus 6 weeks after the preceding recording. **b** S/D curve from a completely paralysed deltoid muscle. **c** S/D curves in a left lateral popliteal nerve lesion in which some reinnervation has taken place. ———— Normal extensor digitorum brevis. – – – – Partially reinnervated extensor digitorum brevis. **d** S/D curves in a left lateral popliteal nerve lesion in which some reinnervation has taken place. ———— Normal extensor digitorum brevis. —·—·—·— Normal peroneus longus. – – – – Partially reinnervated peroneus longus. . . . . . Partially reinnervated extensor digitorum brevis.

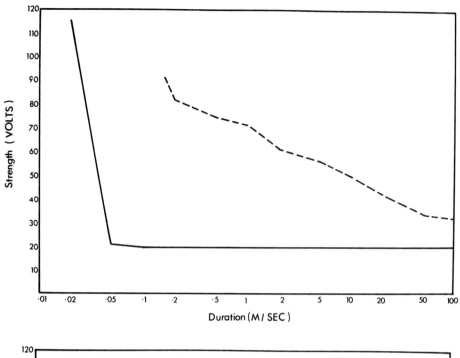

Fig. 32.1(c)

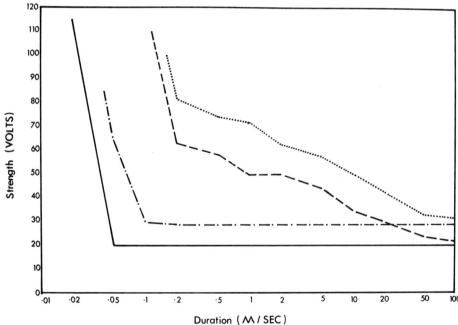

Fig. 32.1(d)

the latter until the denervation strength-duration profile is fully established as described above. The appearance of a kink or discontinuity in the curve is a reliable early sign of denervation (Figs 32. la & b).

The strength duration curve of denervated muscle

In completely denervated muscle the strength duration curve is still continuous but is now characteristic of muscle fibres alone which are less excitable than nerve fibres. Thus responses are only elicited with stimuli of long duration and the necessity to increase the current for stimulation occurs at about 10 milliseconds. The normal duration curve, in the form of a horizontal line rising steeply with stimuli of short duration, is thereby converted into a distinctive steeply rising parabola which is displaced to the right, that is towards the long duration pulses. In other words, the profile of the curve for denervated muscle slopes upwards much more sharply, there is practically no horizontal portion, and the shorter pulse durations do not evoke a response. The rise in current intensity necessary for excitation commences at about 50 milliseconds and is complete at about 1 millisecond (Fig. 32.1b).

The normal and the denervated strength duration curves represent two extremes. A change from one type to the other indicates progressive degeneration or recovery according to the trend of the changes, intermediate types of curve representing varying proportions of the two components.

The strength duration curve during reinnervation

During recovery precisely the reverse occurs. The first sign of recovery is the appearance of a kink or discontinuity in the denervation strength duration curve, which is subdivided into two parts. One has a short time constant characteristic of an appearing nerve fibre response, which depends on the presence of excitable nerve fibres in the muscle, and the other a long time constant characteristic of the muscle fibre response. As recovery proceeds the more rapid component increases and eventually obscures the slower muscle fibre element (Figs 32.1 c,d).

In summary, a continuous curve is found only in normal or denervated muscle, the form of the curve being characteristic for each. The presence of a discontinuity or kink in the curve is evidence that either the muscle is in the early stages of denervation or reinnervation is occurring, the trend of the curve from the normal or the denervated profile indicating the nature of the condition.

Progressive current testing

In S/D determinations the muscle is stimulated by instantaneous shocks which have a rectangular or square wave form and a duration measured in milliseconds. This is an artificial form of stimulation and attempts have been made to imitate the normal contractions of a muscle by using currents in which the stimulus reaches its maximum value slowly, the wave form of the pulse having a period of rise that may be measured even in seconds. Such currents are referred to as progressive currents. Nerve fibres readily adapt to a slowly rising (progressive) current but not muscle tissue. Normally innervated muscle therefore accommodates to progressive current stimulation because of the presence of nerve fibres. On the other hand, denervated muscle loses the capacity to accommodate and so responds to progressive current stimulation of a given duration at much lower thresholds than does the normal muscle. Progressive current testing, therefore, reveals a difference between normal and denervated muscle.

Electromyography

Contractions in normal muscles induced either directly by voluntary effort or indirectly by stimulating the nerve innervating the muscle (stimulation electromyography), are accompanied by muscle action potentials that can be picked up by surface or needle electrodes and recorded by electromyography. The identification and interpretation of abnormal changes in the electromyogram are based on a careful analysis of the characteristic features of the muscle action potential, its shape, amplitude, duration and frequency.

Electromyography is of great value in:

a. detecting denervation;
b. providing useful information relating to the condition of motor nerve fibres as this is expressed in terms of nerve conduction times and velocities;
c. localising nerve lesions;
d. providing a sensitive index of reinnervation;
e. following the course of motor recovery.

The following information is relevant to the use of electromyography as a diagnostic procedure.

1. The role of electromyography is to support and not replace clinical diagnosis.
2. The method is convenient to use and not uncomfortable to the patient.
3. Stimulation electromyography provides a useful method for studying motor conduction times and conduction velocities in nerves from which disturbances of conduction and the site and extent of the lesion may be deduced.
4. The nature and distribution of motor action potentials recorded from muscles in response to voluntary effort and nerve trunk stimulation will reveal whether nerve conduction is normal, partly or completely interrupted, or impaired.
5. A reduction in nerve conduction velocity, an increased terminal latency and a reduction in the number, amplitude and duration of motor unit potentials signify the presence of a lesion impairing conduction.
6. The detection of a few motor unit potentials in the affected muscle or muscles indicates an incomplete lesion in which at least some fibres have escaped injury. This finding is of particular value when the clinical examination has suggested a complete lesion.
7. When a muscle is denervated it fibrillates. This takes the form of fine, rapid, asynchronous rhythmic contractions of muscle fibres that collectively impart a faint continuously rippling movement to the surface of the muscle. This activity is not visible through the skin.

   Fibrillations are accompanied by spontaneous electrical activity that is represented in the electromyogram by characteristic abnormal muscle action potentials. Such fibrillation action potentials provide conclusive evidence of a nerve injury causing Wallerian degeneration.

   Fibrillation potentials diminish in amplitude and frequency with the passage of time but persist as long as contractile elements survive. Fibrillation potentials have been detected in a muscle 15 years after it had been denervated.
8. Persistence of electrical silence in response to voluntary effort and nerve trunk stimulation, followed later by the appearance of spontaneous fibrillation action potentials signifies complete interruption of conduction.
9. Spontaneous fibrillations are characteristic of muscles denervated by nerve lesions in which there is loss of axonal continuity. This is the case with second, third, fourth or fifth degree damage. Electromyography does not differentiate between these categories.
10. In a first degree injury, where axon continuity is preserved but conduction blocked, the affected muscles do not fibrillate.
11. Spontaneous fibrillation potentials are not usually well developed until the 21st day after the injury, though they may be detected earlier or their appearance be delayed.
12. The first signs of reinnervation in a denervated muscle can be detected by this method and the progress of reinnervation and functional recovery in the muscle charted and evaluated.

Limitations of electromyography

Though electromyography offers the earliest evidence of the reinnervation of denervated muscles, the limitations of the method should not be overlooked.

1. Electromyography does not differentiate between nerve severance and lesions in continuity causing Wallerian degeneration.
2. The useful recording range is limited to a centimetre or two surrounding the needle point, while the sites of reinnervation and recovery are at first distributed unevenly through the muscle. On occasions the first fibres to be reinnervated may be electrically inaccessible and so escape detection or be missed by the exploring electrode. To be diagnostically significant recordings should be taken from several sites in order to ensure that, within reason, the electromyograms are representative of the entire muscle. Furthermore, at least several,

if not all, muscles innervated by the nerve should be sampled.

3. Successive examinations are essential to track the course of a deteriorating or recovering lesion. A single examination reveals the state of affairs only at that point in time.
Repeated needle insertions for EMG recording could lead to damage along the needle track.

NERVE CONDUCTION VELOCITY AND CONDUCTION TIME STUDIES

Approximate values for these features are given in Table 32.1.

The contralateral nerve should be used as a basis for determining whether or not these properties are impaired. In this respect it should be noted that rates for the same nerve on the two sides may differ.

Stimulation electromyography is the basis of motor nerve conduction velocity and conduction time studies in which the nerve trunk is stimulated electrically and the muscle action potentials elicited in a selected muscle are recorded. The time interval between the initiation of the nerve impulse at the stimulating electrode and the take-off point of the muscle action potential can be measured by means of suitable recording apparatus. This interval represents the total conduction time. Because the distance between the stimulating and recording electrodes on the surface is only a rough estimate of the distance along the nerve fibres of the nerve trunk, nerve conduction velocity determinations based on these data lack accuracy.

A more acceptable method is to stimulate the nerve trunk, in turn, at two widely separated points along its course while recording the action potentials in a selected muscle in the hand or foot. This gives the total conduction time to the selected muscle on each occasion. Assuming that the

Table 32.1 Motor conduction velocities and latencies

Nerve	Level	Velocity metres/second	Latency milliseconds
Ulnar	Axilla to wrist	55–60	
	Axilla to elbow	56–78	
	Elbow to wrist	54–60	
	Wrist to hypothenar group		2–4
	Wrist to first dorsal interosseous		3–5
Median	Elbow to wrist	50–60	
	Axilla to wrist	60–70	
	Axilla to elbow	60–86	
	Wrist to thenar group		2–5
Radial	Axilla to elbow	62–75	
Femoral	Above knee	63–77	
Sciatic	Buttock to ankle	43–50	
	Above knee	50–57	
	Below knee	43–50	
Tibial	Below knee	33–60	
	Femoral condyles to calf muscles		5.5
	Ankle to abductor hallucis		5–9
Common peroneal	Knee to ankle	43–65	
	Ankle to extensor digitorum brevis		3.5–6

stimulus delay and other factors remain constant, the difference between the two total conduction times becomes the time taken for the nerve impulse to travel between the two points on the nerve. The nerve conduction velocity is then calculated from these data. Measured as it is from the surface, the distance between the two points is again an estimate only but is a closer approximation to the actual distance covered by the nerve impulse.

The data on conduction time and nerve conduction velocity derived by stimulation electromyography relate to the largest calibre and most rapidly conducting motor nerve fibres which have a low threshold to excitation.

These studies provide information of value in:

a. detecting and differentiating between those chronic lesions that disturb nerve conduction, those lesions that block conduction but do not destroy axonal continuity, and those that result in the degeneration of nerve fibres;
b. localising the site of a lesion;
c. following the course of axon regeneration;
d. evaluating the outcome of regeneration.

Potential sources of error when recording and interpreting the results of nerve conduction studies are:

1. Values obtained for nerve conduction times and nerve conduction velocities vary widely from individual to individual. For this reason, when deciding whether or not the conduction time is increased or the conduction velocity slowed, the standard for comparison should be obtained from adjacent normal nerves or the corresponding nerve in the opposite limb.
2. Variations in the distribution of individual nerves.
3. Anomalous innervations.
4. Whether the limb is extended or flexed.
5. Reader error when measuring the distance between two fixed points, and discrepancies between this measurement and the true length of nerve fibres.
6. The age of the subject. Adult values are not reached until about the 5th year; slower velocities are recorded in old age.
7. Temperature. The evidence demonstrates the need to measure conduction rates under standard conditions.
8. Level of the measurement. There is a proximo-distal gradient of conduction velocity in which the rates below the elbow and knee are slower than the rates above those levels.
9. Individual peculiarities in different nerves. Conduction velocities are slower: (a) in motor than in sensory nerve fibres; (b) in the leg than in the arm; (c) in those nerve fibres innervating the most distal muscles in comparison with those innervating more proximal muscles.

Concluding comment

The first signs of returning innervation take the form of: (1) a reduction and finally a cessation of fibrillation potentials and the appearance of re-innervation potentials in the electromyogram; (2) the appearance of two characteristic changes in the profile of the strength duration curve.

A certain number of muscle fibres must be reinnervated before voluntary contractions are possible. At the same time reinnervated fibres that are inadequate in number to meet the needs of voluntary contractions will respond to electrical stimulation. It is for this reason that S/D studies and electromyography detect the reinnervation of muscle fibres in advance of the return of voluntary contractions. However, though these electrical methods provide a reliable guide to the onset of muscle fibre reinnervation, this is not necessarily followed by the return of voluntary movement because muscle fibres may not recover in sufficient numbers for this to occur.

Once voluntary contractions return, from this point onwards these electrical methods cease to serve a useful purpose in the evaluation of motor recovery and function, this role being taken over by the study of voluntary movements which are a more reliable index of useful motor recovery.

Electromyograms, S/D curves and nerve conduction times and velocities are irrelevant in the final analysis of useful motor function. Regardless of what these tell the consultant, what is of prime importance to the patient is useful movement and his ability to handle those daily activities on which his living and his livelihood depend.

MUSCLE BIOPSY

This procedure has a limited use in the diagnosis of nerve injuries. It should be reserved for the difficult and exceptional case when it is necessary to know if muscle fibres are still present in a muscle that has been subjected to prolonged denervation. No recovery is to be expected when muscle tissue is no longer present. Biopsy is rarely indicated within the 1st year of denervation providing denervated muscles have been subjected to appropriate therapy because within this period they retain the capacity to recover and function efficiently following satisfactory reinnervation.

Histological examination of the biopsy specimen provides information on:

1. the state of muscle fibres. The most important information relates to their survival;
2. the nature and distribution of the interstitial connective tissue. Degeneration of muscle fibres and their replacement by connective tissue are a conspicuous feature in long-standing denervation or when treatment of the denervated muscle has been neglected;
3. the state of the endoneurial tubes. Empty endoneurial tubes indicate that regenerating axons are not present in the muscle.

Limitations of muscle biopsy

1. The earliest histological evidence of reinnervation will appear in the area surrounding the motor point which is the area to be avoided when obtaining the biopsy specimen.
2. A biopsy specimen is necessarily restricted to a small sample of the muscle. It may contain no nerve elements and may not be a representative sample of the changes occurring elsewhere in the muscle.
3. Though endoneurial tubes occupied by immature axons are evidence of regeneration this may not be followed by functional

recovery because motor tubes may be occupied by foreign axons that will not contribute to the functional end-result.
4. Because of variations in muscle pathology in different areas in the same muscle, the specimen may not be representative of changes present elsewhere. For this reason the use of single biopsies can provide misleading information about the overall state of the muscle and so are unreliable for deciding when nerve repair is no longer worthwhile.

THE EVALUATION OF MOTOR FUNCTION BASED ON VOLUNTARY MOVEMENTS

This is the most relevant source of information for the evaluation of motor function.

Motor function based on the response to voluntary effort passes through two preliminary phases before the first flicker of movement is possible.

1. The first is palpable or visible contractions of the muscle. Care must be taken to exclude movement transmitted from neighbouring normally functioning muscles. This type of evidence can only be obtained from superficially located muscles.
2. The second is when contractions, though insufficient to move the part, particularly against gravity, become adequate to hold the part in place after it has been passively placed in that position.

The evaluation of motor function as this is expressed in voluntary movements and the actions of individual muscles should take into consideration:

1. The range of movement and the power with which it can be executed. As a routine all movements should be tested against resistance and with the influence of gravity excluded. The range is measured with a protractor and power assessed with spring balances, and the comparison is with the corresponding muscle and movement on the opposite side.
2. The manner in which it is executed. Is the

movement executed strongly, rapidly and efficiently or weakly, slowly and unsteadily?

3. The rate at which fatigue occurs. A muscle and movement that appears to be normal in all other respects may tire more easily and quickly than its counterpart on the normal side.

4. The effect on more complex tasks to which a muscle contributes.

Finally, efficient motor function demands something additional to the ability of individual muscles to contract strongly. It also calls for the restoration of integrated patterns of activity which include the recovery of those sensory mechanisms on which motor performance depends. This is particularly important in the case of the hand, where muscles function as well-integrated and co-ordinated groups in every movement of the digits, combining to give that delicacy, refinement and precision of action that is the basis of manual dexterity and manipulative efficiency. Muscles must, therefore, be reinnervated by axons that are not only adequate in numbers but also of the right functional type and in the appropriate combinations and patterns so that the restored pattern of innervation corresponds as closely as possible to the original. Modified patterns of innervation caused by the loss of some axons and the entry of others into foreign tubes contribute to a residual motor defect.

What we really want to know is how useful and effective a particular prime mover is in executing highly skilled purposive movements involved in the execution of daily tasks, such as lifting a cup, using a knife and fork, writing, shaving, washing, combing one's hair, cleaning teeth, dressing and undressing, cutting with scissors, playing a musical instrument, threading a screw and a host of other daily tasks related to one's routine activities and employment. This point should not be overlooked when devising tests to measure the functional outcome of motor recovery. Such tests are limited only by the ingenuity of the clinician.

Once again, the importance of proprioceptor and other sensory mechanisms in the performance of such skilled acts is emphasised.

The evaluation of motor function for any particular muscle or voluntary movement can be expressed in terms of the following formula. This formula differs in some respects from the one currently in use but it is consistent with the pattern of recovery outlined in Chapter 45.

M0. No palpable or visible contractions and no movement in response to voluntary effort.

M1. Feeble contractions with perhaps a flicker of movement. This recovery is of no functional value.

M2. Feeble movement but not against gravity or any resistance. The muscle may maintain a part in a position into which it has been passively moved.

M3. Movement through a full range against gravity and some but weak resistance.

M4. Movement through a full range and against strong resistance.

M5. Full range and power with isolated testing of the movement. A residual disability in the execution of more complex movements, skilled and non-skilled, in which the muscle participates. Co-ordinated movements are still ill-directed and clumsy and tire more quickly.

M6. Motor function normal in every respect. This is the end result in a second degree injury but is not seen after nerve repair except in the very young.

The strength of the grip and pinch can be measured by suitably calibrated spring devices.

A more precise assessment of motor function can be expressed in terms of the range and power of individual movements measured and compared as a percentage of the corresponding recordings on the sound side. In making such an evaluation, care should be taken to exclude the influences of uninvolved muscles.

These ratings also apply to the lower limb, but in the case of the sciatic nerve there is an additional recovery assessment formula. This also carries a reference to sensory functions which are included here for convenience.

Grade 1. Motor and sensory functions are grossly impaired. There are marked troublesome trophic changes. Severe incapacitating pain is common. If permanent, this condition raises the question of amputation.

Grade 2. Walking is greatly restricted. There is troublesome hypersensitivity of the sole and moderate to severe pain. Despite attention to foot toilet, pressure sores develop but they can be controlled. The disability is sufficiently marked to limit the choice of an occupation.

Grade 3. There is an obvious residual motor and sensory disability that is maximal below the knee. Special shoes and some mechanical aid are necessary to support the arches of the foot and to assist ambulation. There is no disabling supersensitivity of the sole and no pain, but the leg and foot ache after prolonged use of the limb.

Grade 4. Slight generalised or localised residual disability that appears only after long periods of walking or standing. There is no pain and special footwear is not needed.

Grade 5. The limb is normal in every respect.

PART 4. FACTORS COMPLICATING THE EVALUATION OF MOTOR FUNCTION

Many factors complicate the evaluation of motor function, chief among which are the anomalous innervation of muscles and the failure to appreciate the role of trick movements in mimicking and concealing the loss of paralysed prime movers. However, there are others and it is important to identify and understand them so that: (1) false estimates of the nature and extent of the motor disability following nerve injury can be avoided, and (2) when evaluating motor function after nerve repair the recovery due solely to the repair and axonal reinnervation can be distinguished from that effected in other ways.

1. ANOMALOUS INNERVATION OF MUSCLES

If these are not appreciated errors in diagnosis and in the evaluation of end results are inevitable.

Notorious examples in this regard are variations in the innervation of the flexor digitorum profundus and intrinsic muscles of the hand, particularly the thenar group and lumbricals brought about by: (a) communications between the median and ulnar nerves in the forearm and hand, and (b) variations in the distribution of motor branches directly from the median and ulnar nerves.

Details of these variations are provided in *Nerves and Nerve Injuries* (Sunderland 1978, pp 663–669).

Nerve block to reveal anomalous innervations

In order to test whether an anomalous innervation is responsible for the escape of a muscle customarily innervated by the injured nerve, the nerve suspected of providing the anomalous innervation should be blocked by the injection of a local blocking agent. Care should be taken in doing this to ensure that the solution is confined to the nerve under test.

2. TRICK OR SUPPLEMENTARY MOVEMENTS

A patient's ability to execute a movement voluntarily cannot be accepted as infallible proof that the prime mover normally responsible for producing it is functioning. This introduces the question of 'trick' or supplementary movements and the 'trick' or supplementary actions of muscles. These make their appearance only when the normal prime mover is paralysed and their recognition provides reliable evidence that prime movers are involved. If, on the other hand, they escape detection, false estimates of the nature and extent of the lesion will invariably result.

These trick movements may be brought about in the following ways:

a. By the trick action of a muscle. Here the patient retains the ability to execute the movement when the only muscles said by anatomical texts to produce it are paralysed. This involves the active contraction of a muscle that is favourably placed to compensate for the prime mover, but which is only called into action when the latter is paralysed. For example, when the carpal flexors are paralysed the hand can still be flexed against gravity by the abductor pollicis longus.

b. By the contraction of an intact muscle which, by virtue of an accessory slip of insertion into the tendon of the paralysed muscle, can exert a pull on that tendon and thereby simulate the action of the paralysed muscle. Such an example is provided by the slip which the abductor pollicis brevis muscle sends to the extensor pollicis longus. Thus in cases in which the extensor pollicis longus is paralysed the terminal phalanx of the thumb can still be extended by the abductor pollicis brevis innervated by the median nerve.

c. By the tendon action of the paralysed prime mover which is introduced by the contraction of the appropriate antagonists.

There are muscles which, by virtue of their attachments, can move two segments of limb in the same direction. An example of such 'two-joint' muscles is provided by the long flexors of the fingers which flex the fingers and, by their overaction, flex the wrist. Both movements carry the hand and digits in a palmar direction. The length of such a 'two-joint' muscle, however, is usually insufficient to permit a full range of movement in the opposite direction at the joints over which it passes. Thus, full and simultaneous extension of the wrist and fingers leads to tightening of the long flexors of the fingers which then pull the fingers into slight flexion at the interphalangeal joints. The action of a 'two-joint' muscle introduced in this way is referred to as its tendon action, and since it does not involve the active contraction of the muscle, it can operate when the muscle is paralysed. Thus when the long flexors of the fingers are paralysed a variable degree of trick flexion of the fingers can be obtained at the interphalangeal joints by hyper-extending at the wrist. Similarly when the wrist extensors are paralysed some extension of the wrist can be obtained by fully flexing the fingers.

d. By strongly contracting and then suddenly relaxing the antagonists. This permits the

segment displaced to rebound in the direction in which the paralysed muscle would normally displace it, thereby resulting in a movement simulating the action of the paralysed prime mover. Thus in complete lesions of the lateral popliteal nerve pseudo-dorsiflexion of the toes may be obtained by strongly contracting the plantar flexors of the toes and then suddenly relaxing them. This permits the toes to rebound in dorsiflexion.

The significance of these trick or supplementary actions of muscles can only be appreciated by clinical experience.

The following common supplementary movements should not be confused with those movements preserved by the anomalous innervation of muscles.

Nerve divided: Radial
Expected loss of movement:
    Extension of the elbow.
    Extension of the wrist.
    Radial abduction of the wrist.
    Extension of the fingers.
    Extension and radial abduction of the thumb.
Trick or supplementary movements still possible:
    Extension of the elbow under the influence of gravity.
    Extension of the wrist produced by flexion of the fingers and tightening of the passive extensors (Fig. 32.2).

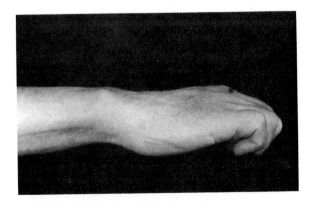

Fig. 32.2 Radial nerve lesion. Extension of the wrist produced by flexion of the fingers which introduces the tendon action of the extensor digitorum communis.

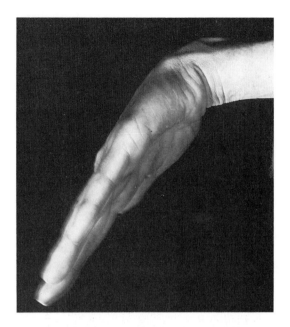

Fig. 32.3 Radial nerve lesion. Extension of the fingers at the metacarpophalangeal joints produced by fully flexing the wrist.

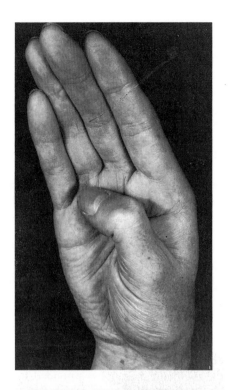

A

Extension of the two terminal phalanges of the fingers by the interossei and lumbricals.

Extension of the proximal phalanges by fully flexing the wrist and pulling on the inert extensor digitorum (Fig. 32.3).

Extension of the terminal joint of the thumb produced by the action of spring back after flexion.

Extension of the two terminal joints of the thumb by means of the tendinous slip that the abductor pollicis brevis gives to the tendon of the extensor pollicis longus. Palmar abduction of the thumb then results in extension of the two terminal phalanges (Figs 32.4 & 32.5).

Nerve divided: Median

Expected loss of movement:

Pronation.

Flexion at the proximal interphalangeal joints of the fingers and of the terminal phalanges of the index and middle fingers.

Flexion of the terminal phalanx of the thumb.

Palmar abduction of the thumb and

Internal rotation of the extended thumb on attempted opposition.

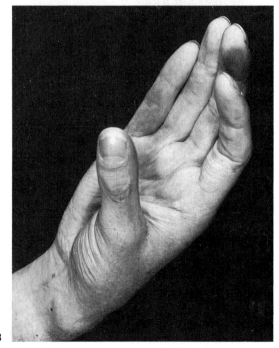

B

Fig. 32.4 Radial nerve lesion. Extension of the terminal phalanx of the thumb produced by the slip passing from the abductor pollicis brevis to the extensor pollicis longus. Extension of the phalanx is here accompanied by palmar abduction of the thumb.

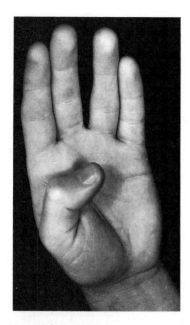

A

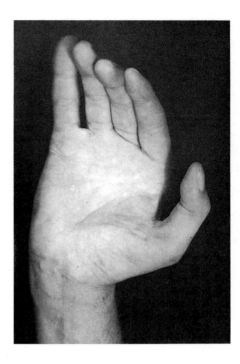

Fig. 32.6 Median nerve lesion. 'Trick' flexion of the terminal phalanx of the thumb produced by extending the wrist and radially abducting the thumb which introduce the tendon action of the flexor pollicis longus.

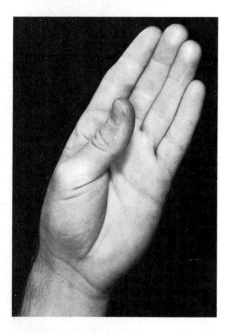

B

Fig. 32.5 Radial nerve lesion. Extension of the terminal phalanx of the thumb as in Fig. 32.4 but in this case the trick movement is not accompanied by palmar abduction of the thumb.

Trick movements still possible:

Pronation. Internal rotation at the shoulder. Brachioradialis will take the forearm to the mid-

prone position from which gravity takes the forearm into pronation. The movement is both clumsy and weak.

The terminal phalanx of the thumb can be flexed by fully extending the wrist and radially abducting the thumb. This introduces the tendon action of the flexor pollicis longus so that the terminal phalanx is pulled into flexion (Figs 32.6 & 32.7).

Flexion of the proximal interphalangeal joints of the ring and little fingers can be effected by the winding up action of the ulnar half of the flexor digitorum profundus innervated by the ulnar nerve.

Flexion of the metacarpophalangeal joint, palmar abduction and opposition of the thumb can be performed by ulnar innervated intrinsic muscles of the hand.

Clumsy palmar abduction of the thumb can be produced by the abductor pollicis longus.

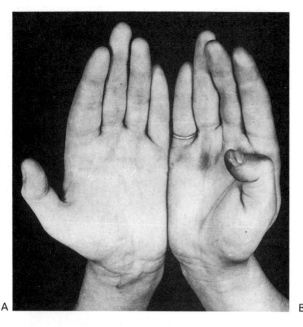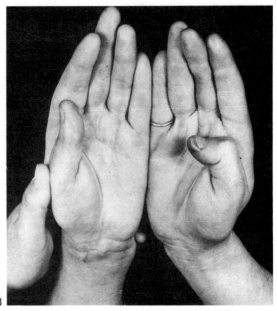

A   B

Fig. 32.7 Median nerve lesion. 'Trick' flexion of the distal phalanx of the thumb produced by radially abducting the thumb and pulling on the inert flexor tendon. This trick movement is not possible if the thumb is held to prevent radial abduction.

Nerve-divided: Ulnar

Expected loss of movement:

Flexion at the distal interphalangeal joint of the little and ring fingers.

Hypothenar elevation on attempted opposition of the thumb and little finger.

Inability to oppose the terminal digital pads of the thumb and the little finger with the latter extended at the interphalangeal joints and flexed at the metacarpophalangeal.

Adduction of the thumb.

Adduction and abduction of the fingers.

Flexion of the metacarpophalangeal joints especially of the ring and little fingers.

Extension of the terminal interphalangeal joints.

Trick movements still possible:

The flexor pollicis longus can compensate for the paralysed adductor pollicis (Figs 32.8 & 32.9).

The extensor pollicis longus acting with the long flexor and alone can function as a supplementary adductor of the thumb (Figs 32.10 & 32.11)

Flexion of the metacarpophalangeal joints can be effected by the 'winding up' action of the flexor digitorum superficialis and of the flexor digitorum profundus serving the index and middle fingers.

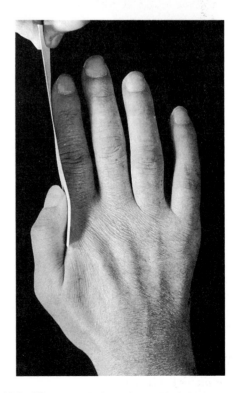

Fig. 32.8 Ulnar nerve lesion. The card is held securely in the first space by the strong contraction of the flexor pollicis longus which has taken over the adductor function of the paralysed adductor pollicis.

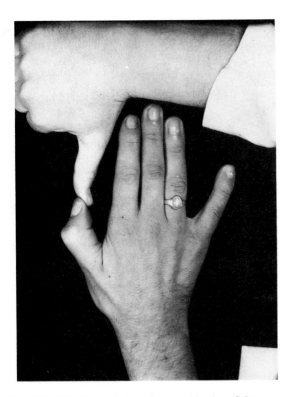

Fig. 32.9 Ulnar nerve lesion. Strong adduction of the thumb by the long flexor and extensor. The flexor has overcome the extensor action of the extensor pollicis longus which, however, is contracting firmly on the flexed phalanx to aid adduction. Observe that the little finger is held abducted.

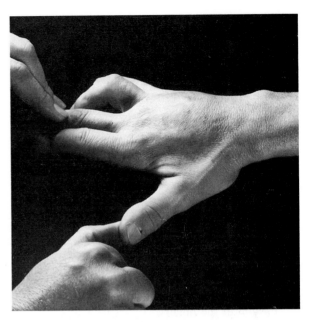

Fig. 32.10 Ulnar nerve lesion. Strong adduction of the thumb by the extensor pollicis longus, the tendon of which is standing out prominently.

Extension of the interphalangeal joints of the fingers can be produced by the common extensor, providing these are prevented from hyperextending the digits at the metacarpophalangeal joints (Fig. 32.12).

The fingers can still be adducted and abducted if flexion and extension, respectively, are permitted.

Adduction and abduction of the index finger may be produced by the extensor indicis and the common extensor to the index finger even when flexion and extension of the digits are prevented.

Abduction of the little finger can be produced by the extensor minimi digit.

Nerves divided: Median and ulnar
Expected loss of movement:
Pronation.
Wrist flexion.

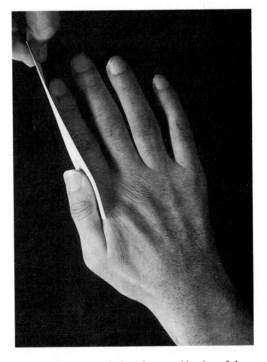

Fig. 32.11 Ulnar nerve lesion. Strong adduction of the thumb by the extensor pollicis longus. Froment's test would here indicate (erroneously) that the adductor pollicis was normal since forced adduction is not accompanied by flexion of the terminal phalanx of the thumb.

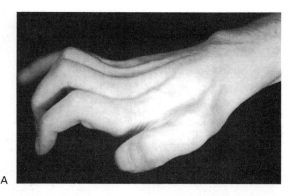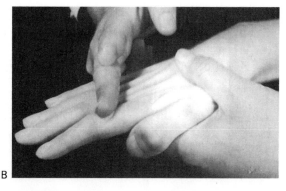

A   B

Fig. 32.12 Lesions of the median and ulnar nerves in the upper arm. Attempts to straighten the fingers resulted in hyperextension at the metacarpophalangeal joints and flexion at the interphalangeal joints. If hyperextension at the metacarpophalangeal joints was prevented, the extensor digitorum could then extend the phalanges at the interphalangeal joints.

Flexion, opposition and adduction of the thumb.

Flexion of the fingers.

Trick movements still possible:

Pronation — see median nerve.

The wrist can still be flexed by the abductor pollicis longus.

The thumb can still be adducted to the radial side of the hand and index finger by the extensor pollicis longus.

The fingers may be slightly flexed by the tendon action of the paralysed long flexors but to do this the wrist must be hyperextended.

Nerve divided: Musculocutaneous

Expected loss of movement:

Elbow flexion.

Trick movement still possible:

Elbow flexion can be strongly performed by the brachioradialis and pronator teres muscles. The pronating action of the latter is greater than the supinating action of the former so that flexion is accompanied by pronation. In complete combined lesions of the radial and musculocutaneous nerves elbow flexion can still be produced by the pronator teres which simultaneously pronates the forearm.

Nerve divided: Axillary

Expected loss of movement:

Shoulder abduction.

Trick movement still possible:

With the passage of time the patient can be trained to abduct the arm to the vertical position by using a combination of the spinati, trapezius, serratus anterior, the clavicular head of pectoralis major, coracobrachialis and the long head of biceps (Fig. 32.13).

Nerve divided: Sciatic

Expected loss of movement:

Flexion of the knee.

Common peroneal division: eversion of the foot, dorsi flexion and inversion of the foot, extension of the toes.

Tibial division: plantar flexion of the foot, inversion of the foot in plantar flexion.

Flexion of the toes.

Trick movements still possible:

Flexion of the knee. The sartorius and gracilis continue to very weakly flex the joint.

Common peroneal nerve:

Dorsi-flexion and inversion of the foot. The slight adduction and inversion produced by the tibialis posterior should not be attributed to the tibialis anterior. If the tibialis posterior is responsible, then there is no associated dorsiflexion of the foot as would occur if the tibialis anterior were contracting. A flicker of dorsiflexion of the foot has been seen to follow strong plantar flexion of the toes. This introduces the tendon action of the digital extensors which in turn leads to feeble dorsi-flexion at the ankle.

Extension of the toes: plantar flexion of the foot introduces the tendon action of the digital extensors while a flicker of extension of the toes

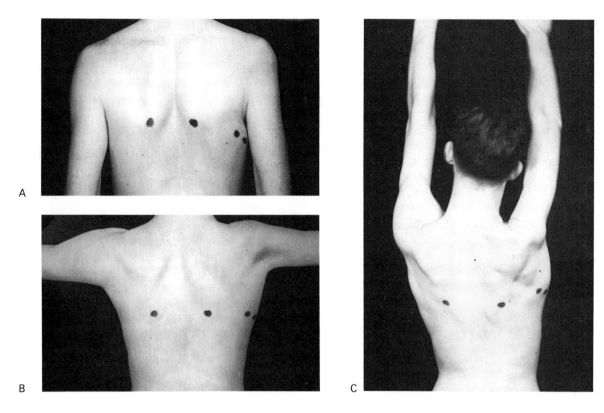

Fig. 32.13 Paralysis of the right deltoid and teres minor. **a** The three dark spots on the right hand side represent, from medial to lateral, the position of the inferior angle of the scapula with the arm at the side, abducted through 90° abducted to the vertical. **b** Arms abducted through 90°. Marked external rotation of the right scapula so that the inferior angle has moved laterally and is now situated beneath the middle spot. The left scapula has undergone only a trace of external rotation. **c** Arms abducted to the vertical position. Further rotation of both scapulae, but the degree of rotation on the right exceeds that present on the left.

may be produced by first strongly contracting the flexors and then relaxing them which permits the toes to rebound in extension.

Tibial nerve:

Plantar-flexion of the foot. Some patients retain the ability to plantar-flex the foot by contracting the peroneus longus. Normally this muscle acts with the other muscles supplied by the common peroneal nerve to give range and variety to combined movements of dorsi-flexion and eversion of the foot. When, however, the normal plantar-flexors are paralysed, their action can be taken over by the peroneus longus.

Flexion of the toes. The toes may be feebly plantar-flexed by strongly dorsi-flexing the ankle, which introduces the tendon action of the digital flexors. If the ankle is immobilised a flicker of flexion of the toes can still be obtained by first strongly extending the toes and then suddenly releasing them. This permits the toes to rebound into a position of plantar-flexion. Pseudo-plantar flexion of the toes may be produced by the claw effect of the long digital extensors. These, owing to absence of the intrinsic muscles, cause hyperextension at the metatarsophalangeal joints and thereby introduce the tendon action of the long flexors.

Nerve divided: Femoral

Expected loss of movement:

Extension at the knee.

Trick movement still possible:

A weak extension effect may be imparted to the knee by the pull of tensor fascia lata.

3. THE ACTION OF GRAVITY

As a routine, movements should be tested against resistance and with the parts positioned to remove the influence of gravity. This is because some movements can still be performed, but not against resistance, when the prime mover is paralysed. This is achieved by relaxing the antagonists and allowing gravity to perform the movement normally executed by the prime mover. For example, the wrist can still be flexed when the normal wrist flexors are paralysed. This is done by relaxing the extensor antagonists and allowing the hand to move into flexion under the influence of gravity. When the triceps is paralysed the forearm can still be fully extended by allowing gravity to perform the movement. Once the influence of gravity is removed the forearm can no longer be extended.

4. TRANSMITTED CONTRACTIONS

There are times when the contractions of normally innervated muscles are transmitted to adjacent paralysed muscles in such a way as to create the misleading impression that the latter are contracting in response to voluntary effort.

5. RUPTURED OR SEVERED TENDONS

When testing motor function it is important not to be misled by the loss of joint movement which is due to the severance of a tendon or tendons. For example, depending on the circumstances of the injury, the inability to flex the terminal phalanx of the thumb could be due to the paralysis of the flexor pollicis longus or to the rupture or severance of its tendon.

6. JOINT STIFFNESS AND SHORTENED ANTAGONISTS

Restrictions on the range of movement due to muscle paresis or paralysis should not be confused with the restriction imposed by joint stiffness and shortened antagonists. For example, as long as the digital extensors remain shortened, digital flexion will be limited in range.

7. HYPERTROPHY OF REINNERVATED MUSCLE FIBRES

A persisting paresis due to incomplete reinnervation may be obscured by the hypertrophy of those muscle fibres that have fully recovered.

8. UNUSUAL DISTURBANCES OF MUSCLE FUNCTION ASSOCIATED WITH NERVE SEVERANCE

Following nerve transection, paralysed muscles sometimes show signs of recovery long before this could be due to the regeneration of axons. For example, following clean severance of the median nerve at the wrist, most or all of the intrinsic muscles of the thumb remain paralysed for approximately 1 week when some commence to contract, feebly at first and then progressively more strongly until finally, 2–12 weeks after the injury, they have either fully recovered or are left with a residual paresis. This anomalous recovery precedes that due to nerve repair and axon regeneration. This phenomenon originally raised the question of whether or not spontaneous recovery could take place in a repaired nerve without the intervention of degeneration followed by regeneration.

Blocking the ulnar nerve during the period of this recovery leads to the paralysis of all the intrinsic thenar muscles, thereby indicating that the early appearance of voluntary contractions in the muscles originally paralysed as a result of the injury is due to an innervation from the uninjured ulnar nerve.

Though it is clear that such early recovery could be due to an ulnar innervation, certain features relating to the paralysis and recovery remain unexplained. Why are the thenar muscles paralysed by severance of the median nerve if they are innervated by an uninjured ulnar nerve, and what is the explanation of the transient nature of the paralysis? These are puzzling features that call for comment.

Four possible explanations could account for this phenomenon:

a. It is well known that some, or more rarely all, of the intrinsic thenar muscles may be doubly innervated from median and ulnar sources. A double innervation of individual muscle *fibres* is unlikely, the accepted distribution being one in which some muscle fibres are innervated by the median nerve and the remainder by the ulnar.

Assuming such an arrangement, it remains to be explained why the ulnar innervated muscle fibres are silenced by severance of the median nerve. The slow recovery under such circumstances could, of course, be due to readjustments, either of a central or peripheral nature, that compensate for the denervation of a quota of the muscle fibres. Such compensatory mechanisms could be modifications to central patterns of activity, the hypertrophy of surviving muscle fibres, and sprouting from the axons of the uninjured nerve that extend to innervate neighbouring denervated muscle fibres and in this way the territory served by the uninjured nerve.

The reinnervation of denervated muscle fibres by invading axon sprouts that bud from neighbouring intact axons requires further consideration. Whether or not such intramuscular axon sprouting occurs in man is not known. Even if it is assumed that such a factor does operate, it could only modify the clinical picture by extending the territory served by the uninjured nerve. This would assist recovery, but obviously fails to explain why the ulnar innervated muscle fibres are rendered inactive in the first place by severance of the median nerve. A further difficulty in accepting such an explanation is that the atypical recovery may involve thenar muscles which, so far as can be judged by nerve block and clinical testing, are innervated solely by the ulnar nerve. Under these conditions there are no denervated fibres to stimulate axon sprouting in the muscle rendered temporarily quiescent as a result of injury.

b. A second possibility concerns the temporary failure of central patterns of activity due to transsynaptic or other disrupting central influences. When a muscle is innervated by both the median and the ulnar nerves it is conceivable that its normal activity is determined by the co-ordinated activity of groups of motor neurons at central levels which combine to innervate and control the entire muscle but by way of different peripheral nerves. These central patterns of activity may be

so delicately integrated that the exclusion of some units, from retrograde neuronal changes following severance of the median nerve, could disorganise and lead to the failure of the entire system. Paralysis of the muscle would follow, some fibres failing because of the severance of axons innervating them, and others because of the temporary arrest of activity in the neurons innervating them. The recovery of neurons, together with central adjustments of a compensatory nature, would be followed by the reappearance of voluntary contractions in those muscle fibres whose function had been temporarily suspended. On the other hand, the recovery of denervated muscle fibres would be delayed until they were reinnervated by regenerated axons.

c. If one is to persist with the claim that a coexisting injury to the ulnar nerve is responsible, then it must be further inferred that only those ulnar nerve fibres innervating the thenar muscles are injured, because there are no other signs of ulnar nerve involvement. Since, however, there is no intraneural fibre localisation at the wrist to justify such an interpretation, it is concluded that the anomalous recovery of the thenar muscles is not due to recovery from a first degree injury of nerve fibres in the ulnar nerve.

d. The explanation that most satisfactorily accounts for this phenomenon is based on the branching of nerve fibres in which the same anterior horn cell supplies axons to a muscle that reach it by way of different peripheral nerves so that each neuron innervates some muscle fibres by way of one peripheral nerve and other muscle fibres by another nerve (Fig. 32.14). This assumes that the axons of anterior horn cells innervating the thenar muscles divide in the medial cord of the brachial plexus or further centrally, one branch entering the ulnar nerve and the other the median, both branches ultimately reaching and participating in the innervation of the same thenar muscle but reaching it over different peripheral nerves. A further possibility is that the same neuron may innervate muscle fibres in different muscles of the thenar group.

The retrograde neuronal changes consequent on the severance of one nerve, in this case the median, are responsible for blocking conduction in

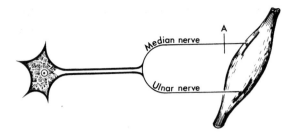

Fig. 32.14 Diagrammatic representation of a muscle innervated by a motor neuron which sends fibres to it, by a process of axon branching, over two peripheral nerves. For simplification only one division of the axon is illustrated and each branch is shown innervating only one muscle fibre.

Severence of the median nerve at *A* leads to retrograde neuronal effects which temporarily arrest conduction in the fibre running in the ulnar nerve. As a result the entire muscle is paralysed. Voluntary activity reappears in the muscle with the recovery of the neuron and the nerve fibre contained in the ulnar nerve trunk. Recovery of the muscle fibres innervated by the severed nerve is delayed until they have been reinnervated by regenerated axons.

the uninjured axon branches that are passing to the thenar muscles by way of the ulnar nerve. The result is paralysis of the thenar muscles, the median supplied muscle fibres suffering as the direct result of severance of the median nerve, and the ulnar innervated fibres being affected indirectly because of the retrograde changes in anterior horn cells whose axons have branched to send one process into the median and another into the ulnar nerve.

Recovery from these retrograde neuronal changes is then followed by two events: (1) by the reversal of the temporary conduction block induced in those axon branches in the ulnar nerve, and (2) the onset of regeneration in the 'sister' branches severed in the median nerve.

9. CONVERSION HYSTERIA

Disturbances of motor function may occur in some cases of conversion hysteria. However these can usually be distinguished from the motor defect that follows a nerve injury. Distinguishing features of the disturbance in conversion hysteria are:

a. the affected muscles and movements do not correspond to the distribution of any particular nerve;
b. the motor defect is not associated with the type of sensory loss that normally occurs with the nerve injury;
c. the motor loss is part of the symptomatic picture of functional disorder;
d. the results of electrodiagnostic testing are inconsistent with motor nerve involvement from a nerve injury.

REFERENCE

Sunderland S 1978 Nerves and nerve injuries, 2nd edn. Churchill Livingstone, Edinburgh, pp 663–669

33. Nerve injury and sensory function

Topics discussed in this chapter include relevant anatomical and physiological considerations, changes in sensory functions caused by nerve injury, testing sensory functions, the sensory examination and documentation and factors complicating the evaluation of sensory functions. The course of sensory recovery after nerve repair is discussed in Chapter 44.

This chapter is not concerned with the more complex and often controversial features of sensory mechanisms and sensory function, as these have been studied by physiological experiments on nerve fibres.

PART 1. GENERAL

TERMINOLOGY

Many of the following definitions are based on the Glossary of Terms issued by the International Association for the Study of Pain.

Protective sensation. This relates to an awareness of and appropriate response to noxious stimuli as represented by pin prick and extremes of temperature above 45°C.

Stereognostic sense or object identification. This is the ability to identify objects by handling them in the absence of visual assistance.

Hoffmann–Tinel's sign. This is the distal tingling in the field of an injured nerve elicited by percussing the nerve to activate and in this way detect the presence of regenerating 'axon' tips. Care should be taken when percussing the nerve to avoid deforming the site of the injury. Percussion should commence at a silent area inferiorly and then be continued upwards following the nerve trunk until a response is elicited.

Paraesthesiae. Unusual, abnormal but not painful, spontaneous or evoked sensations.

Anaesthesia. Insensitivity to all forms of stimulation.

Dissociated anaesthesia. The sensory state in which some sensory modalities survive while others are lost.

Hypo- and hyperaesthesia, hypo- and hyperalgesia. These are cutaneous sensory responses that are abnormal when compared with the responses elicited by applying the same stimuli to the unaffected adjacent skin or corresponding contralateral cutaneous area.

Hypoaesthesia. Diminished sensitivity to all forms of stimulation. Though the term includes painful stimuli, it would be preferable to reserve this term exclusively for tactile and thermal stimuli, painful stimuli being covered by the term hypoalgesia.

Hyperaesthesia. Increased sensitivity to all forms of stimulation. Though the term includes painful stimuli, it would be preferable to reserve this term exclusively for tactile and thermal stimuli, painful stimuli being covered by the term hyperalgesia.

Hypoalgesia. Diminished sensitivity to noxious stimulation.

Hyperalgesia. Increased sensitivity to noxious stimulation.

Pain. This is a subjective sensation which is readily recognisable by, and well known to, the individual but very difficult to define to the satisfaction of all concerned and in a manner likely to be universally accepted. In the words of Thomas Lewis (1942):

'reflection tells me that I am so far from being able satisfactorily to define pain, of which I here write, that the attempt could serve no useful purpose. Pain, like similar subjective things, is known to us by experience and is described by illustration . . . . . to build up a definition in words or to substitute some phrase would carry neither the reader nor myself further.'

While accepting Lewis's admonition, some definition is desirable for the purposes of this text and the following is offered as a compromise. Pain is an unpleasant and disturbing sensory and emotional experience associated with actual, impending or potential tissue damage.

Pain stimulus. One causing pain.

Noxious stimulus. A tissue-damaging stimulus.

Spontaneous pain. Pain occurring in the absence of any external stimulus.

Elicited or evoked pain. Pain occurring in response to an external stimulus disturbing the status quo.

Allodynia. Pain due to a stimulus that is not normally painful when applied elsewhere to the body.

Anaesthesia dolorosa. Pain in an insensitive area or region.

Analgesia. Absence of pain in response to stimulation that should normally be painful.

Causalgia. Severe incapacitating pain following a traumatic nerve lesion and associated with somatic, vasomotor and sudomotor dysfunction.

Dysaesthesia. Any unpleasant abnormal sensation, either spontaneous or evoked. Allodynia hyperpathia and causalgia are all examples of dysaesthesia.

Hyperpathia, Protopathic pain. An extreme form of hyperalgesia and allodynia characterised by the intensity of the pain, faulty localisation, radiation, over-reaction and 'after sensation'. The threshold may be raised but is more often lowered. Hyperpathia is a characteristic component of the causalgia syndrome.

Neuralgia. A nerve lesion causing pain which is intense and intermittent and felt maximally in the distribution of the nerve.

ANATOMICAL AND PHYSIOLOGICAL CONSIDERATIONS

Anatomical

Sensory nerve fibres run in cutaneous branches to reach the skin, and in deep branches that innervate muscles, joints and associated deep structures of the limbs. The nerve fibres of the cutaneous system are arranged in deep and superficial plexuses from which the specialised end organs are innervated and from which free branching occurs to give terminal interlocking patterns of innervation. The tissues deep to the skin also contain free nerve endings together with specialised sensory receptors that differ in structure from those at the surface.

Features of cutaneous innervation are:

1. differences in the structure of receptors that have been related to differences in function;
2. the existence of minor variations in the structure of receptors within the same accepted morphological group that could provide a basis for minor variations in a particular sensory modality;
3. the existence of transition forms among the receptors which throws doubt on the value of attempting too precise a correlation between structure and function;
4. the receptors form a mosaic of discrete spots of sensitivity so that cutaneous sensation is punctate in its distribution;
5. the density of innervation varies from area to area;
6. the pattern of cutaneous innervation is such that each receptor is innervated by several nerve terminals and each nerve terminal innervates more than one receptor. This arrangement permits interactions between stimuli applied to different receptors served by the same nerve fibre.

Physiological considerations

A sensory modality is a subjectively distinctive response to stimulation. The primary sensory modalities described for the skin are touch, pressure, pain, hot and cold and for the deep tissues, pressure, pain and proprioception. These primary modalities may combine to give more complex sensations such as itching and vibration, while variations in the intensity of a given sensation are based on the number of receptors stimulated and are signalled by changes in the frequency and duration of the impulse discharge.

Two hypotheses have been advanced to account for the manner in which different stimuli are distinguished by the sensory receptor apparatus of the skin. According to the first, observed differences in the structure of the receptor end organs are regarded as being of functional significance and each sensory modality has been assigned to a morphologically distinct receptor or group of receptors. A characteristic feature of receptor physiology is that any stimulus which activates the receptor will, regardless of its nature, produce the same subjective response. Each receptor, however, responds to one particular type of stimulus at a much lower threshold than to others. These features impart specificity to the system, each receptor giving rise, on stimulation, to only one specific sensation. Thus receptors function as peripheral analysers of stimuli, encoding them in different discharge patterns for transmission centrally along peripheral nerve fibres.

The second denies any specific relationship between receptor morphology and sensory modality. Here the different types of sensation are attributed to variations in the spatio-temporal pattern of excitation in sensory nerve fibres, the characteristics of the pattern of impulses leaving the skin determining the qualitative aspects of cutaneous sensibility.

While existing knowledge of these fundamental problems still lacks certainty and precision, the pattern of excitation is clearly of importance in determining the nature of the sensory response. At the same time the evidence is also sufficiently strong to justify the conclusion that the mechanisms underlying the ability to distinguish one type of sensation from another also include some measure of receptor specificity.

It may, therefore, be concluded that both neural patterning and receptor specificity are employed in distinguishing between the different sensory modalities.

Sensory nerve fibres

Sensory information picked up by the peripheral receptors is converted into trains of impulses that are transmitted centrally over sensory nerve fibres. These fibres differ in their calibre and conduction properties and each sensory modality is spread over a wide range of fibre calibre, so that no sensory modality is restricted to a particular nerve fibre size. Furthermore, regardless of the nature of the stimulus, the form of the action potential is remarkably constant.

While, therefore, the combination of end organ and sensory fibre imparts a certain specificity to the system, so that each unit is regarded as responding to only one type of sensory stimulus, this specificity cannot be expressed in terms of a particular nerve fibre size.

Information relating to the nature, quality and intensity of the stimulus is transmitted along individual nerve fibres as a pattern of activity or frequency code. This pattern is determined by the velocity of conduction in the nerve fibre, by the time intervals between successive impulses, and by the total duration of the impulse discharge. These features vary according to the particular receptor stimulated, its rate of adaptation and the intensity of the stimulus.

It is not possible, however, to express sensory function simply and solely in terms of the activity in single nerve fibres because sensory receptors, which vary in their arrangement, distribution and threshold to stimulation, are stimulated not singly but in varying numbers and combinations and at different intensities and intervals. This results in complex patterns of activity involving the interaction of many systems. As Walshe (1948) has emphasised:

'Although graduated punctate stimuli may be necessary in the investigation of sensory function, yet such stimuli are not physiological in the sense that the surface of the normal organism under normal conditions does not receive single stimuli of this nature, but more widely distributed and qualitatively multiple stimulations, often affecting simultaneously end organs of diverse kinds.'

Furthermore, though sensory units combine and summate to provide the basis for sensory perception, this does not occur in any simple fashion but involves processes of great complexity.

Central afferent pathways and neuronal pools

Nerve impulses generated at the periphery and conducted centrally as a pattern of activity in sensory nerve fibre systems are transmitted along somato-sensory pathways and through neuronal pools in the spinal cord, brain-stem and thalamus before finally reaching the sensory cortex where conscious awareness of the sensory experience occurs. These central pathways are interrupted by at least two synapses that break them into first, second and third order neuronal units.

Sensory evoked signal patterns are greatly modified as they travel centrally. Synaptic relay centres present many possibilities for the redesign or recoding of sensory evoked signal patterns. Here nerve impulses can, by processes of facilitation and inhibition, be brought together or dispersed, reduced or increased in number, or simply rearranged. In this way the original signal pattern is converted into new patterns of propagated impulses in the succeeding order of neurons. Synaptic relay centres also provide for further modifications by permitting the intermingling of sensory signals from different sensory fibres and receptor systems so that activity occurring elsewhere than in the area stimulated can modify the signal pattern generated by the stimulus.

Of more complexity are those central non-sensory neuronal mechanisms that modify sensory input patterns and activity along sensory pathways. It is now accepted that there is a continual descending influence checking the afferent inflow to the sensory cortex. These appear to be regulatory and directed to eliminating the effects of biologically irrelevant stimuli.

Receptor systems are concerned with the detection and conversion of peripheral sensory events into patterns of propagated impulses that flow into the central nervous system in an unbroken stream and in great profusion. While some systematisation of this information is achieved in terms of receptor specificity, more information reaches the nervous system than is either manageable or significant. Some selective mechanism is, therefore, required to separate the relevant from the irrelevant and, in this way, to control the sensory inflow that is constantly fed into the nervous system from a wide variety of sensory receptors. This could be achieved by modifying receptor sensitivity at the periphery and/or afferent synaptic activity centrally in such a way that irrelevant stimuli become ineffective and the effects of appropriate stimuli intensified.

The possibilities of modifying signal patterns at afferent synaptic centres are almost unlimited. Such centres could function as selective filters to erase irrelevant information from the pattern and to intensify biologically significant messages according to the needs of the moment. Such mechanisms provide the nervous system with a considerable measure of selection and control over the amount and kind of information it receives, though such a function would require that incoming sensory signals be identified and given a significance. How the nervous system recognises a specific stimulus as appropriate or irrelevant is not known, but its ability to do this is presumably based on previous experiences of significant stimuli and the memory patterns to which they give rise.

Thus several variables operate to modify the form of the signal pattern in its passage to the sensory cortex. These processes result in one integrated pattern of information being converted into another, the original pattern being recorded into a form that is functionally more acceptable to the higher centres while, at the same time, preserving the topographical representation of the periphery in the sensory cortex. The particular sensation resulting from a sensory stimulus is, therefore, the product of the activity set up by the peripheral receptor system and that occurring at various levels within the nervous system itself.

The cerebral cortex

Different sensations are, in the final analysis, the property of the sensory cortex because it is here that signal patterns originating at the periphery are finally decoded and translated into a sensory experience.

The spatio-temporal signal patterns, originally generated in a variety of receptor systems at the periphery but modified on their way centrally, are finally discharged into the vast three-dimensional neural networks of the sensory cortex. Here integrative processing takes place in which sensory units work and combine in large numbers against a background of stored information based on past experience. From this activity emerge complex sensations of high discriminative quality. These permit an appreciation of the qualitative aspects of sensation in the form of texture, shape, size, consistency, weight, two-point and temperature discrimination, tactile localisation, the conscious awareness of the position of the various parts of the body in space and relative to one another and an appreciation of the range, rate and direction of movement of a part. Further elaborations of this cortical activity provide the basis for more highly integrated patterns that collectively, and in their most highly developed form, represent the stereognostic sense.

THE VARIABLE NATURE OF THE SENSORY RESPONSE

What ultimately emerges from the sensory cortex as a subjective sensory response or experience is determined initially by the signal pattern generated at the periphery and subsequently by the changes induced in the pattern during its transmission along fibre pathways and across synapses on its way to the cortex.

Variables at the periphery affecting these processes are:

1. The precise size and site of the cutaneous area stimulated and the manner in which the stimulus is applied. Of significance are those variations that relate to the density of cutaneous innervation, and to the number of receptors of different types, sensitivity and rates of adaption that are stimulated, the order in which they are excited, and the intensity of stimulation.
2. The prevailing temperature at the skin surface and the state of the cutaneous circulation, both of which influence functional processes in receptors and nerve terminals.
3. The state of receptor activity as determined by central centrifugal influences.
4. Conditions affecting the conducting properties of nerve fibres as these are expressed in the basic components of the discharge pattern, namely, the velocity of

conduction, impulse frequency and the duration of the discharge.

Cortical factors contributing to processes of analysis and synthesis are: (1) fluctuations in the attention and concentration of the individual, and (2) the state of the memory patterns and the quality of recall at the moment when the incoming pattern is being matched for identification.

For these several reasons, the same stimulus complex does not always produce the same end result. Minor variations in the signal pattern arising in the manner described may be partly or wholly corrected by using information provided from additional and complementary receptor systems such as, for example, vision.

In the absence of such corrective mechanisms the nature of the sensory response to the same stimulus will vary somewhat from time to time because of the impossibility of maintaining the status quo or of recreating precisely the same conditions on subsequent occasions. It is this complication that makes sensory testing so difficult. Because of our inability to control every event in those complex processes that ultimately culminate in a sensory experience, it is not possible to maintain standard conditions in every respect throughout sensory testing, nor is it possible to recreate identical conditions at successive examinations. For this reason nothing is to be gained clinically by resorting to unnecessary detail in testing and evaluating sensory function.

THE HAND AND STEREOGNOSIS

The unique properties of the hand as an important exploring and testing sense organ are based on a wide range and variety of highly skilled digital movements, sensory receptor systems of great informative power, and a cortical representation of great complexity where incoming sensory information is finally integrated and synthesised.

When an object is handled, sensory impressions stream into the cortex from a variety of sensory receptors transmitting information that relates to the size, form, weight, temperature, texture and consistency of the object being handled. In the extensive neuronal networks of the cortex these incoming patterns of activity are involved in a further series of highly integrative processes. From the final synthesis of these data a composite pattern emerges that is matched against memory patterns previously established by training and practice. This is the basis of object identification.

The stereognostic sense is based on experience and practice. If the object is a familiar one recognition will be easy. Clearly, however, a patient will be unable to identify an object of which he has had no prior knowledge, though he may be able to describe its features with some degree of accuracy. If, therefore, the object is a strange one attempts will be made to classify it in terms of existing patterns and the object will be compared with similar objects but not identified.

The thumb, index and middle fingers play the most important part in furnishing information in the process of hand testing. These are all in median nerve territory, and this nerve may be regarded as the major pathway by which sensory information is conveyed centrally from the hand. In this respect the ulnar nerve plays a minor role, its principal contribution relating more to precision and gross grip.

The impairment or loss of tactile, temperature and proprioceptor information from the hand all combine to restrict its usefulness. This is illustrated in patients with lesions of the median nerve in which sensation has been lost but motor function has been preserved. This creates a situation in which the affected thumb and fingers, which are responsible for those many discrete and dexterous movements upon which the skilful handling and recognition of objects depends, can be moved but are insensitive. Under these conditions the patient is unable, without visual assistance, to recognise objects by touch or manipulation. Such patients complain that the hand is useless, or of limited practical use, in the dark or when they are unable to observe what they are attempting to do with it. This disability is not due to a motor defect but is the result of the loss of sensory information from the periphery.

Other defects that come readily to mind are the difficulties experienced in identifying coins handled in the pocket, searching for objects in a crowded handbag, seeking and operating a light switch in the dark, and sweeping coins off a counter with the insensitive ulnar border of the hand in ulnar nerve lesions.

The loss of this information also results in clumsiness and inefficiency that interferes with the highly integrated and skilled digital movements that are part of everyday living and the trade or occupation of the patient: the movements that guide the pen, the instrument and the machine, movements demanded in those myriad day to day tasks associated with dressing and undressing, washing and cleaning one's teeth, combing one's hair, shaving, lifting and holding a cup, using a knife and fork, writing, cutting with scissors, playing a musical instrument, threading a screw, and a host of other daily tasks related to one's routine activities and employment.

While the disabilities that result from the reduction of sensory impulses from the hand have been emphasised, the importance of the informative functions of the sensitive sole and joints of the foot should not be overlooked. When standing and walking sensory impulses stream centrally from the feet that provide information about the nature and stability of the surface with which the feet are in contact, such as its texture, surface irregularities, whether it is firm or soft and so on. Information relating to the orientation in space of the standing subject is additional to, and apart from, that provided by the vestibular apparatus. These important functions associated with standing and walking are affected when sensory recovery in the field of the sciatic nerve is incomplete.

PART 2. CHANGES IN SENSORY FUNCTIONS CAUSED BY NERVE INJURY

A nerve injury may deprive an area of all forms of sensation, or it may result in the distortion of sensory-evoked signal patterns by eliminating some nerve fibres from a complex pattern of sensory innervation, and/or by setting up abnormal impulses in damaged nerve fibres. Such abnormal patterns of activity have greater arousal value and alter the type of sensation that is felt.

Changes in the skin following denervation are described in Chapter 30. Importantly, insensitive skin is prone to injury, the hand and foot being particularly susceptible in this regard.

Changes in sensory functions take the form of:

1. Abnormal sensations or paraesthesiae.
2. Increased sensitivity.
3. Diminished sensitivity.
4. Loss of sensation that may be total or dissociated.
5. Referred sensation and false localisation.

PARAESTHESIAE

These are abnormal disturbing, but not painful, sensations felt in and sometimes beyond the sensory field of the injured nerve. They include intruding sensations of discomfort, numbness, pins and needles, tingling, prickling, aching, warmth, cold and burning. Generally speaking, they are features of progressive, incomplete, or recovering nerve lesions. They are aggravated by cold and by deforming the nerve, particularly at the site of injury.

Abnormal sensations are an expression of abnormal patterns of activity that originate in damaged sensory fibres at the site of the injury, and in sensory neuronal pools that are disorganised as the result of the retrograde disturbances induced by the injury and the arrival of trains of abnormal impulses from the periphery. Sensory information consequently reaches the sensorium in the form of unusual and confused patterns that disrupt normal cortical processes and intrude on consciousness as abnormal sensations.

Paraesthesiae are of two types, spontaneous and elicited. The former arise in the absence of any external stimulus and are based on the abnormal central activity originally created by the injury but which subsequently becomes self-sustaining. Elicited paraesthesiae are set up by pressure or tension on the nerve trunk itself, particularly at the site of the injury.

INCREASED SENSITIVITY. HYPERAESTHESIA AND HYPERALGESIA

These terms are defined on page 305. Here the sensation elicited by the external stimulus is hyperacute rather than different, normal stimuli exciting a sensation of greater intensity than usual. The condition is a feature of cutaneous areas in which sensory recovery is occurring. The hypersensitivity is due to the presence of damaged or immature regenerating nerve fibres, and to abnormal activity at synaptic centres rendered hypersensitive by retrograde neuronal and transsynaptic changes induced by the nerve injury.

DIMINISHED SENSITIVITY. HYPOAESTHESIA AND HYPOALGESIA

These terms are defined on page 305. In this type of sensory defect the distinctive features of individual sensory modalities are retained but each is diminished. The defect may be dissociated or total depending on whether one, some, or all of the modalities are affected.

The fundamental change is one in which the affected cutaneous area is left more sparsely innervated so that the number of fibres activated by a stimulus is reduced. This occurs in some partial nerve lesions, in areas of sensory overlap where one source of sensory supply has been removed, and during the course of sensory recovery following nerve injury.

TOTAL AND DISSOCIATED SENSORY LOSS

In total anaesthesia the affected cutaneous area is insensitive to all forms of sensation. In dissociated sensory loss a particular sensory modality, or modalities, has been removed by selective nerve injury. Analgesia is the absence of a response to a painful stimulus, thermanaesthesia the inability to recognise hot and cold, and tactile anaesthesia the inability to recognise touch.

REFERRED SENSATION AND FALSE LOCALISATION

Normally an individual is capable of localising a point stimulated with a considerable degree of accuracy.

These sensory aberrations have their origin in the rerouting and misdirection of regenerating

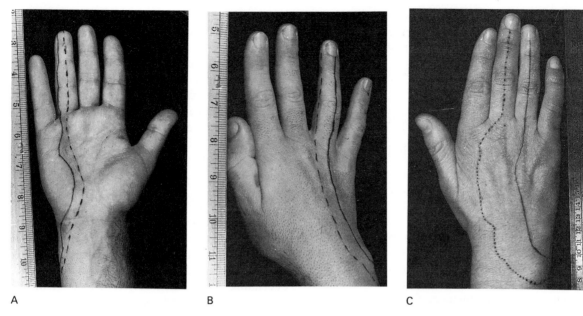

A   B   C

Fig. 33.1 The usual area of altered sensation following division of the ulnar nerve. The marginal zone of hypoaesthesia is between the broken and unbroken lines and, though usually narrow, may be extensive, as is shown in the illustration on the right.

axons that come to reinnervate a cutaneous area that may be some distance from that in which they originally terminated. When these new sensory terminals are stimulated, the sensation is recorded as coming from the old site to which the sensory fibres originally passed, e.g. a touch stimulus applied to the thumb may be felt in the middle finger. Faulty localisation occurring in this way reflects the degree to which the erroneous cross-shunting of axons has occurred during regeneration.

THE NATURE AND DISTRIBUTION OF THE SENSORY DEFICIT FOLLOWING A NERVE INJURY

Following complete severance of a peripheral nerve two cutaneous areas of sensory change can be identified (Fig. 33.1). One is completely insensitive and represents the autonomous zone which is supplied exclusively by the injured nerve. External to this is a fringe area where some sensation is retained but in a modified form. This fringe area receives its sensory innervation from two or more nerves, only one of which has been injured, there-

by resulting in a reduction in the density of innervation. The extent of the defective marginal zone varies for the different sensory modalities.

PART 3. TESTING SENSORY FUNCTION

GENERAL COMMENT

1. Much has been written in recent years about sensory testing and the technical improvements introduced for measuring sensory function (McQuillan et al 1971, Omer 1974, 1975, 1980, 1981, 1983, Daniel et al 1977a,b, Dellon 1978, 1980, 1981, 1983, Mansat et al 1981, Louis et al 1984, Lundborg et al 1986, 1987, Mackin 1988). These tests have been designed and are conducted to put a numerical value on the functional sensibility of the hand — in other words to quantify a function that common knowledge tells us is unquantifiable.

2. Sufficient has been said elsewhere in this chapter to indicate that many complex processes, each of which is subject to variation, are involved in sensory perception and that the latter, though based on information conveyed to the cortex from

peripheral sensory receptor systems, is determined, not by the patterns of impulses leaving the periphery but by the form in which they are ultimately presented to the cortex. Furthermore, sensory signals in their passage between the most remote afferent outposts and the cerebral cortex are exposed to influences that may fluctuate in such a manner that, even though a stimulus applied to the surface at different times may not vary in any respect, it does not necessarily follow that the evoked signal pattern reaching the cortex will be precisely the same on each occasion. All this highlights the ephemeral nature of the activity in sensory systems and explains why the sensory response to a given stimulus may fail to be identified in the same way at successive examinations. It is this ever-changing background to sensory perception, and the many variables involved to which it is not possible to assign a meaningful numerical value, that make the evaluation of sensory functions so difficult. Under such circumstances, as Wilfred Trotter (1941) has reminded us, 'The affectation of scientific exactitude in circumstances where it has no meaning is perhaps the fallacy of method to which medicine is now most exposed.'

It is for this reason that the simplest test methods are all that are required for the evaluation of sensory functions. The more elaborate and complex instrumental methods used by the physiologist in an attempt to assign a numerical value to the various primary forms of sensibility are unsuited for clinical use. Nor is the information they provide any more reliable than that obtainable by simple but more realistic methods.

Despite these difficulties, every precaution should be taken to ensure, by using standard procedures, that those features of sensory testing that are controllable are kept constant at successive examinations. At the same time the test methods employed should be kept within the bounds of practicability.

3. Since convention dictates that peripheral sensation is divisible into the primary sensory modalities of pain, touch, pressure, hot and cold and proprioception, a case can be made for the separate testing of each. However, each sensory modality tested and recorded separately is an unreliable indicator of useful sensory functions, as

this is expressed in terms of the all important functions of sensory discrimination and the stereognostic sense. The latter are the true elements of useful sensory function and should be the central objective of nerve repair. They should be tested and evaluated separately and assessments without reference to them are of little value.

4. The facts of life are such that nobody will use an assessment routine and methods that are too complicated and time-consuming, a grading system that is unnecessarily detailed and documentation that is cumbersome. What is required are simple tests that can be conveniently and easily performed and an assessment routine and a rating system for sensory functions that are practicable, reproducible, and clinically acceptable.

5. For the general surface of the body, tests for cutaneous sensory functions can be confined to the primary sensory modalities because these provide the protective sensory mechanisms that are all that is required of these areas. The situation, however, is very different in the case of the hand. For the hand to function as the efficient information gatherer it is designed to be, a far more complex sensory apparatus is required to provide for the discriminative aspects of sensation and the stereognostic sense which are only of relevance in the case of the hand and the median nerve in particular. This imposes a far more comprehensive and testing routine in the evaluation of sensory functions.

6. Precautions that should be taken when making the assessment are outlined elsewhere (p. 314 and p. 325).

7. When interpreting the data on sensibility and sensory perception it should be remembered that even normal individuals cannot always give accurate answers.

8. Whether or not sensation is altered, and the manner and extent to which it is, is always assessed in terms of the state of sensory function not only in normal neighbouring areas but also at corresponding sites on the opposite side of the body.

9. Of special importance is the end result assessment which is discussed in Chapter 45.

10. There is no evidence that regenerated sensory axons, having reached the skin, can induce the formation of new sensory end organs.

11. The consequences of a regenerating 'axon'

erroneously reinnervating an end organ that differs in type from that which it originally innervated are not known.

12. One might expect the quality of sensory recovery to depend on the density of innervation and the degree to which patterns of innervation have been disturbed by disorderly regeneration. However, Jabaley et al (1976) found that the degree and level of sensory reinnervation present in biopsy material after nerve repair did not, in some patients, match the results of clinical testing or the patient's subjective favourable assessment of the recovery. Clearly an important factor influencing sensory recovery is not so much the amount of nerve tissue present but a patient's ability to exploit whatever innervation is available.

13. Patients do not think in terms of sensory modalities. What is of immediate concern to them are:

   a. whether or not the affected part has protective sensation. The perception of a nociceptor stimulus, and an awareness of some touch and extremes of temperature are adequate to protect a hand or foot from accidental injury;
   b. the ability to use the hand to perform a wide variety of essential daily tasks.

Evaluations of sensory function should be based on these two premises.

14. Mackel and his co-workers (1983a,b, 1985) in their study of mechanoreceptor systems during regeneration in man found that:

   a. Not all types of receptors were reinnervated.
   b. Reinnervated mechanoreceptors were mostly located in the deep tissues and in the palm and proximal phalanges with few in the finger tips where the highest density is normally found. Regenerating sensory axons appeared to have difficulty in reaching the finger tips.
   c. Reinnervated Pacinian corpuscles were not found, which is not surprising since these represent only 12% of the total mechanoreceptor population (Johansson 1978).
   d. The density of reinnervation of the different receptor types correlated with the quality of sensory recovery.
   e. The early stages of reinnervation were characterised by single afferent fibres innervating multiple receptive fields and pronounced fatigue on repetitive stimulation. This was attributed to unstable axon-receptor connections and the transitional properties of immature regenerated axons.

Sensitivity improved with the continuing arrival of more regenerating axons and the progressive maturation of restored axon pathways. This was characterised by:

   i. the shrinkage of large receptive fields from the retraction of some axon sprouts;
   ii. an increase in the size of very small fields due to the branching of axon sprouts to establish connections with neighbouring receptors, and
   iii. the disappearance of multiple receptive fields innervated by a single afferent fibre.

FEATURES OF SENSORY TESTING

These include: (a) the condition under which testing is performed, (b) the selection of tests, (c) the stimulus and (d) the basic components of sensory testing.

The conditions under which testing is performed

The patient should be attentive and aware of the nature of the test. He should be comfortable and relaxed, and free from confusing interruptions and competing sensations. He should be blindfolded or the part to be tested should be appropriately screened from his view. Sensory tests are difficult to conduct and interpret when the part is cold and numb while they are greatly facilitated when the part is warm. Testing should be conducted in a quiet room at a temperature that is comfortable and reproducible.

Adequate time should be allowed for the tests to be performed in an unhurried manner though care should be taken to avoid fatiguing both the patient and the examiner, which is inevitable if the session is too time-consuming and the testing difficult and tedious.

Though the attitude and co-operation of the patient are important in sensory testing, the results obtained also depend on the attitude of the examiner. Where possible, examinations should be conducted by the same person throughout the period of observation.

The selection of tests for evaluating sensory function

The time available in the clinic will usually limit the number of tests that can be usefully employed. The examiner should, therefore, commence the examination with a clear understanding of what can be accomplished within reason and choose his methods and procedures accordingly. Where it is practicable to standardise procedures and the conditions under which they are applied, every effort should be made to do so. Each test should be repeated several times at the same examination before reaching conclusions regarding the state of sensory function. This is to minimise the influence of those variations that could modify the response to a given stimulus.

Because the pattern of cutaneous innervation and the receptor properties of the skin differ from area to area, the observations recorded for one area must, for purposes of evaluation, be compared against those obtained not only from neighbouring unaffected areas but also from the corresponding site on the contralateral side.

The method of applying a stimulus representing a particular sensory modality often involves other modalities simultaneously, for example touch, pressure and temperature. Two sensory experiences are then registered on stimulation. The first is an awareness of a change of state or the recognition that a stimulus has been applied to the skin; this is due to contact. The second relates to the identification of the nature and quality of the stimulus.

Precautions to be taken when testing sensory function are again emphasised.

The stimulus

Two points deserve special mention. Conventional testing for pain sensibility (pinprick) and tactile sensibility (stiff nylon thread) involves the repeated but single application of a point stimulus over the affected cutaneous area. Even though these stimuli can be graded, this is a somewhat artificial way of testing because in any activity, such as when an object is examined between the thumb and fingers, larger cutaneous areas and a vast array of sensory receptors are activated. The acuity of sensory perception demands far more information than can be provided from a point stimulus. For this reason pin scratch or the use of a device that permits several needle points to be applied simultaneously to a test area constitutes a more effective stimulus than single pinpricks. Light stroking with a fine wisp of cotton wool or camel hair brush is also more effective in eliciting a response than is the point application of a von Frey hair or nylon filament. Sensory testing with multiple simultaneous stimuli often elicits a response when a single sharply localised stimulus fails to do so. Others have also found a moving stimulus to be more effective than a static point stimulus (Dellon 1978, 1981, Mackel et al 1983, 1985).

The second point is that movement is an essential component of texture discrimination and object identification, which depend on the repetitive stimulation of a succession of quickly and slowly adapting mechanoreceptors as the object and the skin are moved or rubbed in relation to one another between the thumb and fingers.

The components of sensory testing

The examination of sensory function should be confined to simple procedures using methods which, though they might be considered inadequate for research into sensory mechanisms, are, nevertheless, quite adequate for detecting and evaluating sensory changes and for determining the onset and following the course of recovery.

In all testing, the following precautions should be taken:

a. the object of the test should be explained to the patient before commencing. He should be familiar with objects to be identified if he is to identify rather than describe them;

b. the test should be conducted in the absence of any visual assistance;

c. the time taken to make an identification should be noted and expressed simply as prompt or delayed;

d. for purposes of comparison, tests should be repeated in an identical fashion on the contralateral side.

The tests on which evaluations of sensory functions are based are directed to the following features of the sensory state:

a. *Recognition*. The patient is asked to describe what he feels when a test stimulus is applied. Often with the onset of sensory recovery the patient will indicate in response to a stimulus that he is only aware of a change of state that he is unable to qualify.

b. *Identification*. The patient is requested to identify the stimulus or the object examined.

c. *Localisation*. The patient is requested to indicate the site of application of the stimulus which, for purposes of comparison, should be applied at corresponding sites in the affected and normal limbs. The accuracy of the localisation and the time taken (prompt or slow) in making a decision are recorded. The assessment of the extent and nature of any sensory defect is based on this information.

PART 4. TESTING SENSORY FUNCTION. SPECIFIC TESTS

The conventional and generally accepted methods used for evaluating sensory function include the following.

PINPRICK. PAIN

The sensation elicited by pricking the skin with a sharp pin or needle varies from a feeling of touch to one of sharpness and finally pain. The nature of the response depends on such factors as the strength of the stimulus, the site of application, and the thickness and texture of the skin. When using pin or needle prick to elicit a painful response a distinction should, therefore, be drawn between a sensation of sharpness and pain.

A simple device for pinprick testing is one in which several needles are pushed through a cork disc to cover an area whose dimensions are determined by the size of the test area; a diameter of about 5 mm is generally suitable for the finger tips (Sunderland 1978). The lengths of the needles are adjusted so that the points are applied simultaneously to the skin. Pin scratch is also a more effective stimulus than single pinpricks.

Some regions are more sensitive to pinprick than others and the response shows characteristic changes following denervation and during regeneration.

The importance of pinprick as a test is that if there is no response to a painful stimulus then the part has no protective sensation.

TACTILE APPRECIATION

This can be tested by means of von Frey hairs or Semmes–Weinstein nylon monofilaments of increasing thickness that are calibrated to bend with increasing forces. The filament is applied at right angles to the skin surface and a force applied until the filament just bends. Filaments of increasing bending strength are applied until the patient just feels the stimulus. The surface of the test area is explored in this way.

This test is tedious and time-consuming, is an artificial way of testing cutaneous sensibility and, because of the many variables complicating the interpretation of the results, provides an unreliable metrical expression of the status of light touch. It has no advantages and is now only of historical and academic interest.

Light touch

For touch, a camel hair brush and a wisp of cotton wool are used and the part is tested both by stroking and by fixed contact. For large areas stroking with a finger is just as effective as other methods.

It is important to test separately for moving touch and constant touch. The rapidly adapting sensory fibres are believed to be responsible for transmitting the sensation of moving touch, whereas a constant touch stimulus evaluates slowly adapting fibres. It should be noted that with moving touch the number of receptors activated is greatly increased.

The response to moving touch is simply graded as normal, slightly impaired, greatly impaired or absent.

Tactile localisation

The accuracy of tactile localisation varies according to the method of testing, the region under test, the temperature, the degree of concentration of the individual, and those other variables to which attention has already been directed. Accuracy is highest in the hand and digits and poorest on the dorsum of the trunk.

Pressure sense

Pressure sensibility is tested by pressing a small blunt object to the surface of the skin. There is no sharp line of demarcation between touch and pressure sensibility, the latter gradually replacing the former as the deforming force increases in intensity. Deformation confined to the cutaneous layers of the skin is interpreted as touch, light or heavy in degree depending on the rate of application and the intensity of stimulation. A sensation of pressure occurs when the deforming force involves the deeper tissues.

The manner in which the stimulus is applied will, therefore, influence the precise nature of the sensory response. If the pressure is applied and increased sufficiently slowly the initial sensation is one of touch which is gradually replaced by one of pressure. If, on the other hand, the pressure is developed so rapidly that the deeper receptors are involved simultaneously then the effect becomes one of pressure. In each case a competing temperature sensation may be produced as the test object is applied to the skin. In order to minimise the effects of any accompanying thermal component, the temperature of the test object should be the same as that of the skin surface. Muscles and tendons are sensitive to pressure which may be applied by firmly squeezing them.

When deep receptors are activated by an appropriate stimulus across an anaesthetic superficial cutaneous layer, the sensation elicited is not invariably identified as pressure but may be variously described as one of touch, contact or pressure.

TEMPERATURE SENSE

Sensations of hot and cold are tested by applying the end of heated and cooled cylindrical copper rods with a contact surface of 5 and 10 mm depending on the extent of the area available for testing. The rods are left in broken ice and in water at different temperatures. Since heat loss from the test object occurs rapidly, testing should be limited to brief applications. The time required for the correct identification of the stimulus is noted. Under clinical conditions this method does not permit individual hot and cold spots to be studied separately because the area of skin stimulated is so large that all but summated effects are excluded.

Ice and water at 45°C are usually appreciated and identified without difficulty and such temperatures represent acceptable standards for the simple recognition of cold and heat. An accurate assessment of the finer discriminative features of temperature sensibility is not so easily obtained and requires specialised recording instrumentation. Conduction and convection phenomena at the skin surface, fluctuations in skin temperature, maintaining the temperature of the test object constant throughout the examination, and other differences combine to make it a difficult and time-consuming exercise to obtain precise measurements of the temperature sense at the point of stimulation, and to ensure that the test conditions are identical when one area is being compared with another. For these reasons it is not practicable in the clinic to attempt a detailed analysis of temperature sensibility as a routine procedure. One must be satisfied with recording whether or not the patient can distinguish between hot and cold and the time taken to identify correctly the nature of the stimulus.

PROPRIOCEPTION

Joint and muscle sensibility may be expressed in terms of the ability to recognise, *without visual assistance*, the position of the segments of a limb relative to one another, and to appreciate the direction, degree and rate of movement occurring at a joint.

Position sense is tested by moving the limb segment passively and asking the patient to indicate when movement is first noticed, the direction in which the part is moved and the rate at which it was executed. The movements are carried out smoothly, but at different rates, and always in an identical fashion when the affected and corresponding normal joints are being compared. The direction of quite small angular displacements can normally be appreciated by this simple procedure, which provides approximate threshold values for joint sensibility.

The integrity of the sensory innervation of muscles may also be tested by examining the ability of the patient to detect differences in the weight of objects which the muscle, or muscle group, is called upon to support or raise. This test depends on the ability of the muscle receptors to register differences in the degrees of tension to which they are subjected.

When testing it should not be overlooked that cutaneous receptors, in addition to those of muscles, tendons and joints, also contribute to proprioceptor sensibility.

TACTILE DISCRIMINATION

Clinical tests for tactile discrimination provide the closest correlation with useful functional recovery. This, like other discriminative forms of sensation, is an acquired skill that is improved by training and experience. The simplest test is that in which the patient is asked to distinguish between a sharp and a blunt stimulus.

In the case of the hand the tests are directed to the following.

Two-point discrimination (TPD) testing

The two-point discrimination test has received considerable attention in recent years and for many the classic static TPD remains a standard method for evaluating sensory function.

Two-point discrimination is a measure of the capacity of the cutaneous innervation to resolve two points applied simultaneously to the skin surface in such a way that the cortex recognises two stimuli as opposed to one.

Any device, such as a compass or calipers, that permits the distance between the points of the device to be varied and measured, is suitable for testing two-point discrimination. A simple device for rapid two-point testing is a disc (the Mannerfelt–Ulrich sensitometer) with spokes protruding from the circumference (Thomine 1981, Mackinnon & Dellon 1985). The distances between the fine but blunt points of the spokes are progressively increased around the disc in order to give a range of two-point separation. In this way it is possible, by rotating the disc, to move rapidly through a series of two-point distances. Whether the disc enjoys any definite advantage over easily adjustable calipers is debatable.

The caliper points should be blunt and when applied care should be taken to avoid distorting the skin surface.

The points are first separated by a distance that enables the patient to decide without doubt that he has been touched simultaneously by two points. The points are then brought closer together at successive applications until eventually they can no longer be recognised as two separate contacts. The shortest distance by which two touch stimuli must be separated to be recognised as such is the two-point threshold.

The points are applied so that sometimes two points and sometimes only one make contact with the skin. The two points should always be applied simultaneously and in the long axis of the finger and palm. The applications of double or single stimuli follow a random pattern until there are several observations (say five) for each. Any error in identification should be considered a failure for that distance. On the basis of these findings it is possible to assess sensory acuity.

The two-point threshold varies from individual to individual and one cutaneous area to another, being minimal where the touch receptors are closest, as in the skin of the finger tips, and greatest over the dorsum of the trunk where the receptors are furthest apart. Two-point discrimination also varies considerably from time to time within the same cutaneous area depending on variables already outlined. Thus normal values range from 2 to 4 mm for the digital pads, 5 to

10 mm for the palm and 30 to 50 mm for the forearm and leg. Tactile discrimination becomes defective when two-point discrimination exceeds 6 to 8 mm and is absent with readings exceeding 12 mm.

In a comprehensive and compelling study of two-point discrimination (TPD) Dellon (1978, 1980, 1981, 1983) and his colleagues (1983) demonstrated the decided advantage of the moving two-point discrimination (MTPD) test over static two-point discrimination (STPD). This has been confirmed by others (Poppen et al 1979, Poppen 1980, Louis et al 1984, Hirasawa et al 1985).

The classic STPD test of sensibility is now regarded as an unreliable indicator of the ability of the patient to use his hand (McEwan 1962, Mannerfelt 1962, Vierck & Jones 1969, McQuillan 1970, Krag & Rasmussen 1975, Jabaley et al 1976, Wynn Parry & Salter 1976, Von Prince & Butler 1976, Poppen et al 1979, Schlenker et al 1980).

With MTPD, the two points are drawn along the longitudinal axis of the digit to the terminal digital pad.

Dellon and Munger (1983) from a histological study of finger tip biopsies after nerve repair established a correlation between the MTPD and the rapidly adapting fibre-receptor systems (Meissner's corpuscles), and the STPD and slowly adapting fibre receptor systems (Merkel cells). In a similar study Jabaley et al (1976, 1980) had been unable to find such a correlation and reported that 'No significant correlation was found between the presence of identifiable nerve and receptors in the biopsy and the patient's functional performance'. Ogunro's (1984) findings suggest that with time axon terminals could provide for two-point discrimination of 3 mm.

Finally, Dellon & Kallman (1983) reported the MTPD test as correlating best with the patient's ability to identify objects. If this is so then why not bypass the MTPD test and proceed forthwith with tests to evaluate useful sensory function and the stereognostic sense which are the central objectives of nerve repair?

Though both STPD and MTPD tests put a numerical value on tactile discrimination, which may be useful for purposes of comparison, they are artificial tests that should be replaced by more meaningful methods of evaluating the quality of tactile discrimination and the stereognostic sense and, therefore, useful sensory recovery.

Ridge sensitometer testing

A useful method of testing tactile discrimination, appropriately called the ridge sensitometer test, was first described by Renfrew (1960, 1969) and subsequently developed by Poppen (1980) and his co-workers (1979). The value of the Ridge test lies in the fact that it relies on movement between the skin and surface of the object, thereby generating an array of sensory receptor activity. The device consists of a thin smooth rectangular block of plastic, 13 × 2.0 cm. One surface of the block carries a narrow linear ridge that gradually increases in prominence from zero elevation at one end of the block to a height of 1.5 mm at the other. For the purpose of grading tactile sensibility the ridge is suitably calibrated by dividing the block by transverse lines into eight equal 1 cm segments, the height of the ridge in each segment exceeding that in the preceding segment. The patient is instructed to inform the examiner when, with eyes closed, he first feels an irregularity as the ridge sensitometer is lightly drawn over the surface of the stabilised digit, thereby bringing increasing heights of the ridge into contact with the skin. Normally the elevation is perceived within the first centimetre segment of the ridge. However, the greater the residual sensory defect the higher the ridge before an irregularity is first detected; sensation may be so defective that the patient is unable to detect the ridge.

Though the ridge sensitometer and the MTPD both evaluate moving touch, the former evaluates depth sense detection and the latter distance detection.

The ridge test, though a useful alternative to the MTPD test for measuring tactile discrimination, could, also for the same reason, be omitted from the battery of tests for evaluating sensory recovery.

Miscellaneous tests for tactile discrimination

These involve the detection and identification of embossed printing, Braille characters and Porter's (1966) letters by running the finger across the surfaces. These are good tests.

Vibration sense

This test is the equivalent of subjecting the skin to a rapid succession of brief interrupted stimuli and is directed to the detection of functional rapidly adapting receptors (McQuillan 1971, Daniel et al 1977, Dellon 1981, 1983, Mansat et al 1981, Gelberman et al 1983, Szabo et al 1984, Lundborg et al 1986, 1987). The vibrations are provided by tuning forks calibrated to 30 cps (Meissner corpuscles) and 256 cps (Pacinian corpuscles). Alternatively, the vibrations can be provided by an electrically driven and controllable vibrating head 13 mm in diameter (Bio-Thesiometer: Dellon 1983, Lundborg et al 1986, 1987). According to Dellon this instrument 'neither added new information nor improved information derived from evaluating sensibility with a tuning fork' but Lundborg and his co-workers found it useful and reliable.

Dellon (1983), Gelberman et al (1983), Szabo (1984) and Lundborg et al (1986, 1987) all attach great importance to vibratory sensory testing in detecting reduction of or improvement in sensory acuity, well in advance of information derivable from two-point discrimination testing.

In the test, as used by Dellon, a prong of the tuning fork and not the base is applied to the pulp of the distal phalanx. This means that: (1) the amount of tissue activated is considerable, and (2) the disturbance set up by the vibrations spreads through the tissues and along the finger to reach innervated receptors some distance from the test site.

There are more meaningful ways of testing tactile discrimination. The vibration test along with two-point testing could, despite their convenience, be discarded.

TEXTURE DISCRIMINATION

The ability to appreciate differences in the texture of fabrics and surfaces by the sensations aroused when the object and the skin are rubbed against each other or, as is more commonly the case, when the material is examined between the highly sensitive skin of the thumb and fingers.

It is based on the repetitive stimulation, at different intensities and frequencies, of a succession of touch receptors as the object and the skin are moved or rubbed in relation to one another. The complex patterns of activity generated in this way are integrated and identified centrally as degrees of smoothness or roughness.

Materials of varying grades of smoothness and coarseness are employed for evaluating tactile discrimination. Commonly used for this purpose are cloth samples such as coarse wool, silk, velvet and linen, cards of sandpaper of different grades of coarseness together with a card of the same thickness but with smooth surfaces.

FORM DISCRIMINATION

Based on the identification of objects of different sizes and shapes, e.g. ball, cylinder, cube, ring.

WEIGHT AND CONSISTENCY DISCRIMINATION

Suitable test objects are: wooden spheres, metal ball bearings, and soft rubber balls of the same size.

OBJECT IDENTIFICATION

This is the basis of the 'pick up' test of Moberg (1958, 1962) who has been a persistent advocate for basing the assessment of sensory recovery on the refinements of useful sensory function. In the pick up test objects are identified and the time required to do so correctly recorded. The objects selected for the test are at the discretion of the examiner but should include such common items as: coins of the local currency of different sizes with smooth and milled edges, keys, a safety pin, paper clip, nail, screw, teaspoon, pencil, small comb, lipstick holder, nail file, bottle opener and the various items listed earlier.

Finally, the most decisive test is that based on an individual's capacity to handle a wide range of normal daily tasks in the home and in the workplace, e.g. securely holding a cup, utensil or tool, using cutlery, turning a tap, peeling vegetables and fruit, performing one's toilet (combing hair and brushing teeth). In this regard the patient's subjective assessment of hand function in relation to the performance of his or her normal daily activities is of critical importance.

So far as grading is concerned the best that can be suggested is satisfactory, impaired but manageable, and grossly defective.

In the assessment three additional points should be kept in mind:

1. The patient's ability to execute the various manipulations required for the examination and identification of objects, and to perform a wide variety of daily tasks requires:

   a. good pinch function and precision grip as used for holding a cup, winding a wrist watch, using a pen or pencil, locking and unlocking a door, screwing a nut on a bolt;

   b. strong hand grip as required for opening a door, firmly holding the handle of a tool, carrying a brief case or hand bag, grasping and pulling on a rope.

2. Motor and sensory performance are interdependent.
3. Persisting sensory deficits limit motor performance and reduce stereognostic ability.
4. With median nerve lesions, care should be taken when testing to ensure that a normal ulnar innervated side of the hand is not being used. Only the thumb, index and middle fingers should be used. In the case of the thumb and middle finger, possible extensions and overlaps from the radial and ulnar nerves respectively should be excluded.

ELECTRODIAGNOSTIC TESTS

Sensory nerve conductance testing

This electrodiagnostic method establishes a regenerating nerve's ability to conduct and measures the smallest electrical stimulus that will produce a sensation (Smith & Mott 1986).

The technique involves applying a stimulus transcutaneously to a nerve trunk to activate and thereby detect the presence of regenerating beta sensory fibres in the nerve segment between two skin electrodes. A 10 microsecond pulse is applied to the nerve and its amplitude increased until a propagated impulse induced in the nerve segment

between the electrodes results in the perception of a change of state.

This response can be detected some months in advance of the appearance of signs of sensory recovery detectable by other clinical methods.

The results can be expressed in internationally standardised units. It is a simple, reproducible and reliable method of recording A beta sensory nerve regeneration and for detecting the impending return of sensory recovery. The method, however, gives no clue to the functional outcome of regeneration.

Sensory nerve conduction velocities and latencies

Conduction velocity and conduction time measurements based on evoked sensory nerve potential recording provide valuable information relating to the detection and localisation of nerve lesions, the nature of the lesion and the progress and end result of 'axon' regeneration.

Electrodiagnosis involves the use of specialised equipment, techniques and procedures while the interpretation of results is the province of the specialist. Special texts on the subject should be consulted for detailed information.

Electrical stimulation is the usual source of evoked sensory action potentials, though it is also possible to elicit these potentials in digital nerves by percussing mechanoreceptors at the base of the finger nail.

Electrical stimulation of sensory nerve fibres sets up both orthodromic and antidromic action potentials and both may be used in the study of conduction times and conduction velocities. The siting of the stimulating and recording electrodes permits a study of latency times and conduction rates between the digits and the wrist, the wrist and the elbow, the elbow and the axilla, the toes and the ankle and the ankle and the knee. The median, ulnar, tibial and common peroneal nerves lend themselves to sensory conduction studies because of their superficial location in certain regions and their cutaneous distribution.

Approximate values for sensory nerve conduction velocities and latencies are given in Table 33.1. Rates and latency times vary from individual to individual, which emphasises the need to use

Table 33.1 Sensory nerve conduction velocities (metres/second) and latencies (milliseconds)

Nerve	Level	Velocity	Latency
Median	Index finger to wrist	37–67	2.5–4.0
	Wrist to elbow	43–67	3.8–6.0
	Elbow to axilla	66–70	2.0
Ulnar	Little finger to wrist	37–65	2.2–3.4
	Wrist to elbow	46–65	4–5
	Elbow to axilla	65–69	2.0
Common peroneal	Ankle to knee	33–57	5–9
Posterior tibial	Toe to knee	42–55	
	Toe to ankle	33–48	
	Ankle to knee	44–64	7.0

the contralateral nerve in the same individual as a basis of comparison when deciding whether or not conduction is impaired. Even here the rates on the two sides may normally vary somewhat.

Conduction rates are faster:

1. in the young than in the old;
2. in the arm than in the lower limb;
3. above the knee and elbow compared with more distal levels; the rates are slower in the toe to ankle segment than in the ankle to knee segment;
4. when the part is warmer.

In the case of the median and ulnar nerves:

1. conduction rates in the proximal segments are from 5 to 8 metres per second faster than in the distal segments;
2. digital nerve-wrist conduction times of over 4 milliseconds assume clinical significance;
3. compression of the median nerve in the carpal tunnel results in reduced conduction rates compared with corresponding segments of normal ulnar nerves:

| Median nerve | 31 m/s | Range 21–37 |
| Ulnar nerve | 46 m/s | Range 37–65 |

PART 5. THE SENSORY EXAMINATION AND DOCUMENTATION

Information on the status of sensory function is necessary at three stages in the clinical management of a nerve injury.

1. At the first examination in order to:

   a. identify the nerve injured and to obtain some idea of the severity of the injury, and
   b. establish a baseline for comparisons with subsequent evaluations.

2. At successive clinical examinations in order to determine whether the condition is stationary, improving or deteriorating.
3. At a final examination to establish an end result assessment of sensory function.

The examination of sensory function involves a separate assessment of each of the following features of the sensory state.

The cutaneous distribution of the sensory defect

This is expressed in terms of the autonomous area of total sensory loss and a fringe or marginal zone of impaired sensation. These two areas are carefully charted at each examination in order to detect and trace any change.

To facilitate the recording of data for future reference, the hand, because of its unique properties as an information gatherer, may, for convenience, be zoned into areas such as those shown in Fig. 33.2. This zoning is a modification of that used by Omer (1975, 1980a,b, 1981). It has the advantage that the areas are outlined by skin creases. The digits are numbered from *1* to *5* and

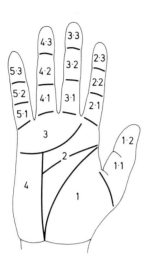

Fig. 33.2 Zoning of the hand and digits for sensory testing.

the phalanges from proximal to distal. For the palm — thenar, hypothenar and palmar areas are outlined and numbered as in the figure.

Elsewhere in the upper limb, and in the lower limb, the affected areas are usually extensive. They should be outlined by skin pencil and recorded on charts for future reference and comparison.

Recognition time

The time taken to respond to a stimulus is recorded simply as prompt or delayed.

Localisation

The ability of the patient to localise the site of a stimulus is recorded as accurate, slightly impaired, grossly impaired, or absent.

The status of peripheral sensibility within the affected area

At each examination attention should be directed to:

1. The state of protective sensation as this is

revealed by the response to pinprick and temperatures greater than 45°C and less than 5°C, all of which are noxious stimuli.
2. The response to:

   a. Pinprick
   b. Static and moving touch
   c. Pressure
   d. Hot and cold
   e. Joint movement

3. Where relevant, the state of texture, form, weight, consistency and temperature discrimination, and object identification.
4. The influence of the sensory defect on motor function, particularly as this relates to manual dexterity and skilled digital movements.
5. A concluding estimate, based on the patient's subjective assessment, of the effect of any residual disability on the overall performance of daily tasks in the household, work place and elsewhere.
6. The state of nerve conduction.
7. The course of sensory recovery. The stages through which sensory recovery passes are discussed in Chapter 44. The reduced sensitivity and poor tactile discrimination after nerve repair are due to incomplete and imperfect reinnervation consequent on the rerouting and misdirection of regenerating axons.

DOCUMENTATION

Patients vary so widely as witnesses and the sensation elicited by each type of stimulus presents such temporal, spatial and individual peculiarities that it is difficult to establish standard grades of sensory function that will encompass all features.

The following is the conventional formula in current use for documenting the status of sensory recovery. It is based on the British Medical Research Council System (Brooks 1954). All testing refers to the autonomous zone.

S0	No recovery
S1	Recovery of deep pain sensibility
S1+	Some superficial pain sensibility
S2	Superficial pain and tactile sensibility

Table 33.2 Sensory functions ratings*

Sensory function examined	Absent	Grossly impaired	Slightly impaired	Normal
Pinprick	P.0	P.1	P.2	P.3
Moving touch	T.0	T.1	T.2	T.3
T° sense	T°.0	T°.1	T°.2	T°.3
Localisation	L.0	L.1	L.2	L.3
Texture discrimination	D.0	D.1	D.2	D.3
Skilled movements required for the pick up test and object identification	M.0	M.1	M.2	M.3
Object identification-stereognosis	S.0	S.1	S.2	S.3

* Note that the symbols used in Table 33.2 to denote sensory ratings do not correspond with those given in the text though they are based on them. They represent a simplified system of recording sensory recovery after nerve repair.

but with some overreaction and inability to localise the stimulus.

S3   As for S2 but no overreaction and some ability to localise.

S3+ As for S3 but with good localisation and some improvement in two point discrimination.

S4   Normal sensibility

This formula fails to convey a meaningful picture of the state of useful sensory function and the role of sensory mechanisms in motor performance. In its place the author proposes the rating system listed in Table 33.2. Static and moving two-point discrimination have been excluded. For the purpose of establishing the ratings shown in Table 33.2, the response to pinprick, touch and temperature has been graded as follows; each part of the autonomous zone is tested separately and with particular reference to the digital pads.

Pinprick

P.0   Cutaneous field anaesthetic

P.1   Awareness of a change of state; usually interpreted as contact and probably due to transmission to deep tissues. The patient is unable to distinguish between the application of the head and point of a pin. The sensation may or may not be localised.

P.2   The patient can distinguish between the application of the head and point of a pin. The latter gives rise to (i) a dullish prick or (ii) an unpleasant sensation, with considerable radiation and false reference.

P.3   Sharp tingling or stinging sensation with some radiation and false reference. The ability to localise, other than to the hand or digit and the leg or foot, is absent.

P.4   A sensation of sharpness with or without some tingling or stinging and with no, or little, radiation. Localisation correct to within 2.0 cm.

P.5   Normal sensation of sharpness and a painful response which is accurately localised.

Moving light touch

T.0   No appreciation of light touch.

T.1   Awareness of a change of state with light touch.

T.2   Light touch gives rise to a radiating tingling sensation and the point of stimulation cannot be localised.

T.3   Light touch just perceptible as such with no localisation other than, in the case of the hand, to the digit, palmar field, or back of the hand, and, in the case of the lower limb, to the leg or foot.

T.4 Light touch appreciated as such, but with diminished acuity. Localisation correct to within 2.0 cm for the palm and digit.

T.5 Normal response to light touch.

Temperature sense

T°0 No temperature sensibility.

T°1 Insensitive to cold and heat except at high thresholds when the sensation elicited is interpreted as painful.

T°2 Temperatures below 15°C and above 45°C are correctly interpreted as cold and hot, respectively. Inside this temperature range the application of the test object elicits a sensation only of touch or pressure.

T°3 Temperatures below 20°C and above 35°C are correctly interpreted as cold and hot, respectively.

T°4 Normal temperature sensibility.

PART 6. FACTORS COMPLICATING THE EVALUATION OF SENSORY FUNCTION

FACTORS OPERATING FROM THE TIME OF THE INJURY

The response to sensory testing, being a subjective business, is influenced by the condition of the patient: whether he is conscious or unconscious, alert or confused, agitated or composed, comfortable or in severe pain, exhausted or refreshed, co-operative or unco-operative. It is impossible to make a reliable assessment of sensory function unless the patient is able and willing to co-operate. Thus an evaluation of sensory function is of no value in a patient who is too ill, too confused by alcohol or too hostile to co-operate.

The age of the patient

At what age have the young acquired a vocabulary, an understanding of events and an attitude that are sufficiently advanced to make them cooperative and reliable witnesses in sensory testing?

This depends on the individual, some being more advanced than others but, in general, evaluating sensory function is likely to contain a high element of error and uncertainty in very young patients.

Sensory testing

Any departure from a standard routine procedure could introduce a source of error when interpreting and finalising an assessment.

The conditions under which testing is conducted.

These are described on page 314 and should be followed if errors in assessing the status of sensory function are to be avoided.

Variations in the cutaneous distribution of individual nerves

Regarding variations in the cutaneous distribution of individual peripheral nerves as a potential source of error, three features call for comment.

a. The area of distribution of a particular cutaneous nerve is subject to individual variations.

b. The area innervated by a particular nerve is normally far greater than that revealed by anatomical dissection. This wider distribution is effected either:

  i. directly by way of microscopic terminal branches of the nerve in question or

  ii. indirectly by way of intercommunications that commonly occur, for example, between the median and musculocutaneous nerves in the upper arm, and the median and ulnar nerves in the forearm and hand.

c. The terminal cutaneous branches of different nerves overlap to a variable but often considerable degree in their distribution. The arrangement means that the area innervated exclusively by one nerve:

  i. is never as great as the anatomical distribution of the cutaneous fibres of that nerve and

ii. varies in extent from individual to individual.

Variations in cutaneous innervation created in these ways are, in turn, the basis of wide, and sometimes confusing, variations in the distribution and nature of the sensory changes that are commonly found, for example, in the hand following injuries of the median and ulnar nerves.

In doubtful cases, blocking the nerve suspected of being responsible for an anomalous innervation will settle the question.

Sensory disturbances in areas not innervated by an injured nerve

A puzzling feature occasionally observed after severance of a major peripheral nerve is the impaired cutaneous sensation in areas external to the territory served by that nerve so that the area of sensory change is much more extensive than would have been expected, even taking into consideration known variations in the branching of peripheral nerves (Sunderland 1952). Thus severance of the ulnar nerve at the wrist is sometimes accompanied by impaired sensation over the entire inner aspect of the forearm, an area normally innervated by the medial cutaneous nerve of the forearm. Sensation is usually rapidly restored in this area whereas, in contrast, recovery in the denervated ulnar field is delayed, and occurs only with regeneration and the entry of new 'axons' into the denervated area in the hand.

Cases of severance of the ulnar nerve at the wrist are particularly suitable for studying this phenomenon because in such injuries the medial cutaneous nerve of the forearm escapes injury or, if it is involved, only the most terminal filaments at the wrist are injured.

There are two explanations to account for the unusual distribution of the sensory loss in these cases.

Sensory fibres are known to branch at proximal levels so that individual neurons innervate larger territories than are customarily attributed to them (Sunderland 1978). It is conceivable that individual posterior root ganglion cells could furnish fibres to the medial cord of the brachial plexus where they divide, one daughter branch entering

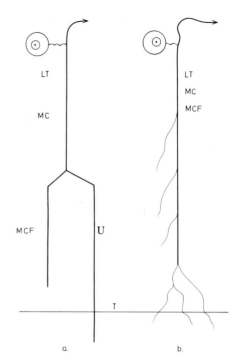

Fig. 33.3 LT = lower trunk of brachial plexus; MC = medial cord of plexus; MCF = medial cutaneous nerve of forearm; U = ulnar nerve; T = level of transection at the wrist.

the ulnar nerve and another the medial cutaneous nerve of the forearm (Fig.33.3a). In this way a neuron serves one cutaneous area over the medial aspect of the forearm and another in the hand. Collectively, these neurons could account for the entire cutaneous area served by the medial cutaneous nerve of the forearm and the ulnar nerve.

Thus the correct picture of the peripheral sensory nervous system is not of single fibres going to discrete well-defined terminations, but of fibres whose complex branching means that: (a) the territory served by a neuron is more extensive than the terminal branching of a nerve trunk at the periphery would indicate, and (b) widely separated tissues can be brought under the influence of one neuron

Following severance of the ulnar nerve at the wrist, the retrograde neuronal changes could be sufficiently severe to silence the entire affected neuronal system. This would affect conduction in that branch of a nerve fibre contained in the uninjured medial cutaneous nerve of the forearm and in this way lead to the impairment of sensation over the medial aspect of the forearm, in other words, in an area served by a peripheral nerve that had not been damaged.

The recovery of neurons from these retrograde effects would be reflected at the periphery in two ways. Firstly, by regenerating axon sprouts emerging from the proximal stump of the severed ulnar nerve. Signs of recovery would be delayed until the arrival of these regenerating processes in the ulnar field. Secondly, conduction would return in the uninjured branches of the affected neurons, thereby resulting in the early and rapid restoration of sensation in the cutaneous area served by the medial cutaneous nerve of the forearm. The pattern of recovery in the hand and over the medial aspect of the forearm is consistent with this interpretation.

It could, of course, be argued that, alternatively, severance of terminal fibres of the medial cutaneous nerve at the wrist could be followed by retrograde changes in the parent neurons of sufficient severity to silence them. The impaired sensation over the medial aspect of the forearm would then suggest that individual fibres of this nerve were branching at proximal levels, some daughter branches innervating the inner aspect of the forearm with others continuing on to the wrist to be severed at that level (Fig.33.3b).

Thus one explanation involves a pattern of distribution in which a neuron supplies two separate areas over different peripheral nerves while, in contrast, the other depends upon an arrangement in which the 'axon' of individual neurons distributes filaments, by extensive branching, over the entire medial aspect of the forearm. The weight of evidence favours the former because following severance of the entire ulnar nerve trunk at the wrist, the retrograde neuronal changes are likely to be more severe and more extensive than those occurring after severance of the fine terminal filaments of the medial cutaneous nerve of the forearm in the same injury at the wrist.

However, whatever the arrangement, our uncertainty and the necessity to speculate on these matters does direct attention to the need for more precise information about the branching of nerve fibres.

The extension of such a concept to other nerves and other cutaneous areas may account for many of the unusual sensory phenomena that accompany some nerve injuries, and for some minor injuries being followed by unexpectedly widespread effects.

Conversion hysteria

Anaesthesia and other disturbances of cutaneous sensation are common in conversion hysteria. However they have certain characteristics that distinguish them from the sensory changes associated with peripheral nerve damage.

a. The affected area does not correspond to the anatomical distribution of a peripheral nerve but has a glove or stocking distribution.
b. The sensory defect is not associated with any loss of function. Providing there is no motor disability the patient is easily able, with closed eyes, to execute the discrete movements involved in examining an object for which an efficient cutaneous sensation is indispensible.
c. They are not associated with trophic changes.
d. They are never a predominant or isolated sign but are part of a symptomatic picture of functional disorder. The important point is that the clinician can increase and consolidate the symptom by taking an interest in it and making frequent tests. One should take into consideration that, if the examiner inadvertently concentrates his attention and testing on a cutaneous area corresponding to the distribution of a peripheral nerve, then the patient may oblige by identifying that as the affected area.

FACTORS DEVELOPING SOME TIME AFTER THE INJURY

1. Hoffmann–Tinel's sign

In eliciting the sign, care should be taken at all times to ensure that the nerve is stimulated below the site of the injury or repair without disturbing either.

It should be noted that, though an advancing Hoffmann–Tinel sign indicates the progression of sensory 'axon' tips down the nerve, it provides no clue as to whether or not they are in endoneurial tubes that will lead them to the skin, nor does it provide any evidence of the numbers regenerating. While the sign indicates that axons are regenerating it is not a reliable measure of *useful* regeneration.

2. The error of attributing shrinkage of the cutaneous anaesthetic area to axon regeneration

Some shrinkage of the autonomous cutaneous area of total sensory loss is often observed to take place in the absence of any regeneration and it is important not to attribute this type of sensory improvement to the entry of regenerating sensory processes into the denervated area.

Pollock (1919, 1920) and Pollock and Davis (1933) attributed this shrinkage to the slow recovery of the threshold to stimulation of uninjured nerve fibres of the marginal zone of overlap. However, the reason for the postulated temporary impairment of conduction in these particular fibres was not explained.

Two explanations have been advanced to account for the reduction in the affected cutaneous area. One is based on the growth of neighbouring intact nerve fibres into the denervated skin and the other on the recovery of sensory neurons from retrograde changes induced by the nerve injury.

Livingston (1947), Leonard (1973) and Inbal et al (1987) have attributed the gradual and progressive shrinkage to invasion of the denervated skin by sprouting from sensory terminals of neighbouring uninjured nerves.

Presumably, nerve section disturbs an equilibrium to which neighbouring intact nerve terminals respond by sprouting. The rate and extent of this growth is determined by the success with which the sprouts find pathways that facilitate their growth. Nerve fibre sprouting and reinnervation occurring in this way are not usually sufficiently extensive to restore sensation to large areas of denervated skin, though occasionally this may occur to a remarkable degree (Livingston 1947).

There is considerable experimental support for this interpretation (Weddell et al 1941, Gutmann & Guttmann 1942, Guth 1956, Burgess et al 1974, Brenowitz & Devor 1981, Brenan 1983, Kinnman & Aldskogius 1986). The accounts of Devor et al (1979), Diamond & Jackson (1980) and Diamond (1981) gave qualified support to the concept. Horsch (1981) was unable to demonstrate such collateral sprouting of 'mechanoreceptor axons.'

Alpar and Brooks' (1978) report of their long term results of ulnar to median nerve pedicle grafts includes an interesting incidental observation that some sensation returned in the ulnar field which they could only attribute to ingrowth from the regenerating cutaneous fibres in the median nerve. Their patients refused nerve block.

Similar views on the shrinkage of the anaesthetic area have been expressed more recently by Waris et al (1983) when they wrote:

Are there nerves normally present in areas of overlap that don't function until there is a loss of nerve function in an adjacent area, or do nerves grow into these areas in the same way as sweat glands in a skin graft are reinnervated.

Care should be taken at all times to exclude, by appropriate nerve blocking procedures, this type of sensory improvement being attributed to regeneration in a repaired nerve.

Phenomena based on retrograde neuronal disturbances and nerve fibre branching

The manner in which this factor could complicate the evaluation of sensory function can be best explained by reference to Fig. 33.4.

Individual sensory neurons could, by fibre branching, send branches to the adjacent cutaneous areas over separate peripheral nerves, where some overlapping of 'daughter' fibres could take place. Though hundreds of sensory neurons would be involved, the changes that would follow division of a peripheral nerve will be described in terms of two sensory neurons.

Consider two adjacent cutaneous areas AY and BX with an area of overlap XY. The process of neuron N^1 branches to send fibres to the periphery over two peripheral nerves PN^1 and PN^2. The nerve fibre in PN^1 is distributed over areas AX and XY, i.e. area AY, while that coursing in PN^2 is distributed over areas BY and YX, i.e. BX. The

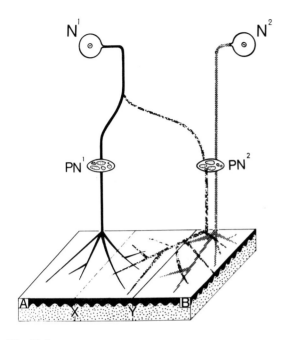

Fig. 33.4

1. The area BY, originally rendered hypoaesthetic by the nerve injury, recovers completely because it is now fully innervated by N^1 and N^2.
2. The marginal anaesthetic zone, XY, shows some recovery but only becomes hypoaesthetic because the only functioning fibres are those from N^1 reaching the area over PN^2.

The anaesthetic area AX remains unchanged because the fibre branch innervating it has been severed in PN^1. Signs of returning function only appear in this area when it is reached by new sensory processes regenerating along PN^1.

The overall effect is one in which the anaesthetic area shrinks from AY to AX, a previously anaesthetic area XY becomes hypoaesthetic, while sensory function is fully restored in area BY which was previously hypoaesthetic. All these changes occur without any ingrowth of sensory fibres.

process of neuron N^2 passes to the periphery in PN^2 and is distributed only to BY.

This arrangement means that:

1. Area AX is innervated solely from N^1 by way of PN^1.
2. Area XY receives sensory fibres from two different peripheral nerves, PN^1 and PN^2, though the nerve fibres are part of the same neuron N^1.
3. Area BY is innervated by nerve fibres contained in PN^2, though these fibres are derived from two sources, N^1 and N^2.

Severance of nerve trunk PN^1 results in retrograde effects in neuron N^1 which arrest sensory function over the entire peripheral field served by it. As a result, area AY becomes anaesthetic but area BY, which adjoins AY, is rendered only hypoaesthetic because it is still partly innervated by neuron N^2.

With the recovery of N^1, conduction returns in the fibre branch running in PN^2 and, with this recovery, sensory function returns in the cutaneous area which it serves. This brings about two changes at the periphery:

Sensory phenomena based on central mechanisms

Immediately following a nerve injury, the pattern and density of cutaneous innervation in an area of sensory nerve overlap could be so modified, and retrograde neuronal and transsynaptic disturbances so severe, that the sensory cortex is temporarily unable to interpret the altered signal patterns reaching it so that a stimulus in the area of sensory overlap now fails to elicit a response. With the passage of time stimuli from the area in question, to which the cortex was previously unresponsive, could come to elicit a response that would be registered as diminished sensation. Thus a partially denervated area previously insensitive to a stimulus would now respond, not because of any recovery at the periphery but because of readjustments to central mechanisms.

Finally, in evaluating the end result it is also important not to overlook the fact that the residual sensory disability consequent on incomplete and imperfect axon regeneration can be improved by re-training directed to increasing the patient's ability to use, to greater advantage, new and altered patterns of sensory innervation.

The basis for this continued improvement is, presumably, adaptive readjustments to flexible central neuronal patterns that permit the more effective use of altered sensory signal patterns reaching them from the periphery. As a result, the patient learns to recognise and identify an altered profile of sensory impulses and to relate the new sensations to a past event. With the passage of time the well motivated patient has a remarkable capacity for improving the quality of the recovery.

It is difficult to put a time limit on this last phase of recovery, depending as it does on a further set of factors such as the general attitude, intelligence, patience, perseverance and motivation of the patient. But it is a slow process that can certainly extend into the 5th year, and in some patients probably extends beyond that time. This is only an expression of the old adage that 'practice makes perfect'.

REFERENCES

Alpar E K, Brooks D M 1978 Long term results of ulnar to median nerve pedicle nerve grafts. The Hand 10: 61

Brenan A 1983 Collateral innervation of skin by C-fibres following nerve injury in the rat. Journal of Physiology (London) 338: 59P–60P

Brenowitz G L, Devor M 1981 Reinnervation of rat glabrous hindpaw skin by collateral sprouts following denervation by sciatic nerve section. Anatomical Record 199: 37A

Brooks D M 1954 Open wounds of the brachial plexus. In: Seddon H J (ed) Peripheral nerve injuries. Her Majesty's Stationery Office, London, p 420

Burgess P R, English K B, Horsch K W, Stensaas L J 1974 Patterning in the regeneration of type 1 cutaneous mechanoreceptors. Journal of Physiology (London) 236: 57

Daniel C R, Bower J D, Pearson J E, Holbert R D 1977a Vibrometry and uremic peripheral neuropathy. Southern Medical Journal 70: 1311

Daniel C R, Bower J D, Pearson J E, Holbert R D 1977b Vibrometry and neuropathy. Journal Mississippi State Medical Association 18: 30

Dellon A L 1978 The moving two-point discrimination test. Clinical evaluation of the quickly adapting fiber/receptor system. Journal of Hand Surgery 3: 474

Dellon A L 1980 Clinical use of vibratory stimuli to evaluate peripheral nerve injury and compression neuropathy. Plastic and Reconstructive Surgery 65: 466

Dellon A L 1981 Evaluation of sensibility and re-education of sensation in the Hand. Williams and Wilkins, Baltimore

Dellon A L 1983 The vibrometer. Plastic and Reconstructive Surgery 71: 427

Dellon A L, Kallman C H 1983 Evaluation of functional sensation in the hand. Journal of Hand Surgery 8: 865

Dellon A L, Munger B L 1983 Correlation of histology and sensibility after nerve repair. Journal of Hand Surgery 8: 871

Devor M, Schonfeld D, Seltzer Z, Wall P D 1979 Two modes of cutaneous reinnervation following peripheral nerve injury. Journal of Comparative Neurology 185: 211

Diamond J 1981 The recovery of sensory function in skin after peripheral nerve lesions. In: Gorio A, Millesi H, Mingrino S (eds) Post-traumatic nerve regeneration. Raven Press, New York, p 533

Diamond J, Jackson P C 1980 Regeneration and collateral sprouting of peripheral nerves. In: Jewett D L, McCarroll H R (eds) Nerve repair and regeneration: its clinical and experimental basis. Mosby, St Louis, p 115

Gelberman R H, Szabo R M, Williamson R V, Dimick M P 1983 Sensibility testing in peripheral nerve compression syndromes. An experimental study in humans. Journal of Bone and Joint Surgery 65A: 632

Guth L 1956 Regeneration in the mammalian peripheral nervous system. Physiological Reviews 36: 441

Gutmann E, Guttmann L 1942 Factors affecting recovery of sensory function after nerve lesions. Journal of Neurology, Neurosurgery and Psychiatry 5: 117

Hirasawa Y, Katsumi Y, Tokioka T 1985 Evaluation of sensibility after sensory reconstruction of the thumb. Journal of Bone and Joint Surgery 67B: 814

Horsch K 1981 Absence of functional collateral sprouting of mechanoreceptor axons into denervated areas of mammalian skin. Experimental Neurology 74: 313

Inbal R, Rousso M, Ashur H et al 1987 Collateral sprouting in skin and sensory recovery after nerve injury in man. Pain 28: 141

Jabaley M E, Burns J E, Orcutt B S, Bryant W M 1976 Comparison of histologic and functional recovery after peripheral nerve repair. Journal of Hand Surgery 1: 119

Jabaley M E, Dellon A L 1980 Evaluation of sensibility by microhistological studies. In: Omer G E, Spinner M (eds) Management of peripheral nerve problems. Saunders, Philadelphia, p 954

Johansson R S 1978 Tactile sensibility of the human hand: receptive field characteristics of mechanoreceptive units in the glabrous skin area. Journal of Physiology (London) 281: 101

Kinnman E, Aldskogius H 1986 Collateral sprouting of sensory axons in the glabrous skin of the hind paw after chronic sciatic nerve lesion in adult and neonatal rats: a morphological study. Brain Research 377: 73

Krag K, Rasmussen K B 1975 The neurovascular island flap for defective sensibility of the thumb. Journal of Bone and Joint Surgery 57B: 495

Leonard M H 1973 Return of skin sensation in children without repair of nerves. Clinical Orthopedics and Related Research 95: 273

Lewis T 1942 Pain. Macmillan, New York, p v

Livingston W K 1947 Evidence of active invasion of denervated areas by sensory fibers from neighboring nerves in man. Journal of Neurosurgery 4: 140

Louis D S, Greene T L, Jacobson K E et al 1984 Evaluation of normal values for stationary and moving two-point discrimination in the hand. Journal of Hand Surgery 9A: 552

Lundborg G, Lie-Stenström A K, Sollerman C et al 1986 Digital vibrogram: a new diagnostic tool for sensory testing in compression neuropathy. Journal of Hand Surgery 11A: 693

Lundborg G, Sollerman C, Stromberg T, Pyykkö J 1987 A new principle for assessment of vibrotactile sense in vibration induced neuropathy. Scandinavian Journal of Work and Environmental Health 13: 375

McEwan L E 1962 Median and ulnar nerve injuries. Australian and New Zealand Journal of Surgery 32: 89

Mackel R, Brink E E, Wittowsky G 1983a Transitional properties of afferents reinnervating mechanoreceptors in human glabrous skin. Brain Research 276: 339

Mackel R, Kunesch E, Waldhör F, Struppler A 1983b Reinnervation of mechanoreceptors in the human glabrous skin following peripheral nerve repair. Brain Research 268: 49

Mackel R, Brink E E, Wittkowsky G 1985 Properties of cutaneous mechanosensitive afferents during the early stages of regeneration in man. Brain Research 329: 49

Mackin E J 1988 Sensibility evaluation. In: Tubiana R (ed) The hand. Saunders, Philadelphia, Vol 3, p 489

Mackinnon S E, Dellon A L 1985 Two-point discrimination tester. Journal of Hand Surgery 10A: 906

McQuillan W 1970 Sensory recovery after nerve repair. Hand 2: 7

McQuillan W M, Neilson J M, Boardman A K, Hay R L 1971 Sensory evaluation after median nerve repair. The Hand 3: 101

Mannerfelt L 1962 Evaluation of functional sensation of skin grafts in the hand area. British Journal of Plastic Surgery 15: 136

Mansat M, Delprat M, Delprat J M 1981 The vibrometer. An electromagnetic transducer as an attempt to examine sensibility of the hand in quantitative terms. The Hand 13: 202

Moberg E 1958 Objective methods for determining the functional value of sensibility in the skin. Journal of Bone and Joint Surgery 40B: 454

Moberg E 1962 Criticism and study of methods for examining sensibility of the hand. Neurology 12: 8

Ogunro G 1984 Restoration of sensibility to the thumb by the technique of digital nerve advancement. Journal of Hand Surgery 9A: 440

Omer G E 1974 Sensation and sensibility in the upper extremity. Clinical Orthopaedics 104: 30

Omer G E 1975 Evaluation of an acute traumatic peripheral nerve injury. In: Michon J, Moberg E (eds) Traumatic nerve lesions of the upper limb. Churchill Livingstone, Edinburgh, p 45

Omer G E 1980a Sensibility testing. In: Omer G E, Spinner M (eds) Management of peripheral nerve problems. Saunders, Philadelphia, p 3

Omer G E 1980b Sensory evaluation by the pick up test. In: Jewett D L, McCarroll H R (eds) Nerve repair and regeneration: its clinical and experimental basis. Mosby, St Louis p 250

Omer G E 1981 Physical diagnosis of peripheral nerve injuries. In: Frykman G K (ed) Symposium on peripheral nerve injuries. The Orthopedic Clinics of North America 12: 207

Omer G E 1983 Report of the Committee for Evaluation of the Clinical Result in Peripheral Nerve Injury. Journal of Hand Surgery 8A: 754

Pollock L J 1919 Overlap of so-called protopathic sensibility as seen in peripheral nerve lesions. Archives of Neurology and Psychiatry Chicago 2: 667

Pollock L J 1920 Nerve overlap as related to the relatively early return of pain sense following injury to the peripheral nerves. Journal of Comparative Neurology 32: 357

Pollock L J, Davis L 1933 Peripheral nerve injuries Hoeber, New York

Poppen N K 1980 Clinical evaluation of the von Frey and two-point discrimination tests and correlation with a dynamic test of sensibility. In: Jewett D L, McCarroll H R (eds) Nerve repair and regeneration. Its clinical and experimental basis. Mosby, St Louis p 252

Poppen N K, McCarroll H R, Doyle J R et al 1979 Recovery of sensibility after suture of digital nerves. Journal of Hand Surgery 4: 212

Porter R W 1966 New test for finger tip sensation. British Medical Journal 2: 927

Renfrew S 1960 Aesthiometers. Lancet 1: 1011

Renfrew S 1969 Finger tip sensation. A routine neurological test. Lancet 1: 396

Schlenker J D, Kleinert H E, Tsai T 1980 Methods and results of replantation following traumatic amputation of the thumb in sixty-four patients. Journal of Hand Surgery 5: 63

Smith P J, Mott G 1986 Sensory threshold and conductance testing in nerve injuries. Journal of Hand Surgery 11B: 157

Sunderland S 1952 Disturbances of sensation occurring in an area not innervated by the severed nerve. Brain 75: 585

Sunderland S 1978 Nerves and nerve injuries. Churchill Livingstone, Edinburgh

Szabo R M, Gelberman R H, Williamson R V et al 1984 Vibratory sensory testing in acute peripheral nerve compression. Journal of Hand Surgery 9A: 104

Thomine J M 1981 The clinical examination of the hand. In: Tubiana R (ed) The hand. Saunders, Philadelphia, Vol. 1, p 616

Trotter W 1941 The collected papers of Wilfrid Trotter. Oxford University Press, London, p 160

Vierck C J, Jones M B 1969 Size discrimination on the skin. Science 163: 488

Von Prince K, Butler B 1976 Measuring sensory function of the hand in peripheral nerve injuries. American Journal of Occupational Therapy 21: 385

Walshe F M R 1948 Critical studies in neurology. Churchill Livingstone, Edinburgh, p 26

Waris T, Rechardt L, Kyösola K 1983 Reinnervation of human skin grafts. A histochemical study. Plastic and Reconstructive Surgery 72: 439

Weddell G, Guttmann L, Gutmann E 1941 The local extension of nerve fibres into denervated areas of skin. Journal of Neurology, Neurosurgery and Psychiatry 4: 206

Wynn Parry C B, Salter M 1976 Sensory re-education after median nerve lesions. Hand 8: 250

34. What can nerve trauma tell us about pain mechanisms?

SOME HISTORICAL CONSIDERATIONS

The thrust of this section is to direct attention to the importance of neuropathological, as opposed to neurophysiological, phenomena in the genesis of neurogenic pain mechanisms.

Today, as it has been in the past, physiological considerations continue to dominate the study of pain mechanisms and it is of more than passing interest to look back on why this should be so.

The first conspicuous landmark in this saga of pain mechanisms did not come until the second half of the last century. Prior to 1850 no information was available on the microstructure of nerves. This only came with the invention of the compound microscope and the introduction, in the second half of the last century, of staining techniques by Gerlach, Nissl, Waldeyer, Weigert, Marchi, Golgi and Cajal and many others which revealed for the first time the more detailed structural features of nerve fibres. However, it was not until 1878 that it was possible for Ranvier to write the first definitive text on the histology of the nervous system. These new techniques revealed, inter alia, a considerable range in nerve fibre calibre. However, the association of nociception with fine nerve fibres and inhibition with large fibre activity did not come until much later.

In a series of experimental masterpieces towards the close of the 19th century Sherrington introduced the term synapse and gave experimental reality to inhibition. In *'The Integrative Action of the Nervous System'*, based on the Silliman Lectures and first printed in 1906, he wrote: 'We do not yet understand the intimate nature of inhibition . . . its seat is certainly central, and in all probability is, as argued above, situated at the points of synapsis'. Importantly he also demonstrated that inhibition is an active process and not the simple absence of activity. From this time on excitation, inhibition and the synapse were to dominate neurological thinking.

The next major landmark was provided by Henry Head in 1905. Without going into any detail, Head's observations on returning cutaneous sensation after the repair of transected nerves led him to postulate the existence of two distinct and separate systems of cutaneous nerve fibres. These he called protopathic and epicritic. The protopathic was phylogenetically the older of the two, was served by its own type of fibre and was protective in its essential functions. The epicritic was of more recent origin, provided the refinements of cutaneous sensation, was served by its own specific type of nerve fibre and exerted an inhibitory effect on the protopathic.

Protopathic sensation was the type first elicited in a previously anaesthetic cutaneous area and was characterised by an exquisite sensitivity to pinprick that produced intense, widely radiating, non-localisable pain. This was attributed to the earlier arrival of protopathic fibres that regenerated at a faster rate than epicritic fibres. The restoration of normal sensation was delayed until the arrival of the more slowly regenerating epicritic fibres that exerted an inhibitory effect on the protopathic elements.

This duality was continued into the central nervous system where the protopathic system was assigned to a special pathway, the spinothalamic tract, and a special terminal centre, the thalamus. The epicritic system was assigned to the dorsal columns of the cord, the sensory lemnisci and thalamus with terminals in the postcentral sensory cortex.

Head was no histologist and wisely refrained from attempting any correlation between these two systems and fibre size. This was provided by Ranson in a series of papers between 1908 and 1915 in which histological evidence was documented linking protopathic sensation with nonmyelinated nerve fibres and the small cells of dorsal root ganglia. It was not until almost 50 years later that Gerard (1951) and Bishop and his associates (1933, 1955, 1959, 1960) provided experimental support for the concept that the phylogenetically older protopathic system is served by fine fibres and the more recently acquired epicritic system by large fibres.

The next major advance came when Erlanger and Gasser (1924, 1937) adapted the electronoscillograph to study and analyse the compound action potential of the nerve impulse. Refinements of this method have since proved to be a valuable tool in the hands of the experimental physiologist. From their studies, Erlanger and Gasser considered that a correspondence between fibre size and the characteristics of the matching action potential record permitted a classification of nerve fibres into three groups, A B and C. This grouping was subsequently expanded to four by Bishop and Heinbecker (1930).

Erlanger and Gasser (1937) found that it was 'impossible to tell from the size of a peripheral fiber what its central characteristics are going to be' and Gasser (1935) was careful to point out that the fibres serving different sensory functions must be widely distributed through various fibre sizes, a view later endorsed by others (Lewis and Pochin 1938, Sinclair and Hinshaw 1950, 1951, Sinclair 1967).

Fifty years on there is, as yet, no unequivocal evidence, even with intrafascicular recording techniques, to prove that stimulation can be confined to a single nerve fibre and that this stimulation gives rise to a particular sensation.

Over the years physiologists have, however, been reluctant to abandon the concept of functional specificity in relation to nerve fibre size, though today it has become the practice to talk of nerve fibres responding to noxious stimuli and not of pain fibres.

In 1951, Gerard returned to the concept of a dual peripheral system when he wrote that the fast conducting fibres were inhibitory and postulated that 'when the larger fibres fail the small pain fibres, no longer modulated in the cord, carry up and into consciousness the excessive and distorted awareness of pain.' Note that pain has now been assigned to fine fibres and inhibition to large fibres.

Further support for the concept of a dual system came 2 years later when Landau and Bishop (1953) reported that after selectively blocking the A delta fibres, the pain elicited by stimulating C fibres was greatly increased. Again pain is assigned to fine fibres, and an implied inhibitory action for A delta fibres is clear.

At this point in time, the position as regards pain mechanisms in the peripheral nervous system was one in which two separate systems were involved, one composed of fine fibres conveying noxious stimuli centrally and a second composed of large fibres that normally exerted an inhibitory influence over the first. In other words, pain, in at least some respects, was a release phenomenon.

In 1942 Wortis et al introduced the term fibre dissociation to account for the painful symptoms associated with certain toxic metabolic polyneuropathies. In the absence of histological confirmation, the assumption was that the condition had resulted in the preferential loss of large calibre nerve fibres.

At the close of the 1950s Noordenbos's clinical studies on painful nerve injuries led him to conclude that large heavily myelinated nerve fibres are more susceptible to injury than fine fibres with little or no myelin. True to physiological tradition he then took the further step of claiming that causalgia was the result of the reduction or loss of the inhibitory action of large fast conducting nerve fibres which facilitated the passage of slow impulse nociceptor activity centrally.

To cap this physiological saga, Melzack and Wall in 1965 came up with the Gate Control Theory that incorporated inhibitory mechanisms and opposing roles for large and fine calibre nerve fibres.

On the face of it, the proposition of a dual sensory fibre system in which one exercises an inhibitory influence over the other seems reasonable and well-authenticated experimentally, and could well provide the peripheral setting for pain mechanisms. At the same time it should be noted that throughout these deliberations, the approach to the study of pain mechanisms has been exclusively physiological. Nowhere is there any reference to the possibility that nerve fibres could, for any one of a number of reasons, be subjected to pathological changes that could disturb their functional properties to the point of causing them to function abnormally. And yet there is substantial clinical evidence to support the thesis that neuropathological phenomena do play a role in pain mechanisms and in a manner that challenges the undisputed validity of physiological theory as the sole basis of pain mechanisms.

1. Head's subdivision of the somatosensory system into protopathic and epicritic components did not pass unchallenged. The theory was criticised at its inception by Trotter and Davies (1909), Boring (1916) and Sharpey-Schafer (1927), who repeated Head's experiments on self-inflicted nerve injury and came up with a very different explanation. They denied the existence of two separate protopathic-epicritic fibre systems for sensory perception. Instead they found that the experimental findings were more in keeping with a gradual return from anaesthesia through hypoaesthesia to normal sensation. The changing quality of sensation was due not to the separate arrival in the skin of two different fibre systems but to the gradual conversion of one form of sensation into another by successive stages in the regeneration of the same nerve fibres.

    This introduced for the first time the concept that pathological changes could alter the functional properties of nerve fibres.

    Personal observations on recovering sensation after nerve injury and nerve repair, and in skin flaps, fully confirm the earlier observations of Trotter and Davies and Sharpey–Schafer.

2. Fine axons do not regenerate at faster rates than thick axons as was postulated by Head. All regenerating axons when they reach the periphery are fine and unmyelinated and structurally have the features of C fibres. This explains the plethora of fine nerve endings in the early stages of reinnervation and the early hypersensitivity of the reinnervated skin and its 'protopathic' qualities. It is only when the fine regenerated axons of the larger fibres progressively remyelinate and increase in thickness that the quality of the sensory recovery improves.

3. If large sensory fibre activity does exert an inhibitory influence over that in fine C fibres, then nerve lesions in which large fibres are lost but fine C fibres survive could be expected to be painful. This is believed by many to be the genesis of the painful nerve lesion in the carpal tunnel syndrome and causalgia (see later).

Finally, the first suggestion that neuropathological changes could be at work in pain mechanisms we owe to Livingston (1938, 1944, 1948) who, in his thought-provoking writings on pain mechanisms, suggested that causalgia was the functional expression of self-sustaining abnormal activity in the internuncial neuronal pool of the spinal cord, created in some unexplained way by the peripheral nerve injury. At that time, while working on central neuronal reactions to severe trauma to peripheral nerves, it occurred to the author that the disorderly activity generated in the internuncial pools of neurons, as postulated by Livingston, could be a consequence of retrograde neuronal pathology (Sunderland and Kelly 1948, Sunderland 1976a,b, 1978).

The contents of this chapter are devoted to an examination of these matters. As mentioned at the beginning, the thrust of this historical outline has been to emphasise that in any consideration of the genesis of pain mechanisms, thinking should not be limited to physiology but should be widened to recognise the importance of neuropathological phenomena.

INTRODUCTION

With the exception of the rare sufferer from congenital indifference to pain, every person knows what pain is. However, though pain is easily recognised it is difficult to define and, while most writers on the subject have attempted to establish an acceptable definition, their efforts add little to our understanding of the problem. I shall not, therefore, be diverted by another such attempt but agree with Thomas Lewis (1942) when he wrote:

reflection tells me that I am so far from being able to satisfactorily to define pain of which I here write, that the attempt could serve no useful purpose. Pain, like similar subjective things, is known to us by experience and is described by illustration . . . to build up a definition in words or to substitute some phrase would carry neither the reader nor myself further.

Despite the rapidly growing literature on pain, and prolific as recent advances in this field have been, there are still areas where uncertainty persists, many questions to which we have yet to find acceptable answers, and many issues that are the subject of continuing disagreement and controversy. One of our difficulties is that animal experiments still dominate the investigation of pain. While this is understandable and inevitable it is unfortunate because, though such experiments do provide important clues, they will not produce the final answers. Pain is a human and personal experience and the limitations of animal experiment in such a situation must be obvious. In this respect we would do well to remember that valuable information is still to be obtained by the intelligent and persistent clinical investigator with the capacity to recognise in unusual clinical situations those unique experiments by which Nature reveals its secrets. In such a situation it is reasonable to ask 'What can nerve lesions tell us about pain mechanisms?'

This explains the clinical bias in the design of this chapter, for it is at the clinical level that we should be seeking clues that will lead us to a better understanding of the genesis and nature of the pathophysiological disturbances that are the basis of the painful sequelae of peripheral nerve lesions which sometimes become the dominant clinical feature of the injury. The chapter is not concerned per se with nerve lesions as clinical entities but rather with what they can tell us about the genesis of painful states in general.

The title of this chapter, 'What can nerve trauma tell us about pain mechanisms?', is based on the curious clinical finding that trauma to nerve trunks is seldom painful despite the fact that all peripheral nerves contain large numbers of fine calibre nerve fibres that, contemporary teaching tells us, are associated with nociception.

Thus, when equally extensive wounds with and without nerve involvement are compared, the pain is usually due to wounding of the general tissues, e.g. skin, subcutaneous tissues, muscle, bone and joints, and is unrelated to the co-existing nerve trunk injury. When pain is due to injury to the nerve it is either a fleeting incident at the time the injury was inflicted or makes an appearance only with regeneration when an exquisitely sensitive neuroma develops at the site of injury, the cutaneous field previously insensitive becomes hyperalgesic and there is tenderness and aching in recovering muscles.

In contradistinction to the painless nerve injury, some nerve lesions are habitually painful.

These clinical curiosities raise some interesting questions.

1. Why should some nerve lesions be painful and others free of pain?
2. What is the pathophysiological basis of the painful nerve lesion and in what respects does it differ from that of the painless lesion?
3. What is the nature of the neurogenic mechanism or mechanisms, responsible for the painful state?

Before proceeding to an examination of these questions, a brief reference will be made to certain generalisations that have a bearing on what is to follow.

1. There is a popular misconception that compressing a nerve is painful. However, a normal nerve may be compressed to the point of conduction failure and even grossly deformed without pain. This was well known to Waller (1862) and to Head (1896), who wrote 'pressure on nerve trunks causes numbness and tingling, but not superficial tenderness.' Striking the ulnar nerve behind the medial epicondyle causes paraesthesiae,

but not pain, to shoot into the ulnar side of the hand. Pain and tenderness are local and the victim vigorously rubs the elbow, not the hand. Though accompanied by paraesthesiae, chronic ulnar nerve lesions at the elbow often appear and progress quite painlessly. Radial crutch and sleep palsy develop painlessly despite the fact that the radial nerve contains a substantial number of cutaneous sensory fibres (Chapter 8). The patient with a late radial nerve palsy complicating a fractured humerus also complains not of pain but of a wrist drop. Pressure palsies of the common peroneal nerve at the neck of the fibula caused by an ill-fitting plaster cast develop insidiously and are only revealed when the cast is removed and the foot drop becomes apparent. Lindahl (1946, 1966) has also reported paresis and sensory defects without pain following compression of lumbar nerve roots in tuberculous spondylitis.

Though compressing normal nerves is painless, the effects of mechanical deformation are very different once the nerve is injured. Damaged nerve fibres then constitute a focus for the generation and discharge of abnormal trains of abnormal impulses centrally, either spontaneously or in response to other factors that disturb the status quo.

2. A distinction should be drawn between:

a. spontaneous pain at rest and elicited or provoked pain that requires an external stimulus or some movement of the limb to cause it;
b. local tenderness of a nerve trunk and pain referred to its peripheral distribution. Involvement of the nervi nervorum provides an explanation for the local tenderness and pain from local pressure on the nerve, while distally referred pain is due to involvement of distally destined nerve fibres traversing the injured segment of the nerve and damaged at that site.

3. Damage to the major process of a nerve cell results in changes in the cell body and related trans-synaptic changes in nerve cells with which it is synaptically related. The severity of these changes is influenced by, inter alia, the proximity of the lesion to the cell body and the severity of the deforming force. Thus a local injury to a peripheral nerve may affect whole groups of neurons and produce widespread central effects.

4. Discrete physiological functions may be served by fibres with a considerable range of fibre diameter so that cutaneous sensory functions are not dependent on fibre size (Gasser 1935, 1943, Lewis and Pochin 1938, Sinclair and Hinshaw 1950, 1951a,b). However in the case of nociception there is a bias towards non-myelinated and finely myelinated nerve fibres.

Though a variety of painful nerve injuries is available for the study of these issues, those selected for consideration are:

1. The median nerve lesion in the carpal tunnel as an example of a painful chronic compartment compression lesion.
2. Painful spinal nerve involvement in the intervertebral foramen as a painful nerve injury based on friction trauma and fibrosis.
3. Causalgia.

These three groups have been chosen because each presents unique features that have been particularly useful in studying the genesis and modus operandi of pain mechanisms.

THE PAINFUL MEDIAN NERVE LESION IN THE CARPAL TUNNEL

This painful nerve lesion has been selected:

1. to illustrate the role and significance of regional anatomical factors in the genesis of pain mechanisms;
2. to dispute a popular misconception that the pain in this condition is invariably a consequence of the physical deformation of nerve fibres caused by nerve compression in the carpal tunnel;
3. to introduce a new pathogenic factor in pain mechanisms, namely one based on ischaemia of normal nerve fibres (Sunderland 1976b).

From a study of the literature on the carpal tunnel syndrome it would appear that the preferred explanation for the pain in this condition is based on the physical deformation of nerve fibres caused by repeated compression of the median nerve in the carpal tunnel (Ochoa 1980). Support for this belief comes from experimentally produced compression nerve lesions in which the nerve fibres at the edges of a compressed nerve segment showed a characteristic pattern of nodal intussusception and paranodal demyelination. In these lesions the thick nerve fibres were reported as suffering earlier and to a greater degree than fine fibres. Though never explicitly stated, the inference is that, with the nerve fibre dissociation created in this way, the inhibitory influence that large fibre activity exerts at central levels on ongoing fine fibre activity is removed. This leaves the latter free to summate to levels that, according to the Gate Control Theory, could provide the essential mechanism for the painful state.

While this might appear to be a plausible explanation for the genesis of the pain in the carpal tunnel syndrome there are several reasons why it should be rejected. When these are examined, the physical deformation of median nerve fibres is found to be an unlikely cause of the pain.

An alternative explanation has been proposed to account for the development of a nocigenic mechanism in the carpal tunnel syndrome. This is based on ischaemia of median nerve fibres secondary to chronic compartment compression of the median nerve in the carpal tunnel.

The pathophysiology of this painful nerve injury is fully discussed elsewhere (Chapter 17) and that account should be consulted for this information.

A final question: is the pain in the carpal tunnel syndrome a release phenomenon based on selective nerve fibre dissociation, due to the early failure of large fibres, or is it due to the direct effect of ischaemia on nociceptor nerve fibres, or both?

If the conventional belief that thick myelinated nerve fibres suffer earlier and to a greater degree than the fine fibres is correct, then this could account for nerve fibre dissociation favouring fine fibres.

However, it is not uncommon for pain in the early stages of the condition to be unaccompanied by any objective evidence of sensory dysfunction, which would be unusual if the large fibres were the first to suffer. Moreover, despite the localisation and vulnerable position of the motor fasciculi in relation to the flexor retinaculum, and the large calibre of motor fibres, pain often precedes signs of motor nerve fibre involvement. This rather suggests that the pain is due to the direct involvement of nociceptor fibres, a view supported by the finding that, in the median nerve at the wrist, fine nerve fibres greatly outnumber all others, by a factor of 3 or 4 to 1.

When all the evidence is critically examined, one is forced to conclude that the offending mechanism responsible for the pain associated with compression of the median nerve in the carpal tunnel is due, at least in the initial stages, to an impaired blood supply to nerve fibres and not to their structural deformation.

PAINFUL SPINAL NERVE LESIONS SECONDARY TO PATHOLOGICAL DEVELOPMENTS IN THE CERVICAL AND LUMBAR INTERVERTEBRAL FORAMINA

The pathogenesis of this painful nerve lesion has been fully discussed in Chapter 19, which should be consulted for details. The nerve lesion is usually attributed to compression of the nerve in an entrapment situation. However, all is not what it seems to be and, again, anatomical considerations are crucial to an understanding of the genesis of these painful lesions. Accordingly, the proposition that nerve compression is the responsible offending agent needs to be examined in relation to the regional anatomical features of the foramen.

When this is done it will be found that the genesis of the painful spinal nerve lesion in the foramen is not quite the same in the cervical and lumbar regions.

1. In the cervical region the cause is not nerve compression but friction trauma causing nerve fibre damage, an inflammatory reaction, reactionary fibrosis, ischaemia of nerve fibres, and the fixation of the damaged nerve segment by adhesions with the consequent loss of mobility and increased vulnerability to traction deformation.
2. In the lumbar region the cause could be the mechanism described in (1) above, nerve compression, or a combination of the two.

CAUSALGIA

Causalgia is the most interesting, and distressing, of all painful nerve lesions and is worthy of special and detailed study because it provides important clues to the genesis and modus operandi of pain mechanisms.

Causalgia has achieved universal acceptance because it was coined by one of the masters of medicine and because it is a brief and expressive name for a little understood syndrome.

In many respects causalgia was an unfortunate choice in that the literal meaning of the term is 'burning pain' (Greek kausos, heat + algia, pain). However, this is a generic term and relates to only one, and not the most commanding, feature of the pain to which Weir Mitchell originally attached the name.

From the way in which the term causalgia is being interpreted and used in the literature today it is clear that it is now being applied indiscriminately to a variety of different painful lesions, presumably on the grounds that in each the pain has a burning quality. As a consequence, causalgia has come to mean different things to different people. Be that as it may, our concern here is not with semantics. However, the misuse of the term inevitably leads to misunderstanding and confusion, and to avoid this the condition to which causalgia is applied should always be explicitly defined.

Whatever mechanism is advanced to account for causalgia it should relate to, and be consistent with, the following distinctive clinical features of the condition.

The wounding mechanism

1. Causalgia shows a preference for the median, ulnar, lower trunk of the brachial plexus and sciatic (tibial) nerves.
2. There is a much higher incidence of causalgia with injuries above the elbow and knee, that is in the proximal part of the limb.
3. The injury is caused by high velocity missile wounding.
4. The injury is sustained under conditions of extreme stress.

The nerve injury

1. The nerve is rarely severed and loss of function is temporary.
2. Recovery occurs spontaneously and ultimately reaches a degree that contraindicates excision of the damaged segment of the nerve followed by nerve suture.

Characteristic features of the pain

1. The onset is often immediate.
2. The development of trophic changes and hyperpathia in the peripheral distribution of the injured nerve.
3. The pain is initially confined to the hand or foot but may spread beyond the distribution of the injured nerve.
4. The pain may be spontaneous, fluctuate in severity and persist in the absence of any stimulus originating in the injured limb. Its outstanding feature is that it causes intense suffering.
5. While the pain is often described as having an intense burning quality it is important to note that it may be defined in other terms, e.g. tearing, boring, intense aching, lancinating, like a corkscrew or nail being driven into the palm or the foot.
6. A particularly significant feature of the pain is that attacks are provoked or the pain intensified, by a wide range of stimuli:

Somatic	A jar to, or movement of, the limb. A fly alighting on the foot.
Auditory	A loud noise, an explosion or the sound of aircraft. Scraping the sole of a shoe on the floor.
Visual	Bright sunlight. Switching on the light in a darkened room.
Emotional	Excitement of a game or sporting event. Watching an exciting movie. Receiving bad news.

Temperatures and barometric changes

It is as if the entire central nervous system is acutely hypersensitive. It is this abnormal hypersensitivity to all forms of stimuli that converts the unfortunate victim into a recluse and ultimately a complete nervous wreck.

Potential sources of pain-producing activity

Though, in any painful nerve lesion, the injured segment of the nerve is normally the source of the pain-producing activity, it is conceivable that pain-producing mechanisms could develop in the affected peripheral tissues or centrally in the neuraxis. It is, therefore, important to distinguish between the pathology of the offending nerve lesion and the neurogenic mechanisms responsible for the pain. As we shall see, a study of causalgia has been particularly revealing in confirming that disturbed central mechanisms may become the source of the pain in some nerve injuries.

THE INJURED SEGMENT OF THE NERVE AS THE SOURCE OF PAIN-PRODUCING ACTIVITY

The injured segment of the nerve or the proximal stump of a severed nerve is, of course, the logical place to commence the search for a pain-producing focus and the mechanisms that activate it. Potential sources of pain-producing pathology in the injured segment include:

The ends of severed nerve fibres and regenerating axons
Neuromas
Nerve fibre cross-talk
Ephaptic synapses
Altered axon-Schwann cell relationships
Nerve fibre dissociation
Involvement of the injured segment in adhesions
Ischaemia
The action of algesic agents

The ends of severed nerve fibres and regenerating axons

The pain-producing focus in most painful nerve injuries is concealed in a matrix, composed essentially of fibroblasts, Schwann cells, collagen and blood vessels, that contains the traumatised ends of severed nerve fibres along with a disorganised and tangled meshwork of bare, or inadequately sheathed, regenerating axons that branch and rebranch in patternless confusion. These regenerating axons may be: (i) diffusely distributed through the injured segment of the nerve, the surrounding tissues and any attached adhesions, or (ii) compacted into a swelling or neuroma, at the end of the proximal stump of a severed nerve, at the site of damage to a nerve remaining in continuity and at the site where a severed nerve has been repaired.

Regardless of the particular form and arrangement taken by these neural elements, they may be unduly sensitive to any disturbance of the status quo whether it be mechanical, ischaemic or chemical in nature. As long ago as 1930 Adrian had shown that the excitability at the end of a severed nerve is sufficiently high to generate spontaneous discharges and that, in this respect, sensory nerve fibres are more effective impulse generators than sectioned motor fibres. However, Wall & Gutnick (1974), in a further study of such ongoing activity, found that it only occurred under special conditions such as, for example, when the nerve was allowed to dehydrate or the calcium level of the damaged axons was greatly reduced.

Neuroma formations

Neuromas vary in size and consistency depending on their vascularity and the amount and density of each of their major constituents (Chapter 23).

There is now much evidence to the effect that the severed axons in the neuroma that develops on the proximal stump of a severed nerve are the site of ongoing spontaneous activity.

In the present context of the painful nerve lesion, two additional features of neuromas are of special interest.

  i. Not all neuromas are painful. Why some should be exquisitely sensitive and painful while others are insensitive, even in the same individual, remains obscure. Perhaps sensitivity is influenced by the extent to which the aberrant regenerating axons acquire protective insulating sheaths. It is usually the small hard nodule that is insensitive, presumably because the aborted axons are few in number, have well-developed insulating sheaths and are well-protected by an overproduction of fibrous tissue which forms the major component of the neuroma.

On the other hand, large soft neuromas appear to be the principal offenders, probably because they are mainly composed of highly sensitive bare and immature axons and their terminals.

ii. In the case of painful neuromas, the pain is not spontaneous but must be elicited either by direct pressure or indirectly by movements that disturb the neuroma via adhesions.

Nerve fibre cross-talk and ephaptic synapses

Additional pathology implicated in nocigenic processes at the site of injury includes the formation of ephaptic synapses and changes affecting the insulating properties of the nerve sheath, thereby permitting interactions between nerve fibres. The overall effect of these changes is to expose nerve fibres to cross-stimulation so that activity in one group of nerve fibres may now influence and interfere with conduction in neighbouring fibres. It is usually assumed that the interaction is between sympathetic and nociceptor fibres, the former driving the latter to frenzied activity.

Uncertainty still surrounds the formation of artificial synapses and structural changes in nerve fibres that destroy their insulating properties. Nor is it known if such phenomena occur in man.

Changes in the relationship established between Schwann cells and nonmyelinated axons

In a normal nerve it is common for a Schwann cell to envelop several nonmyelinated axons, though each axon is separated and isolated from its neighbours by a fold of Schwann cell cytoplasm. However, in neuromas the relationship between a Schwann cell and its nonmyelinated axons is different in that the intervening folds of Schwann cell cytoplasm are missing so that bare axons are now in direct contact (Sakurai, personal communication). Such an altered relationship would favour

'cross talk' interference between axons and the formation of artificial synapses. However, the relationship would only have relevance to pain if the axons in contact were nociceptors and postganglionic sympathetics.

Nerve fibre dissociation

On the assumption that large fibres are more susceptible to injury than fine fibres, it has been claimed that in causalgia the former have suffered maximally while the latter have escaped. Fibre dissociation originating in this way would favour uninhibited fine fibre activity which is regarded by some as the basis of the painful state. Though this concept appears to have some attractive features, it is based on assumptions that lack convincing support.

Disturbances activating nocigenic mechanisms

Having established the structural background to nocigenic mechanisms in the damaged nerve segment, the next step is to consider the means by which such mechanisms are activated to produce pain. These include mechanical deformation, ischaemia, temperature and barometric changes and algesic agents.

Mechanical deformation. Mechanical deformation is usually caused by locally applied pressure, friction, or traction. The risk of subjecting a neuroma, the damaged segment of the nerve, or the site of a repair, to pain-producing traction deformation is greatly increased when those parts are fixed by adhesions to freely moving surrounding structures. In such a situation external neurolysis may be sufficient to relieve pain.

Ischaemia. It is important to note that the provocative stimulus may involve not the structural deformation of nerve fibres, but vascular complications that expose normal, as well as damaged, nerve fibres to ischaemia to which both are extremely sensitive. The risk of abnormal axons being threatened by ischaemia is greatly increased when local blood vessels are damaged and a co-existing fibrosis interferes with transport mechanisms.

Temperature and barometric changes. Regarding the influence of changes in temperature and barometric pressure, it is well known that cold and a falling atmospheric pressure may aggravate or precipitate attacks of pain. Just how this is brought about is not known but it could be due to a direct effect on neurogenic mechanisms or to a secondary effect by way of circulatory changes.

Algesic agents. It is known from a study of postinjection nerve injury that some chemical agents have a direct pain-producing effect on nerve fibres. There is also experimental evidence to show that abnormal changes in the impulse generating properties of free nerve terminals may be initiated by a range of algesic substances that are conveyed to the damaged nerve segment by way of the circulation or are produced locally as the result of tissue damage and activity at sympathetic nerve endings.

THE CUTANEOUS TISSUES AS A SOURCE OF PAIN-PRODUCING MECHANISMS.

The affected cutaneous tissues in painful nerve lesions are receiving increasing attention as a potential source of pain-producing mechanisms, particularly when they are oedematous, poorly vascularised, and are the site of trophic changes.

The belief that cutaneous tissues are the site of pain-producing mechanisms is based on the following considerations:

1. Regenerating immature nerve terminals arriving in the cutaneous tissues are extremely sensitive to mechanical deformation, ischaemia, temperature changes and algesic agents. This is the basis of the hyperalgesia and hyperpathia that develop in the initial stages of the reinnervation of the skin and may persist. This pain is not spontaneous but must be elicited.
2. The formation of artificial synapses between sensory and sympathetic nerve endings.
3. Cutaneous nociceptor endings are claimed to be particularly sensitive to algesic agents (substance P, prostaglandins, bradykinin, serotonin, noradrenaline). These agents are either conveyed to the affected cutaneous tissues by the circulation or are released there in response to:

    a. antidromic activity in sensory nerve

fibres generated at the site of the nerve lesion by chronic irritation and/or activity at ephaptic synapses;
    b. vasomotor effects due to irritation of vasoconstrictor fibres in the injured segment of the nerve;
    c. increased activity in sympathetic nerve fibres with the release of noradrenaline at their endings;
    d. venous and lymphatic stasis from disuse that promote the formation and accumulation of metabolites that lower the threshold of nerve endings to algesic influences.

The belief that cutaneous tissues are the site of pain-producing mechanism is consistent with the following clinical observations:

    i. The hyperalgesia and hyperpathia that are present in the initial stages of cutaneous reinnervation.
    ii. The burning quality of the pain is regarded as evidence of a cutaneous origin.
    iii. An isolated report that the pain is occasionally relieved by blocking the nerve below the lesion. This observation requires confirmation.
    iv. The co-existence of hyperpathia and trophic changes affecting cutaneous tissues. These trophic changes are secondary effects of disuse and immobolisation of the limb imposed by the severity of the pain. They are maximal in the hand or foot and take the form of venous and lymphatic stasis, oedema, atrophy of the skin and nails, osteoporosis and joint stiffness and ankylosis. These trophic changes are believed to promote the formation of:

    a. artificial synapses between sensory and sympathetic nerve endings, and

    b. metabolites that lower the threshold of nociceptor nerve endings to algesic influences.

    v. The effectiveness of guanethidine therapy (β blockers) and sympathetic nerve blocks in relieving pain, particularly hyperpathia. The beneficial effect of these procedures is attributed to:

a. interrupting the release of noradrenaline;
b. correcting troublesome vasoconstriction;
c. improving the circulation and in this way also facilitating the removal of algesic substances from the tissues;
d. eliminating ephaptic synapses that have developed in the cutaneous tissues.

COMMENT

From what has been said, it is clear that, if the injured segment of the nerve and/or the cutaneous tissues are sites of pain-producing mechanisms, this would require an intact sympathetic innervation and functioning sensory feedback system in the injured nerve. While this condition is satisfied in some patients, it is absent in others where there is incontrovertible evidence that these sites could not possibly have been the source of the nocigenic activity. This evidence is based on the following observations. How, for example, are we to account for the pain that is present and persists when there can be no sensory feed-back from the periphery and the cutaneous tissues have been deprived of their sympathetic innervation because:

1. the nerve has been severed at the time of the injury;
2. the lesion is physiologically complete;
3. the injured nerve segment has been resected;
4. the nerve has been blocked, pharmacologically or surgically, proximal to the lesion.

Peripherally located nocigenic mechanisms could not be responsible:

1. when the onset of pain is immediate or occurs long before the pathological changes held to be responsible for the painful state could have developed;
2. when causalgia complicates total nerve root avulsion injuries of the brachial plexus, the limb then being isolated from the central nervous system;
3. for phantom limb causalgia which occurs in the absence of the cutaneous tissues of the amputated limb;
4. when the pain is described in terms other than burning such as crushing, stabbing, agonising, deep aching and likened to a corkscrew being driven into the foot or palm of the hand. These terms would suggest a deeply seated mechanism.

Finally, identifying the injured segment and the cutaneous tissues as sites of the pain-producing activity fails to explain why some nerve lesions are painful and others are not, particularly when the pathology in the two groups appears to be identical.

From all that has been said, neither the injured segment of the nerve nor the denervated tissues could be the source of pain-producing activity in severe causalgia.

Faced with this impasse, the search for the mechanism responsible for the severe intractable pain of causalgia, that persists in the absence of any sensory input from the limb, must be extended into the central nervous system.

PAIN-PRODUCING MECHANISMS IN THE CENTRAL NERVOUS SYSTEM

In 1944, Livingston suggested that causalgia was the functional expression of self-sustaining abnormal activity in the internuncial neuronal pool of the spinal cord, created in some unexplained way by the peripheral nerve injury.

At that time, while working on the central neuronal reactions to severe trauma to peripheral nerves, the author proposed that the disorderly activity generated in the internuncial pools of neurons, as postulated by Livingston, was a consequence of this retrograde neuronal pathology (Sunderland and Kelly 1948, Sunderland 1976, 1978). There was nothing new about the existence of these central neuronal effects because it had been known since the turn of the century that the distress or death of sensory ganglion cells caused by severe injury to a peripheral nerve induces a trans-synaptic reaction in dorsal horn neurons with which they are synaptically related. There is now much contemporary physiological and pathological evidence confirming this sequence of events.

Could it be that the loss of some dorsal horn neurons, and the failure of others to recover completely, impair and disorganise neuronal systems and patterns in such a manner, and to such a degree, as to create an intraspinal focus of abnormal activity? Importantly, the intraspinal changes and disturbances originating in this way, in turn, initiate a trans-synaptic chain reaction inducing similar changes along transmission pathways and through transmission centres as far centrally as the cortex itself, where causalgia is the functional expression of the terminal effects of this disordered activity on the sensorium. In this way a local injury to a peripheral nerve may come to produce widespread central effects.

At this point it seemed reasonable to suggest that the pathological changes induced in this way provide the essential framework for a centrally located nocigenic mechanism (Sunderland 1976).

It is surprising, however, that most contemporary workers have ignored the significance of central pathological changes and have, instead, concentrated on nerve fibre physiology, facilitation and inhibition, the gate control theory, and nerve fibre imbalance and dissociation. It is only recently that these central changes in neuronal systems have commenced to receive the long-overdue recognition they deserve.

Spontaneous impulse generation in dorsal root ganglia after peripheral nerve section is now well documented in the literature (Denny Brown et al 1973, Kirk 1974, Govrin-Lippmann and Devor 1978, Ochoa and Torebjörk 1980, Wiesenfeld & Lindblom 1980, Korenman and Devor 1981, Nystrom & Hagbath 1981, Scadding 1981, DeSantis & Duckworth 1982, Wall & Devor 1983, Burchiel 1984, Burchiel, Wyler & Heavner 1986). And there is now experimental data confirming that the activities of whole groups of central neurons may be affected as a result of retrograde changes to peripheral nerve injury (Eccles 1957, 1964, Eccles et al 1959, Loeser & Ward 1967, Thulin 1961).

Just how widespread these effects may be is illustrated by the following case history of a patient whom I was able to investigate more than 30 years ago.

A jockey was involved in a riding accident in which he sustained a fracture of the mid-thoracic spine with complete and permanent paraplegia. He subsequently developed a persistent distressingly severe pain in a phantom left foot. Despite the traumatic transection of the cord, a cordotomy was performed in another clinic to relieve his pain, presumably on the grounds that the damaged segment of the cord was the site of abnormal pain-producing activity. This cordotomy was ineffective. Subsequently the patient was referred to the neurosurgeon with whom I was working at the time. Mahoney's paper on cortical excision for the relief of intractable pain had been published the year before and, on the basis of his experience, it was decided to excise the leg area of the sensory cortex in the hope of relieving the pain. This was done under local anaesthesia. As the cortex and subjacent white matter representing the leg area were being removed, the patient volunteered the information: 'What a relief to get rid of that pain.' And his last words on leaving the theatre were: 'It is just wonderful. I just hope that it will stay like

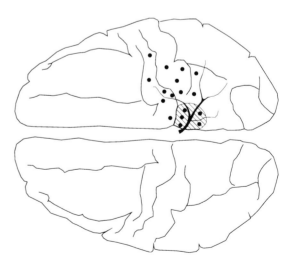

Fig. 34.1 Diagram illustrating the area (shaded) of the postcentral sensory cortex removed. This included the leg area on the medial aspect of the hemisphere. The dots mark the cortical sites stimulated. A large superior cerebral vein that crossed the leg area complicated the cortical ablation.

it.' The diagram (Fig. 34.1, p. 344) made at the time illustrates the area excised and the points stimulated during the operation. Regrettably, the relief was only temporary for after a few months the pain returned with its old intensity.

If a term is to be applied to the distorted neuronal patterns and systems within the central nervous systems and the disturbances to which they give rise, then Turbulence Hypothesis seems to be appropriate. It is certainly one which is consistent with the following characteristic clinical features of causalgia.

1. The persistence of causalgia after isolating the injured nerve segment and the affected peripheral tissues from the central nervous system.
2. Causalgia occurring in patients following avulsion of all nerve roots of the brachial plexus.
3. The much higher incidence of causalgia following high nerve injuries due to wounding by high velocity missiles. The severity of the retrograde neuronal changes is known to be proportional to the severity of the injury and its proximity to the cell bodies.
4. The instantaneous onset of pain at the time of the injury.
5. While the abnormal impulse generating properties of the injured nerve segment and affected peripheral tissues may play a part in precipitating, augmenting, and perpetuating this abnormal central activity, the essential feature of causalgia becomes a disorganised intraspinal focus of hyperexcitability that continues to discharge spontaneously in the absence of any normal or abnormal input from the affected limb. This would account for the spontaneous pain in causalgia.
6. The spreading distribution of the pain. The pain gradually extends beyond the limits of the territory served by the injured nerve and so comes to have a much wider distribution. This occurs as the central disturbance gradually spreads to involve wider and wider areas of the cord.
7. The waxing and waning of the spontaneous pain is a reflection of fluctuations in the level of activity in the central hyperactive foci.
8. In most patients pain gradually subsides and finally disappears, presumably as neurons recover from the retrograde reaction caused by the nerve injury.
9. Anything that increases activity in the nervous system will precipitate an attack of pain or aggravate pain already present. An endless variety of stimuli fall into this category. These have been outlined on page 339. It is this acute abnormal hypersensitivity to all forms of stimuli that converts the unfortunate victim into a recluse and ultimately a complete nervous wreck.

SYMPATHETIC NERVOUS SYSTEM AND THE PAINFUL NERVE LESION

A final point in this saga of painful nerve lesions concerns the possible role of the sympathetic nervous system in their production. Reflex sympathetic dystrophy is excluded from consideration here because this painful condition is a consequence of an injury to tissues other than nerve trunks. This gives it a separate identity.

The grounds for implicating the sympathetic nervous system in nocigenic mechanisms are based on two observations:

1. the dramatic relief that usually follows blocking the sympathetic innervation to the affected limb either by pharmacological or surgical means;
2. the beneficial effects of guanethidine therapy which are attributed to blocking the release of noradrenaline at sympathetic nerve endings.

If one concedes that the sympathetic nervous system is involved, as one must on the evidence, then the next step is to explain the nature of that involvement.

The sympathetic nervous system has been causally associated with painful nerve lesions in several ways:

1. The interruption of aberrant sensory fibres traversing sympathetic ganglia on their way

centrally. The existence of such aberrant fibres has never been convincingly demonstrated.

2. Vasomotor effects, based on the irritation of vasoconstrictor fibres in the damaged segment of the nerve, could be responsible for adversely affecting the nutrition of tissues, thereby promoting the formation and accumulation of pain-producing metabolites.

3. The formation of ephaptic synapses and pathological changes affecting the insulating properties of the nerve sheath in the damaged segment of the nerve could permit cross-talk interference between sympathetic and nociceptor fibres.

4. The release of noradrenaline in the damaged segment of the nerve, or in a neuroma, is claimed to aggravate abnormal ongoing activity in the impulse generating properties of fine free axon terminals (Wall & Gutnick 1974a,b, Govrin-Lippmann & Devor 1978, Devor & Janig 1981, Korenmann & Devor 1981, Devor & Bernstein 1982, Blumberg & Janig 1984). However, axons allowed to regenerate into mesothelial chambers did not exhibit such ongoing activity (Danielsen et al 1986).

5. The formation of ephaptic synapses between sympathetic and sensory nerve endings in the affected cutaneous tissues is believed to be facilitated when these tissues are oedematous and are poorly nourished by a stagnant circulation.

6. The increased release of noradrenaline at overactive sympathetic nerve endings is claimed to increase the activity of sensory receptors perhaps already hypersensitised by the nerve injury.

There is no doubt that sympathectomy, pharmacological or surgical, and guanethidine therapy are usually, though not always, effective in relieving the pain but just how this is brought about remains unclear.

It should be noted that this causal relationship carries the proviso that sympathetic and sensory feedback pathways should be functionally intact, although this mandatory prerequisite is not always satisfied as, for example, when the pain is unrelieved by sympatectomy and when causalgia complicates total rupture and avulsion injuries of the brachial plexus that isolate the limb from the nervous system. Additional incompatible evidence is provided by (1) the immediate onset of the pain long before those pathological changes held to be responsible for the offending mechanism could develop, and (2) the painful nerve lesion that is physiologically complete.

When all the evidence is assembled and critically analysed, involvement of the sympathetic nervous system appears to be clear enough in some painful nerve lesions but not so in others. Furthermore, a convincing explanation for the dramatic relief that often follows sympathectomy still eludes us and the precise role of the sympathetic nervous system in the genesis and operation of pain mechanisms remains very much a mystery.

Concluding comments

In bringing this chapter to a close, it can be said that much can be learned about the genesis and modus operandi of pain mechanisms from a clinical study of painful nerve lesions.

Summarising, the following key points are of particular significance in this respect:

1. In any individual case it is important to ascertain if, and how, regional anatomical features could be involved in pain-producing processes. For example, such factors do play a significant role in the production of painful lesions of the median nerve in the carpal tunnel, of the spinal nerve in the intervertebral foramen, and of other nerves in entrapment situations.

2. The pathophysiological basis of the painful state after peripheral nerve injury follows no constant pattern.

3. Though the essential pathology in the injured segment of a painful nerve lesion is a hypersensitive disorganised meshwork of unsheathed, or inadequately sheathed, regenerating axons and free axon terminals, it is clear that other pathogenic elements could also be involved. Co-existing accessory elements take the form of:

(a) adhesions that fix the nerve to its bed thereby increasing its vulnerability to traction deformation, and (b) an impaired blood supply to the injured nerve segment caused by direct injury to local blood vessels, and a surrounding fibrosis.

4. Pain mechanisms may be based, not on the physical deformation of nerve fibres, but on vascular complications that subject them to ischaemia.

5. Nerve fibre dissociation in which fine fibres survive and large fibres are eliminated is rejected as a cause of causalgia.

6. Nocigenic systems are activated by mechanical deformation, ischaemia, algesic agents and temperature and barometric changes.

7. The study throws no light on the controversial role of ephaptic synapses and defects in the insulating properties of nerve sheaths in the genesis of nocigenic mechanisms other than to reveal that these structural changes could not have been contributing elements in some painful nerve lesions.

8. While the injured segment of the nerve and the affected cutaneous tissues, particularly the former, are the locus operandi of pain mechanisms in most painful nerve lesions, there is convincing evidence that, in others, e.g. causalgia, the mechanisms responsible for the pain are located within the central nervous system and that these abnormal impulse generators can discharge spontaneously and quite independently of any peripheral influence. It is therefore important to distinguish between the pathology of a lesion and the neurogenic mechanisms responsible for the pain.

9. Central mechanisms are based on the retrograde and trans-synaptic neuronal reaction to nerve injury and involve pools of neurons and afferent transmission pathways extending from the spinal cord to the cerebral cortex.

10. While the development of central nocigenic mechanisms appears to be the outcome of acute and severe trauma to a peripheral nerve, it is conceivable that peripheral nerve involvement causing longstanding chronic pain could, with the passage of time, promote the same sort of central changes that are responsible for the severe, intractable and incapacitating pain of causalgia.

11. Because the nocigenic mechanism could be located in one or more of these sites, local, peripheral and central, it is important, in any individual case, to determine which is at fault. Failure to do this means that therapy is likely to remain ill-directed and the outcome uncertain. Under these conditions it will be impossible to remove treatment from the thraldom of empiricism.

12. The dramatic relief that often follows sympathetic blocking procedures is compelling evidence that the sympathetic nervous system is in some unexplained way involved in pain mechanisms. At the same time it should not be overlooked that there are painful nerve lesions in which the possibility of any contribution from the sympathetic nervous system can be confidently excluded. The role of the sympathetic nervous system in the genesis and operation of pain mechanisms remains unclear.

13. The influence of a psychologically and emotionally unstable personality in the genesis of pain mechanisms is well authenticated. This leads one to ask if there is such a state or condition of the body as a Pain Diathesis in which the injured tissues and the central nervous system react in a special way in certain individuals that makes them more susceptible to painful sequelae. At the same time, the contribution of psychic factors in *true* causalgia needs to be treated with considerable caution.

Harassed by continuous pain and lack of sleep, the patient, after a time, may become a nervous wreck. If seen at this stage by an enthusiastic clinician with a psychosomatic bias, he may have his mind probed in a search for 'psychic trauma'. And the practitioner who suspects a psychogenic cause seldom fails to uncover a confirmatory history. Some physicians and surgeons, finding it difficult to appreciate the fact that these patients suffer intensely, are ever on the alert for evidence which may suggest that they are dramatising or exaggerating their symptoms. To adopt such an attitude is, in fact, to commit a grievous error; apart from the serious mistake in diagnosis, a great injustice is being done to the patient in attempting to lay upon him both the blame for being ill and the responsibility for curing himself. The patient is the only witness we have, and if he says he has pain there are no grounds on which we can contradict him.

Many who try to explain such pains upon a psychogenic basis seem to have made no clear distinction between the perception of pain that is present and the imagining of pain that is not there. There is, of course, a cortical element in every act of perceiving pain, even as there is a cortical element in perceiving a sight or a sound. But the fact that the observer cannot personally confirm the patient's act of perception (as he can confirm the sound that he also hears, which the patient describes) sometimes causes him to regard the pain as somehow less real than other more material perceptions, and to believe that it can be relieved by the patient's mental efforts.

EPILOGUE

If the reader has followed the arguments advanced in this presentation he will rightly conclude that the data that have accumulated from this examination of painful peripheral nerve injuries leave many questions unanswered.

Furthermore, though it has been possible to identify a number of structural changes that could function as abnormal impulse generators, and a variety of influences, physical and others, that could disturb the status quo and provoke a painful response, it has not been possible to settle the vexed question of why some nerve injuries are painful and others are not, particularly when the wounding mechanisms, and the nature and pathology of the nerve injury appear to be the same in each case.

However, some synthesis of the available information is not out of place, if only to provide a challenge to the imagination and to experimental initiative directed to new and more fruitful lines of investigation.

REFERENCES

Adrian E D 1930 Effects of injury on mammalian nerve fibres. Proceedings of the Royal Society B 106: 596

Bishop G H 1959 Relationship of fibre size and sensory modality. Journal Nervous and Mental Disease 128: 89

Bishop G H 1960 The relation of nerve fibre size to modality of sensation. In: Montague W (ed) Advances in biology of skin, Volume 1. Cutaneous innervation. Pergamon Press, New York, p 88

Bishop G H, Clare M H 1955 Organisation and distribution of fibers in the optic nerve of the cat. Journal of Comparative Neurology 103: 269

Bishop G H, Heinbecker P 1930 Differentiation of axon types in visceral nerves by means of the potential record. American Journal of Physiology 94: 170

Bishop G H, Heinbecker P, O'Leary J L 1933 The function of the non-myelinated fibers of the dorsal roots. American Journal of Physiology 106: 647

Blumberg H, Janig W 1984 Discharge pattern of afferent fibres from a neuroma. Pain 20: 335

Boring E G 1916 Cutaneous sensation after nerve division. Quarterly Journal of Experimental Physiology 10: 1

Burchiel K J 1984 Spontaneous impulse generation in normal and denervated dorsal root ganglia: sensitivity to alpha-adrenergic stimulation and hypoxia. Experimental Neurology 85: 257

Burchiel K, Wyler A, Heavner J E 1986 Peripheral and central nervous system. In: Methods of animal experimentation. Academic Press, New York, p 217

Danielsen N, Shyu B C, Dahlin L B, Lundborg G, Andersson S 1986 Absence of ongoing activity in fibres arising from proximal nerve ends regenerating into mesothelial chambers. Pain 26: 93

Denny Brown D, Kirk E J, Yanagisawa N 1973 The tract of Lissauer in relation to sensory transmission in the dorsal horn of spinal cord in the macaque monkey. Journal of Comparative Neurology 151: 175

DeSantis M, Duckworth J W 1982 Properties of primary afferent neurons from muscle which are spontaneously active after a lesion of their peripheral processes. Experimental Neurology 75: 261

Devor M, Bernstein J J 1982 Abnormal impulse generation in neuromas: electrophysiology and ultrastructure. In: Culp W J, Ochoa J (eds) Abnormal nerves and muscles as impulse generators. Oxford University Press, New York, p 363

Devor M, Janig W 1981 Activation of myelinated afferent ending in a neuroma by stimulation of the sympathetic supply in the rat. Neuroscience Letters 24: 43

Eccles J C 1957 The Physiology of nerve cells. Johns Hopkins Press, Baltimore

Eccles J C 1964 The physiology of synapses. Springer, Berlin

Eccles J C, Krnjevic K, Miledi R 1959 Delayed effects of peripheral severance of afferent nerve fibres on the efficacy of their central synapses. Journal of Physiology (London) 145: 204

Erlanger J, Gasser H S 1924 The compound nature of the action current of nerves as disclosed by the cathode ray oscillograph. American Journal of Physiology 70: 624

Erlanger J, Gasser H S 1937 Electrical signs of nervous activity. Oxford University Press, London

Gasser H S 1935 Conduction in nerves in relation to fiber types. In: Sensation: its mechanisms and disturbances. Proceedings of the Association for Research in Nervous and Mental Disease. Williams & Wilkins, Baltimore 15: 35

Gasser H S 1943 Pain-producing impulses in peripheral nerves. Pain. Proceedings of the Association for Nervous and Mental Disease. Williams & Wilkins, Baltimore 23: 44

Gerard R W 1951 The physiology of pain: abnormal neuron states in causalgia and related phenomena. Anesthesiology 12: 1

Govrin-Lippmann R, Devor M 1978 Ongoing activity in severed nerves: source and variation with time. Brain Research 159: 406

Head H 1896 On disturbances of sensation with especial reference to the pain of visceral disease. Brain 19: 153

Head H 1905 The afferent nervous system from a new aspect. Brain 28: 99

Kirk E J 1974 Impulses in dorsal spinal nerve rootlets in cats and rabbits arising from dorsal root ganglia isolated from the periphery. Journal of Comparative Neurology 155: 165

Korenman E M D, Devor M 1981 Ectopic adrenergic sensitivity in damaged peripheral nerve axons in the rat. Experimental Neurology 72: 63

Landau W, Bishop G H 1953 Pain from dermal, periosteal and fascial endings and from inflammation. Archives of Neurology and Psychiatry Chicago 69: 490

Lewis T 1942 Pain. Macmillan, New York, p v

Lewis T, Pochin E E 1938 Effects of asphyxia and pressure on sensory nerves of man. Clinical Science 3: 141

Lindahl O 1946 Om ischiassjukdomens patogens. Svensk Läkartidning. 51: 2389

Lindahl O 1966 Hyperalgesia of the lumbar nerve roots in sciatica. Acta Orthopaedica Scandinavica 37: 367

Livingston W K 1938 Post-traumatic pain syndromes. An interpretation of the underlying pathological physiology. Western Journal of Surgery Obstetrics and Gynaecology 46: 341, 426

Livingston W K 1944 Pain mechanisms. A physiological interpretation of causalgia and its related states. Macmillan, New York

Livingston W K 1948 The vicious circle in causalgia. Annals of the New York Academy of Sciences 50: 247

Loeser J D, Ward A A 1967 Some effects of deafferentation on neurons of the cat spinal cord. Archives of Neurology (Chicago) 17: 629

Melzack R, Wall P D 1965 Pain mechanisms: a new theory. Science 150: 971

Noordenbos W 1959 Pain. Elsevier, Amsterdam

Nystrom B, Hagbath K E 1981 Microelectrode recordings from transected nerves in amputees with phantom limb pain. Neuroscience Letters 27: 211

Ochoa J 1980 Nerve fiber pathology in acute and chronic compression. In: Omer G E, Spinner M (eds) Management of peripheral nerve problems. Saunders, Philadelphia, p 487

Ochoa J L, Torebjörk H E 1980 Paresthesiae from ectopic impulse generation in human sensory nerves. Brain 103: 835

Ranson S W 1908 The architectural relations of the afferent elements entering into the formation of the spinal ganglia. Journal of Comparative Neurology 18: 121

Ranson S W 1911 Non-medullated nerve fibres in the spinal nerves. American Journal of Anatomy 12: 67

Ranson S W 1913 The course within the spinal cord of the non-medullated fibers of the dorsal roots. A study of Lissauer's tract in the cat. Journal of Comparative Neurology 23: 259

Ranson S W 1914 The tract of Lissauer and the substantia gelatinosa. American Journal of Anatomy 16: 97

Ranson S W 1915 Unmyelinated nerve fibers as conductors of protopathic sensation. Brain 38: 381

Scadding J W 1981 The development of ongoing activity, mechanosensitivity and adrenaline sensitivity in severed peripheral nerve axons. Experimental Neurology 73: 345

Sharpey-Schafer E 1927 Recovery after severance of cutaneous nerves. Brain 50: 538

Sherrington C 1947 The integrative action of the nervous system. University Press, Cambridge, p 193

Sinclair D 1967 Cutaneous sensation. Oxford University Press, London

Sinclair D C, Hinshaw J R 1950 Sensory changes in procaine nerve block. Brain 73: 224

Sinclair D C, Hinshaw J R 1950 A comparison of the sensory dissocation produced by procaine and by limb compression. Brain 73: 480

Sinclair D C, Hinshaw J R 1951a Sensory changes in nerve blocks induced by cooling. Brain 74: 318

Sinclair D C, Hinshaw J R 1951b Sensory phenomena in experimental nerve block. Quarterly Journal of Experimental Psychology 3: 49

Sunderland S 1976a Pain mechanisms in causalgia. Journal of Neurology, Neurosurgery and Psychiatry 39: 471

Sunderland S 1976b Nerve lesion in the carpal tunnel syndrome. Journal of Neurology, Neurosurgery and Psychiatry 39: 615

Sunderland S 1978 The painful sequelae of injuries to peripheral nerves. In: Nerves and nerve injuries. Churchill Livingstone, Edinburgh, p 377

Sunderland S, Kelly M 1948 The painful sequelae of injuries to peripheral nerves. Australian and New Zealand Journal of Surgery 18: 75

Thulin C-A 1961 Electrophysiological study of consecutive changes of feline ventral root reflexes during degeneration and regeneration following peripheral nerve section. Experimental Neurology 4: 531

Trotter W B, Davies H M 1909 Experimental studies in the innervation of the skin. Journal of Physiology (London) 38: 134

Wall P D, Devor M 1978 Physiology of sensation after peripheral nerve injury, regeneration and neuroma formation. In: Waxsman S G (ed) Physiology and pathobiology of axons. Raven Press, New York, p 377

Wall P D, Devor M 1983 Sensory afferent impulses originate from dorsal root ganglia as well as from the periphery in normal and nerve injured rats. Pain 17: 321

Wall P D, Gutnick M 1974a Properties of afferent nerve impulses originating from a neuroma. Nature 248: 740

Wall P D, Gutnick M 1974b Ongoing activity in peripheral nerves: the physiology and pharmacology of impulses originating from a neuroma. Experimental Neurology 43: 580

Waller A 1862 On the sensory motory and vasomotory symptoms resulting from refrigeration and compression of the ulnar and other nerves in man. Proceedings of the Royal Society 12: 89

Wiesenfeld Z, Lindblom U 1980 Behavioural and electrophysiological effects of various types of peripheral nerve lesions in the rat: a comparison of possible models for chronic pain. Pain 8: 285

Wortis H, Stein M H, Joliffe N 1942 Fibre dissociation in peripheral neuropathy. Archives of Internal Medicine 69: 222

35. Nerve injury and sympathetic function

GENERAL CONSIDERATIONS

Sympathetic nerve fibres are an important component of peripheral nerves, innervating a wide range of tissues and serving a wide variety of functions. By virtue of their effects, they have been classified as vasomotor, sudomotor and pilomotor fibres. This chapter is concerned only with damage to postganglionic fibres and not with the consequences of involvement of the preganglionic components.

Vasoconstrictor fibres act on the smooth muscle of the wall of blood vessels. In this way they regulate and control the flow of blood to the skin and muscles, delicately adjusting the circulation to meet the functional demands of tissues as these vary during the various phases of activity. Further regulatory mechanisms are provided by elaborate arterio-venous communications that are also under sympathetic control. Sympathetic nerve fibres innervate sweat glands and regulate the production of their secretions. They activate the arrectores pili muscles of the skin, causing the erection of hairs and the goose flesh effects at the surface of the body.

Vascular changes, the erection of hairs and sweating have been associated with separate vasomotor, pilomotor and sudorific fibre systems. Whether this functional specificity is a property of the nerve fibre itself, whether it is solely attributable to the end organ with the nerve fibre merely participating as an activating agent, or whether it is a shared activity is not known. For this reason the consequences of misdirected regeneration, such as would occur with the regeneration of vasomotor fibres to sweat glands, are uncertain.

The activities of structures innervated by sympathetic nerves are controlled in two ways. The first involves neural mechanisms mediated over sympathetic nerves and the second a non-neural factor in the form of chemical and humoral agents elaborated at the periphery or circulating in the blood. It is therefore important to recognise that the denervation of structures supplied by sympathetic nerves does not render them completely inactive, for they continue to respond in an autonomous manner to persisting local non-neural influences. Thus denervated vessels remain sensitive to noradrenaline and sweat glands to pilocarpine.

Interference with the sympathetic innervation of a part produces conspicuous changes in sweat secretion and in the vascularity and nutrition of the denervated tissues. Methods for detecting the involvement of sympathetic nerve fibres in nerve injuries are based on alterations in sweat secretion.

Interference with the vascularity and nutrition of the denervated tissues results in the development of trophic disturbances and changes that are discussed in Chapter 30.

Features of significance in relation to sympathetic nerve fibres are:

1. They are fine in calibre and are mostly nonmyelinated, though some postganglionic fibres are finely myelinated.
2. They innervate blood vessels, glands and hair muscles of the skin by way of the cutaneous nerves, and deeper structures by way of the deep branches of the main nerve trunks.
3. The major distribution of the postganglionic fibres to the limbs is by way of nerve

trunks in which they are intermingled with somatic motor and sensory fibres.

4. Most of the sympathetic nerve fibres to the limbs are destined for the hands and feet.

5. Some peripheral nerves contain more sympathetic fibres than others. This is particularly so for those nerves that supply the hand and the foot, namely, the median, sciatic and tibial nerves, and to a lesser degree the ulnar nerve. It is for this reason that lesions of different peripheral nerves produce variable sympathetic effects at the periphery. Thus lesions of the radial and musculocutaneous nerves are associated with minimal sympathetic changes, whereas such changes are particularly marked in lesions of the median, sciatic and tibial nerves where they take the form of trophic changes affecting the hand and foot, and particularly the digits.

6. Sympathetic nerve fibres have the same peripheral distribution as the branch of the peripheral nerve which contains them. Thus the cutaneous areas of sensory and sympathetic loss correspond. Centrally there is an autonomous area surrounded by a marginal zone where sympathetic responses are present but diminished.

7. The skin and subcutaneous tissues are richly endowed with sympathetic fibres that branch and intertwine to form complicated plexuses.

8. Postganglionic fibres pass from the ganglionated sympathetic trunk, spinal nerves and limb plexuses to form peri-arterial plexuses that serve the major vessels only as far distally as about the mid level of the upper arm and thigh. Additionally above this level, and solely below it, the vessels are innervated by vasomotor branches from peripheral nerve trunks. These branches leave at successive, but irregular, levels to reach and descend along the vessel for a variable distance before its innervation is taken over by the next branch. The last vasomotor branches are those from the digital nerves to the digital vessels.

9. The collateral branches of preganglionic axons establish synaptic relationships with several postganglionic sympathetic neurons both in the same and neighbouring ganglia. This means that localised activity centrally could lead to widespread sympathetic changes at the periphery. The repeated branching of sympathetic fibres at the periphery contributes to the further diffusion of sympathetic influences and provides for axon reflexes which are a feature of peripheral sympathetic mechanisms.

10. The preganglionic sympathetic neurons of the lateral grey column of the spinal cord are subject to influences originating in the spinal cord, basal centres of the brain and the cerebral cortex itself. This permits abnormal activity occurring elsewhere in the nervous system to spread to sympathetic neurons, thereby creating disturbances in sympathetic function at the periphery.

11. The sympathetic neurons and their processes appear to lack any organised arrangement, activity producing general rather than discrete effects at the periphery although localised adjustments are possible to meet local functional demands. Thus the sympathetic nervous system is designed to produce, as easily and as rapidly as possible, generalised and widespread reactions to meet vital necessities, all critical stresses evoking a response on the same general plan.

THE EFFECTS OF SYMPATHETIC DENERVATION

Following section of a peripheral nerve the vessels in the denervated area fully dilate and the part becomes warmer. Sweating is abolished and the goose flesh effect seen in the skin with cooling does not appear. Despite these characteristic changes, the denervated tissues continue to respond to local non-neural influences to which, under certain conditions, they may even become hypersensitive. This is reflected in the increased sensitivity of denervated smooth muscle to circulating noradrenaline which is secreted in response to numerous stimuli such as emotion and cold. Under these conditions exposure of the denervated area to cold results in vasoconstriction. These non-neural responses are not usually present immediately following the injury but take some days to develop.

REGENERATIVE PROCESSES AND RECOVERY PHENOMENA

We know surprisingly little about the regeneration of postganglionic fibres. The pattern of recovery following peripheral nerve injuries supports the general conclusion that the regeneration of these fibres follows essentially the same pattern as that recorded for somatic nerves.

Signs of returning sympathetic function in the form of vasomotor, sudomotor and pilomotor responses are not necessarily due to the regeneration of sympathetic axons. Non-neural mechanisms continue to evoke responses in denervated structures and care should be taken not to confuse these with the appearance of recovery in sympathetic pathways.

FACTORS INFLUENCING THE EXTENT AND QUALITY OF THE FUNCTIONAL RECOVERY

Axon branching

Sympathetic patterns of innervation do not demand the same precise and accurate restoration of nerve fibre connections as are required for the restoration of highly specialised somatic functions. For this reason the budding and collateral sprouting of sympathetic axons that occur during regeneration are likely to be more effective in compensating for the loss of some axons than is the case with somatic fibre regeneration.

The erroneous entry of axons into foreign endoneurial tubes

Regenerating sympathetic axons will enter functionally unrelated endoneurial tubes and pass along them to the periphery. Conversely, somatic axons will regenerate into and along sympathetic endoneurial tubes.

The maturation of regenerated sympathetic nerve fibres

The calibre and myelination of somatic nerve fibres vary in a manner that has functional significance and which involves complex processes additional to axon growth during regeneration. Postganglionic nerve fibres are, on the other hand, of fine calibre and are either non-myelinated, which applies to the majority, or very finely myelinated. With such a simple structure it might reasonably be expected that the maturation of regenerated sympathetic axons would be a more simple and rapid process and less subject to those modifications that adversely affect somatic function.

The constitution of the new as opposed to the original pattern of innervation

In the case of somatic systems, the degree of correspondence between the original and the restored patterns of innervation determines the extent and quality of motor and sensory recovery. The circumstances are not the same in the case of the regeneration of sympathetic fibres.

The manner in which the new arrangement after regeneration of sympathetic axons departs from the original depends on those factors that lead to the elimination of some axons and the misdirected growth of others which deprives them of any functional significance. The functional consequences of such residual defects should not be as damaging as would be the case for somatic functions because sympathetic effects, being of a more generalised character, require less complicated nerve patterns than those needed to provide for the wide range and quality of sensory and motor function. Thus arterioles and sweat glands perform precisely the same function in each case, no matter where they are located. It is not necessary, therefore, for regenerating sympathetic axons to re-establish connections with the same precision so long as the connections are functionally appropriate and are in sufficient numbers. Thus the restoration of vasomotor and sudomotor functions does not require the reconstitution of a complex pattern of innervation, or the participation of central adjustments, but only the reinnervation of vessels and sweat glands.

Defects in regeneration may, however, reach a degree that results in instability, irregularities or a loss in sympathetic functions in the affected region. Whether it is essential that vasoconstrictor fibres go to vessels, sudomotor fibres to sweat glands and pilomotor fibres to the arrectores pili muscles or whether there is complete non-specificity and interchangeability in this respect is not known. If such specificity should exist then the abnormal rerouting of axons could have more serious consequences.

Compensatory mechanisms

These could operate by way of axon budding and the extension of sprouts from neighbouring unin-jured sympathetic axons into the denervated area.

The pattern of recovery

The growth of postganglionic axons and the re-establishment of effective peripheral connections proceeds proximo-distally so that the denervated area is gradually reduced and sympathetic re-sponses are correspondingly restored. Such recovery closely follows that associated with the sensory reinnervation of the skin. The hypersen-sitivity of denervated blood vessels to noradrenaline is gradually reduced as regeneration proceeds.

THE EFFECTS OF PERMANENT SYMPATHETIC DENERVATION

The effects of depriving a limb of its sympathetic innervation are without effect on sensory function, as observations on patients with sympathectomised limbs will testify. When, however, the sympathetic loss is associated with a residual sensory loss, the nutrition and vitality of the denervated region are in jeopardy and trophic changes under these con-ditions are common.

Importantly, the loss of sweating, which leaves a dry skin, deprives it of the ability to resist the movement of an object across its surface which is an essential element in the efficient performance of many daily manual tasks, particularly those in-volving a strong grip.

TESTING SYMPATHETIC FUNCTION

Two methods used clinically for determining the distribution of any impairment or loss of sym-pathetic function are based on the presence or absence of the moisture, due to sweating, at the surface of the skin (Sunderland 1978). They are the colorimetric sweating test and the electrical skin resistance test. The former depends on dyes in a powder base which have an affinity for water, and which change colour in the presence of skin moisture. The electrical skin resistance test is based on the resistance of the skin to the passage of a weak current. This resistance varies according to the state of sudomotor function. Sweating lowers skin resistance while dry unsweating skin greatly increases it. Both are objective tests and give useful information about the condition of sympathetic nerve fibres.

Some regions of the body sweat more readily and profusely than others, and some individuals more so than others; such variation should be kept in mind when conducting the tests.

The sympathetic fibres innervating the skin are incorporated in peripheral nerve trunks and are distributed by their cutaneous branches to the su-perficial and deep cutaneous plexuses from which the sudomotor fibres finally pass to the sweat glands. The arrangement is one in which the sudomotor and sensory nerve fibres in a peripheral nerve have the same cutaneous distribution so that, following a nerve injury, the areas of altered sweating and sensation will correspond.

The colorimetric and skin resistance tests, which reflect changes in sweat gland activity, are particularly useful for detecting nerve injuries, for outlining the limits of altered cutaneous sen-sibility, and for following the course of recovery as regeneration proceeds. Furthermore, because the tests do not depend on subjective sensations they have added value in cases of suspected malingering or where the testing of sensory func-tion presents special difficulties.

Colorimetric tests

Finger print test

The method most commonly used was introduced by Moberg (1958, 1960) for the study of median and ulnar nerve function in nerve injuries. The test is not concerned with the total area of sympathetic loss but only with the sudomotor function of the terminal pads of the digits. For this reason its use is, for all practical purposes, restricted to the median and ulnar nerves.

The test is based on a colour change in which finger prints are taken on specially prepared paper strips. These strips are either impregnated with a dye combination which changes colour in the presence of moisture (iodine-starch test) or which can be subsequently processed in such a way as to stain chemical substances in the sweat secretion which have been transferred from the finger pad to the paper when the finger print was taken (ninhydrin test).

Ninhydrin test

This method is based on the colour change produced when certain amino acids are stained by a ninhydrin solution. The stainable amino acids on which the test depends are the products of sweat gland activity and are not derived elsewhere at the skin surface.

Moberg has reported a close correspondence between sudomotor function, as determined by these methods, and certain specialised tactile functions so that improvement in the quality of the prints, in the form of increasing clearness, is a reliable indicator of improvement in sensation. Others, however, have been unable to establish any correlation between the return of sudomotor activity and the functional value of the restored sensation (Stromberg et al 1961; Önne 1962).

Colorimetric methods are unsuitable for rapid day-to-day testing. They should be replaced by electrical skin resistance testing, which is by far the best and most useful of the methods available for evaluating the status of sympathetic function. In addition, it clearly defines the area of sensory loss.

The electrical skin resistance test.

The resistance of the skin to the passage of an electric current is determined by its moisture content, so that the resistance is lowered by sweating which is produced by sympathetic activity but is greatly increased in areas of dry unsweating skin. The latter occurs when sympathetic activity is depressed (as on cold days) and after the skin has been deprived of its sympathetic innervation.

Because the transition from an area of high resistance (denervated skin) to an area of low resistance (normal skin) is very sharp, measurements of skin resistance provide valuable information relating to the sympathetic innervation of the skin. Observations of this nature commenced with Fere as long ago as 1888 and the method has since been developed and used by others (Sunderland 1968; Buratti 1972; Egyed et al 1980; Swain et al 1985; Wilson 1985; Smith & Mott 1986).

Instruments, called dermometers, have been designed to detect and measure skin resistance as an index of the moisture content of the skin. As the electrical resistance increases, the current flow through the circuit is reduced and in practice it is the reduction in current flow which is measured. By this method, areas of sympathetic loss can be isolated from their normal surroundings and charted with accuracy. The instrument consists of fixed and exploring electrodes, a source of current, a microammeter, a switch and a rheostat to provide variable resistances.

Dermometry offers a simple, convenient, practical, rapid and effective method for outlining areas of completely and partially denervated skin. The method has a decided advantage over colorimetric testing in that it is more accurate, takes less time and gives quantitative information.

Direct observation of sweating

Sweating may be directly observed by means of a plus 20 ophthalmoscope lens and this has been used for the evaluation of sudomotor function in nerve injuries.

Thermography

Thermography is the process of recording thermal images, the emission of heat normally radiated from tissues being detected by a heat sensor. There is now a growing literature on the use of thermography as a diagnostic and investigative tool in a variety of conditions.

Human skin is an excellent natural emitter of infrared radiation which can be recorded and used to give a quantitative temperature map of the skin. The temperature of a part is largely determined by the amount of blood flow, variations in which will, consequently, lead to asymmetries in the intensity of heat emissions and so to abnormalities in the thermographic pattern.

The loss of the sympathetic innervation when a peripheral nerve is transected results in transient vasodilatation in the denervated skin, which becomes temporarily flushed and warm, and this change can be detected by thermography. This technique is capable of giving an objective evaluation of sympathetic nerve fibre involvement and, therefore, of nerve trunk damage but offers no advantages over the other methods of testing sympathetic function. Thermography remains a research tool and has no place in the routine clinical examination of nerve injuries.

OBSERVATIONS

Studies of cutaneous sympathetic innervation using colorimetric and skin resistance methods have provided the following information:

1. The transition between areas of abnormally high and normally low skin resistance is gradual, and not abrupt, and is represented by a zone or band approximately 2–10 mm in width.
2. The area of altered skin resistance coincides with the area of cutaneous sensory change. The area of abnormally increased resistance corresponds to the area of autonomous sensory loss, and the band representing the gradual transition from abnormal to normal responses matches the zone of sensory overlap and diminished sensation.
3. Colorimetric investigation of sweat secretion shows that sweating is absent only within the autonomous sensory area of the affected nerve; in the marginal zone of sensory overlap, sudomotor function is present though diminished.
4. Because of this correspondence, the skin resistance test provides useful supplementary information concerning the state of sensory function, particularly under conditions where sensory testing is difficult and giving conflicting information. Thus in the case of suspected malingering the test is of more value than conflicting subjective reporting by the patient.
5. The onset of regeneration may be recognised and its progress followed by charting the progressive reduction in the dimensions of the area of high skin resistance.
6. In partial nerve lesions, due either to incomplete damage or partial recovery, discrepancies between the results of sensory testing and skin resistance studies are to be expected. Thus, in partial nerve injuries, the sensory and sympathetic fibres will be affected in different combinations and proportions, with the severity of damage varying from fibre to fibre. Such differences would be reflected throughout regeneration. In recovering injuries, the onset of regeneration and the course of recovery may not coincide in the two sets of fibres, the common skin area being reinnervated irregularly and at different rates by the different fibres.
7. Discrepancies in the sensory and sympathetic findings might suggest either a partial nerve injury or regeneration in a recovering lesion. Care should, however, be taken in interpreting this type of information.
8. The presence of some sweating in the cutaneous field of a nerve known to have been injured does not necessarily indicate a partial injury or returning function. In some cases the degree of overlap from neighbouring uninjured nerves is so extensive that the peripheral sympathetic effects of complete nerve section are subtotal rather than total. Procaine blocking of the uninjured nerve responsible for the overlap will resolve this difficulty.

REFERENCES

Buratti G 1972 Electrodiagnosis of denervation of skin. The Hand 4: 68

Egyed B, Eory A, Veres T, Manninger J 1980 Measurement of electrical resistance after nerve injuries of the hand. The Hand 12: 275

Fere C 1888 Note sur des modifications de la résistance électrique sous l'influence des excitations sensorielles et des émotions. Comptes rendu hebdomadaires des séances et Mémoires de la Société de Biologie 40: 217

Moberg E 1958 Objective methods for determining the functional value of sensibility in the hand. Journal of Bone and Joint Surgery 40B: 454

Moberg E 1960 Evaluation of sensibility in the hand. Surgical Clinics of North America 40: 357

Önne L 1962 Recovery of sensibility and sudomotor activity in the hand after nerve suture. Acta Chirurgica Scandinavica Supplement 300: 1

Smith P J, Mott G 1986 Sensory threshold and conductance testing in nerve injuries. Journal of Hand Surgery 11B: 157

Stromberg W B, McFarlane R M, Bell J L et al 1961 Injury of the median and ulnar nerves, 150 cases with an evaluation of Moberg's ninhydrin test. Journal of Bone and Joint Surgery 43A: 717

Sunderland S 1968 Nerves and nerve injuries, 1st edn. Churchill Livingstone, Edinburgh, p 517

Sunderland S 1978 Nerves and nerve injuries, 2nd edn. Churchill Livingstone, Edinburgh, p 466

Swain I D, Wilson G R, Crook S C 1985 A simple method of measuring the electrical resistance of the skin. Journal of Hand Surgery 10B: 319

Wilson G R 1985 A simple device for the objective evaluation of peripheral nerve injury. Journal of Hand Surgery 10B: 324

The clinical management of nerve injury and repair

36. The history of nerve repair

'All honour to those who go first even if those who come later go further.'

The history of the repair of severed nerves is a long, complicated and somewhat tortuous story which remains incomplete. However, some of the phases through which it has passed are identifiable and worthy of comment in the context of current attitudes to nerve repair.

Nerves had been identified as such, and distinguished from tendons, as long ago as the 3rd century BC, by Herophilus, who also traced nerves to the spinal cord and separated them into motor and sensory components.

Regarding the repair of severed nerves, history is silent until Galen (131–201 AD), who had described the entire peripheral nervous system up to and including the digital nerves, reported that he had seen and heard that severed nerves had been sutured with incredible results. However, there is nothing in his writings to suggest that he, himself, ever used the procedure. In fact the traditional Hippocratic teaching of those times doubted that nerve healing occurred.

Though there is a reference to nerve suture by Paul of Aegina (625–690), the first clear reference to the suture repair of a severed nerve is attributed to the Persians but these accounts were short on detail (Rhazes 850–932 and Avicenna, Ali Abu Ibn Sina 980—1037).

If the contents of the surviving medical manuscripts of the Middle Ages are any guide to established practice of those times, then it would appear that the suture of severed nerves was rarely undertaken. Mention of it was made by Saliceto (1210–1277), by Lanfranchi (1296) the founder of French surgery, and by his distinguished pupil, Guy de Chauliac (1300–1368), the most celebrated authority on surgery in the 14th century, and by Leonard of Bertapaglia (1380–1463).

Leonard merits special attention because, unlike his predecessors whose writings contain only passing references to nerve injuries and their treatment, he devoted an entire chapter in his *Chirurgica* to the subject (Ladenheim 1989). However, nowhere in his writings is there any reference to operative detail or surgical techniques. This was undoubtedly due to his firm belief that these could not be learnt from books but only by serving an apprenticeship under the tutelage of an experienced surgeon and by observing and assisting him in his craft. He wrote 'You must accompany and observe the qualified physician, seeing him work before you yourself practice, for, by observing terrible accidents, you will discern the methods employed by those who treat them and thus attain the perfection of the masters.' He also shrewdly observed that 'There are many who read but do not comprehend' and he was getting close to the Renaissance attitude and spirit with his comment: 'Trust incompletely anything cited by authority unless it can be explained by experiment or by reason.' These astute observations are as relevant today as they were 5 centuries ago.

It is interesting to speculate on why the repair of nerves was rarely undertaken in mediaeval times and why opinion was actively opposed to it. This is particularly unexpected at a time when physicians were familiar with the sensory loss and flaccid paralysis accompanying nerve injury, and when such injuries must have been common, bearing in mind the frequent and favoured use of the lance, the sword, the rapier and the dagger. Possible explanations offered by the present writer are based on the following five considerations:

1. Nerve suture was, presumably, initially advocated in the mistaken belief that the simple restoration of structural continuity of the nerve trunk would result in the restoration of function, as was the case with most other tissues. Such an expectation is understandable in the absence of any knowledge of the internal structure of nerve trunks or of the complexities of nerve regeneration. In any event it was a belief that was to persist for another 5 centuries.

2. There is nothing in the records to indicate that these mediaeval practitioners were aware that recovery did not immediately follow nerve suture but was delayed for considerable periods. Unaware of the significance of long-term evaluations, it would be reasonable for the surgeon to conclude, in the absence of any improvement shortly after the operation when the patient was still under observation and the wound had healed, that nerve suture was a worthless undertaking.

3. Throughout these mediaeval manuscripts there are repeated references to wound infection, the formation of pus and the treatment of the suppurating wound. The disastrous consequences of closing suppurating wounds were well known. Priority was accordingly given to measures to clean wounds and to promote sound healing. For this purpose preference was given to the use of an extensive variety of empirically selected therapeutic preparations in the form of ointments, salves, potions, poultices, unctions, plasters and the like.

4. Though surgeons were well aware of the difference between nerve and sinew (tendon), it must have been difficult at times to distinguish between them where inspection was limited to the existing laceration because of an unwillingness to extend the wound in order to facilitate identification. Even today it is not unknown for a nerve to be unwittingly sutured to a tendon and vice versa — understandable in the past but inexcusable today.

5. The belief that nothing was to be gained by suturing the nerve was probably supported by the observation that occasionally some improvement occurred despite the fact that no attempt had been made to repair the nerve.

Whatever the reason for the mediaeval surgeon's opposition to nerve suture he could be forgiven for concluding, on the evidence available to him, that the outcome was the same regardless of whether or not the nerve ends were reunited. From this he further concluded that this practice was not only an unrewarding exercise but, by interfering with the wound, could also be a life-threatening one. On both counts nerve suture was without benefit to either the patient's well-being or the surgeon's reputation.

Despite the efforts of some surgeons, notably Ferrara (1608) and Arnemann (1787), to keep alive the concept of nerve suture, the conventional opposition to this procedure, so evident in the Middle Ages, was to persist well into the 19th century, gaining additional support from de la Roche (1778) with his comment that, even though the ends of a transected nerve can join and form a scar, the nerve loses permanently the ability to produce movement. And even as late as 1846, Virchow wrote that persisting gaps over 10 cm in length between the nerve ends were sometimes followed by 'unbelievable' recovery. These observations carried implications that were damaging, though for different reasons, to the cause of those advocating nerve suture.

Real progress came at the close of the 18th century with the thought-provoking observations of Cruikshank (1795), who showed that anatomical continuity of a severed nerve could be restored by healing, and that 'the reunited nerve had been restored in its function'. Cruikshank's observations were confirmed by Haighton (1795) and later by Prévost (1827), Müller (1838) and Steinrück (1838). Others at that time favouring nerve suture were Flourens (1828) and Baudens (1836). Though convinced that recovery followed nerve reunion, none of these writers could have suspected that the recovery was due to axon regeneration because little was known of the structure of nerve fibres at that time and nothing of the process of axon regeneration. Their experiments did, however, convincingly demonstrate that nerve reunion could occur after nerve transection and be followed by recovery, and that an interval elapsed between the two events.

The entire picture was to change dramatically in the second half of the 19th century as the result of a series of momentous and far-reaching developments which, inter alia, turned the tide in favour of nerve repair. Crucial among these developments were improvements to the compound microscope and the introduction of greatly improved stains and staining techniques which revealed the finer structural details of nerve fibres and nerve trunks. This information, in turn, paved the way for a study of the reaction of axons to nerve trunk transection and so to the phenomena of Wallerian degeneration and axon regeneration.

Nerve fibres had been described as tubular structures by Dutrochet in 1824. In 1838 Remak identified non-myelinated nerve fibres, reported them arising from sympathetic ganglion cells, and was probably the first to mention a myelin sheath for nerve fibres. A year later Schwann (1839) added the Schwann cell component to the sheath. Subsequently, the finer details of the histological features of nerve fibres were steadily provided by the new staining techniques of Gerlach (1858) and Nissl (1894) with their basic aniline dyes, Waldeyer (1891) with his haematoxylin for staining axis cylinders, Golgi (1883, 1886, 1907) with his silver impregnation methods, Apathy (1897) with his gold staining technique, and Weigert (1882, 1885) and Marchi & Alghieri (1885) with their methods for staining myelin.

By 1865 it was possible for Deiters to provide a histological picture of the nerve cell and in 1875 for Ranvier to write the first definitive text on the histology of the nervous system.

From this intense laboratory activity two issues of commanding interest emerged which were to remain at the root of neurological thinking for the remainder of the 19th century. The first concerned the nature of the structural relationship existing between nerve cells and the second the mechanism of axon regeneration. Each of these was, in turn, the source of conflicting beliefs and interpretations that defied resolution until the close of the century.

THE RELATIONSHIP BETWEEN NERVE CELLS

Only a passing reference will be made to the controversy surrounding the structural relationship obtaining between nerve cells because it does not touch directly on the subject of nerve repair. Briefly there were two conflicting views on this histological feature. Kölliker (1853, 1861) had earlier postulated that each nerve cell is a separate and structurally independent entity so that the nervous system is composed of a system of discontinuous units. This became known as the 'neurone doctrine' or theory when Waldeyer introduced the term neurone in 1891.

The opposing view was expressed in the nerve net or reticular theory which was championed by such distinguished investigators as Gerlach (1858), Weigert (1882), Golgi (1883, 1886, 1907), Apathy (1897), Bethe (1901) and Held (1897, 1907, 1909, 1929). They postulated that the terminals of the processes of different nerve cells form a continuous nerve net. The controversy surrounding this subject continued into the 20th century when it was finally settled by the convincing investigations of Cajal (1908, 1913, 1928, 1952, 1954) and Ross Harrison (1910). For a full discussion of this subject the reader should consult *Neuron Theory or Reticular Theory* by Ramon y Cajal (1954).

AXON REGENERATION

The controversy generated throughout the 19th century by the concept of axon regeneration is specially relevant to the subject of nerve repair. The key to the treasure house of axon regeneration and nerve repair was provided in 1795 in a paper by Cruikshank, in which he reported the results of experiments which showed that the ends of a severed nerve could reunite by way of what appeared to be nerve tissue and be followed by recovery after a delay which suggested 'regeneration' of the nerve. These observations, which had far-reaching implications, were confirmed by others and are referred to in an earlier section (p 362). The use of the term 're-generation' in this context is, however, unclear because Cruikshank likened it to the healing of bone. Moreover, the regeneration of axons could not have been suspected because, at that time, no information was available on the microstructure of nerves. However, the observation that the ends of a severed nerve could reunite and be followed by recovery had two important consequences: (1) it set in train the search for the biological processes and mechanisms responsible for the recovery, and (2) it restored confidence in the value of nerve suture as a therapeutic procedure and led to a renaissance in nerve repair.

It is clear from a study of the sequence of events that followed in the 19th century that progress was dependent on two further developments. One of these involved those crucial histological enquiries that revealed details of the structural features of nerve fibres. The other was the experimental investigations of Waller (1850, 1852, 1892), who convincingly demonstrated that, following nerve transection, the nerve fibre left attached to the parent cell survived whereas that portion separated from it underwent degenerative changes that came to be known as Wallerian degeneration. From this observation it was correctly concluded that recovery required the restoration of axonal continuity with the periphery. However, there was a diversity of opinion on the precise manner in which this occurred and the ensuing controversy was to continue unabated throughout the remainder of the 19th century.

One view attributed recovery to the growth of the surviving axon tips from the proximal nerve stump and their passage down the nerve trunk, finally restoring axonal continuity with the periphery. Principal support for this theory came from the classical embryological investigations of His (1879, 1890) which revealed that axons developed as extended outgrowths from developing neuroblasts. Despite this evidence, axon growth down the nerve was not the preferred explanation at that time. This was accorded to the peripheral theory which postulated that surviving cells along the separated distal length of the nerve elaborated new axons and myelin sheaths which later became attached to surviving nerve fibres in the proximal nerve stump. This was consistent with the belief that nerve fibres developed embryologically from the alignment and union of individual cells, a view supported by the cellular theory enunciated by Schwann in 1839. This claim

carried great weight despite the convincing evidence to the contrary provided by His.

The peripheral theory also received support from experimental investigations in which the speed of recovery following nerve reunion was interpreted as confirming this concept (Schiff 1854; Bruch 1855; Lents 1856; Philipeaux and Vulpian 1859). More importantly, the theory received considerable and continuing support from clinical surgery. Reference has been made earlier to the return to favour of nerve suture, largely as the result of Cruikshank's pioneering investigations. With the case for nerve suture securely established, accounts of nerve repair with so-called successful results appeared in increasing numbers (Flourens 1828, Baudens 1836, Paget 1863, Laugier 1864, Létiévant 1873, Langenbeck 1876, 1883, Heuter 1883, Markoe 1885, Rawa 1885). In many of these patients the onset of recovery was reported as occurring with such rapidity as to exclude axon growth as the responsible mechanism. However, with the advantage of hindsight, it seems clear that such rapid recoveries were almost certainly due to the misinterpretation of clinical findings and were, in fact, unrelated to events taking place in the sutured nerve (Chapters 32 and 33). In any event, regardless of misleading errors introduced in this way, this interpretation continued to dominate laboratory and clinical thinking until the close of the century. It was strongly supported by Kennedy in a comprehensive critical review of the subject in 1897 and 1898, and as late as 1901 by Balance and Stewart in their influential publication *The Healing of Nerves* when they unhesitatingly declared their adherence to the peripheral theory.

However, the tide was about to turn again and a strongly held theory superceded. This might have happened earlier if accounts of Cajal's discoveries on nerve regeneration had not been confined to the little-read Spanish literature. In his publications, he recorded observations which convincingly and conclusively showed that regenerating axons were outgrowths of single neurons and that they did not originate in cell chains or protoplasmic bridges as claimed by adherents of the peripheral theory. His views became more widely known and accepted only in the first years of the 20th century. The peripheral theory was further disproved by Ross Harrison's (1910) transplantation studies on regenerating nerves in tadpoles which confirmed the correctness of the views expressed earlier by His and Cajal.

In his monumental and comprehensive writings on nerve growth and nerve regeneration at the turn of the century, Cajal advanced the hypothesis that a chemotropic substance was elaborated by target tissues that exerted an attractive and directional influence on growing axon tips. Soon after, Forssman (1900), applying this hypothesis to the growth of regenerating axons between the ends of a severed nerve, introduced the term neurotropism to the literature.

In respect to nerve repair, this concept of neurotropism was open to two interpretations. It could have been used to argue against the need for reuniting the nerve ends on the grounds that neurotropic influences would effect the desired nerve reunion and recovery. This would also explain the recovery recorded when a severed nerve had not been repaired. On the other hand, the concept could have been used to strengthen the case for nerve suture, since reuniting the nerve ends would enhance the neurotropic effect by bringing the proximal nerve end to the source of the stimulus.

This pro and con argument never arose because Cajal's hypothesis remained buried in the Spanish literature and by the time it did surface it could have applied equally to the two theories of nerve regeneration referred to earlier and so would have elicited little further interest.

The realisation that neurotropism might hold the key to the quality of functional recovery after nerve repair, and the manner in which it could do so, came only 50 years later. This subject is of such importance to nerve repair that a special chapter is devoted to it (p. 115).

At this point it is of interest to assemble the principal legacies which laboratory workers and clinicians of the nineteenth century passed on to the next century.

1. The value of nerve suture was firmly established and the procedure fully vindicated.

   Various methods were devised for approximating and reuniting the ends of a severed nerve but they all had one common and single objective, namely to restore nerve trunk continuity in the mistaken belief that nature and nerve regeneration would then do the rest. Such expectations were not unreasonable because, at that time, the internal structure of nerves was unexplored territory and no information was available on the complex anatomical arrangements and physiological mechanisms that play such a decisive role in nerve regeneration. Providing this essential information has been the major contribution of the 20th century to nerve repair.

2. The neurone doctrine was confirmed and the reticular theory convincingly disproved.

3. The recovery following nerve repair was shown to be the result of axon regeneration as represented by the continuous growth of axon tips down the nerve, thereby reconstituting new axon pathways to the periphery.

4. Confirmation of the existence of a chemotropic factor, elaborated in the distal stump of a severed nerve, that assisted recovery by attracting regenerating axon tips to and into the nerve stump.

5. The events of the 19th century also offered convincing proof of the substantial contributions that laboratory techniques and investigations can make to the practice of the healing services.

6. The clear demonstration of the need to create and maintain a continuing dialogue between laboratory scientists and clinicians in order to foster the exchange of experiences, thoughts and ideas between groups that would not otherwise come together. This is necessary in order to ensure that each is kept informed about what the other is attempting to do, thereby avoiding unnecessary delays in the application of new knowledge to clinical situations and problems.

THE 20th CENTURY

The situation prior to and during World War I was one in which nerves were still regarded as simple cord-like structures. These, when severed, were repaired by simply restoring continuity in the expectation that nerve regeneration would then restore function. While it is true that for most severed tissues and structures, once some form of mechanical repair has been effected, natural processes attend to the return of function, the surgeon failed to appreciate that he could expect no such reward for his services in the case of nerve repair. That factors far more complex than the simple restoration of nerve trunk continuity and nerve regeneration were involved was not even suspected.

Though the 1914–1918 war years brought a sharp increase in the numbers of nerve injuries, the wounded were not segregated for special consideration and attention, nor was the situation one to encourage research into improving the generally poor results of nerve repair.

The most serious problem posed by these battle injuries was the size of the gaps to be closed in order to effect end-to-end union of the nerve ends. These gaps were much greater than those seen in civilian practice because of:

1. the greater destructive effects on tissues of missile wounding, and
2. prolonged wound infection which increased the amount of nerve tissue requiring resection at the nerve ends before reaching tissue favourable for repair. This, in turn, greatly increased the gap to be reduced in order to reunite the nerve ends.

The disastrous record of nerve grafting to close large gaps left the surgeon with no option other than to employ extreme measures to restore nerve trunk continuity. This more often than not subjected both the nerve and the suture line to considerable tension either at the time of the repair or post-operatively. As a consequence, suture line failure was common and the overall results of repair under such adverse conditions were decidedly poor.

What lessons had been learned during the war years were soon forgotten as surgeons returned to civilian practice and patients with nerve injuries not only declined in numbers but were also widely scattered among the surgical profession. As a result, these patients never accumulated in suf-

ficient numbers in any one clinic or consulting room to excite the investigational instincts of the surgeon. Infection remained a problem, nerves were still regarded as simple cord-like structures, and procedures to close large gaps under considerable tension were still preferred to nerve grafting. Under these conditions it should come as no surprise that the results of nerve repair continued to be disappointing.

However, towards the end of this period there emerged the first of the serious attempts to seek a clearer understanding of the complex processes involved in nerve regeneration and nerve repair.

As with so many advances in the surgery of trauma, it was World War II which set the stage for the first great break-through in nerve repair. Importantly, those war years again saw the accumulation of even greater numbers of servicemen with peripheral nerve injuries but, on this occasion, with a difference. For the first time these patients were referred to special centres created for the specific purpose of ensuring that they would not only receive specialist attention but would also be available for thorough investigation and study.

The means of effectively controlling wound infection by antibiotics was an outstanding achievement, while studies at a basic level revealed the complexities of the internal structure of nerves and with it came the realisation that the restoration of continuity is only the first step in the restoration of function. The latter was now shown to be influenced by a host of complex and variable structural arrangements and physiological processes operating central to, at and below the site of the repair. Of particular importance among the many factors which were found to complicate and adversely affect recovery were those that resulted in both disorderly regeneration and the loss of regenerating axons at the suture line, so that the restored pattern of innervation was both imperfect and incomplete in comparison with the original.

From these studies a clearer picture of the central objective of nerve repair finally emerged, namely to reduce the loss of axons which occurs during regeneration and to assist regenerating axons to re-establish *useful* functional connections with the periphery, so that the new pattern of innervation approximated as closely as possible to the original. This, in turn, laid the foundations for the development of procedures and techniques directed to these ends. Innovatory amongst these was the suggestion that microsurgical techniques might be used to improve the repair of severed nerves (Sunderland 1945, 1953). However, for various reasons surgeons were slow to recognise the significance of the data emerging from basic studies and to take advantage of information made available from this source. It was not until the 1960s that the feasibility of employing microsurgical techniques in the repair of nerves was taken up and applied clinically.

Briefly, the transition from the period of enlightenment to the period of technical achievement and exploitation came:

1. when the significance of the data made available from basic studies finally filtered through to the clinical level;
2. with the realisation that nerve repair involved far more than the simple restoration of nerve trunk continuity;

3. with the recognition that the repair of nerves had become a highly specialised undertaking, demanding a detailed knowledge of the internal anatomy of nerves and regenerative processes and calling for great technical skill and experience, meticulous observance of atraumatic techniques, and the use of operative methods, instruments and suture materials specially designed for this type of work;
4. with the application of microsurgical techniques to the repair of nerves;
5. with the emergence, in particular, of hand and plastic surgery as recognised specialties and, with this, a more adventurous approach to the treatment of mutilating injuries.

It is these developments that form the background and substance of the contents of this section of the book.

REFERENCES

Apathy S 1897 Das leitende Element des Nervensystems und seine topographischen Beziehungen zu den Zellen. Mittheilungen aus dem Zoologischen Station zu Neapel. 12: 495

Arneman J 1787 Versuche über die Regeneration der Nerven. Vandenhoeck et Ruprecht. Göttingen

Avicenna (980–1037) See Greener

Ballance C A, Stewart P 1901 The healing of nerves. Macmillan, London

Baudens J B L 1836 Clinique des Plaies d'Armes à Feu. Baillière, Paris

Bethe A 1901 Ueber die Regeneration peripherischen Nerven. Neurologisches Zentralblatt 20: 720

Bruch C 1855 Über die Regeneration durchschnittenen nerven. Zeitschrift für Wissenschaftliche Zoologie 6: 135

Cruickshank W 1795 Experiments on the nerves, particularly on their reproduction and on the spinal marrow of living animals. Philosophical Transactions of the Royal Society of London 80: 177

Deiters O F K 1865 Untersuchungen über Gehirn und Rückenmark des Menschen und der Säugetiere. Vieweg, Braunschweig

de la Roche F G 1778 Analyse des fonctions du système nerveux. Villard and Nouffer, Geneva

Dutrochet R J H 1824 Recherches anatomiques et physiologiques sur la structure intime des animaux et végétaux et sur leur mobilité. Baillière, Paris

Ferrara G 1608 Nuova Selva di Cirurgia Divisia in tre Parti. S. Combi, Venice

Flourens P 1828 Expériences sur la réunion on cicatrisation des plaies de la Moelle épinere et des nerfs. Annales des Sciences Naturelles 13: 113

Forssman J 1900 Zur Kenntniss des Neurotropismus. Ziegler's Beiträge zur Pathologische Anatomie 27: 407

Galen C Quoted by Leonard of Bertapaglia

Gerlach J 1858 Microskopische Studien aus dem Gebiete der menschlichen Morphologie. Enke Erlangen

Golgi C 1883 Recherches sur l'histologie des centres nerveux. Archives Italianne de Biologie 3: 285

Golgi C 1886 Studi sulla fina anatomia degli organi centrali del sistema nervoso. Hoepli, Milan

Golgi C 1907 La dottrina del neurone. Teoria e fatti. Archivio di Fisiologia 4: 187

Guy de Chauliac On wounds and fractures. Translated and published by W A Brennan 1923

Greener O C 1930 A treatise on the Canon of Medicine of Avicenna, incorporating a translation of the First Book. Luzac, London

Haighton J 1795 An experimental enquiry concerning the reproduction of nerves. Philosophical Transactions of the Royal Society London. 85: 519

Harrison R G 1910 The outgrowth of the nerve fiber as a mode of protoplasmic movement. Journal of Experimental Zoology 9: 787

Held H 1897 Beiträge zur Struktur der Nervenzellen und ihrer Fortsätze. 2° Abhandlung. Archiv für Anatomie Physiologie und Wissenschaftliche Medizin. Anatomische Abteilung Supplement Band S 204

Held H 1907 Kristische Bemerkungen zu der Verteidigung der Neuroblasten — und der Neuronentheorie durch R y Cajal. Anatomischer Anzeiger 30: 369

Held H 1909 Dei Entwicklung des Nervengewebes bei den Wirbeltieren. Barth, Leipzig

Held H 1929 Die Lehre von den Neuronen und vom Neurocytium und ihre heutiger Stand. Fortschritte der naturwissenschaftliche Forschungen. Neue Folge Heft 8

Heuter K 1883 Die allgemeine Chirurgie. Vogel Verlaz, Leipzig

His H 1897 Ueber die Anfänge des peripherischen Nervensystems. Archiv für Anatomie Physiologie und wissenschalftliche Medizin. Anatomische Abteiling S 456

His W 1890 Histogenese und Zusammenhang der Nervenelemente. Archiv für Anatomie, Physiologie und wissenschaftliche Medizin. Anatomische Abteilung Supplementum Band S 95

Kennedy R 1897 On the regeneration of nerves. Philosophical Transactions. Royal Society London 188: 257

Kennedy R 1898 Degeneration and regeneration of nerves: an historical review. Proceedings Royal Philosophical Society Glasgow 29: 193

Kölliker R A 1853 Manual of human histology. Translated and edited by G Buck & T Huxley. Sydenham Society, London

Kölliker R A 1861 Entwicklungsgeschichte des Menschen und der höheren Tiere. Engelman, Leipzig

Ladenheim J C 1989 Leonard of Bertapaglia: On nerve injuries and skull fractures. Futura, New York

Lanfranchi G 1934 In: Garrison F H An introduction to the history of medicine, 3rd edn. Saunders, Philadelphia, p 145

Langenbeck B 1876 Verhandlungen der deutschen Gesellschaft für Chirurgie (Fünfter Congress), p 111

Langenbeck B 1883 Secundäre directe Ischiadicusnacht $2\frac{1}{2}$ Jahre nach der Verletzung. Deutsche Zeitschrift für Chirurgie 23: 341

Laugier C 1864 Séance de l'Académie des Sciences (Paris) Gazette des Hôpitaux 37: 297

Lents E 1856 Beiträge zur Lehre von der Regeneration durchschnittenen Nerven. Zeitschrift für wissenschaftliche Zoologie 7: 145

Leonard of Bertapaglia. On nerve injuries and skull fractures. Translated by Ladenheim J C. Futura, New York, 1989

Létiévant E 1873 Traité des Sections Nerveuses. Baillière, Paris

Marchi V, Alghieri G 1885 Sulle degenerazione discendenti consecutive a lesioni della corteccia cerebrale. Revista sperimentale di freniatria e medicina legale delle alienazioni Mentale 11: 492

Markoe T M 1885 Secondary nerve suture. Annals of Surgery 2: 181

Müller J 1838 Elements of physiology. Translated by W Baly. Taylor & Walton, London

Nissl F 1894 Uber eine neue Untersuchungsmethode des Centralorgans speziell zur Feststellung der Localisation der Nervenzellen. Neurologisches Zentralblatt 13: 507

Paget J 1863 Lectures on surgical pathology delivered at the Royal College of Surgeons. Revised and edited by W Turner. Longman, London, 1: 282

Paul of Aegina. The seven books. Translated by F Adams. Sydenham Society, London, 1844–1847

Philipeaux J, Vulpian A 1859 Note sur des expériences démontrant que les nerfs séparés des centres nerveux peuvent après être altérés complètement se regénérer tout en demeurant isolés de ces centres et recouvrir leurs propriétés physiologiques. Comptes Rendus Hebdomadaires des Séances de l'Acadèmie des Sciences 59: 507

Prévost J L 1827 Über die Wiedererzeugung des nervengebewebes. Froriep's neue Notizen 17: 113

Ramon y Cajal S 1908 Studien über Nervenregeneration. Leipzig

Ramon y Cajal S 1913–14 Estudios sobre la degeneración y regeneración del sistema nervosa. Madrid

Ramon y Cajal S 1928 Degeneration and regeneration of the nervous system. Translated and edited by R M May. Oxford University Press, London

Ramon y Cajal S 1952 Histologie du Système Nerveux de l'homme & des vertébrés. Instituo Ramon y Cajal, Madrid

Ramon y Cajal S 1954 Neuron theory or reticular theory Translated by M U Purkiss & C A Fox. Instituto Ramon Y Cajal, Madrid

Ranvier L A 1875 Traité Technique d'Histologie. Savy, Paris

Rawa A L 1885 Ueber die nervennaht. Wiener medizinische Wochenschrift 35: 368

Remak R 1838 Observationes anatomicae et microscopicae de systematis nervosi structura. Reimerianis Berolini

Rhazes. Quoted in Leonard of Bertapaglia

Schiff M 1854 Sur la régénération des nerfs et sur les altérations qui surviennent dans les nerfs paralysés. Comptes Rendus Hebdomadaires des Séances de l'Académie des Sciences 38: 448

Schwann T 1839 Mikroskopische Untersuchungen über die Übereinstimmung in der Struktur und dem Wachstum der Tiere und Pflanzen Reimer, Berlin

Steinrück C O 1838 De nervorum regeneratione Decker Berlin. Abstracted in Schmidt's Jahrbücher der in- und ausländischen gesammtem Medicin 1840 26: 102

Sunderland S 1945 The intraneural topography of the radial, median and ulnar nerves. Brain 68: 243

Sunderland S 1953 Funicular suture and funicular exclusion in the repair of severed nerves. British Journal of Surgery 40: 580

Virchow R 1846 Die krankhaften Geschwulste. Hirschwold, Berlin

Waldeyer W 1891 Über einige neuere Forschungen im Gebiete der Anatomie des Zentralnervensystems. Deutsche medizinische Wochenschrift 17: 1213, 1244, 1267, 1287, 1331, 1352.

Waller A V 1850 Experiments on the section of the glosso-pharyngeal and hypoglossal nerves of the frog, and observations of the alterations produced thereby in the structure of their primitive fibres. Philosophical Transactions. Royal Society of London 40: 423

Waller A V 1852 Nouvelle méthode anatomique pour l'investigation du système nerveux. Georgi, Bonn

Waller A V 1892 Nouvelles recherches sur la régénération des fibres nerveuses. Comptes Rendus Hebdommadaires des Séances de l'Académie des Sciences 34: 675

Weigert C 1882 Über eine neue Untersuchungsmethode des centralnervensystems. Zentralblatt für medizinischer Wissenschaften. 20: 753

Weigert C 1885 Eine Verbesserung der Haematoxylin — Blutlaugensalz-methode für das Centralnervensystem. Fortschritte der Medizin 3: 236

37. The principles of non-surgical treatment

Despite recent work on axon regeneration (Chapter 15) there are no proven measures or procedures that will hasten the onset of regeneration or accelerate the growth of regenerating axons along the nerve. Treatment is, therefore, confined to preventing the development of those complications at the periphery, due directly or indirectly to denervation, that will seriously threaten the restoration of function in structures that will ultimately be reinnervated. This introduces for consideration both the objectives of treatment and the procedures directed to achieving them.

Bearing in mind the prior needs of co-existing injuries to other structures, such treatment should be commenced immediately the affected parts are accessible and it is permissable to proceed.

The simplest therapeutic procedures that satisfy well established principles are just as effective as those requiring more complicated, time demanding and costly equipment.

To be effective physiotherapy requires the continuing co-operation and interest of the patient. It is difficult to justify persevering with treatment in a patient who is lacking in intelligence, devoid of any motivation or interest, and indifferent to the outcome.

The patient should be encouraged and trained to become his own therapist. Treatment requiring supervision and a demanding routine should not be continued any longer than is absolutely necessary.

There will be few occasions when supervised treatment should be extended beyond 3 months after the onset of recovery and then only in the case of the hand.

Because a muscle may act as a prime mover, antagonist, synergist or fixator, it may take on different roles in different movements and in this way contribute to many more voluntary acts than are usually ascribed to it when only its function as a prime mover is under consideration. In this way the most unexpected muscles may be trained to compensate for muscles that have ceased to act. This means that:

a. muscles whose nerve supply is intact may perform movements that are so similar to those normally produced by the paralysed muscle that involvement of the latter may escape recognition, and
b. retraining may be used to exploit the supplementary actions of some muscles in order to compensate for others that have been permanently paralysed.

Objectives. The key objectives of treatment are the maintenance of denervated muscles, joints and periarticular structures, and skin in an optimal condition pending reinnervation, and the prevention of deformities. After the reappearance of voluntary movements, the emphasis changes to remedial training directed to increasing the range, power and quality of integrated movements, and the range and quality of discriminative sensibility and the stereognostic sense.

Procedures. The care of denervated tissues involves a balanced and judicious combination of two contrasting procedures. On the one hand, immobilisation in a functionally sound position is required to prevent the formation of deformities and to maintain paralysed muscles in a position of rest. On the other, massage and exercises are required to promote blood flow through muscles and to preserve the free movement of tendons and joints.

THE CARE AND TREATMENT OF DENERVATED MUSCLES

Here treatment is directed to the preservation of denervated muscle tissue. This is accomplished by:

1. Protecting the affected parts from exposure to cold which aggravates the degenerative changes occurring in denervated skin and muscle.
2. Protecting paralysed muscles from injury because denervation renders them particularly sensitive to trauma. Paralysed muscles should at all times be handled gently, particularly during massage and passive exercises, and splinting should be carefully supervised to prevent damage from pressure and friction.
3. Stimulating the arterial, venous and lymphatic circulation through the denervated regions. This reduces the incidence and severity of trophic changes, prevents oedema and generally improves the nutrition of tissues. Vascular and lymphatic stasis occur with:

   a. the inactivity imposed by the paralysis of muscles and/or immobilisation of the part;
   b. dysfunction in denervated vasomotor systems;
   c. exposure to cold, and
   d. damage to the major vessels to the limb where this is an additional complicating factor.

Conditions that reduce blood flow through denervated muscles accelerate atrophy, and encourage muscle fibre degeneration, fibrosis and the development of contractures. Vascular and lymphatic stasis, and the nutritional changes to which they give rise, also lead to an increase in tissue fluid which, as the result of inactivity, accumulates in tissue spaces. From there it slowly gravitates to, and collects in, dependent regions. This fluid softens poorly nourished tissues that subsequently undergo fibrosis and develop adhesions. Tendon sheaths become thickened and involved in adhesions that restrict their free running. Adhesions in fascial planes impair the free movement of muscles over one another, and intramusclar fibrosis results in muscle contractures. The organisation of diffused blood and any inflammatory reaction add to these complications.

4. Maintaining paralysed muscles at rest and protecting them from being overstretched or permanently shortened by interstitial fibrosis. The paralysis of muscles leaves other forces unopposed that tend to deform the system. Forces released in this way are represented by gravity, pressures and tensions acting externally on the parts (e.g. incorrect splinting), and internal forces in the form of muscle spasm and muscle imbalance from the overaction of normally innervated antagonists. The influence of gravity tends to be overlooked but should be counteracted in every case. Unless these deforming forces are neutralised they result in:

   a. lengthening of paralysed muscles;
   b. shortening of their antagonists;
   c. joint deformity.

If the deforming forces and the changes to which they give rise are not corrected, further complications appear in the form of fibrosis, muscle contractures, joint stiffness and ankylosis. These impart a permanency to the changes that prejudices the restoration of function following satisfactory reinnervation.

For some paralysed muscles, overstretching may be periodically relieved by the action of gravity and the activity of unaffected muscles. Where no such natural relieving mechanism is available, failure to ensure relaxation by suitable splinting will inevitably lead to overstretching of paralysed muscles by the action of unopposed forces. This, in turn, leads to the development of irreducible contractures in the now shortened antagonists and to the lengthening of those that are paralysed. On the other hand, if a paralysed muscle is left immobilised in a shortened position, the ensuing fibrosis will fix it in that position while the now overstretched antagonists will remain lengthened.

In either event, following satisfactory reinnervation, the range of movement possible will be restricted and impaired.

Joints should always be immobilised in a position of rest and relieved at regular intervals to allow paralysed muscles to be passively exercised.

5. Preventing the development of joint deformities and their fixation by muscle contractures and ankylosis. Deformities develop as the parts take up a position which is determined by the redistribution of forces introduced by the paralysis of some muscles, the unopposed action of others and the continuing influence of gravity.

An abnormal position may be unaffected by surviving movements and, if left uncorrected, the periarticular changes and shortened antagonists ultimately convert a reducible into a fixed deformity.

6. Accelerating the restoration of function and power in muscles after reinnervation.
7. Assisting re-education in the absence of complete reinnervation.
8. Planning and conducting re-educational training programmes directed to improving the quality of the sensory recovery and to offsetting the effects of any residual sensory deficit.

All these therapeutic activities demand skilled supervision for several hours daily and the untiring interest of the patient in his own treatment and welfare.

Procedures directed to maintaining denervated muscles in an optimum condition so that following reinnervation they will function efficiently

These cover a wide range but, in general, are based on the need to maintain an effective blood flow through the muscles, to protect their fibres from cold and mechanical injury and to preserve a full range of movements at joints.

Massage and movement

1. Movement is the first essential in maintaining the blood supply to, and circulation through, the affected parts. Massage and movement in the form of passive and active exercises improve the circulation by assisting venous return and by reducing venous and lymphatic stasis and any associated oedema. The pull on paralysed muscles within their fascial sheaths by the contractions of neighbouring muscles also assists in driving blood from them.
2. Constantly maintaining a full range of passive movement at all joints assists in preventing tendons from becoming adherent and counteracts the development of crippling contractures, deformities and joint stiffness.

It is important that the massage and movements should be gentle, because denervated muscle fibres are particularly susceptible to mechanical injury which accelerates atrophy and leads to degeneration.

Warmth

Exposure to cold makes additional demands that cannot be satisfied by an already impaired circulation. As a result, denervated muscle fibres suffer more acutely, and more fail to survive and are replaced by fibrous tissue. In applying heat to improve the circulation precautions should be taken to ensure that insensitive regions do not sustain thermal injury.

Bandaging

Where appropriate, compression bandaging may be used to limit venous congestion, oedema, and effusions. This bandaging should be sufficiently firm to control any swelling but not too tight to still further embarrass an already defective circulation.

Electrotherapy

While this does not entirely prevent denervation muscle atrophy, it is said to slow the process. It is doubtful if anything is to be gained by continuing electrical stimulation beyond the onset of voluntary motor recovery because, from this time onwards, muscle contractions induced by voluntary effort are far more effective in restoring muscle power than contractions produced artificially.

The role of electrotherapy in treatment is discussed in Chapter 28.

Procedures to maintain paralysed muscles in a position of rest and to prevent the formation of deformities

Splints and mechanical appliances are used to assist motor recovery by:

1. resting paralysed muscles in a position to prevent overstretching;
2. preventing or correcting deformities which, if left untreated, would become fixed by ankylosis and muscle contractures, and
3. supporting joint systems that have been left unprotected and weakened by the paralysis of supporting muscles and the softening of ligaments and capsular tissues.

In this way both muscles and joints are maintained under optimal conditions pending re-innervation and the restoration of function.

The splint

In order to achieve the desired objectives, splints or related appliances should meet the following requirements:

1. They should be of a design that meets the particular needs of each patient. They should be properly applied and their use carefully supervised.
2. Splinting should be dynamic and not static. The device should:

   a. permit free movements at the joints by not hindering the activity of normally innervated muscles and, therefore, the voluntary use of the part;
   b. prevent the unrelieved stretching of paralysed muscles and the development of deformities. This is achieved by neutralising the unopposed action of antagonists and gravity.

3. Splinting should be reviewed at regular intervals and the splint modified as the occasion demands.

4. Splints should be constructed of materials that are light, durable, easily cleaned, and cheap to replace should this become necessary. Finally, there are those mechanical appliances and splints with spring devices that have certain advantages over the fixed mould. These are so designed that the spring device substitutes for the paralysed muscles. Mechanical devices that meet these requirements have been described by Wynn Parry and his associates (1970, 1973).

5. Regardless of the material used or the particular design selected, the splint should:

   a. be comfortable and easily managed by the patient;
   b. not press on soft tissues, particularly over bony areas and regions traversed by nerves, nor should it constrict paralysed muscles since these are unduly sensitive to trauma;
   c. support joints and muscles in such a way as to prevent the overstretching of paralysed muscles and the development of deformities. Muscles particularly at risk are those in which gravity and the unopposed action of strong antagonists lead to overstretching. Care should be taken, especially during the night, to ensure that paralysed muscles are retained in a slightly relaxed position. For example, the paralysed extensors of the foot in lateral popliteal nerve lesions are readily overstretched if the weight of bedclothing is allowed to force the foot into plantar flexion;
   d. be conveniently applied and easily removed, so that the affected regions can be freed at regular intervals for physiotherapy and other forms of treatment.

6. Splints should not interfere with the mobility of the digits. The importance of leaving the thumb and fingers supported but accessible for free and frequent manipulations cannot be overemphasised.

The position of immobilisation

From studies of the effects of muscle shortening and stretching on the changes occurring in paralysed and recovering muscles there is sufficient evidence to indicate that:

a. overstretching delays and limits the recovery of useful function following reinnervation. At the same time, immobilisation in an excessively relaxed position leads to interstitial fibrosis, contractures and permanent shortening;
b. careful and efficient splinting to ensure a neutral or slightly relaxed position for the paralysed muscles is the least damaging to muscle fibres.

The danger of unrelieved immobilisation

Immobilisation to prevent the overstretching of paralysed muscles and the development of deformities from the unopposed action of other forces should never be carried to excess. The harmful effects of prolonged and unrelieved immobilisation on muscles rendered inactive are discussed in Chapter 28. Immobilisation reduces blood flow and lymphatic drainage which, in turn, are partly if not solely responsible for:

1. increasing the severity of the atrophic processes and encouraging degeneration and fibrosis in denervated muscles;
2. delaying the onset and progress of recovery following reinnervation, and
3. favouring the development of tendon adhesions and periarticular fibrosis that restrict movement.

In order to counteract these adverse effects, splinting should not be too tight and the splint should be removed at frequent and regular intervals to permit massage, exercise and other appropriate remedial procedures aimed at improving the circulation through the denervated tissues. Muscles should not be immobilised for long periods. If extensive immobilisation of the limb is unavoidable then at least the thumb and fingers should be left accessible because the metacarpophalangeal and interphalangeal joints are especially liable to become stiff if they are kept

fixed, and stiff fingers are slow to regain their mobility. These conditions are easier to prevent than to cure and it is well to remember that a deformed and rigid hand or foot will not function even if reinnervation is complete.

CARE AND TREATMENT OF JOINTS AND PERIARTICULAR STRUCTURES

Involvement of the joint capsule and ligaments in the pathological processes introduced by denervation weakens joints and makes them less resistant to deforming forces. In the chronic stages, the changes take the form of fibrous ankylosis that results in joint stiffness or an irreducible deformity. In addition, sensory loss deprives the denervated regions of protective mechanisms, thereby rendering them more susceptible to trauma. Joint injury therefore occurs more frequently and easily when the joint and associated tissues are insensitive and have been weakened by softened ligaments and the paralysis of muscles. Such injuries increase the effusion of fluid in and about the joint and in this way aggravate fibrosis and the formation of restrictive adhesions.

The limitations on mobility imposed by these complications, and their adverse effect on the quality of the recovery that is possible following reinnervation, are frequently of a greater degree and importance than the actual paralysis of muscles.

Treatment should be directed to:

1. preserving a free and full range of joint movements and free running tendons by maintaining the mobility of tendons and joints so that the former are not allowed to become restricted by adhesions and the latter are prevented from becoming stiff and ankylosed. The importance is stressed of maintaining at all times a free and full range of movements within the limits imposed by any co-existing bone or joint injury;
2. supporting insensitive joint systems that have been weakened by the softening of ligaments and the paralysis of muscles. This is particularly important after sciatic and medial popliteal nerve lesions which

denervate the weight-bearing joints of the foot. The denervated foot deserves the same careful attention as the affected hand, for the deformities and disabilities of the foot that develop and persist as sequelae of nerve injury are difficult to correct;

3. preventing the development of irreducible joint deformities by a judicious combination of splinting, aimed at overcoming the action of unopposed antagonists, and exercises planned to maintain a full range of movement at the affected joints. While the development of deformities and their fixation should be prevented by appropriate splinting and physiotherapy, the dangers of unrelieved immobilisation should be emphasised for this is the most common cause of irreducible deformity formation, tendon adhesions and periarticular fibrosis.

THE CARE OF DENERVATED SKIN

Here treatment is directed to the preservation of denervated insensitive skin.

Insensitive skin is particularly vulnerable to injury, especially that of the hands and feet. The skin should be kept clean and protected from pressure, friction and contact with hot objects. Advice to the patient, though simple, is nevertheless important and should not be overlooked. The patient should be warned against the dangers of:

1. injury from handling hot and sharp objects;
2. even trivial injuries to the feet. The sole is dry as well as insensitive in sciatic and medial popliteal lesions. Shoes, conventional or surgical, should be comfortable and well fitting, and socks should not carry darns or rough soles which will rub on dry insensitive areas and damage them. The risk of burns from hot water and hot water bottles should be explained;
3. careless treatment of the nails which are common sites of trophic disturbances;
4. exposure to cold. This is particularly important in the case of the hands and feet, and when the circulation has been still further embarrassed by the ligation of the major arterial channel to the limb. The

affected hand should be protected with a glove or mitten; both the glove and the hand should be warmed before the glove is used;
5. incorrectly applied splinting that leads to pressure and friction.

MEASURES DIRECTED TO THE REFINEMENTS OF FUNCTIONAL RECOVERY. SENSORY RE-EDUCATION

Useful and purposeful voluntary movements require the integrated and co-ordinated action of many muscles working in groups and combinations, and functioning as prime movers, antagonists, synergists and fixators.

The proper performance of movements also depends on the orderly and well regulated manner in which muscle fibres within a muscle, and muscles within a functional group, are recruited and co-ordinated to perform the desired movement.

The regulatory mechanisms concerned with these activities are based on central patterning; the more precise and delicate the movement, the more complicated the action patterns involved. These patterns are established by previous training and practice, the time and effort spent in perfecting and reinforcing a movement determining the precision and skill with which it is performed.

The restoration of useful and purposeful movements clearly demands far more than the recovery of individual muscles, depending as it does on the restoration of those complex integrated, specialised and regulated patterns of activity, both motor and sensory, that obtained before the injury. The degree to which motor function is impaired is determined by the extent to which the patterns of innervation have been modified and disorganised by the nerve injury and during the course of regeneration.

So far, the emphasis has been on the restoration of motor function. However, proprioceptor feedback mechanisms play a key and essential role in the creation and subsequent control and regulation of voluntary movements. They keep the cortex continually informed of what is taking place at the periphery so that, where necessary, appropriate central adjustments can be made to ensure that the willed movement is performed smoothly and accurately.

A critical factor affecting the quality of motor recovery is, therefore, the extent to which sensory mechanisms are left defective by faulty sensory reinnervation. Thus much of a residual motor inco-ordination and clumsiness may be based on a sensory defect rather than muscle weakness. On the other hand, though the immobilised hand and digits can feel, localise and recognise simple stimuli, objects must be handled, as well as felt, in order to increase the range of discriminative sensibility and to permit the accurate identification of objects.

Finally, there is another side to sensation, namely sensibility itself. Providing anatomical sensory reinnervation has reached an appropriate level, remedial training programmes should be directed to increasing the range and quality of discriminative analysis and the stereognostic sense using simple repetitive exercises, first under visual guidance and then in its absence. In this way the patient learns to recognise and identify an altered profile of sensory impulses and to relate these new sensations to past experience.

Also worthy of note is the development and persistence in some patients of hyperalgesia and hyperpathia in the cutaneous field of the nerve that severely restrict the use of the hand or foot. This complication may require a programme of intensive desensitisation.

Measures aimed at hastening full restoration of function, as distinct from improving voluntary contractions in individual muscles, are concerned with those final processes on which satisfactory motor performance, and sensory discrimination and the stereognostic sense, depend. As we have seen, these represent the most complex aspect of recovery, involving as they do the restoration and reconditioning of intricate patterns of activity.

Programmes of sensory re-education directed to improving the quality of both motor and sensory function following nerve repair have made a late arrival in the therapeutic arena. Movements and motor function were the front runners and little regard was originally paid to the fundamental principle that motor and sensory functions are interdependent. This early neglect was reflected in the literature of the day. To the best of the author's knowledge the first writings in English devoted specifically to sensory re-education were those of Wynn Parry in 1966. Today the situation is very different. The importance of sensory re-education is now generally recognised and appreciated, and many articles and texts on the subject are now available (Wynn Parry 1966, 1973, 1986, Wynn Parry et al 1970, Weeks and Wray 1973, Dellon et al 1974, Almquist 1975, Fallet 1975, Mansat & Delprat 1975, Wynn Parry & Salter 1976, Dellon et al 1977, Maynard 1977, Bell 1978, Curtis 1978, Fess 1978, Curtis & Dellon 1980, Dellon 1980, 1981, Dellon & Jabaley 1982). In essence, the role of re-educational programmes is to train the patient to use to the greatest advantage what innervated tissue is available to him as the result of incomplete and imperfect reinnervation. In this respect it follows the fundamental principle that repetition and practice make perfect.

The most persistent and intensive treatment should be reserved for the hand, where this final phase of recovery demands all the refinements of physiotherapy and occupational therapy. No other part of the body possesses a greater range of purposive voluntary movements than does the hand and these may respond to remedial training to a remarkable degree. The methods employed include a wide range of remedial, re-educational and vocational exercises and counselling services that, basically, are planned to encourage the patient to obtain, by his own concentration and efforts, the widest possible range and variety of movements from his reinnervated muscles. In this respect perseverance and practice make perfect.

The complete and rapid recovery of motor skills is to be expected after first and second degree injuries where the pattern of innervation is not disturbed by the injury or by the regenerative processes associated with it. Difficulties arise when reinnervation is incomplete and defective. As a result, re-education, vocational training, and rehabilitation become more time consuming, difficult and often less rewarding exercises. The extent to which re-educational therapy can lead to central readjustments of a beneficial nature remains unclear, though there is good evidence that training may restore some original skills by utilising alternative pathways and readjusting central mechanisms.

THE DURATION OF TREATMENT

Treatment should be intensive in the initial stages, but when recovery is well advanced and the patient active, costly and time-consuming forms of physical therapy become an unnecessary luxury. By this time the average patient should have acquired sufficient knowledge of the elementary principles underlying the treatment of his condition to accept responsibility for those simple forms of therapy that exercise paresed muscles and prevent periarticular adhesions and fibrosis. Excluding the exceptional case, these conditions obtain in all patients with first and second degree injuries.

However, the situation is very different following nerve repair where the onset of recovery is delayed, rarely progresses regularly and uninterruptedly, and the eventual functional outcome is unpredictable. In the initial stages treatment is directed to maintaining the denervated parts in the best possible condition pending their reinnervation and in preventing the formation of restrictive adhesions and joint deformities. For these reasons it is necessary after nerve repair to persevere with supervised treatment over longer periods.

Regarding supervised programmes of sensory re-education, there is no point in commencing these until the functional outcome has become clearer and motor and sensory function have recovered to a degree that makes the effort worth while.

How long should such treatment be continued from the time of its inception? Supervised programmes of sensory re-education cannot go on forever bearing in mind costs, the demands on the time and effort of both patient and therapist, and its relevance beyond a certain point in time. Moreover, not all patients are suitable for intensive sensory re-educational training. Here the patient is all important, his motivation, intelligence, willingness to learn and perseverance. The price of sustained improvement is constant practice, for it is a matter of common knowledge that what is gained is so easily and rapidly lost by neglect and indifference. Supervised treatment should be limited to less than 6 months depending on the circumstances. An integral and important segment of the re-educational process should be to train the patient to be his own therapist.

THE RESIDUAL DISABILITY

The residual disability that persists when regeneration and the restoration of function fall far short of completion may be sufficiently severe and disabling to require further treatment. This raises for consideration such matters as the use of corrective mechanical devices, tendon transplantation and other reconstructive procedures, and even the question of amputating a severely and permanently denervated limb. The corrective and reconstructive procedures of plastic and orthopaedic surgery are not, however, the concern of this presentation. For this information the reader is referred to standard texts devoted to those subjects.

REFERENCES

Almquist E E 1975 The effect of training on sensory function. In: Michon J, Moberg E (eds) Traumatic nerve lesions of the upper limb. Churchill Livingstone, Edinburgh, p 53

Bell J A 1978 Sensibility evaluation. In: Hunter J M, Schneider L H, Mackin E J, Bell J A (eds) Rehabilitation of the hand. Mosby, St Louis

Bell J A 1983 Sensibility testing: state of the art. In: Hunter J M, Schneider L H, Mackin E J, Callahan A D (eds) Rehabilitation of the hand, 2nd edn. Mosby, St Louis

Curtis R M 1978 Sensory re-education after peripheral nerve injury. In: Fredrick S, Brody G S (eds) Symposium on the neurological aspects of plastic surgery. Mosby, St Louis, p 47

Curtis R M, Dellon A L 1980 Sensory re-education after peripheral nerve injury. In: Omer G, Spinner M (eds) Management of peripheral nerve injuries. Saunders, Philadelphia, p 769

Dellon A L 1980 Evaluation of sensibility and re-education of sensation. In: Mansat M (ed) Proceedings: Symposium on Upper Extremity Sensory Problems, June 1980

Dellon A L 1981 Evaluation of sensibility and re-education of sensation in the hand. Williams & Wilkins, Baltimore

Dellon A L, Jabaley M E 1982 Re-education of sensation in the hand following nerve suture. Clinical Orthopaedics 163: 75

Dellon A L, Curtis R M, Edgerton M T 1971 Re-education of sensation in the hand following nerve injury. Journal of Bone and Joint Surgery 53A: 813

Dellon A L, Curtis R M, Edgerton M T 1974 Re-education of sensation in the hand following nerve injury. Plastic and Reconstructive Surgery 53: 297

Dellon A L, Curtis R M, Edgerton M T 1977 Program for sensory re-education in the hand following nerve injury. In: Marshall E (ed) Hand rehabilitation. Sammon, Brookfield, p 110

Fallet G H 1975 Physiotherapy and functional rehabilitation after lesions of the peripheral nerves. In: Michon J,

Moberg E (eds) Traumatic nerve lesions of the upper limb. Churchill Livingstone, Edinburgh, p 55

Fess E E, Harmon K S, Strickland J W et al 1978 Evaluation of the hand by objective measurement. In: Hunter J M, Schneider L H, Mackin E J et al (eds) Rehabilitation of the hand. Mosby, St Louis

Mansat M, Delprat J 1975 Reeducation de la sensibilité de la main. Annales Medecine Physique 18: 527

Maynard J 1977 Sensory re-education after peripheral nerve injury In: Hunter J, Mackin E, Schneider L et al (eds) Rehabilitation of the hand. Williams & Wilkins, Baltimore

Weeks P M, Wray C B 1973 Management of acute hand injuries. Mosby, St Louis, p 302

Wynn Parry C B 1966 Rehabilitation of the hand, 1st edn. Butterworths, London

Wynn Parry C B 1966 Diagnosis and after-care of peripheral nerve lesions in the upper extremity. Journal of Bone and Joint Surgery 48A: 607

Wynn Parry C B 1973 Rehabilitation of the hand, 3rd edn. Butterworths, London

Wynn Parry C B 1986 Sensation. Journal of Bone and Joint Surgery 68B: 15

Wynn Parry C B, Salter M 1976 Sensory re-education after median nerve lesions. The Hand 8: 250

Wynn Parry C B, Harper D, Fletcher I et al 1970 New types of lively splints for peripheral nerve lesions affecting the hand. The Hand 2: 31

38. Neurolysis. Mobilisation. Transposition. Painful neuromas

These procedures may be necessary during the course of nerve repair. They may also be undertaken independently where an injured nerve is left in continuity but the integrity of nerve fibres is threatened, where recovery is arrested or prevented, and where a painful neuroma calls for surgical attention.

PART 1. NEUROLYSIS

The pathology, distribution and consequences of neural fibrosis are discussed in Chapter 24, which should be consulted before reading this section.

Neurolysis, in one form or another, comes up for consideration in the surgical management of nerve injuries when troublesome neural fibrosis develops as a consequence of a nerve injury due to physical or chemical trauma, ischaemia or leprous neuritis.

Trauma of increasing severity affects in turn the tissues constituting the bed of the nerve, the superficial epineurium surrounding the nerve trunk, the interfascicular connective tissue and finally the perineurium and intrafascicular tissues.

Neurolysis is the process of freeing the nerve from its bed by removing restrictive adhesions attaching it to surrounding structures, and by resecting constrictive scar tissue from around and within the nerve.

The rationale of neurolysis is generally believed to be the freeing of nerve fibres from the constrictive effect of fibrous tissue that is responsible for preventing or arresting recovery, or for impairing or distorting conduction in nerve fibres. However, there is good reason for believing that fibrosis also impairs the blood supply to nerve fibres and therefore their nutrition (p. 217). This means that during neurolysis, nothing should be done that would further imperil the blood supply to the involved segment of the nerve.

Before proceeding to discuss this procedure attention is directed to certain fundamental principles that should be kept constantly in mind:

1. Neurolysis should always be performed under magnification.
2. Neurolysis should not be undertaken unless electrical stimulating and recording facilities are available for testing the status of nerve conduction through the affected segment.

   Before freeing the nerve trunk from constrictive scar tissue, the nerve should be stimulated proximal to the affected segment in order to ascertain if evoked potentials can be detected further distally or if there is any response in muscles innervated by the nerve. This is necessary for two reasons:

   a. Muscles that are not responding to voluntary effort may contract when the nerve trunk is directly stimulated. Such a finding is of prognostic significance, indicating as it does that immature regenerating axons have reached the periphery and that recovery is impending.
   b. Immature nerve fibres are especially vulnerable to mechanical deformation. In the process of freeing the nerve trunk from scar tissue, no matter how gently and carefully the separation is effected, immature fibres may suffer a transient conduction block. If stimulating the nerve trunk is deferred until after the nerve has been freed, it would then fail to reveal the presence of nerve fibres that

were conducting prior to neurolysis. Failure to elicit a response could then be erroneously interpreted as evidence pointing to failed regeneration.

3. The nerve is never approached directly through scar tissue but is first clearly identified above and below the site of involvement, following which it is then traced in both directions through this tissue. Branches given off in this region, or traversing the scar, should be identified and carefully preserved during the dissection.

4. Care should be taken at all stages to avoid damaging the blood supply to the nerve. The major nutrient vessels run in the superficial epineurium on the surface of the nerve and more deeply in the interfascicular epineurium. These, however, are the very tissues that the surgeon seeks to remove in external and internal neurolysis. It is not possible to remove all epineurial scar tissue without destroying the blood supply to the treated section of the nerve. There is, of course, always the possibility that revascularisation might be facilitated during healing by an ingrowth from neighbouring vessels.

5. Healing may result in the development of further troublesome fibrosis. The value of 'protective' wrappings to prevent this remains a controversial question. Such wrappings restrict revascularisation of the nerve from the tissues constituting the nerve bed. Moreover, the belief that such wrappings will prevent an ingrowth of damaging fibroblasts from external sources is misplaced because replacement fibrosis comes from epineurial fibroblasts left behind and these will be free to multiply within the wrapping. Such wrappings should, however, reduce the incidence of troublesome adhesions that reform to attach the nerve to its bed.

Wrappings, if they are used, should provide a minimal harmful reaction and should be reserved for the unusual case where local conditions, such as a poor bed, indicate that a covering is desirable. Thin silastic sheeting appears to be reasonably well tolerated by surrounding tissues and will remain the preferred material for the time being.

6. Good spontaneous recovery may still occur despite a high degree of scarring (Woodhall et al 1956).

7. Neurolysis is only justified if the replacement scar is less damaging than that originally present.

EXTERNAL NEUROLYSIS

Types of external neurolysis include:

Simple	The nerve trunk is freed by dissecting away adhesions attaching it to its bed and by separating it from surrounding scar tissue.
Epineurotomy	This involves splitting the thickened fibrotic superficial epineurium by a longitudinal incision with the intention of decompressing the contained fasciculi.
Epineurectomy	Resecting the thickened fibrotic superficial epineurium surrounding the nerve. It may be total or subtotal.

1. Where the damage is maximal in the surrounding tissues of the nerve bed, a minor nerve injury may become converted into something more serious as encircling scar tissue that follows healing contracts around the nerve, constricts it and impairs its blood supply.

2. Where the superficial epineurial tissue is involved the nerve trunk may be:

   a. encircled by scar tissue that is, however, loosely attached to its surroundings;
   b. firmly attached to its bed and neighbouring structures by adhesions, and/or
   c. buried in scar tissue.

This scar tissue may be localised or extend a variable, but sometimes considerable, distance along the nerve. It varies in density and may or may not constrict the nerve.

When the nerve is bound down by adhesions it is subject to repeated deformation during movements. Traction on the nerve produced in this way is a common source of pain which, if this be the sole cause of the pain, will be relieved by neurolysis.

Intact branches from proximal levels are often buried in the scar tissue which is matted about the parent trunk and these should be preserved. A neighbouring nerve trunk that has escaped injury may also be traversing the scar tissue and should be avoided when the damaged nerve is being freed. This critical phase of the operation is greatly facilitated by repeatedly exploring the tissue with the stimulator as dissection proceeds.

All stages of the procedure should be carried out with the greatest gentleness and care, due consideration being given to preserving the blood supply to the nerve trunk lest the isolated section be converted into an ischaemic strand of fibrous tissue. All bleeding and oozing points should be delicately but effectively controlled in order to prevent the re-formation of fibrous tissue and the creation of a new set of complications to threaten the nerve.

In certain regions nerve trunks are intimately associated with major vessels which may be involved with them in dense scar tissue through which fine vessels pass from the parent artery to the nerve. When freeing the nerve particular care should be taken to avoid damaging the artery. Initially neurolysis is confined to that aspect of the nerve which is not attached to the vessel. If the nerve and vessel are so firmly adherent that continued attempts to completely free the former would endanger the vessel then neurolysis should be terminated. If spontaneous recovery is not yet overdue, and the local pathology favours the possibility of it occurring, there should be no further interference with the nerve trunk. Only rarely will one be justified in sacrificing the main artery to the limb in order to preserve continuity of the nerve trunk. Where, on the other hand, the clinical findings and local conditions make surgical repair of the nerve mandatory, further treatment of the lesion then follows the general lines discussed in Chapter 42.

INTERNAL NEUROLYSIS

Types of internal neurolysis include:

Simple	Resecting the deep interfascicular epineurium with the object of releasing individual fasciculi from interfascicular scar tissue. It may be total or subtotal.
Fasciculotomy	Splitting the perineurium with the object of decompressing the fasciculus.
Fasciculectomy	Resecting the perineurium from around the fasciculus with the object of decompressing its contents.

Fasciculotomy and fasciculectomy are contraindicated, except in selected cases of leprous neuritis (Carayon 1962, Enna 1974, 1980).

Intrafascicular neurolysis, attempting to free individual nerve fibres from surrounding endoneurial scar tissue, is not a practicable procedure and should be discouraged.

The extent and density of intraneural scarring is not easy to estimate. However, the nature of the scar tissue revealed during external neurolysis usually gives some indication of the severity of the internal damage. Dense paraneural scar tissue that defies safe and easy dissection from the nerve bed and leaves the surface of the nerve with a thickened sheath is an ominous sign.

Intraneural fibrosis adversely affects nerve fibre function by:

1. constricting fasciculi and nerve fibres, thereby interfering with axon transport systems and blocking conduction in those fibres that are still in continuity or have regenerated;
2. interfering with nutrient vessels so that the blood supply to nerve fibres is impaired;
3. interposing unfavourable tissue between the intrafascicular capillaries and the Schwann cell basement membrane and in this way impairing the diffusion and transport of nutrient materials from capillaries to nerve fibres;
4. delaying and obstructing the advance of regenerating axons;

5. creating an impenetrable barrier to regenerating axons.

Internal neurolysis is directed to releasing individual fasciculi from interfascicular scar tissue in the expectation that this will restore the environment of nerve fibres to its original state.

With regard to internal neurolysis it should be noted that:

a. endoneurial fibrosis, which is particularly damaging, cannot be dealt with surgically;
b. breaching the perineurium represents a serious threat to the contents of a fasciculus. This allows, inter alia, epineurial fibroblasts to invade the fasciculus where thicker collagen fibres are deposited, thereby adding to the severity of the fibrosis. This is because epineurial fibroblasts produce thicker and more collagen fibres than do those of endoneurial tissue (p. 47);
c. decompressing constricted fasciculi in an attempt to improve an impoverished intrafascicular circulation is the most that can be expected of internal neurolysis. The procedure should, therefore, be confined to the careful removal of epineurial scar tissue;
d. internal neurolysis, even when confined to the epineurium, carries the following risks:

  i. destruction of fine fascicular intercommunications;
  ii. further damage to the intraneural nutrient vessels and to the microvascular circulation;
  iii. scar tissue may reform that is as harmful or more damaging than the original.

Technically, internal neurolysis is a more difficult and hazardous procedure than external neurolysis, involving as it does the removal of interfascicular scar tissue and the freeing of individual fasciculi.

Great care must be exercised at all stages of the dissection to avoid damaging the fine interfascicular communications which should not be mistaken for adhesions. Again, because many of these communications are of microscopic dimensions and are not always distinguishable from the scar tissue in which they are running, the risk of severing them is great indeed and the procedure should only be attempted under magnification. A further complication is introduced if the fine interfascicular vascular network is damaged to a degree that results in haemorrhage or ischaemia, both of which promote further scarring. However, improved microsurgical techniques have reduced, but not eliminated, the risks of internal neurolysis. The danger of destroying fascicular cross-communications and important intraneural vessels must be kept constantly in mind.

Whether gentle interfascicular injections of warm saline serve a useful purpose in breaking down constricting scar tissue and in reducing the adverse effects of epineurial scarring remains uncertain. Experience suggests that it is no substitute for careful and thorough intraneural exploration. Where the nature of internal scarring contra-indicates internal neurolysis, the intraneural injection of fluid will prove no more successful in disrupting scar tissue. On the other hand, the method may give some indication of the density and extent of the interfascicular scarring in that if the injection fluid does not readily enter the nerve, flow between bundles and separate them, then it is unlikely that internal neurolysis will prove more effective.

Under no circumstances should the *perineurial sheath* of fasciculi be breached nor should saline be injected inside the fasciculus. Both result in further damage to nerve fibres.

Intrafascicular scarring presents a serious problem, for it is evidence of a third degree injury of some severity in which scarring has followed the destruction of some axons and is, in turn, constricting and blocking the regeneration of others. Under these conditions internal neurolysis is of no value and, bearing in mind the conditions existing inside fasciculi, it may do further harm by aggravating the lesion and destroying additional numbers of surviving fibres.

Internal neurolysis is a potentially dangerous procedure. However, providing it is performed under magnification and is confined to the gentle and cautious removal of epineurial scar tissue with due regard to preserving the integrity of fasciculi and vessels, then it can be effective in recreating conditions that favour axon regeneration and the restoration of conduction in intact pathways. This, however, is not always possible and if the dissection is carelessly performed the effects can be catastrophic.

Intraneural neurolysis continues to be controversial. Gentili et al (1981) have reported that it is without adverse effects on nerve fibres. According to others the procedure confers no advantages on regeneration (Tazaki 1983, Mackinnon & Dellon 1986, 1988), while a third group has shown that such surgical intervention results in the recurrence of paraneural and intraneural fibrosis that may be even more of a problem than that which was originally present (Rydevik et al 1976, Frykman et al 1981, Lundborg 1988).

Clinically, internal neurolysis has its advocates (Matchabelli 1945, Bateman 1962, Carayon 1962, Brown 1969, 1972a,b, Brown 1970, Samii 1972, 1976, Bonola 1973, Curtis & Eversman 1973, Kahl et al 1973, Zhu et al 1985, Sakurai & Miyasaka 1986) but others have expressed reservations and cautionary views on the use of the procedure (Kline & Hackett 1975, Seddon 1975, Sunderland 1978, Wilgis 1979, Lundborg 1988).

Sakurai and Miyasaka (1986), from their study of neural fibrosis and neurolysis, decided that neurolysis of the brachial plexus should not go beyond the resection of external scar. Elsewhere, they favour internal neurolysis limited to a longitudinal epineurotomy in order to preserve blood vessels. It would appear from their account, however, that they would not hesitate to open the perineurium longitudinally.

HOW EFFECTIVE IS NEUROLYSIS

There are occasions when the onset of recovery is believed by the inexperienced to be unduly delayed. Premature exploration then reveals a nerve in continuity but involved at the site of wounding in scar tissue that appears to be constricting the nerve in a manner interpreted as being responsible for blocking conduction or hindering regeneration. When neurolysis is performed under these conditions and is immediately followed by recovery it is only natural that the improvement should be attributed to the surgical procedure which, it is assumed, has removed a barrier to axon regeneration and recovery.

The value of neurolysis in these cases is, however, questionable because the pattern of recovery associated with it is often one in which structures recover in a manner that is precisely the same as that observed when spontaneous regeneration takes place in the absence of any surgical interference. It is, therefore, possible that neurolysis in these cases has merely preceded delayed but normal regeneration that would, in any event, have resulted in recovery.

Many of the dramatic recoveries claimed for neurolysis are undoubtedly due to the mistaken belief that signs of spontaneous recovery are to be expected much earlier than is the case and that a delayed onset is indisputable evidence of a mechanical block in the form of constricting scar tissue. However, the onset of recovery in lesions in continuity may be delayed for quite long periods and then progress in a normal fashion to completion.

Thus regeneration may be well advanced but not evident at the time of the neurolysis. In Omer's (1974) experience neurolysis proved to be effective in 60% of the cases in which it was thought to be indicated. However, when those cases were excluded in which the neurolysis could have been a coincidental and unnecessary element in the subsequent recovery, the success rate was reduced to 36%.

Credit, however, can be claimed for neurolysis under the following conditions:

1. When recovery follows so quickly after the operation and involves such widespread areas of the peripheral field at or about the same time that it cannot be explained by the growth of axons to the periphery. This, generally speaking, is the pattern of recovery following a first degree or conduction block injury. This recovery may be evident within a few days of the operation. There are two explanations to account for this unusual pattern of recovery.

a. There are those first degree injuries that will show no recovery from simple conduction block until the agent responsible for the block has been removed. This is the type of injury that is classified as a complicated first degree injury in Chapter 25.

b. In the second group, the nerve has sustained

a second degree injury in which axons have already regenerated to the periphery, but conduction along the restored pathways is blocked by constricting scar tissue at the site of injury. Immediately this block is removed, conduction is rapidly restored in the affected fibres, and with it signs of recovery appear at the periphery. Such an explanation is supported by the finding that strong electrical stimulation above the scar may produce feeble muscular contractions at the periphery when no response can be obtained from voluntary effort. Some days after freeing the nerve, however, all muscles in the peripheral field are contracting voluntarily.

2. When spontaneous recovery is already long overdue at the time of the neurolysis and there is further delay subsequent to operation before signs of recovery appear, the onset and progress of the latter then being consistent with the growth of axons to the periphery following their release from constricting scar tissue by neurolysis.

3. Finally, there are those cases in which recovery that has been proceeding normally is suddenly arrested. Should neurolysis be followed by immediate resumption of improvement, then it is reasonable to attribute this to the neurolysis.

Frequently, uneasiness over what appears to be a long delay in the onset of recovery leads to exploration and neurolysis. When this is followed by orderly reinnervation that is undoubtedly due to axon growth, but which occurs too early to be accounted for by the regeneration of axons released from constriction, the neurolysis must be regarded as having been premature. Such a scenario indicates that spontaneous regeneration was already well advanced at the time of the operation but had not yet had sufficient time to reveal itself.

Two further points of interest relating to neurolysis are:

a. when neurolysis is responsible for the recovery it is usual for sensory fibres to recover before motor;
b. the aged are not excluded from the benefits of neurolysis (Levine & Spinner 1971).

ADVERSE EFFECTS OF NEUROLYSIS

Neurolysis carries the risks of:

1. injury to the nutrient arterial system of the nerve;
2. injury to fasciculi;
3. the division of fine intercommunications between fasciculi;
4. a recurrence of troublesome paraneural and intraneural fibrosis that is even more of a problem than that which was originally present.

THE INDICATIONS FOR NEUROLYSIS

Neurolysis is undertaken:

1. To relieve pain by removing:

   a. adhesions that fix the nerve to its bed so that the injured segment is pulled on during movements, and
   b. constricting scar tissue that is deforming nociceptor fibres and impairing their blood supply.

2. To assist regeneration and hasten recovery by freeing the nerve from adhesions and scar tissue that are believed to be obstructing or delaying the growth of regenerating axons or blocking conduction in nerve fibres.
3. When regeneration that is progressing satisfactorily is suddenly arrested.
4. When a nerve has been unnecessarily and prematurely explored and is found to be in continuity but surrounded by scar tissue. The opportunity should be taken to free the nerve. It is difficult in these cases to evaluate the contribution of the neurolysis to the spontaneous recovery that follows.
5. Following unsatisfactory recovery after nerve repair the question arises as to whether or not scar tissue involving the suture site is responsible for arresting recovery. The nerve should be explored and encircling scar tissue carefully removed.
6. In the treatment of leprous neuritis (Carayon 1962, Enna 1974, 1980).
7. To free the median nerve and its fasciculi from scar tissue in the carpal tunnel. Just

how effective is neurolysis in patients with median nerve involvement in the carpal tunnel syndrome? Clearly, having opened the tunnel, there is merit in delicately freeing the nerve from surrounding scar tissue and adhesions that attach it to neighbouring structures.

The median nerve receives no newly entering nutrient arteries in the carpal tunnel. Those present have all come from above and below the flexor retinaculum. Moreover the major nutrients are all contained in the superficial epineurium and interfascicular tissues and every care should be taken to preserve them when undertaking any surgical procedure on the nerve in the carpal tunnel.

If major longitudinally aligned nutrient arteries are a visible and prominent feature of the superficial epineurium after decompressing the canal by dividing the retinaculum, then it would be unwise to proceed to a total excision of superficial epineurial scar tissue. The procedure should be confined to freeing the nerve of adhesions and performing an epineurotomy, rather than an epineurectomy, the scarred sheath being split longitudinally in order to avoid cutting across major nutrient vessels.

It is the role of internal neurolysis in the treatment of this median nerve lesion that is in question. Curtis & Eversman in 1973 recommended the removal of the interfascicular scar in those patients in whom there was a well-established motor and sensory loss, the objective being to release the incarcerated fasciculi from the constrictive effects of scar tissue. Since then, the practice has been uncritically and rapidly adopted by many others. In many respects, internal neurolysis is based on a misunderstanding of the pathogenesis of this lesion. This is discussed in Chapter 17. Recapitulating, initially the lesion has a vascular basis and is not the result of the direct mechanical compression deformation of fasciculi and nerve fibres. It is caused by ischaemia consequent on compression forces developing within the carpal tunnel. This

ischaemia compromises the supply of blood and nutrients to the nerve and promotes a reaction in the connective tissue elements. Fibrosis developing in this way still further embarrasses the circulation. Scarring originating in this way first involves the epineurium but, as the pressure in the tunnel continues to increase, the deepening ischaemia rapidly extends to involve the intrafascicular tissues. The resulting endoneurial fibrosis is most damaging to nerve fibres and, once established, is irreversible and irremediable. Opening the fasciculi by dividing the perineurial sheath is not the answer, except in the treatment of leprous neuritis.

The most destructive lesion threatening the structural and functional integrity of nerve fibres develops inside the fasciculi and progresses until their contents are replaced by fibrous tissue. Until nerve fibres can be individually decompressed without interfering with their blood supply, this complication will remain beyond the reach of the enterprising surgeon. That is a prize that has yet to be won.

In the meantime the best that can be done is to avoid worsening the condition. Policy should be directed to anticipating these developments by decompressing the tunnel immediately objective signs of sensory and motor involvement are detected.

Internal neurolysis to free fasciculi in the median nerve lesion of the carpal syndrome remains a questionable procedure because:

a. it disregards the pathogenesis of the lesion;
b. it is impossible technically to perform the procedure effectively without damaging nutrient vessels and fasciculi and interfascicular linkages. The risk of still further compromising the blood supply to nerve fibres is considerable and this adds to the fibrosis which is the main offender;
c. when the motor and sensory loss are well-established, the pathology is located inside as well as external to the fasciculi

and is irreversible and irreparable. Internal neurolysis is without effect on this lesion once it is well-established;

d. clinical studies comparing the results of carpal tunnel decompression with and without internal neurolysis indicate that neurolysis achieves no more than simple decompression of the tunnel (Rhoades et al 1985a,b, Gelberman et al 1987). The author shares the view of those many others who believe that extensive internal neurolysis is contraindicated in the treatment of the median nerve lesion in the carpal tunnel syndrome;

8. To remove constrictive scar tissue resulting from the unintentional injection of tissue destructive agents into the nerve. The nerves most at risk are the radial nerve on the outer aspect of the mid upper arm and the sciatic nerve in the gluteal region, two common sites for the administration of therapeutic injections. However, no nerve is safe if it is in injection territory.

PART 2. MOBILISATION

Free and extensive mobilisation of nerves is frequently required in peripheral nerve surgery in order to permit transposition of the nerve to a new bed or to join widely separated nerve ends without tension. This may require freeing the nerve from its bed over considerable distances. This in turn may necessitate the separation of branches from the parent nerve and the sacrifice of some branches and nutrient vessels. The effect of these procedures on the nerve trunk is not without risk.

THE STRIPPING OF BRANCHES

The distance for which a branch may be safely stripped without damaging fasciculi is determined by the intraneural length over which the fascicular group representing the branch maintains its individuality and can be readily separated from the nerve. Estimates of these distances for different nerves are available (Sunderland 1945).

Deceptive features that make it difficult to decide with confidence how far a branch can be stripped without damaging fibres are:

1. individual and unpredictable variations in the distances within the nerve over which a branch fascicular group remains as a completely independent system before engaging in plexus formations with neighbouring fasciculi composed of fibres from other branches;
2. the microscopic but significant intercommunications involved in this process. Fascicular linkages are often so fine that they cannot be detected by the unaided eye.

The apparent ease with which a branch may sometimes be separated can be dangerously misleading, the dissection frequently resulting in an artificial separation with the destruction of fine fascicular intercommunications. For these reasons it is essential, when mobilising the nerve, to ensure that branch stripping is no more extensive than is absolutely necessary and the separation itself should be carefully performed under magnification. Whether a branch should be sacrificed to facilitate mobilisation depends on the judgement of the surgeon and the importance of the branch.

THE BLOOD SUPPLY TO THE NERVE

Mobilisation usually necessitates division of some nutrient arteries, the number sacrificed depending on the spacing of such vessels along the nerve. Fortunately each peripheral nerve is abundantly vascularised throughout its entire length by a succession of vessels which, by their repeated division and anastomosis on and within the nerve, outline an unbroken longitudinal intraneural vascular net (Chapter 10). A distinctive feature of this pattern is the considerable overlap of supply between the nutrient arteries entering at different levels. It is also common to see one or several longitudinally arranged macroscopic arterioles on the surface of large peripheral nerves. These superficial channels, which are of variable but often considerable length, are reinforced at intervals by new arteriae nervorum. Anastomotic systems created in this way make it unlikely that any nutrient artery will dominate the intraneural circulation in any particular segment of a nerve; possible exceptions are the median artery and the artery to the sciatic nerve. It is well established that nerves may be mobilised for considerable distances without disturbing the intraneural circulation. However, when the mobilised nerve is severed distally, the collateral circulation feeding it from below is eliminated. This sets a critical limit of 6–8 cm for the length that can be safely mobilised. Despite this observation, nerves may be carefully separated from surrounding tissues for distances of at least 20 cm and yet, when divided distally, the cut end of the long mobilised proximal section continues to bleed. For example, during transposition anterior to the humeral epincondyle, the ulnar nerve may be safely mobilised over corresponding distances. The ulnar nerve has been freed from the axilla to the wrist without causing ischaemia (Bristow 1941). Despite these clinical observations it would be wise to avoid unnecessary mobilisation and to keep within the recommended critical limits in order to preserve the intraneural circulation, thereby ensuring the best available blood supply to any suture line.

In the event of the loss of one or more entering nutrient vessels, the circulation is maintained by the large longitudinal anastomosing channels on the surface of the nerve. Should the latter be interrupted, vascularisation of the nerve then depends solely on the collateral circulation established by the vessels within the nerve and these are not always as large as those on the surface. The manner in which the arteriae nervorum should be divided when mobilising the nerve is important. The essential feature in the procedure is the preservation of the superficial longitudinal arterial system. Reference to Figure 38.1 will make this point clear. The superficial vascular pathway will be preserved if regional nutrient vessels are divided as far from the nerve as is practicable (at point *a*) in order to avoid the anastomotic ascending and descending branches contributed by them to the superficial longitudinal arterial system. If the nerve is roughly and carelessly dissected or stripped from its bed, the delicate channels are likely to be torn at the site where they enter the nerve (at point *b*), thereby interrupting superficial systems on the surface and embarrassing the intraneural circulation. This complication is less

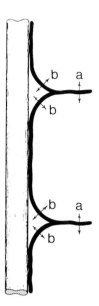

Fig. 38.1

likely to arise if there are several superficial longitudinal channels, since this increases the chances of one or more surviving to maintain the circulation.

Should a large nutrient vessel be torn or inadvertently divided at the surface of the nerve, it may retract into the epineurium and cause troublesome haemorrhage, while attempts to secure the vessel may damage fasciculi. Such complications can be avoided by the planned ligation of vessels at some distance from the nerve and a knowledge of the regional sources of supply to the nerve is of value in this respect.

If a peripheral nerve is being mobilised under tourniquet control nutrient arteries may be severed and retract unnoticed within the nerve. These may bleed postoperatively and lead to scarring which subsequently endangers regenerating axons. Since quite large vessels, both on and within the nerve, may be severed when preparing nerve ends for repair, it is advisable to release the tourniquet during this procedure in order to determine whether any substantial 'bleeders' are presenting at the nerve ends. If haemorrhage reaches proportions that require attention, any but the most delicate attempts to secure the severed vessels will inevitably damage fasciculi. Failure to control extensive bleeding at and about a suture line may aggravate scarring, which introduces an additional hazard to useful regeneration. Capillary bleeding is usually controlled by the suture, but even here post-operative oozing may lead to complications.

Intraneural haemorrhage may reach considerable proportions in the sciatic nerve where the main intraneural channels are often of large calibre. This may be one of the factors responsible for severe changes occurring in the nerve following trauma that leaves the nerve in continuity. Occasionally fusiform swellings at the site of injury are partly the result of the organisation of haematomas that have separated the fasciculi.

PART 3. TRANSPOSITION

Transposition is undertaken:

1. to provide a new and more favourable bed for a repaired nerve or an injured nerve left in continuity;
2. to give a shorter course to the periphery in order to:

   a. relieve an injured nerve in continuity or a repaired nerve from the abnormal tension introduced during a full range of joint movement, and
   b. enable separated nerve ends to be united.

A study of the effects of transposition in patients with nerve lesions in continuity indicates that these procedures arrest the deterioration of function and assist recovery. Thus transposition of the ulnar nerve anterior to the medial humeral epicondyle for the cure of traumatic neuritis caused by repeated tension and friction behind the epicondyle during elbow movement arrests and reverses the progressive deterioration in ulnar nerve function, and often results in distinct improvement.

It is difficult to assess the value of transposition in the case of nerve suture because, with so many factors operating throughout regeneration to affect the end-result, improvement could be due to factors that coincide with, but are unrelated to, the transposition. There is, however, sufficient evidence to show that the procedure is without

harmful effects, while the observation that it is often associated with distinct improvement suggests that it assists recovery.

PART 4. SURGICAL TREATMENT OF PAINFUL NEUROMAS

Neuroma formation and the histopathology of neuromas are discussed in Chapter 23. Painful neuromas are represented among those that develop:

1. on an injured nerve that is left in continuity;
2. at the suture site of a repaired nerve;
3. at the proximal end of an irreparably severed nerve;
4. at the proximal end of severed nerves in an amputation stump.

Before proceeding to a consideration of each of these categories some general features of painful neuromas call for comment. A puzzling feature is that all are not painful. Why some should be painful and others insensitive, even in the same individual, remains a mystery. If we had an answer to this question we would be a little closer to deciding what is required to convert a painful into a non-painful neuroma. In the author's experience:

1. large soft neuromas are more likely to be painful than the small hard nodules;
2. neuromas on cutaneous nerves and mixed nerves in which sensory fibres predominate, such as the median and posterior tibial, are more likely to be painful;
3. neuromas on nerves in continuity are usually less painful than those on the proximal stump of a severed nerve;
4. neuroma pain is elicited and not spontaneous, requiring as it does some physical, chemical or vascular stimulus to provoke a painful response. The offending stimulus is usually:

   a. pressure from an ill-fitting prosthesis, firm or gentle palpation or pressure generated during limb movements, or
   b. traction deformation introduced by adhesions and joint movement. This information provides a clue to the

measures to be taken in the surgical treatment of painful neuromas.

Treatment

The first step in the treatment of a painful neuroma is to flood the neuroma and surrounding tissues with a local anaesthetic. A course of this treatment usually brings only temporary relief on each occasion but the exceptional case may obtain permanent relief.

However, the subject matter of this section is not the treatment of pain but the treatment of a neuroma that is painful.

Regarding surgical procedures on painful neuromas, the treatment of those located on the proximal stump of an irreparably severed nerve and those of amputation stumps differs from the treatment of a tender painful neuroma on a nerve in continuity. These varieties will be considered separately.

Criteria for surgical intervention

These are: (1) the failure of conservative measures to cure or relieve the pain; (2) failed recovery in an injured nerve left in continuity.

The objectives

Since neuroma pain is not spontaneous but evoked, surgical treatment should be directed to satisfying two principal objectives: (a) to remove the neuroma from a pressure-bearing area or one exposed to repeated trauma; (b) to free the neuroma from adhesions that attach it to moving parts thereby relieving it of repeated deformation during limb movements.

TREATMENT OF THE PAINFUL NEUROMA ON A NERVE IN CONTINUITY

Decision making in the case of a neuroma, painful or not, on a nerve in continuity presents a problem because of the difficulty of predicting what effect the neuroma will have on recovery by way of delaying, obstructing and confusing axon regeneration (see Chapter 40). What can be said is that the presence of a neuroma, while foreshadow-ing incomplete recovery, is not incompatible with an acceptable degree of spontaneous recovery and one of an order surpassing that obtainable by nerve suture.

A painful neuroma on a nerve in continuity with acceptable function is not a justification for excision and suture. Nerve repair may be followed by a suture site neuroma that is as large as, or even larger, and more troublesome than the one that was removed.

The problem of a neuroma on a nerve in continuity is the unpredictability of the outcome. Accordingly, surgical intervention should be deferred until spontaneous recovery can be excluded. In this respect it is important to remember that the onset of such recovery may be delayed for several months. Ample time should therefore be allowed for this to occur before deciding whether or not to resect the neuroma and repair the nerve.

Meanwhile some information may be obtained by:

1. *Palpating the neuroma.* The soft smooth neuroma and lateral nodule are favourable signs, whereas the firm to hard neuroma indicates dense fibrosis and a poorer prognosis. An elongated fusiform neuroma may represent a reaction to haemorrhage into interfascicular tissues or friction trauma and not a break in continuity of fasciculi.
2. *Eliciting Hoffmann–Tinel's sign (HTS).* Where the nerve is composed solely of sensory fibres, an advancing HTS is a useful guide to the presence of regenerating axons and their movement down the nerve. However, in the case of a mixed nerve, the sign is unreliable because sensory axons may be growing down motor endoneurial tubes and motor down sensory. The limitations of the HTS in these circumstances should not be overlooked.
3. *Electrodiagnostic testing.* Kline and others have written extensively on the evaluation of the neuroma in continuity by using electroneuromyographic methods to detect and follow the growth of axons down the nerve. These methods have proved to be a valuable tool for this purpose, but they require the services of skilled personnel well

versed in the application of the techniques and experienced in interpreting the results (Kline & De Jonge 1968, Kline et al 1969, Kline & Nulsen 1972, Kline & Hackett 1975, Terzis et al 1976, 1980, Kline 1980, 1982, Bedeschi 1988, Terzis 1988).

If and when the nerve is finally explored steps should be taken before resecting the neuroma to confirm the absence of regeneration by:

1. completing the electroneuromyographic profile of the nerve, and
2. comparing the size of the nerve above and below the neuroma. Reference has been made elsewhere (p. 85) to the changes occurring in a nerve below a lesion when continuity is lost. An atrophied nerve trunk below the neuroma indicates a lesion that is not regenerating.

A painful neuroma on a nerve in continuity should be treated conservatively in the first instance. Such neuromas often become less sensitive with the passage of time and there should be no premature surgical intervention that would jeopardise spontaneous recovery.

Where there is an acceptable degree of functional recovery but a disabling tender painful neuroma remains, the nerve should be explored and the neuroma: (1) freed from adhesions or scar tissue that have been subjecting it to traction deformation during limb movements, and (2) where the option exists, transferred to a more suitable bed and protected site away from a pressure bearing area.

In the absence of useful recovery the neuroma should be resected and the nerve sutured or grafted with the object not only of relieving the pain but also of obtaining a favourable result.

TREATMENT OF THE PAINFUL SUTURE LINE NEUROMA

The risk of a painful neuroma developing at the suture site can be minimised by obtaining good fascicular apposition at the nerve ends during end-to-end repair. Troublesome neuromas are more likely to develop when fascicular tissue at the proximal nerve end is opposed to interfascicular

epineurial tissue in the distal stump into which regenerating axons will grow, branch and ramify, and Schwann cells and fibroblasts will multiply to form an enlargement at that site. This is particularly likely to occur where the fasciculi are well separated by a large amount of interfascicular epineurial tissue and the fascicular patterns at the nerve ends as expressed in terms of the size, number and arrangement of the fasciculi are dissimilar.

Once a painful troublesome suture line neuroma has developed, further management depends on such information as:

1. whether or not the nerve can be transferred to a new site where the neuroma is protected from compression and traction;
2. whether or not recovery in the field of the repaired nerve is negligible or has reached an acceptable level. Proceeding to a secondary repair involves sacrificing the recovery that has already occurred without any guarantee that function will be improved and a troublesome neuroma will not re-form (Chapter 40).

It is again emphasised that adequate time should always be allowed for regeneration to occur lest the neuroma be resected and the nerve resutured or grafted prematurely. At the time of the repair, whenever it is performed, biopsy material from the neuroma and new nerve ends should be taken and prepared for histological examination. The results will either reassure or dismay the surgeon.

THE TREATMENT OF A PAINFUL NEUROMA ON THE PROXIMAL STUMP OF AN IRREPARABLY SEVERED NERVE

In these cases the neuroma should be resected and repair attempted by nerve grafting. If this is not possible then the neuroma should be treated as outlined in the following section.

TREATMENT OF PAINFUL AMPUTATION STUMP AND RELATED NEUROMAS

Treatment of a painful neuroma in this category is undertaken:

1. as a preventative measure when: (a) nerves

are severed at the time of an amputation, and (b) a cutaneous nerve, e.g. the sural, is being removed for autografting;

2. at a later date when previous attempts to prevent neuroma formation have been unsuccessful;

3. the neuroma occupies the proximal stump of an irreparably injured nerve.

The treatment is essentially the same for all and is covered in the following passages.

Today a wide range of physical methods, chemical agents, materials and surgical techniques is available for the treatment of painful neuromas, including the transplantation of the nerve end into a variety of available tissues (Sunderland 1978). More recently, fascicle ligation (Battista et al 1981) and cross-uniting nerve ends by suture have been added to the list. Wood and Mudge (1987) have treated painful neuromas following amputation by cross-uniting the stump of the median and ulnar nerves with the object of confining regenerating axons to the anastomotic nerve loop. In one of five patients the anterior interosseous stump was joined to the stump of the superficial radial nerve. They claim that the patients reported an 80–90 per cent reduction in the pain. However, this procedure does not eliminate the possibility of a painful suture line neuroma developing at the site of the cross-union.

All these methods are based on a common objective which is to prevent, or at least curtail and constrain, the growth of regenerating axons at the nerve end. This is an objective that is difficult to achieve bearing in mind the unlimited capacity of axons to regenerate.

Meanwhile the subject continues to attract attention without materially altering the situation (Laborde et al 1982, Dellon et al 1984, Mass et al 1984, Mackinnon et al 1985, Dellon & Mackinnon 1986). As Tupper (1986) has so perceptively observed, all methods give about 80 per cent good results. So why not settle for the simplest method?

The need to devise an effective and dependable way of preventing the formation of a painful neuroma raises some interesting questions.

A neuroma represents a concentrated circumscribed mass of fine bare axon terminals in which the painful response to a deforming stimulus is likely to be maximal. At the same time the methods currently available to prevent the formation of painful neuromas are designed to regulate axon regeneration and to confine growing axons to the nerve end. However, would it not be better to deregulate axon regeneration by implanting the nerve end directly into muscle, or into a tissue plane between muscles, thereby allowing regenerating axons to become widely dispersed and lost in tissues instead of attempting to confine and concentrate them at the nerve end? The terms axon regulation and axon deregulation appear to be appropriate to cover these two situations.

Axon regulation

This method adheres to the old and well-entrenched principle of pulling the nerve down, cleanly cutting it short and, after treating and capping the nerve end, allowing it to retract into a pressure-free bed.

There is no procedure that is consistently successful in preventing a troublesome neuroma from re-forming. Each has had, and continues to have, its advocates. Simple ligation at two levels, 1 cm apart, combined with the use of a chemical coagulant before finally enclosing the stump in a silastic cap, seems to offer the best prospect of success. Regardless of the method adopted, care should always be taken to isolate the nerve stump from a pressure-bearing area. However, after taking all these precautions some failures must be expected.

The great obstacle to success is firstly, the tremendous capacity of axons to regenerate and secondly, the cellular reaction and fibrosis that follows any form of interference with the nerve end. This reaction provides a framework for regenerating axons which absorbs them and so distorts their growth that a relatively circumscribed mass appears which enlarges until the activity of axons is fully spent. Thus any procedure involving the nerve end will not necessarily prevent regeneration, while it inevitably contributes to the formation of a matrix that provides the basis for the formation of a neuroma when regenerating axons reach it. That each method has its failures and successes is almost certainly due to chance and to the participation of unidentified factors that govern the growth and interaction of tissues and the sensitivity of bare axon terminals.

Though regenerating axons may force their way through dense fibrous tissue, the normal perineurium presents an impenetrable barrier to their passage. When designing methods to control neuroma formation at nerve ends, the importance of the normal perineurial sheath in confining the growth of axons within fasciculi does not appear to have been widely appreciated. Procedures will succeed only if they seal severed fasciculi and, in this way, prevent the escape of regenerating axons into the neighbouring connective tissue where their disorderly growth is responsible for the formation of the neuroma. Technically, the effective and permanent sealing of the fasciculi presents difficulties that have yet to be overcome.

Axon deregulation

Here the time-honoured practice is followed of pulling the nerve down and cutting it short. Without any further treatment, the nerve end is allowed to retract into a well-protected site, or is implanted into muscle or into a fascial plane between muscles. Again it is imperative that the nerve end should not be located in a pressure bearing area.

Only continued trials will reveal which of the two methods is the more reliable in preventing the formation and reformation of painful neuromas.

REFERENCES

Bateman J E 1962 Trauma to nerves in limbs. Saunders, Philadelphia, p 168

Battista A F, Cravioto H M, Budzilovich G N 1981 Painful neuroma: changes produced in peripheral nerve after fascicle ligation. Neurosurgery 9: 589

Bedeschi P 1988 Intraoperative electroneuromyographic investigation of peripheral nerve lesions. In: Tubiana R (ed) The hand. Saunders, Philadelphia, 3: 446

Bonola A 1973 Indications et technique de la neurolyse interne au microscope d'opération. In: Orthopaedic Surgery and Traumatology, Proceedings of the 12th Congress of the International Society of Orthopaedic Surgery and Traumatology Tel Aviv 1972. Excerpta Medica, Amsterdam, p 343

Bristow W R 1941 Injuries to peripheral nerves. British Medical Journal 1: 373

Brown B A 1969 Internal neurolysis in treatment of traumatic peripheral nerve lesions. California Medicine 110: 460

Brown B A 1972a Sciatic injection neuropathy — treatment by internal neurolysis. California Medicine 116: 13

Brown B A 1972b Internal neurolysis in traumatic peripheral nerve lesions in continuity. Surgical Clinics of North America 52: 1167

Brown H A 1970 Internal neurolysis in the treatment of peripheral nerve lesions. Clinical Neurosurgery 17: 99

Carayon A 1962 La neurolyse fasciculaire — application aux lésions nerveuses péripheriques en continuité (Trauma, lépre, tumours) Journal Chirurgie Paris 83: 435

Curtis R M, Eversmann W W 1973 Internal neurolysis as an adjunct to the treatment of the carpal tunnel syndrome. Journal of Bone and Joint Surgery 55A: 733

Dellon A L, Mackinnon S E 1986 Treatment of the painful neuroma by neuroma resection and muscle implantation. Plastic and Reconstructive Surgery 77: 427

Dellon A L Mackinnon S E, Pestronk A 1984 Implantation of sensory nerve into muscle: preliminary clinical and experimental observations on neuroma formation. Annals of Plastic Surgery 12: 30

Enna C D 1974 Neurolysis and transposition of the ulnar nerve in leprosy. Journal of Neurosurgery 40: 734

Enna C D 1980 The management of leprous neuritis. In: Omer G E, Spinner M (eds) Management of peripheral nerve problems. Saunders, Philadelphia, p 742

Frykman G K, Adams J, Bowen W W 1981 Neurolysis. The Orthopaedic Clinics of North America 12: 325

Gelberman R H, Pfeffer G B, Galbraith R T, Szabo R M, Rydevik B 1987 Results of treatment of severe carpal tunnel syndrome without internal neurolysis of the median nerve. Journal of Bone and Joint Surgery 69A: 896

Gentili F, Hudson A R, Kline W G, Hunter D 1981 Morphological and physiological alterations following internal neurolysis of normal rat sciatic nerve. In: Gorio A, Millesi H, Mingrino S (eds) Post-traumatic peripheral nerve regeneration: experimental basis and clinical implications. Raven Press, New York, p 183

Kahl R I, Samii M, Willebrand H 1973 Clinical results of perineural fascicular neurolysis. Proceedings of the German Society for Neurosurgery Modern Aspects of Neurosurgery International Congress Series. Excerpta Medica, Amsterdam 4: 209

Kline D G 1980 Evaluation of the neuroma in continuity. In: Omer G E, Spinner M (eds) Management of peripheral nerve problems. Saunders, Philadelphia, p 450

Kline D G 1982 Timing for exploration of nerve lesions and evaluation of the neuroma — in continuity. Clinical Orthopaedics and Related Research 163: 42

Kline D G, De Jonge B R 1968 Evoked potentials to evaluate peripheral nerve injury. Surgery, Gynecology and Obstetrics 127: 1239

Kline D G, Hackett E 1975 Reappraisal of timing for exploration of civilian peripheral nerve injuries. Surgery 78: 54

Kline D G, Nulsen F E 1972 The neuroma in continuity. Surgical Clinics of North America 52: 1189

Kline D G, Hackett E F, May P R 1969 Evaluation of nerve injuries by evoked potentials and electromyography. Journal of Neurosurgery 31: 128

Laborde K J, Kalisman M, Tsai T M 1982 Results of surgical treatment of painful neuromas of the hand. Journal of Hand Surgery 7A: 190

Levine J, Spinner M 1971 Neurolysis in elderly patients. Clinical Orthopaedics 80: 13

Lundborg G 1988 Nerve injury and repair. Churchill Livingstone, Edinburgh, p 105

Mackinnon S E, Dellon A L, Hudson A R, Hunter D A 1985 Alteration of neuroma formation by manipulation of its microenvironment. Plastic and Reconstructive Surgery 76: 345

Mackinnon S E, Dellon A L 1986 An experimental study of treatment methods for chronic nerve compression. Journal of Hand Surgery 11A: 759

Mackinnon S E, Dellon A L 1988 Evaluation of microsurgical internal neurolysis in a primate median nerve model of chronic nerve compression. Journal of Hand Surgery 13A: 345

Mass D P, Ciano M C, Tortosa R et al 1984 Treatment of painful hand neuromas by their transfer into bone. Plastic and Reconstructive Surgery 74: 183

Matchabelli A N 1945 The treatment of causalgia by the operation of 'fasciculation'. Khirurgiya Moscow 4: 46

Omer G E 1974 Injuries to nerves of the upper extremity. Journal of Bone and Joint Surgery 56A: 1615

Rhoades C E, Mowery C A, Gelberman R H 1985a Results of internal neurolysis of the median nerve for severe carpal tunnel syndrome. Journal of Bone and Joint Surgery 67A: 253

Rhoades C E, Gelberman R H, Botte M J, Szabo R 1985b The results of carpal tunnel release with and without internal neurolysis of the median nerve for severe carpal tunnel syndrome. Journal of Hand Surgery 10A: 62

Rydevik B, Lundborg G, Nordborg C 1976 Intraneural tissue reactions induced by internal neurolysis. Scandinavian Journal of Plastic and Reconstructive Surgery 10: 3

Sakurai M, Miyasaka Y 1986 Neural fibrosis and the effect of neurolysis. Journal of Bone and Joint Surgery 68B: 483

Samii M 1972 Die operative Wiederherstellung verletzter Nerven. Langenbecks Archiv für Klinische Chirurgie 332: 355

Samii M 1976 Intraneurale Neurolyse des Nervus medianus beim Karpal Tunnel Syndrome. Hand Chirurgie 8: 117

Seddon H 1975 Surgical disorders of the peripheral nerves, 2nd edn. Churchill Livingstone, Edinburgh, p 280

Sunderland S 1945 The intraneural topography of the radial, median and ulnar nerves. Brain 68: 243

Sunderland S 1978 Nerves and nerve injuries, 2nd edn. Churchill Livingstone, Edinburgh, p 499

Tazaki K I 1983 An experimental study on the repair of peripheral nerve lesions — subacute compression neuropathy and neurolysis. Journal of the Japanese Orthopaedic Association 57: 1821

Terzis J K 1988 Electrophysiological techniques in surgery of peripheral nerves serving the hand. In: Tubiana R (ed) The hand. Saunders, Philadelphia, p 438

Terzis J K, Dykes R W, Hakstian R W 1976 Electrophysiological recordings in peripheral nerve surgery: a review. Journal of Hand Surgery 1: 52

Terzis J K, Daniel R K, Williams H B 1980 Intraoperative assessment of nerve lesions with fascicular dissection and electrophysiological recordings. In: Omer G E, Spinner M (eds) Management of peripheral nerve problems. Saunders, Philadelphia, p 462

Tupper J W 1986 Discussion of paper by Dellon A L & Mackinnon S E 1986 Journal of Plastic & Reconstructive Surgery 77: 437

Wilgis E F S 1979 Internal neurolysis. American Academy of Orthopaedic Surgeons Symposium on Microsurgery. Mosby, St Louis, p 170

Wood V E, Mudge M K 1987 Treatment of neuromas about a major amputation stump. Journal of Hand Surgery 12A: 302

Woodhall B, Nulsen F E, White J C, Davis L 1956 Neurosurgical implications. In: Woodhall B, Beebe G W (eds) Peripheral nerve regeneration: a follow-up study of 3656 World War II injuries. V A Medical Monograph Government Printing Office, Washington D C, p 569

Zhu S-X, Lu S, Yao J et al 1985 Intrafascicular decompression in the treatment of causalgia with special reference to the mechanisms. Annals of Plastic Surgery 15: 460

39. Factors influencing the quality of the recovery after nerve repair

Nerve repair, to be undertaken with any prospect of success, requires an appreciation of the physiological requirements for complete recovery, a knowledge of the anatomical features that are essential to meet those requirements, the recognition of the many factors affecting regeneration and functional recovery and an understanding of the manner in which they produce their effects, particularly those of an adverse nature.

Of particular concern are the unpredictable results of peripheral nerve surgery, even when repair is performed by experienced and skilled personnel under the most favourable conditions. The results are often good but too often they are disappointing and sometimes decidedly bad, the number of unsatisfactory recoveries increasing as critical standards for testing function are applied. What is the explanation of this unpredictability? Are the failures due to conditions imposed by the wounding, to the characteristics of the nerve injury itself, to faulty technique when performing the repair, to structural features at the suture line, or to other factors that the surgeon is unable to control?

Many factors are now known to influence axon regeneration and the quality of the recovery after nerve repair. Some operate from the time of the injury, some develop with the passage of time in denervated tissues while others are introduced later during the repair of the nerve and subsequently during axon regeneration and the reinnervation of peripheral tissues. Within this framework they operate central to, at, and distal to the site of the repair.

Most of these factors have been referred to, but in a disconnected way, in earlier chapters. Here the opportunity has been taken to draw them together.

PART I. FACTORS OPERATING CENTRAL TO THE LESION

RETROGRADE NEURONAL CHANGES

The essential feature of regeneration in peripheral nerve fibres is the outgrowth of axons to replace the processes that have perished as a result of the injury. Such regeneration requires the survival of the nerve cells whose axons have been injured.

Following section of a nerve fibre some neurons remain unaffected, others undergo profound changes that culminate in disintegration, while an intermediate group shows a retrograde reaction of varying severity that is partly or fully reversible.

1. These retrograde neuronal effects, and the trans-synaptic changes associated with them, adversely affect regeneration and limit recovery by (i) reducing the number of axons available for regeneration, (ii) impairing the function of restored pathways, and (iii) modifying patterns of activity and in this way reducing their efficiency.

2. The effects are more severe after high than after low lesions and are directly proportional to the severity of the causative injury. The greater retrograde reaction following injury close to the cord is also related to the fact that all the fibres of the nerve trunk are involved whereas with peripheral injuries those fibres leaving by more proximal branches escape.

3. Additional trauma to the proximal stump

during the preparation of nerve ends for repair aggravates the retrograde effects, particularly when a careless and rough technique is employed. Nerve tissue should be treated at all times with the greatest respect.

4. The effects are more serious in sensory than in motor neurons. Sensory recovery is therefore slower and less satisfactory than motor recovery.

5. Variations in the severity of the retrograde neuronal reaction, as this is reflected in degeneration, delayed and incomplete recovery, and persistent trans-synaptic effects, may be responsible for variations in:

   a. the distance for which Wallerian degeneration extends centrally in the proximal stump;

   b. the onset of regeneration. Increases in the severity of the retrograde reaction result in increased delays in the onset of recovery;

   c. rates of axon regeneration which are slower after nerve repair than after injuries recovering spontaneously;

   d. the extent and quality of the recovery.

THE REGENERATIVE POWER OF NEURONS THAT SURVIVE SEVERANCE OF THEIR AXON

Surviving neurons retain the capacity to regenerate functionally efficient pathways for at least a year and there is evidence that this capacity persists for even longer periods. Whether this desirable property is retained indefinitely remains unknown.

CENTRAL FACTORS INFLUENCING THE CONVERSION OF THE RESTORED PATHWAY INTO A FUNCTIONALLY EFFICIENT FIBRE SYSTEM

The maturation of restored pathways, on which depends the full restoration of their functional efficiency, involves morphological changes of a highly complex nature such as myelination and the restoration of the calibre of the fibre. Any factor that restricts these processes will permanently impair the function of the new fibre.

Central influences that adversely affect the conversion of the restored pathways into an efficient fibre system operate at neuronal levels in the following ways:

1. Incomplete recovery of the neuron from retrograde or trans-synaptic effects could reduce its capacity to restore a regenerated axon to its original diameter and degree of myelination.

2. Axon sprouting during regeneration increases the number of processes controlled by the neuron. By dissipating its resources, this may prevent the cell from exerting its full influence on any one fibre. It is conceivable that axon branching may reach such abnormal proportions that the maturation of pathways is seriously impaired.

3. The length of a regenerating axon may be a factor affecting maturation and its capacity to function efficiently. During regeneration the axon of an originally short nerve fibre may enter an endoneurial tube originally occupied by a long fibre. When this occurs it is known that the regenerating axon will grow the full length of the endoneurial tube which it enters. In this way a neuron originally controlling the activities of a short fibre is now called upon to administer to the needs of a process of considerable length, and it is conceivable that it may be unable to satisfy these additional needs.

PART 2. FACTORS OPERATING AT THE LEVEL OF THE REPAIR

These include factors influencing the passage of axons through the interfacial tissue and their entry into the distal stump, fasciculi and functionally related endoneurial tubes (Fig. 39.1).

FACTORS INFLUENCING THE PASSAGE OF AXONS THROUGH THE INTERFACIAL TISSUE

Structural features of the interfacial tissue

1. This tissue must be sufficiently strong to maintain permanent apposition of the nerve

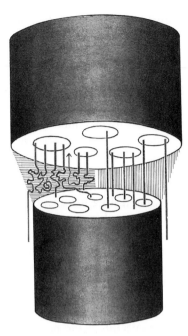

Fig. 39.1 Diagrammatic representation of factors operating at the suture line which prejudice useful regeneration: discrepancies in the dimensions and fascicular patterns of the nerve stumps and structural features of the junctional tissue which obstruct or hinder the orderly advance of regenerating axons.

ends. This strength is provided by its collagen content.

2. The tissue between the nerve ends is never as suitable a medium for the growth of axons as are endoneurial tubes.

3. Having emerged from the proximal nerve end, the direction taken by regenerating axons is determined by the structural features of the interfacial tissue.

4. Varying as it does in the density, arrangement and amount of its collagen content, the interfacial tissue represents a region where axons may be obstructed, misdirected and delayed in their passage distally.

5. Resistance is minimal when the collagen fibres are arranged in the longitudinal axis of the nerve and in parallel strands along which axon tips can glide freely and easily in the right direction.

6. Resistance to the passage of regenerating axons is maximal when the collagen fibres are densely packed and irregularly arranged. These irregularities also cause axons to twist and turn and to be misdirected as they advance.

7. Axons branch on their way through the interfacial tissue. Whether this is due to a stimulus provided by obstruction or to other factors is not known.

This branching increases the potentialities for recovery by:

a. compensating for the loss of some axons due to retrograde changes and the failure of others to enter endoneurial tubes, and

b. providing a variety of seekers to explore the best available route to endoneurial tubes. Such sprouting may, however, reduce the quality of the recovery, not only by overloading neurons but also by adding to the erroneous cross-shunting of axons. Another disadvantage is that during regeneration multiple sprouts from either a single or different axons may enter the same tube simultaneously. Only one of these ultimately survives, though the reason for this is unknown, nor has it been determined whether the surviving axon is that which first reaches peripheral tissues or that which is most closely associated anatomically and functionally with the tube. In any event, the occupation of one tube by axons from different neurons and the ultimate atrophy of all but one axon adds to the fibre loss that occurs during regeneration.

Little direct information appears to be available as to whether or not multiple sprouts from the same axon can, on entering different tubes, each survive and grow distally. That such may occur, however, is supported by the observation that peripheral nerve fibres normally divide as they travel peripherally. Such regeneration may, however, complicate recovery by leading to a dissipation of the energies of the neuron over several pathways so that it is unable to direct the normal activity of any one of them. Whether adjustments can occur to compensate for this is not known.

Many of the fibre pathways recreated in these ways would certainly bear no relationship to the original fibre pattern. The wasteful regeneration arising as the result of two or more axons finding their way into the one tube is less likely to occur, however, when the tubes are small and able to admit only one process. For this reason the multiple filling of a single tube is more likely to occur when repair is executed at a time before the tubes have atrophied unduly.

FACTORS INFLUENCING THE ENTRY OF AXONS INTO THE DISTAL STUMP

The relative dimensions of the nerve ends

Having traversed the bridging tissue, axons must next enter the distal stump if they are to reach the fasciculi and their contained endoneurial tubes. Whether they will do this or not largely depends on the relative dimensions of the opposed nerve ends.

Important generalisations in this respect are:

1. the denervation atrophy of fasciculi in the distal stump increases progressively until the 4th month beyond which the cross-sectional area remains essentially unchanged;
2. with atrophy of the distal stump by as much as 50–60 per cent, the discrepancy between the two nerve ends is then such that many regenerating axons would pass outside the distal stump (p. 85);
3. the fascicular and epineurial tissue may be so proportioned at the site of the repair that, despite marked denervation atrophy of the fasciculi, the overall reduction of the cross-sectional area of the distal stump is small. The general appearance of the nerve ends would then suggest that satisfactory end-to-end union is possible. The situation, however, is not as favourable as might appear because any pre-existing disparity in the fascicular patterns at the nerve ends will have been accentuated by the fascicular atrophy in the distal stump, the arrangement being one that favours the growth of axons into the interfascicular tissues instead of into fasciculi (p. 34). Only a cross-sectional analysis of biopsy material taken from the nerve ends during their preparation for nerve repair will reveal the extent of this unfavourable feature.

FACTORS INFLUENCING THE ENTRY OF AXONS INTO THE FASCICULI OF THE DISTAL STUMP

New axons, if they are to reach and reinnervate peripheral tissues, must first enter the fasciculi of the distal stump which alone contain the endoneurial tubes that will guide them back to peripheral connections. Axons that grow into the interfascicular epineurial tissue of the distal stump end blindly there and add only to the size and tenderness of the neuroma that develops at that site. This is wasteful regeneration.

The entry of regenerating axons into fasciculi depends on the fascicular patterns at the nerve ends, the cross-sectional area of the trunk occupied by the fasciculi and the degree to which denervated fasciculi have atrophied.

The fascicular patterns at the nerve ends

Only with clean transection will the fascicular patterns at the nerve ends correspond. The loss of even a short length of the nerve, either by injury or in the preparation of the nerve ends for repair, leaves the nerve ends with dissimilar patterns. This means that, when the nerve ends are united, fascicular non-correspondence at the nerve ends will result in the wasteful regeneration of many axons into the interfascicular tissue of the distal stump.

The cross-sectional area of the nerve trunk occupied by fasciculi

In general, the fasciculi of human nerves are large and compactly arranged in some regions, and small and widely separated in others.

Despite the dissimilarity of the fascicular patterns at the nerve ends, the chances of obtaining reasonable fascicular apposition are increased when the fasciculi are large, few in number and are tightly packed. There is then less interfascicular tissue into which regenerating axons may regenerate. Conversely, when the fasciculi are numerous, small, and widely separated by a large amount of epineurial tissue, the chances are greatly increased of fascicular tissue being opposed to interfascicular tissue. The total effect is that more axons go astray so that recovery is less complete and the prognosis consequently worse.

Denervation fascicular atrophy

Owing to the denervation fascicular shrinkage referred to earlier, the chances of restoring useful connections with the fasciculi of the distal stump diminish progressively over the first 4 months, after which the conditions remain substantially the same. Because the number of endoneurial tubes remains unchanged, fascicular shrinkage must lead to the tubes occupying a smaller area of the nerve end. As a result, fewer regenerating axons will reach them than would have been the case had they continued to occupy their original area.

FACTORS INFLUENCING THE ENTRY OF REGENERATING AXONS INTO APPROPRIATE ENDONEURIAL TUBES

There are no neurotropic factors to attract motor and sensory axons into endoneurial tubes, let alone regenerating axons into their old or functionally appropriate tubes (Chapter 16). Their entry occurs in a random fashion influenced only by the manner in which they traverse the bridging tissue and arrive at the face of the distal nerve end. As a consequence, some axon tips find their way into foreign endoneurial tubes while others fail, for one reason or another, to reach the fasciculi of the distal stump. Factors that influence the restoration of functionally useful connections under these circumstances include the order in which axons approach the distal stump, the nerve fibre composition of the nerve trunk, and the number of nerve fibres representing individual branches and their fascicular distribution at the level of the repair.

The order in which axons approach the distal stump

Some axons may reach and compete for the tubes before others have an opportunity to do so. This is because:

1. all axons do not commence regenerating simultaneously owing to the fact that, in any

injury, the trauma sustained by individual nerve fibres varies;

2. following severance of a nerve the fibres of the proximal stump are involved in a retrograde degeneration that extends centrally for different distances in different fibres. Consequently, all axons do not commence sprouting at the same level, which means that some have longer distances to travel than others before reaching the distal stump. The factors controlling the extent of this central degeneration in individual fibres are unknown but they are related to the severity of the injury;

3. the tissue at the suture line is rarely uniform so that some axons may encounter obstacles that delay their passage to the distal stump. As result of their later arrival, these will be at a disadvantage in the competition for endoneurial tubes.

The number of nerve fibres corresponding to individual branches and the nerve fibre composition of the nerve trunk

The number of nerve fibres at the suture level corresponding to individual branches has an important bearing on the effectiveness of regeneration because the quality of recovery depends on the number of axons reaching their destination and the degree to which they restore the original pattern of innervation. If the fibres of a particular branch are numerous, there is more chance of some of their regenerating axons reaching corresponding endoneurial tubes; a factor contributing to this would be the multiple budding of axon sprouts. When, on the other hand, the fibres to a branch are few in number and scattered through the fasciculi their chances of establishing correct continuity when competing for endoneurial tubes would be correspondingly reduced.

Peripheral nerves may, in a general way, be subdivided into two main categories:

1. Those containing a mixture of motor and sensory nerve fibres for the skin, deep structures and, importantly, proprioceptor fibres for muscles and joints.

2. Those composed of cutaneous nerve fibres

only, e.g. the digital nerves and the named cutaneous nerves of the limbs such as the superficial radial and saphenous nerves. The erroneous cross-shunting of axons into foreign endoneurial tubes, which leads to imperfections in reinnervation and impaired recovery, is of much greater significance when a nerve is of the mixed motor and sensory variety compared with one composed solely of cutaneous fibres.

The composition of a nerve trunk in terms of motor and sensory fibres therefore becomes a relevant factor in influencing the quality of the recovery of the nerve repair. As might be expected, nerves in which motor fibres predominate are more likely to show better motor than sensory recovery and the reverse would obtain where sensory fibres greatly outnumber the motor. This is one of the reasons why the results of nerve repair are less satisfactory when a mixed nerve, composed of motor and sensory fibres in about equal numbers, has been repaired at levels where the fibres are intermingled.

At the wrist about 90 per cent of the fascicular cross-sectional area of the median nerve is occupied by sensory fibres and about 10 per cent by the fibres for the thenar muscles. At this level, the fibres for individual terminal branches are also well localised in separate fasciculi or groups of fasciculi. Above the elbow, where the fibres of other branches are included, the terminal sensory fibres occupy about 60 per cent of the fascicular cross-sectional area of the nerve, and the terminal motor about 5 per cent. Furthermore, at proximal levels, the fibres from the different terminal branches are also intermingled and widely dispersed over the fasciculi. Similar conditions obtain in the case of the ulnar nerve where the values for the sensory and motor components at the wrist are approximately 55 and 45 per cent, respectively, while the corresponding values above the elbow for the hand branches are 35 and 28 per cent.

This feature explains why sensory recovery in the hand is usually superior after nerve repair at the wrist compared with repair at proximal levels. The proportional representation of motor and sensory fibres in the median and ulnar nerves at the wrist also accounts for the better median sensory,

as opposed to motor, recovery after repair at that level, and the less satisfactory overall recovery in the ulnar nerve unless the motor and sensory fascicular groups are identified and repaired separately.

The arrangement of nerve fibres at the suture line

Nerve fasciculi are, in general, of two types and both occur together at the same level. There are those that are composed solely of fibres from one branch. Others contain fibres from several different sources in varying combinations and proportions. The outcome of regeneration at levels where the branch fibre localisation is sharp and where the fibres from all or several branches are mixed calls for separate consideration. Naturally intermediate patterns occur but they do not·materially affect the discussion.

Where individual branch fibres are sharply localised in separate fasciculi regenerating axons are more likely to enter correspondingly related tubes, providing fascicular apposition is suitable and the axons are not diverted unduly from their course during their passage through the bridging tissue.

On the other hand, where fibres from several different sources are intermingled the entry of axons into original or functionally related tubes is complicated by such factors as the growth of axons through the bridging tissue, axon branching, the numbers of fibres representing different branches, and denervation atrophy of the endoneurial tubes.

FACTORS OPERATING BELOW THE LEVEL OF THE REPAIR

Factors operating in the nerve pathway below the lesion may influence the course of regeneration and the quality of the recovery by impeding the growth of axons and their conversion into functionally efficient fibre systems.

Normally the products of degeneration have been removed and the macrophages have departed within 30 days; over this period such products do not hinder the advance of axons (p. 94). On occasions, both debris and cells could, perhaps, persist in a form that might conceivably impede the passage of axons but the conditions under which this complication might operate in individual fibres are still undefined.

Denervation atrophy of endoneurial tubes

The lumen of each endoneurial tube commences to shrink as the breakdown and removal of myelin and axoplasm nears completion. The fibres are affected in proportion to their diameters, the largest being reduced to endoneurial tubes of variable diameter, the largest of which, from the third month onwards, rarely exceed 3 μm. After the various phases of degeneration have been completed the contents of the endoneurial tubes are entirely the product of Schwann cell proliferation.

Whether or not this endoneurial tube shrinkage has an adverse effect on the maturation of restored axon pathways is by no means clear.

This atrophy does not necessarily slow the descent of regenerating axons. Furthermore, complete, or very good, restoration of function in human muscles can occur following periods of denervation of at least a year. Within this period either the maturation of the nerve fibres is not hindered, or their failure to recover their original diameters is of little, if any, significance.

Though the point at which denervation atrophy of the tubes finally impairs recovery is not known, the changes occurring during at least the 1st year of denervation do not assume significance in impeding those developments in the restored pathways that convert them into functionally efficient pathways.

Factors that affect the efficiency of restored pathways

The efficient utilisation of reinnervated muscles and skin depends on the efficiency of the newly restored fibres. This includes the restoration of their histological and physiological characteristics and their capacity to contribute in an orderly and efficient manner to patterns of activity.

Factors contributing to the impaired efficiency of restored pathways include:

1. persistent neuronal defects;
2. the overloading of neurons as a result of the

branching of regenerating axons so that each neuron ultimately reinnervates a larger field than it originally served;
3. the uncompleted development of restored pathways.

The loss of branches in the wound owing to direct damage or avulsion from the nerve trunk or muscle

The manner in which this complication adversely affects recovery requires no elaboration.

FACTORS INTRODUCED BY THE DENERVATION OF MUSCLES

Factors responsible for the incomplete recovery of muscles are those that lead to a reduction in:

1. *The number of muscle fibres*. Muscle fibres survive denervation for several years providing they are well cared for, loss by degeneration assuming significance only when treatment is neglected and the muscle is kept immobilised, exposed to cold, subjected to trauma and its circulation impaired (Chapter 28).

Prolonged neglect of the peripheral tissues prior and subsequent to repair provokes the development of irreversible changes that are prejudicial to recovery, while non-neural injuries may contribute to the residual disability. Where such complications have been allowed to develop it should not be surprising if repair ends in failure regardless of the number of axons that regenerate and reach their destination.

2. *The number of reinnervated muscle fibres*. Some muscle fibres are never reinnervated because of:

a. a reduction in the number of axons reinnervating the muscle owing to:

   i. the retrograde degeneration of some neurons;
   ii. the failure of some axons to enter functionally related endoneurial tubes in the distal stump;

b. the failure of some axons to re-establish continuity with their old end plates and their inability to form new ones owing to extensive intramuscular fibrosis.

3. *The efficiency of reinnervated muscle fibres.* This could be due to:

a. the incomplete maturation of restored axon pathways and a consequent reduction in their efficiency;
b. axons that fail to re-connect with their old end-organs form new end-organs that are probably less efficient;
c. the failure of satisfactorily reinnervated muscle fibres to recover completely owing to persisting irreversible changes in the fibre;
d. intramuscular changes such as fibrosis that impair the co-ordinated activity of groups of muscle fibres;
e. distortion of the pattern of innervation which results from the loss of some axons and the erroneous cross-shunting of others at the suture line.

The quality of useful recovery depends not only on the numbers of nerve fibres reinnervating muscles, and the degree to which the structural features of both nerve and muscle fibres are restored, but also on the restoration of patterns of innervation involving both motor and sensory fibres of diverse sizes and functions. Residual disturbances of function arising in this way can often be improved by appropriate remedial training.

Changes developing within muscles that are directly attributable to denervation do not assume significance within at least the 1st year of denervation, providing the muscles are maintained in good condition by physiotherapy. It is emphasised that muscle fibre degeneration and fibrosis become a serious factor limiting recovery only when the denervated region is immobilised, exposed to cold and is deprived of treatment designed to maintain the circulation and to prevent venous and lymphatic stasis. This factor should never be underestimated in treatment. By adopting measures to prevent the development of these complications the surgeon takes advantage of one of the few ways available to him of improving the quality of the recovery.

PART 4. MISCELLANEOUS FACTORS

FACTORS INTRODUCED BY THE INJURY

In general, when a nerve is cleanly transected by broken glass, knives or other sharp penetrating objects, nerve repair can be expected to give a result that is far superior to any that is obtainable following severe wounding by a missile, traction or a gross mutilating injury. This is because with more severe wounding:

1. a much greater length of the nerve is destroyed. This reduces the chances of a successful repair by introducing unfavourable conditions at the nerve ends for repair and by creating a gap that can only be closed under unacceptable conditions or by nerve grafting;
2. the retrograde neuronal changes are more severe in the latter;
3. complications such as extensive soft tissue damage, bone injury and infection may necessitate delaying nerve repair for longer periods than are desirable;
4. gross tissue destruction and the residual scarring often leave a poor bed for the suture line. The loss of a normal muscular bed and the unavailability of a more favourable alternative site reduce the prospects of a good recovery.

THE SIGNIFICANCE OF THE INTERVAL BETWEEN INJURY AND REPAIR

Considerable delays in the repair of severed nerves may be inevitable for any one of a number of justifiable reasons. Awaiting signs of spontaneous recovery when this is to be expected may also involve delays of up to 6 months. Do such delays adversely affect the quality of the recovery when nerve repair is ultimately required?

While it is undoubtedly true that the quality of the recovery deteriorates as the interval between the injury and the repair increases, there is the difficulty of evaluating this factor when others that are known to influence the outcome have not been and cannot be excluded.

That late repairs do not, in general, fare as well as those undertaken earlier should not be surprising because many of the harmful effects attributed to delay have their origin not in the delay itself but in the severe wounding that is responsible not only for delaying the repair but also for introducing such complications as the destruction of greater lengths of the nerve, suture line tension, infection, increased scarring and an unsatisfactory bed for the suture line, and longer periods of immobilisation required for the treatment of co-existing injuries involving other structures in the wounded limb.

Relevant observations are:

1. Repair undertaken a year or more after the injury is sometimes followed by surprisingly good recoveries, while early repair within a few months of the injury may be associated with a disappointingly poor result.
2. Denervated muscle and skin retain the capacity to function efficiently again following reinnervation after long periods of denervation providing:

   a. these structures are maintained in good condition by appropriate therapy and
   b. axons can be directed in sufficient numbers to their original, or functionally similar, end-organs.

3. Within at least the first 12 months:

   a. the capacity of the central stump to regenerate is retained and the subsequent rate of growth of the regenerating axons is not affected;
   b. the distal stump will receive and transmit axons in a manner that does not differ greatly from that observed when repair is undertaken immediately or after only a short delay;

4. The quality of the recovery appears, on superficial examination, to depend not so much on when but on how well the nerve is repaired and the conditions of wounding.

Despite the foregoing, avoidable delay in repairing the nerve is highly undesirable for the following three reasons.

1. Despite the occasional exceptional recovery, the overall picture indicates a decline in the quality of the recovery as the interval between injury and repair lengthens, and particularly when this exceeds 6 months.
2. Delays are of particular significance as regards the nerve below the repair where it is clear that the chances of restoring useful

connections slowly deteriorate over the first 4 months, after which conditions remain substantially the same.
3. Delay in repairing the nerve increases the time for which the treatment of peripheral tissues, muscles, tendons and joints must be continued and supervised. The greater the delay the greater the risk of denervated tissues being neglected or inadequately treated. This increases the chances of contractures and deformities developing that limit the mobility of joints and the function of muscles after they have been reinnervated. Early repair shortens the period of disability and, all other things being equal, results in better recovery.

There is no doubt that the sooner a severed nerve can be repaired and the denervated distal section of the nerve and peripheral tissues reinnervated the better. Nothing is to be gained and much is to be lost by unnecessarily delaying repair.

THE METHODS, MATERIALS AND TECHNIQUES OF NERVE REPAIR

The methods, materials and technique employed to repair the nerve are matters of some significance. Thus the results of end-to-end nerve repair without undue tension will be far superior to those obtainable from nerve grafting. The criteria for selecting an epineurial or group fascicular repair should be carefully observed and adhered to lest they be misapplied with a consequently poorer result.

The role of microsurgery should be clearly understood. Conventional epineurial repair requires only low magnification. Group fascicular repair requires higher magnification and a more demanding technique. Further details are provided in Chapters 42 and 43.

THE SIGNIFICANCE OF THE LEVEL OF THE REPAIR

High nerve repairs fare less well than those at distal levels for the following reasons:

1. the intensity of the retrograde neuronal reaction varies inversely with the distance of the

injury from the cell. Amputation of a substantial part of the axoplasm threatens the survival of the cell and has serious consequences for its recovery and its capacity to regenerate the lost part of the axon. One would therefore expect the consequences of a high injury to be more serious than those following a low injury, the loss of axoplasm being greatest in the case of those nerve fibres that innervate the peripheral parts of the limb.

2. After high repairs recovery in the small distal muscles is less frequent, and when it occurs is inferior to that recorded for the proximal muscles because:

a. the nerve fibres innervating proximal muscles are more numerous, occupy a greater cross-sectional area of the nerve and are more localised at the repair site than the branch fibres destined to innervate structures at distal levels.

After high repairs regenerating axons representing distal muscles are at a distinct disadvantage in the competition for endoneurial tubes. After repairs in the lower half of the upper arm, the proximal muscles recover better because the nerve fibres representing the branches to the forearm muscles are still localised in the nerve, whereas at higher levels they are scattered and intermingled with one another and with the remaining fibres of the nerve trunk. In contrast, above the elbow, the different branch fibre systems for the hand are widely represented and intermingle in the fasciculi, the fascicular distribution being one that favours the misdirection of axons into foreign endoneurial tubes.

b. proximal muscles often combine as prime movers in executing coarse movements and so may be regarded as constituting a functional unit. For this reason the reinnervation of one member of the group by nerve fibres originally innervating another does not greatly disturb the pattern. The two heads of gastrocnemius and soleus, the hamstring group, the peronei, and the extensors of the wrist are examples in point.

In contrast, the intrinsic muscles of the hand are concerned with complex and discrete movements in which each muscle has a specific role to play. Consequently, any distortion of the pattern of innervation consequent on disorderly axon regeneration to these muscles would be reflected in a corresponding disorganisation of well integrated and co-ordinated patterns of activity. This, in turn, would seriously limit the restoration of function.

After high repairs, recovery is better in the case of the larger proximal muscles controlling simple movements, while the smaller distal muscles concerned with more delicate functions never recover to the same degree.

3. The greater distance to be covered by regenerating axons and their slower rate of growth at distal levels mean that distal muscles remain denervated for longer periods. This allows more time for the development of those denervation changes in tissues that limit the restoration of function following reinnervation.

4. After high nerve repairs it is the proximally-innervated muscles that recover completely or nearly so, while recovery in the distal muscles is far inferior. This has been attributed by some to the longer period for which the latter have been denervated. This is an unlikely explanation. In the first place the quality of the recovery in the distal muscles after immediate or early suture is still inferior to that recorded for the proximal muscles after delayed repair, despite the fact that the former have often been denervated for much shorter periods than the latter. Secondly, conditions are more favourable for recovery in the proximal than in the distal muscles for the following reasons.

a. In proximal injuries the neurons innervating the distal segment of the limb are the most severely affected by retrograde disturbances.

b. The nerve fibres supplying the proximal muscles occupy a greater cross-sectional area of the nerve and are more sharply localised at proximal levels than the fibres destined for structures further distally. In the competition for endoneurial tubes after high repair the regenerating axons representing the distal muscles are at a distinct disadvantage.

c. The consequences of loss of axons and disorderly reinnervation are more serious for the distal muscles than the proximal. It is stressed that the foregoing comments have relevance only when muscles have been maintained in good condition by appropriate therapy. Neglect by way of unrelieved immobilisation and exposure to cold leads to deformities and, by encouraging vascular and lymphatic stasis within the muscle, promotes the degeneration of fibres and the development of fibrosis that seriously curtail function when reinnervation occurs. There is no doubt that the texture of human muscles neglected in this way is changed and that, other things being equal, the quality of the recovery in them is inferior to that occurring when the muscles have been suitably treated.

THE SIGNIFICANCE OF MOBILISING THE NERVE

Mobilising the nerve and transposing it to permit tension free end-to-end union and to provide a favourable bed for the nerve is without adverse effect on regeneration, providing the mobilisation is carefully performed with due regard to preserving the blood supply to the nerve.

THE SIGNIFICANCE OF GAP DISTANCE BETWEEN THE NERVE ENDS

The quality of the recovery deteriorates as the distance between the nerve ends increases. Long gaps adversely affect recovery by:

1. increasing the difficulty of effecting satisfactory end-to-end union and introducing the additional hazards of tension, postoperative stretching and suture line separation;
2. increasing the difficulty of restoring correct axial relationships at the nerve ends;
3. adding to the problem of adjusting for discrepancies in branch fibre fascicular arrangements at the nerve ends. This factor is responsible for increasing the loss of regenerating axons into interfascicular tissues and foreign endoneurial tubes;

4. introducing the problem of having to decide when to abandon end-to-end union in favour of grafting.

In addition, long gaps are usually associated with more severe wounding where infection may be a problem, nerve repair is unavoidably delayed and the repaired nerve is left occupying a scarred and unsatisfactory bed. These are all factors that reduce the quality of the recovery. It is, therefore, not surprising that long gaps are usually associated with poorer recoveries.

THE SIGNIFICANCE OF INFECTION AND THE CONDITION OF THE NERVE BED

Infection and residual scarring in a healed wound adversely affect nerve repair and the quality of the recovery by adding to the pathological changes at the nerve ends, and by leaving an unsatisfactory bed for the suture line.

Infection

This often necessitates delaying the repair and the poorer recovery associated with this combination could be due to the delay rather than the infection. Modern wound treatment has, however, largely eliminated the serious consequences of prolonged and crippling suppuration.

Infection produces its harmful effects in several ways.

1. Should the wound become infected postoperatively it destroys the integrity of the suture line.
2. It involves the nerve stumps in a spreading neuritis. This increases the length of the nerve stumps involved in an intraneural fibrosis that obliterates the internal structure of the nerve. The ensuing fibrosis converts the elastic perineurium and endoneurium into dense fibrous tissue that lacks elasticity.
3. The sequelae of infection increase the length of the nerve stumps involved in extraneural scarring thereby adding to the amount that needs resection in order to expose tissue that is suitable for end-to-end union and regeneration. The overall effect of extending

the resection is to increase the gap to be closed and all that this implies.

The bed for the repaired nerve

The scarring that follows soft tissue damage and infection may leave the repaired nerve with an unsatisfactory bed. Though transposition to a new and more satisfactory site, preferably of uninjured muscle, is usually possible, this can not always be found, and the suture line may be left unprotected under conditions that lead to its involvement in further scarring and adhesions. This, in turn, may result in increased fibrosis at the suture line which obstructs or retards the growth of regenerating axons, the development of a tender bulb and/or scar, and pain on movement from the deformation caused by adhesions.

A scarred bed also impairs the revascularisation of the suture line, or nerve graft, by vessels normally derived from that source.

Though an unsatisfactory bed is an undesirable feature of the repair, and likely to contribute to a poor result, it would seem that the most harmful effect of infection and scarring is an increased delay in repairing the nerve and an increase in length of the nerve requiring resection when preparing the nerve ends for repair.

THE SIGNIFICANCE OF CO-EXISTING INJURIES

Bone injury

Nerve and bone injuries are often associated. The same mechanism may be responsible for both, or the nerve may be ruptured as the bone ends are violently separated or transfixed by a spur of bone, both of which require repair of the nerve.

The presence of a healed fracture does not adversely affect regeneration providing the repaired nerve is not left riding across the rough surface of callus.

Vascular injury

Combined nerve–artery damage is most common in the proximal part of the limb and in the ulnar nerve at the wrist. Such injuries are usually associated with more severe wounding and the loss of greater lengths of the nerve. These characteristics of the injury are all known to be associated with poorer results and, combined as they are with other co-existing variables, it is difficult to evaluate the significance of arterial damage as a factor influencing nerve regeneration. What evidence is available suggests that the results of nerve repair are improved if a severed artery is repaired at the same time as the nerve.

THE SIGNIFICANCE OF A PERSISTING NON-NEURAL DISABILITY

When assessing the end-results of nerve suture with a view to evaluating the relative importance of the many different factors that influence regenerative processes and the quality of the recovery, care should be taken to identify and exclude those non-neural complications that are limiting the quality of the end result.

TREATMENT

There have been repeated references elsewhere to the overriding importance of maintaining the denervated parts in the best possible condition pending reinnervation. This point is stressed in the present context because no matter how satisfactory neurological recovery may be, this can be of little value to a patient if mobility of the affected parts has been permanently lost. The quality of the recovery is, therefore, largely determined by the measures adopted to: (1) prevent irreversible changes developing in denervated muscles that will impair their function following reinnervation; (2) preserve a complete and free range of movement at joints; and (3) prevent the formation of contractures and restrictive adhesions. It is important to recognise the contribution that physiotherapy, occupational therapy and remedial training programmes can make to the restoration of useful motor and sensory functions. Finally, there are those additional factors of a psychological nature that affect re-educational training and the social and occupational rehabilitation of the patient.

THE AGE OF THE PATIENT

Over the adult range, the age of the patient appears to be without effect on the course of regeneration and the quality of the end result. However, clinical experience teaches us that the recovery in children is far superior to that seen after nerve repair in adults (see Sunderland 1978 for references). All recent writers who refer to this subject are agreed on this point. The results of nerve repair are, all other things being equal, so uniformly and consistently superior in children as to justify the conclusion that the recuperative powers in the young are greater than those of adults. According to Almquist and Eeg–Olofsson (1970, 1975), the better clinical results in the young are based on the greater adaptability of the central nervous system at that age rather than to better axon regeneration.

THE SURGEON

A peripheral nerve is a complex structure and the restoration of anatomical continuity of a severed nerve is only the first step in a long chain of complex processes that are directed to the re-establishment of useful axonal connections with the periphery and those further changes that ultimately culminate in complete functional recovery of reinnervated tissues. The great challenge to nerve surgery is to promote the restoration of those nerve fibre-end-organ relationships on which normal function depends and it is this, and this alone, that determines the success or failure of nerve repair.

The number of factors that operate in any individual case to affect the useful regeneration of axons, the proper reinnervation of tissues and the complete restoration of function have been outlined in this chapter. Admittedly, much of the available information is in the form of over-simplifications of exceedingly complex processes, but it does permit an appreciation of those major factors that combine on the one hand to assist recovery and on the other to prevent, arrest or delay it. There will always be some unavoidable causes of failure, but it is essential that the surgeon should be aware of their existence even if he is unable to do much about them nor should he fail

to recognise and deal with those that can be avoided or corrected. The decisions to be taken in any individual case place the surgeon in a position where he, in fact, becomes the key variable in determining end results. If his sole objective is merely to unite the nerve ends and leave the rest to chance he will more often fail in his task than succeed. Nor is there room for the rough, ill-informed and careless technician.

THE PATIENT. THE PSYCHOLOGICAL PHASE OF RECOVERY

In earlier sections the focal point of attention has been the nerve lesion, regenerative processes, re-innervation, the restoration of function, and the various factors that contribute to improving or reducing the overall quality of the recovery. These cover the anatomical and physiological phases of repair that might be regarded as representing neurological recovery. Such recovery, however, only sets the stage for those additional adjustments to restored motor and sensory mechanisms that convert a reinnervated but useless part into one that is of practical value to the patient. Complete neurological recovery is not complete functional recovery and the gap between the two is bridged by what might be regarded as the final or psychological phase that determines whether the reinnervated part will be useful or not.

A residual disability that is crippling to one patient may be of little significance to another, and two patients with essentially the same motor and sensory loss may report differently on the useful-ness of the part. To the skilled craftsman or musician whose activities demand a high degree of digital dexterity even a minor ulnar nerve deficit may represent a serious disability, whereas the same, or an even greater, deficit would pass un-noticed by a manual labourer — one would report a useless hand and poor recovery and the other a useful hand and a good recovery. In other words, the quality of the recovery must be interpreted in an entirely different manner from that based on the standard clinical testing of motor and sensory function directed to particular muscles and the state of individual modalities of sensation. The important factors are now those that determine the social and occupational rehabilitation of the patient.

This introduces for consideration a wide spectrum of psychological and sociological factors ranging over such features as the motivation, interests and attitudes of the patient and those of his medical advisers; whether he is co-operative or unco-operative as a patient; whether or not the dominant limb is affected; the presence of any residual discomfort, disturbing paraesthesiae or pain; the particular demands of his occupation, profession, hobbies, sporting or other interests and the extent to which the patient is handicapped in this respect; his educational level, social environment and family relationships; problems associated with compensation and possible litigation, and finally such personal qualities as perseverance, determination and patience. Recovery is generally a slow, prolonged and tedious business and it is during the long months of treatment that the personality of the patient asserts itself and determines whether he is going to make the most of his neurological recovery. Some will devote considerable time and effort to retraining while others will remain indifferent and apathetic to all measures to assist them. To some the reinnervated part will remain useless and the disability one to be exploited. To others the disabled hand or leg will represent a challenge and be made to serve some useful purpose.

Also of importance is the interest and attention given to the patient, for only too often his indifference and disinterest and an unsatisfactory functional recovery are but a reflection of the inadequate attention and treatment he has received.

These factors assume considerable significance in the final evaluation of what has been recovered and what has been permanently lost. This subject, however, is limitless and raises issues that are outside this presentation other than to stress that they are all part of the total picture. The nerve lesion is not an isolated event confined to a limb and it can not be dissociated from the patient to whom it belongs.

COMPENSATORY MECHANISMS

There are mechanisms that compensate in some measure for faulty regeneration and the incomplete and imperfect reinnervation following nerve repair. Some operate during the course of regeneration and the reinnervation of the periphery, while others become effective only after these processes have been completed.

Mechanisms operating at the interface between the nerve ends

The degeneration of some neurons and the persistance of severe defects in others reduce the potential for the production of new axons. This loss may be offset by the multiple sprouting of individual axons of surviving neurons, but whether this operates in a useful way is unknown. It is possible that such indiscriminate branching could:

1. adversely affect regeneration by increasing the competition for endoneurial tubes and, in one way or another, aggravating the occupation of endoneurial tubes by foreign or functionally unrelated axons, and
2. lead to a dissipation of the energies of the neuron over several pathways, with the result that the cell is unable to direct the normal regeneration of any one of them. It is possible, however, that surviving neurons could undergo a compensatory hypertrophy in response to overloading at the periphery which would enable them to extend their control over a greater peripheral field.

Mechanisms operating at the periphery

The loss of some muscle fibres and the reduced efficiency of others may be offset by the 'use' hypertrophy of those fibres that have fully recovered. After partial nerve root section surviving nerve terminals in a muscle sprout and reinnervate adjacent denervated muscle fibres. This, of course, does not apply when a nerve trunk has been severed and repaired.

On the sensory side, there is the questionable possibility that the denervated area may be reduced by ingrowths from the sensory terminals of adjacent intact cutaneous nerves, while the sensory overlap from neighbouring intact nerves takes on a new significance (p. 328).

Finally, in the absence of reinnervation, functional adjustments may partly compensate for the residual motor disability by the development of substitution movements. Thus the trick or supplementary actions of muscles may be trained to compensate for a movement that has been lost by the permanent paralysis of another muscle or muscles.

Mechanisms generated centrally

It is well established that improvement can continue long after axon regeneration and reinnervation have been completed. How is this effected?

After allowing for the use-hypertrophy of muscle fibres as a late contributing factor, it is clear that, with the passage of time, continued improvement cannot be attributed to peripheral adjustments. Further improvement must involve the reorganisation of central mechanisms that are sufficiently flexible to respond to remedial training and practice in a manner permitting the motivated patient to utilise incomplete and imperfect patterns of motor and sensory innervation to greater effect. Continued improvement is, therefore, based on the capacity of the central nervous system to adjust to a new situation in order to meet new needs and demands.

The concept of flexible and adjustable central neural circuits being responsible in this way is supported by:

1. the success of remedial therapy after tendon transfers in which muscles normally producing one particular action can be trained to perform others;
2. the remarkable recoveries that occur after nerve repair in children. Such recoveries are rarely seen in adults despite the fact that regenerating axons are subjected to the same hazards in both. The superior results in the young are not due to a more effective regeneration and maturation of axons but are best accounted for by the intervention of some central factor.

Though these clinical observations strongly favour the existence of some central factor participating in the recovery process to improve function, and one of greater potential in the young than in the adult, they throw no light on the mechanisms by which this might be effected. One way in which recovery might be improved is by the creation of new processes by the neurons whose axons have been severed, the establishment of new synaptic relationships, and a rearrangement of central neuronal circuitry, all as a continuum of the retrograde response to the peripheral injury. To be functionally effective this new system requires the 'fine-tuning' that only retraining and the unbroken effort on the part of the patient can provide. This remains, of course, an oversimplificated and obscure explanation for what are obviously exceedingly complex phenomena.

PART 5. GENERAL COMMENT

It is apparent from this overview that the course of regeneration and functional recovery after nerve repair are complicated by many factors, each of which varies from patient to patient and from incident to incident. These operate at all levels along the pathway from the neuron to the tissue innervated by it, and they are so inextricably interwoven that it is impossible to isolate and evaluate each individually.

This illustrates the enormous complexity of the task of determining in what proportion each of the various factors contributes to the outcome of nerve repair and is responsible for any residual defect.

However, despite the impossibility of isolating each factor for separate study it is clear that some affect the course of regeneration and the quality of recovery more seriously than others. The principal offenders appear to be those that result in:

1. the loss of regenerating axons from:

   a. retrograde neuronal degeneration;
   b. the failure of regenerating axons to reach the distal stump owing to:
   (i) unfavourable tissue reactions at the suture line, (ii) suture line failure, and (iii) disparities in the size of the nerve ends caused by atrophy of the distal stump;
   c. the wasteful regeneration of axons into the interfascicular tissue of the distal

stump owing to fascicular mismatching at the nerve ends;

d. the entry of axons into functionally unrelated endoneurial tubes. This is influenced by such factors as the number of axons destined for individual branches and the extent to which they are localised at the level of the repair.

2. impaired functioning of restored pathways owing to residual neuronal defects, the incomplete maturation of regenerated fibres and the ability of denervated muscles to function efficiently after reinnervation;

3. disorganisation of the original pattern of innervation which is modified by the loss of some nerve cells and nerve fibres and the erroneous cross-shunting of axons into foreign endoneurial tubes;

4. the development of irreversible changes in denervated structures that limit recovery following reinnervation. The readiness with which complications develop in neglected structures, particularly in some patients who appear to show idiosyncrasies in this regard, emphasises the importance of maintaining the parts in the best possible condition throughout the period of denervation.

Within the 1st year of denervation changes developing in the nerve below the transection do not necessarily delay or prevent at a later date the conversion of a restored axonal pathway into a functionally efficient fibre. Over the same period, skin and denervated muscles also retain the capacity to function efficiently on reinnervation, providing they are reached by regenerating axons in sufficient numbers, in appropriate combinations, and from appropriate centres. This, however, only applies to denervated muscles that are maintained in an optimal state by physiotherapy.

Finally, there are those many other factors that contribute, favourably or adversely, to the outcome of the repair as this is expressed in terms of the quality of the recovery. Such factors include the skill and experience of the surgeon, the nature of the injury, the gap distance to be closed, the method, materials and technique employed to repair the nerve, the delay in repairing the nerve,

the level of the repair, the nature of the bed available for the repaired nerve, the effect of mobilising and transposing the nerve, the age of the patient, the psychological, occupational and sociological background of the patient and the duration and nature of pre- and post-operative conservative treatment.

Some compensatory adjustments are available to offset the adverse effects of those factors that combine to impair regeneration and mar recovery. In this regard the role of axon branching during regeneration is uncertain. The disorganisation of patterns of innervation arising as the result of faulty regeneration may be corrected by functional adjustments to neural circuitry in the central nervous system. On the motor side the hypertrophy of satisfactorily reinnervated muscle fibres balances the loss of others. On the sensory side areas of cutaneous sensory loss may be reduced by the ingrowth of sensory 'axon' sprouts from the sensory terminals of normal neighbouring cutaneous nerves while the overlapping cutaneous innervation from another nerve takes on a new significance (p. 328).

An analysis of the many variables that combine to reduce the quality of the recovery after nerve repair makes it obvious why the outcome is so uncertain and so often disappointing. However, some encouragement is to be gained from the knowledge that the nervous system possesses tremendous recuperative powers.

In the search for ways of improving the results of nerve repair, it is necessary to distinguish those factors that can be modified, corrected or controlled and those that are beyond our reach, for it is on the former that efforts should be concentrated because they provide the only means available to us of removing the uncertainty from nerve repair and improving recovery.

The importance of the continuing care of denervated tissues at all stages is again emphasised.

If any reliability is to be claimed for prognosis and decision-making in nerve repair it is essential that these activities should be based on a clear understanding of the several factors that influence recovery and the manner in which each exerts its influence.

Caution should also be exercised when evaluating any innovation introduced to improve results.

Such assessments will be inconclusive unless all factors influencing the extent and quality of the recovery are taken into consideration. Additional emphasis is given to this point when it is remembered that it has not yet been possible to assign to some factors their relative importance in the repair process. This subject will assume considerable importance when the end-results of large numbers of nerve repairs come to be analysed to settle controversial issues relating to nerve regeneration and nerve repair. The interpretation of end-result evaluations is too often open to the criticism that investigators have been preoccupied with certain factors to the exclusion of others that may, in fact, have been of greater significance in influencing the quality of the recovery.

REFERENCES

Almquist E, Eeg-Oloffsson O 1970 Sensory nerve conduction velocity and two point discrimination in sutured nerves. Journal of Bone and Joint Surgery 52A: 791

Almquist E, Eeg-Oloffsson O 1975 An electrical and clinical follow-up of nerves sutured at different ages. In: Michon J, Moberg E (eds) Traumatic nerve lesions of the upper limb. Churchill Livingstone, Edinburgh, p 61

Sunderland S 1978 Nerves and nerve injuries, 2nd edn. Churchill Livingstone, Edinburgh, p 587

40. Decision making in the clinical management of nerve injury and repair

Decision making is an inevitable and crucial part of the clinical management of nerve injury, being involved at all stages before, during and after the actual repair.

DECISION MAKING AND THE DIAGNOSIS OF NERVE INJURY

The first decision on which management policy is based concerns the identification of the nerve injured, the level of the injury and a provisional estimate of the nature and severity of the injury. This information is provided in Chapter 31.

The second step is to confirm or exclude first degree damage where spontaneous recovery is inevitable, rapid and complete (Chapters 13 and 25). This can be done on the basis of: (1) the nature of the wounding mechanism; (2) the characteristic clinical features of such an injury; and (3) electrodiagnostic evidence.

WHAT SHOULD BE DONE WHEN A CONFIRMED FIRST DEGREE LESION FAILS TO SHOW SIGNS OF RECOVERY WITHIN THE ALLOTTED TIME?

Most lesions will have recovered within a month, with recovery following a characteristic pattern. If there are no signs of recovery by the 6th week the nerve should be explored and a neurolysis performed.

When assessing the value of neurolysis in these cases, the possibility of unusual but still normal delayed spontaneous recovery should be considered.

WHEN SHOULD A CLOSED NERVE INJURY BE EXPLORED AS A DIAGNOSTIC PROCEDURE?

1. A nerve should be explored immediately local conditions are favourable as an early diagnostic procedure to confirm the pathology when there are grounds for suspecting nerve severance or an irreparable injury. Such is likely to be the case:

a. after severe stretch injuries;
b. when the position of a spike of fractured bone suggests direct damage to the nerve;
c. with wounding due to penetrating injuries caused by sharp objects;
d. wounding with a fracture caused by missiles or shell fragments;
e. close range shotgun wounding.

2. A nerve should be explored:

a. when the level, nature, and severity of the injury are such that to await spontaneous recovery would involve unduly long delays. Should nerve repair subsequently become necessary such delays would prolong treatment unnecessarily and could prejudice the end result. Examples are provided by a sciatic nerve injury in the buttock and median and ulnar nerve injuries in the axilla;
b. when function is steadily deteriorating;
c. when recovery that has been progressing satisfactorily with conservative treatment is suddenly arrested. This applies particularly where the recovery has not yet reached a useful degree;
d. when spontaneous recovery is overdue despite reports stating that the nerve had been observed to be in continuity;

e. when the functions lost as the result of partial lesions or incomplete recovery are of major functional significance, whereas those retained are of relatively little value to the patient;

f. as an exploratory procedure in the treatment of painful states. Exploration carries the following reservations:

  i. Even in skilled hands, the possibility exists of unavoidably damaging intact nerve fibres and branches when resecting scar tissue.

  ii. The danger to be avoided during early exploration is the temptation to interfere with nerves that would recover if left undisturbed. Early exploration will often reveal a nerve that is in continuity but showing pathological changes that do not, however, pose a threat to successful spontaneous regeneration and recovery.

3. Normal delays in the onset of spontaneous recovery should be taken into consideration when assessing the value of neurolysis.

WHAT SHOULD BE DONE WHEN EXPLORATION REVEALS A NERVE IN CONTINUITY?

Deciding when to resect a lesion in continuity depends on whether adequate time has been allowed for spontaneous recovery to occur.

When adequate time has not been allowed for spontaneous recovery to occur

This represents premature exploration. Though the status of a nerve lesion is usually clarified by exploration, there are occasions when, short of gross disorganisation, it is impossible to assess the effect of the lesion on the regenerative capacity of the nerve and the likely outcome of a 'wait and see' policy. The dilemma then is whether to resect and suture with the expectation of an average result or to await spontaneous recovery with an unknown result but one that could be far superior to the best achievable by suture. Uncertainty stems from the knowledge that:

1. though the nerve may appear or feel normal, favourable external features may conceal severe pathology within the nerve.

2. clinical experience has shown that what appears on inspection to be damage is not incompatible with a degree of spontaneous recovery that is superior to the results achievable by nerve suture.

3. the histological examination of material from premature resections has shown that 'neuromas in continuity' and other evidence of severe damage are not necessarily incompatible with good regeneration that would probably have resulted in a degree of recovery superior to that achievable by suture (Woodhall et al 1956). This is an endorsement of the views expressed by Spielmeyer (1918), who wrote that nerve lesions were being resected that would have recovered spontaneously had they been left alone.

The continuity of an exposed nerve should be respected and an apparently damaged segment never resected too hastily. Resection should be deferred until the situation is clarified by the appearance or non-appearance of signs heralding spontaneous recovery. Three months is an insufficient interval for this purpose, lesions within 10–15 cm of the first muscle to be reinnervated requiring 4–6 months.

Nerve conduction studies should be conducted and a nerve that is involved in scar tissue and adherent to neighbouring structures should be carefully freed by neurolysis. Following this the wound should be closed without any further interference.

When spontaneous recovery is overdue

Nerve conduction studies are now necessary. If the damaged segment is not conducting, and the nerve below is silent, then the damaged segment should be resected and further surgical treatment planned on the size of the gap to be closed.

WHAT SHOULD BE DONE WHEN THERE IS A NEUROMA ON A NERVE IN CONTINUITY?

This subject is discussed in Chapter 38, page 389.

WHEN SHOULD EXPLORATION OF AN INJURED NERVE BE DEFERRED?

Exploration should be deferred when:

1. the nerve injury has the hallmarks of first degree damage;
2. the wounding mechanism suggests a lesion in continuity with every prospect of spontaneous recovery;
3. the nerve was observed in continuity in the wound at the time of the original injury;
4. the clinical findings point to partial, as opposed to complete, interruption of conduction;
5. signs of spontaneous recovery are already evident;
6. recovery is progressing satisfactorily, even if slowly;
7. radiological examination excludes the likelihood of direct damage to the nerve between, or by the ends of, a fractured bone.

WHEN IS NERVE REPAIR NO LONGER WORTHWHILE?

For one reason or another a severed nerve may have escaped attention for many years. This makes it necessary to know the maximum delay that is compatible with an acceptable degree of recovery if the nerve were repaired, and the manner and extent to which considerable delays are harmful to regeneration and functional recovery.

Nerve repair is justified as long as neurons retain the capacity to regenerate a new axon, conditions in the distal stump present no impenetrable obstacle to regenerating axons, and the denervated tissues have survived in a condition that will enable them to respond efficiently if they are satisfactorily reinnervated. Because the available data are so incomplete it is not possible to provide answers to these questions with any confidence.

The capacity of severed axons to sprout

Neurons of human nerves retain the capacity to sprout new axons for several years, but for exactly how long is not known.

Axon regeneration in the distal stump following prolonged denervation

In general, after 6 months the overall results of nerve repair steadily deteriorate with increasing delays in the repair.

While it is generally true that the chances of obtaining a satisfactory recovery after nerve repair decline with the passage of time there is no doubt that, even after many years, regenerating axons retain a remarkable capacity to grow and force their way successfully to the periphery along atrophied endoneurial tubes.

Regarding the end result, so many adverse factors contribute to an impaired recovery in any individual case that it is impossible to assign a specific value to the time element. All that can be said is that, on occasion, acceptable recoveries can occur after repair has been delayed for many years, though these occasions become less frequent as the delay lengthens. However, at what point failure is inevitable is not known.

Trial (1985) has reported a good result (S3, M3-4) following repair of the ulnar nerve in a 15-year-old boy in which the interval between division and repair was 9 years. More of this type of information is needed before it will be possible to determine the delay beyond which nerve repair is destined to fail.

For what period can denervated human muscles survive and subsequently function on reinnervation?

The capacity of human muscles to recover on reinnervation following prolonged denervation is discussed in Chapter 29. Good, and sometimes complete, restoration of function may occur in muscles denervated for at least a year, providing axons can be directed in sufficient numbers to their original or functionally similar end organs, and that the quiescent muscle has been maintained in the best possible condition by appropriate therapy. The earlier the reinnervation, however, the better the chances of recovery. Though delay ultimately introduces changes that combine to limit the effectiveness of reinnervation, there is no information as to the point at which these changes become irreversible.

The maximal delays observed clinically that are compatible with some recovery

The quality of the recovery deteriorates continuously after the 6th month, by which time the unsatisfactory results are beginning to outnumber the satisfactory ones. However, only after operations performed during the 3rd year do negative results predominate. Yet worthwhile recoveries may occasionally be obtained in nerves repaired 2–4, or even 9 (Trial 1985), years after injury. It appears that no interval is too long to preclude the possibility of some recovery after repair providing muscles, tendons, joints and the cutaneous tissues have been maintained in a condition that will enable them to respond suitably when regenerating axons reinnervate them in sufficient numbers and in the appropriate combinations.

When should all thought of repairing a nerve be abandoned is a question to which it is not yet possible to give a dogmatic answer.

DECISION MAKING IN ACUTE NERVE LESIONS OF UNDISCLOSED PATHOLOGY

Where the condition of the injured nerve is not known it is important to decide, as a matter of urgency, whether or not recovery is likely to occur spontaneously. This is necessary because a severed nerve should be repaired with the least possible delay or irreparable damage recognised and other remedial procedures undertaken.

A single clinical examination will not disclose whether the loss of function is due to nerve severance or to a lesion that has left the nerve in continuity, though there are three ways in which this information may be obtained:

1. From a study of the nature and severity of the wounding mechanism.
2. By repeated clinical examinations to detect

the onset of spontaneous recovery. The nerve is explored immediately signs of recovery become overdue.
3. By exploring the damaged segment of the nerve. This gives decisive information but it may be necessary to delay the exploration because of the condition of the wound, serious coexisting injuries to other structures or for other reasons.

The nature of the wounding mechanism

Generalising, it can be said that:
1. most closed nerve lesions will be of first or second degree severity;
2. most missile injuries cause second degree damage;
3. complete loss of function from sharp penetrating objects is most likely the result of nerve severance;
4. lesions associated with fractures are usually of the first or second degree variety, but when the bone has been fractured by a missile the nerve has probably been severed.

The closed injury

Nerve lesions caused by an acute closed injury to a limb are due to compression and/or traction, the deforming force acting across and/or along a length of the nerve. The injury may, therefore, produce a localised lesion or one that involves a considerable length of the nerve. Common within this group are those lesions accompanying closed fractures and joint injury. Here the nerve has been damaged by the original force, by deformation resulting secondarily from separation of the bone ends and angulation at the site of injury, or by rough and careless manipulation during reduction.

Nerve damage in closed injuries ranges in severity from transient interruption of conduction to puncture of the nerve by a spike of bone, rupture from stretch or, more rarely, to severance from blunt trauma that does not break the skin. Most, however, are of the first and second degree variety, recover spontaneously and carry a good prognosis. This is particularly so when the nerve lesion is associated with a closed fracture.

Traction injuries carry the gravest prognosis,

though even here it is well to remember that many represent only mild involvement and the serious ones are fortunately not common.

Excluding cases of damage from severe traction, most nerve lesions in closed injuries recover spontaneously. It is therefore advisable to defer exploration until spontaneous recovery has had an opportunity to reveal itself. Signs of spontaneous recovery point to the nerve being in continuity. Exploration is then no longer indicated, providing recovery proceeds in a normal manner.

It is possible to estimate when the onset of recovery should be expected from a knowledge of latent periods, rates of regeneration and the distance from the site of the nerve lesion to the first muscle or muscles to be reinnervated. A descending Hoffmann–Tinel's sign is of doubtful value unless the injured nerve is composed solely of sensory fibres, when it assumes some significance. If favourable signs fail to appear as estimated, it is assumed that the nerve has been divided and treatment is planned accordingly. The period of uncertainty should not be prolonged beyond a point where it could rightly be argued that further delay in repairing the nerve could prejudice the quality of the recovery. This explains why it is important to ascertain the condition of the nerve in high lesions as soon as possible and why, in these cases, exploration of the nerve should preferably be undertaken without delay (e.g. the sciatic injury in the buttock). Where, however, spontaneous recovery can be expected with confidence the situation is best met by setting an arbitrary waiting limit of 4–6 months depending on the level and severity of the lesion.

When there is any reasonable doubt about the state of the nerve, and particularly where the clinical history and findings point strongly to nerve severance, it would be wise to explore the nerve without further delay as part of the diagnostic exercise.

The open wound

Open wounds vary from simple penetrating injuries and lacerations, causing minimal damage to tissues, to extensive wounding with gross destruction of soft tissue, compound fractures and/or joint injury, and tearing of vessels. Further complica-tions are infection and delayed healing that terminate in formidable scarring. Regardless of the nature of the wound and the mechanism responsible for it, there is no doubt that the chances of a nerve being severed are greatly increased in this type of wounding. At the same time it is remarkable, and a measure of the tensile strength and mobility of nerves, how often a nerve escapes or sustains damage that leaves it in continuity and from which it subsequently recovers spontaneously. The severity of the wound, therefore, provides no reliable clue to the condition of the injured nerve. A small penetrating injury from a sharp object may sever the nerve, whereas complicated wounding with gross destruction of tissue may leave it in continuity.

In civilian accidents the most common nerve injuries are those caused by puncture and cutting from sharp objects. Here the loss of nerve function is likely to be due to nerve division and, for this reason, the injury should always be considered one of nerve severance until proven otherwise by exploration.

It should also be noted that considerable delays in the onset of spontaneous recovery by no means exclude the possibility of complete recovery.

Regarding permissible delays to allow for spontaneous recovery, the nature of the wounding mechanism, the wound, the level of the injury and the particular nerve involved provide useful information on what to expect. Two to 5 or 6 months will cover all eventualities except in the case of high lesions in the axilla and buttock, where immediate exploration is justified.

WHEN SHOULD A NERVE THAT IS KNOWN TO HAVE BEEN SEVERED BE REPAIRED?

The simple answer to this question is: immediately local conditions are considered favourable for repair. It is the decision as to when local conditions are to be adjudged favourable that invites debate. In this respect injuries fall into two groups, complicated and uncomplicated.

Uncomplicated nerve severance

At one end of a scale of trauma is the clean transection, simple laceration, or puncture wound from a sharp object, and seen within a few hours of the injury. With this type of wounding the nerve and neighbouring tissues have been cleanly severed, tissue loss is minimal, the state of the wound suggests that residual scarring is unlikely to be a problem and wound infection is preventable by appropriate antibiotic therapy. The injury is, in fact, comparable to that inflicted by the surgeon when he enters the region at a later date and prepares the nerve ends for repair.

Under these favourable conditions the nerve should be repaired as soon as possible, within 12 hours of the injury with something of the order of a further 24 hours' grace if conditions warrant it. Staff skilled and experienced in the treatment of nerve injuries and facilities should be available to perform a prompt and technically sound repair.

The following advantages may be claimed for primary repair under the conditions specified:

1. Since there has been no crushing of tissues but only clean severence, there is negligible tissue loss so that:

   a. little, if any, preparatory trimming of the nerve ends is required;
   b. extensive mobilisation and translocation are not necessary to effect end-to-end union of the nerve ends;
   c. the nerve ends can be easily drawn together and reunited without unacceptable tension;
   d. the loss of only a few millimetres of nerve leaves the opposing ends with corresponding fascicular patterns which makes it easier to align them correctly when they are opposed. Unnecessarily sacrificing tissue when preparing the nerve ends for repair widens the gap to be closed and almost certainly disturbs fascicular relations to a degree that adds to the loss of regenerating axons at the suture line.

2. The nerve ends can be found easily, little extension of the wound being required to locate them. When a nerve is severed, the ends retract in the surrounding connective tissue where, if left undisturbed, they become fixed in a shortened position as healing proceeds and scar tissue forms. The nerve ends may also become lost in scar tissue, which adds to the difficulty of locating them at a later date. In addition, bulbs that form at the nerve ends also increase the amount of preparatory trimming of the nerve stumps required to obtain favourable conditions for an end-to-end union at a later date. All this adds to the distance separating the nerve ends. Though extensive mobilisation to bring them together is, if carefully executed, a harmless procedure, suture under tension is a common cause of suture line failure.

   Primary repair has particular advantages in the case of nerves in the hand and digits, where immediate repair gives good results whereas delay creates conditions that complicate repair at a later date.

3. Electrical scanning techniques can be applied to the nerve ends to assist in the identification and matching of fasciculi and groups of fasciculi. This advantage is lost 72 hours after the transection.

4. Immediately following a clean transection injury the epineurium provides an adequate, but not too secure, base for sutures. This is an advantage in that the sutures will pull out if too much tension is required to bring the nerve ends together. The epineurium is much thicker and stronger 3–5 weeks after the injury. There is then the temptation when sutures are holding well to finish with harmful tension at the suture site.

5. Reasonable limb positioning, if required to effect satisfactory union, does not adversely affect repair or aggravate scarring.

6. Repairing the nerve with the least possible delay reduces the time for which peripheral tissues are denervated and the period for which the patient is incapacitated.

7. Primary suture should obviate the need for any further surgery. Should resuture become necessary, the second operation is made technically easier in that the first repair prevents retraction of the nerve ends and, in doing so, reduces the gap to be closed.

The protagonists for early secondary repair, regardless of the nature of the wounding, maintain that such a policy takes the surgical treatment of nerve injuries out of the hands of the inexperienced casualty surgeon and makes the repair an elective procedure performed by an experienced specialist.

While a good secondary repair is far more likely to give a satisfactory result than a badly performed primary repair, the results from a well executed primary repair are even better. Primary suture should clearly be reserved for those cases where the conditions of wounding justify it and where capable and experienced staff are available.

One concluding thought regarding primary nerve repair. Having accidently severed a nerve in the course of an operation, or following the resection of a tumour, when should the nerve be repaired? Is there a surgeon who would advocate a delay of 3 weeks?

Complicated nerve severance

At the other end of a scale of trauma is the acute severe wounding that has resulted in the bruising and destruction of tissues and a contaminated wound that heals slowly and leaves extensive residual scarring. The severed nerve has rarely been cleanly divided, a segment of variable length has usually vanished, and the nerve ends are bruised and ragged. Co-existing injuries to bones, joints, tendons and/or vessels are common.

Under these unfavourable conditions primary repair of the nerve is contraindicated for the following reasons.

1. The nerve ends are ragged and contused and, within a few days of the injury, are the site of an acute inflammatory reaction. This leads to marked oedematous swelling of the epineurium and converts it into soft and friable tissue. At this time, fine adhesions are also forming and commencing to bind the nerve ends to neighbouring traumatised tissues.

Nerve suture is sheath suture and to be effective it depends on a strong, healthy epineurium that will hold sutures securely. The soft and friable epineurium at the contused ends of a freshly divided nerve makes suturing difficult and cannot be relied on to maintain effective union. This predisposes to postoperative separation of the nerve ends.

2. The damage caused by high velocity missiles in particular often extends for considerable distances, both proximally and distally. At this early stage, the extensive longitudinal intraneural damage may not be visible externally and more of the nerve is usually damaged than is apparent. Under these conditions the preparation of the nerve ends for repair is likely to be inadequate because it is rarely possible to estimate the extent and severity of the intraneural damage adjacent to the nerve ends with sufficient accuracy to decide how much of each should be resected in order to reach tissue that will: (a) aid healing and give the strongest possible union at the suture line and (b) later facilitate the passage of regenerating axons across the suture line.

The inability to determine the true limits of the damage means uniting nerve ends under conditions that will inevitably terminate in extensive fibrosis at that site.

3. Where a length of the nerve has been destroyed, the gap may be difficult to close if primary repair is attempted. Where the risk of infection remains high, it is not permissible to extend the wound in order to mobilise and transpose the nerve in order to gain sufficient length to allow union without undue tension. The excessive tension required to bring the nerve ends together adds to the technical difficulties of the repair and, with a weakened epineurium, makes it difficult to maintain union. The combination of tension and weakness at the suture line is a common cause of failed repair.

4. The scarring associated with healing of the tissues of the nerve bed may involve the suture site in adhesions and a constrictive fibrosis that will later: (a) obstruct and retard the advance of regenerating axons, and (b) attach the nerve to its bed so that it is subjected to traction during limb movements. This may result in the development of a tender painful scar and troublesome paraesthesiae.

5. Repair should not be performed in an infected field or where the risk of infection is great, nor in one in which the tissue damage has precipitated reactions that increase the prospect of

extensive scarring. It should be delayed until a clean, healthy bed is available for the nerve and the surgeon can dictate the terms of the repair.

6. High quality nerve repair under these conditions is both difficult and time consuming and should not be performed under emergency conditions where the surgeon is compelled to work under pressure and the patient is in a poor condition.

The high incidence of failure after primary repair with this type of wounding is due to intraneural scarring at and adjacent to the suture line, the involvement of the nerve at this site in paraneural fibrosis and adhesions, and suture line separation owing to tension and the unsatisfactory condition of the epineurium that cannot be relied on to hold sutures. The nerve should not be repaired until the wound is soundly healed. The nerve ends should be secured under very light tension to surrounding tissues with a few temporary holding sutures in order to prevent their further separation from retraction, and during wound healing and postoperative limb movements. Radio-opaque suture materials have the advantage of serving as markers that will assist in planning the closure of the gap at a later date.

Some are opposed to the use of anchoring sutures on the grounds that they are unnecessary and may increase the fibrosis about the nerve. The procedure, however, has the advantage of simplifying repair at a later date. If the sutures hold, gradual postoperative stretching will also produce some lengthening of the nerve, and the nerve ends are also more readily located. The technical difficulties of a secondary repair are thereby reduced.

The optimum time for nerve repair after complicated wounding

The earliest possible time when nerve repair can be undertaken depends on the condition of the wound. This is generally most favourable for repair 3–5 weeks after the injury when:

a. the state of the nerve trunk in relation to the surrounding tissues representing the nerve bed can now be clearly defined;
b. the intraneural changes that are incompatible

with good union and useful regeneration are now more clearly delineated from normal tissue. This permits a more accurate evaluation of the ultimate limits of intraneural fibrosis, unfavourable tissue being trimmed away until the arrangement offers prospects of a good recovery;
c. mobilisation and transposition in order to overcome nerve gaps may now be safely undertaken so that the nerve ends can be united under the most favourable conditions possible;
d. the epineurium is thicker and stronger. This facilitates suturing and gives a more secure and reliable union at the suture line;
e. the repair can be planned and carried out in an unhurried manner as an elective procedure;
f. the parent neurons are still in an optimal condition for regeneration.

An unconvincing argument in support of delaying nerve repair until the 3rd week is based on the false claim that this allows time for the endoneurial tubes to be cleared of the products of Wallerian degeneration which, it is believed, obstruct the advance of regenerating axons.

However, after second degree injuries, regenerating axons grow down the nerve below the lesion earlier and more rapidly than after suture. Such axon tips must contend with the same products of degeneration despite which regeneration proceeds smoothly and recovery is always complete. The presence of such debris does not hinder the growth and advance of regenerating axons.

The case for delaying the repair following complicated wounding can be fully justified on clinical grounds alone and does not require misleading biological argument to support it.

WHEN AND HOW SHOULD A LIMB BE EXTENDED WHEN IT IS FLEXED TO PERMIT END-TO-END NERVE REPAIR?

1. Joint flexion increases the slack in the nerve and so relieves tension. Reference has been made elsewhere (Chapter 12) to the normal relationship of nerves to the flexor aspect of joints which

prevents them becoming overstretched during limb movements. The only two exceptions are the ulnar nerve at the elbow and the sciatic nerve at the hip. Even here the ulnar can be transposed to the flexer aspect of the joint, but no such relief can be provided for the sciatic.

2. Where mobilisation, rerouting and acute joint flexion are all required to bring the nerve ends together, and even then only under obvious tension, end-to-end union should be abandoned in favour of grafting.

3. A limb should never be maintained in acute flexion. The permissible range for nerve repair should not exceed 30° for the wrist and no more than 90° for the elbow and knee. Even within these ranges only the slightest tension should be used to bring the nerve ends together. Orf (1978) has gone even further. From a careful study of the critical resection length and gap distance in peripheral nerves (see next section) he has concluded that the practice of flexing neighbouring joints to effect end-to-end union should be discontinued. In arriving at this conclusion he was influenced by:

a. the now greatly improved results of nerve autografting that make it an acceptable alternative to suture under tension, and
b. the need to avoid harmful tension at the suture line and elsewhere along the nerve at all costs. If joint flexion is required to effect end-to-end union then it is inevitable that harmful tension will be introduced when the limb is straightened. Orf further states that mobilisation and transposition, as auxiliary measures to close a gap, are only justifiable if they are not excessive and are not accompanied by joint flexion. However, some joint flexion is now such a well entrenched practice in nerve repair that it is unlikely to be abandoned.

4. The healed suture line has the same tensile strength as the rest of the nerve 4–6 weeks after repair.

5. When the limb is extended not only is the suture line in jeopardy but there is also the risk of traction damage at other levels. The postoperative fixation of the suture line to its bed by adhesions also reduces the tolerance of the nerve to traction.

6. The suture line should be safe with slight flexion, slight tension and very gradual postoperative straightening of the limb. The rate of extension should be very slow indeed, the slower the better, but in these matters one must be reasonable. Extension is commenced 4–6 weeks after the repair. The nerve will adjust to gradual extension providing it takes place sufficiently slowly. Abrupt forcible extension will assuredly cause traction damage either at the suture line or elsewhere along the nerve.

Achieving full extension should take about 3 weeks at the wrist and 4–6 weeks at the elbow and knee.

WHEN SHOULD END-TO-END REPAIR BE ABANDONED IN FAVOUR OF SOME ALTERNATIVE METHOD OF RECONSTRUCTING THE NERVE — THE CRITICAL GAP DISTANCE

This subject remains one of debate and controversy. Some regard *any* tension at the suture line as having an adverse effect on the outcome and do not hesitate to resort to grafting when the gap in a nerve exceeds 1–2 cm. Others, however, believe that larger gaps can be safely repaired by end-to-end union.

Clearly some flexibility is to be expected in the gap distance beyond which end-to-end union is contraindicated, depending as it does on the particular conditions prevailing in any individual case. It is this, and the conflicting information available, that introduce an element of uncertainty in decision-making. Until more precise and reliable information is available on this subject, the decision as to when end-to-end union should be abandoned in favour of some other method of repair will remain a matter of clinical judgement and experience based on some relevant and helpful guide lines.

Definitions

The term critical resection length has been introduced to refer to the length of a segment of a nerve in continuity that, when excised, would jeopardise the end result if the nerve were repaired by end-to-end suture (Orf 1978). It is a term that is not used in this text.

Nerve defect. This is the amount of the nerve destroyed and not the distance ultimately separating the nerve ends. With a clean transection the fascicular patterns at the nerve ends will correspond despite the gap created by their elastic recoil. However, when a segment of more than 1 cm of a nerve has been destroyed, the fascicular patterns at the nerve ends will no longer correspond in every respect.

The gap distance. This term is favoured because it is the gap that must be corrected during the repair of the nerve. It comprises the length of nerve destroyed by the injury or excised, the degree to which the nerve ends have retracted and the amount of each sacrificed in preparing them for the repair.

As the distance between the nerve ends increases a point is ultimately reached when acceptable coaptation is no longer possible. This is the critical gap distance and it determines the point at which end-to-end repair is abandoned in favour of some alternative method of repair.

General comment

1. When considering the distance between the nerve ends that can be safely closed by slight and gentle stretching, mobilisation, transposition and limb flexion, a careful distinction should be drawn between gaps that it is possible to close anatomically, without regard to the outcome, and those unions that are compatible with functional recovery. It is the functionally optimal and not the anatomically maximal gap that can be closed that should concern the surgeon.

2. A nerve trunk is an elastic structure which explains why, following transection, the nerve ends retract and become separated. Because of this elasticity the retracted nerve ends can be easily drawn together again and held by sutures. Some data relating to gaps created by retraction are given in Table 40.1.

The contribution of nerve end retraction to the critical gap distance varies depending on such factors as the size of the nerve, its fascicular structure, and particularly its perineurial content, its mobility in relation to neighbouring structures and points of fixation along its course, and the position of joints. In the case of nerves crossing the flexor aspect of the joint, separation of the nerve ends is least with full flexion and greatest when the limb is fully extended. However, the reverse obtains for the ulnar and sciatic nerves, for these cross the extensor aspect of the elbow and hip joint, respectively.

3. Gaps that can be closed without prejudicing recovery depend on information relating to:

a. Correlations between gap length and the quality of the recovery. Short nerve grafts certainly do well, but whether they consistently do better than a well-executed epineurial repair under identical conditions remains to be seen. It should never be forgotten that:

   i. though two suture lines without tension are preferable to one suture line under considerable tension, one suture line

Table 40.1 Data relating to retraction gaps in nerves

Source	Nerve	Retraction gap in mm
Koschitz–Kosic 1960	Dog sciatic	40
Millesi 1973	Rabbit sciatic	8–12
Orf 1978	Rabbit sciatic Rat sciatic	Limb flexed 6.6 ± 1.5 Limb extended 15.5 ± 2.5
Stevens et al 1985	Rat sciatic	5.2–9.2 Average 7.2
McQuillan 1965	Human	10
Petrov & Solarov 1965	Human sciatic	40
Sunderland (personal observations)	Human — median and ulnar	10–20 depending on factors given in the text

with slight tension is an even more
acceptable form of repair;

ii. the optimal revascularisation of a nerve
graft presents greater problems than the
optimal revascularisation of a single
suture site;

iii. nerve autografting involves the sacrifice
of another nerve, sometimes with
unpleasant consequences.

b. The tensile strength and elasticity of nerves
and an understanding of the changes
occurring in them during elongation. This
information is of considerable importance
because stretching the nerve is the simplest
and, therefore, the first measure adopted to
close the gap, while some stretching is also
introduced when other methods are
employed to reconstruct the nerve. The
elastic properties of peripheral nerves, the
elongation possible within their elastic range,
and the nature and distribution of the
pathological changes developing in a nerve
as it is stretched to and beyond the elastic
limit are discussed in Chapters 12 and 18.
The relevant properties of nerves in the
present context are:

i. the nerve is free to elongate in its bed
unless fixed by tissue or adhesions, or is
rendered inelastic by intraneural fibrosis;

ii. after the normal slack and undulations
in a nerve trunk are taken up, the nerve
behaves as an elastic structure over a
range of elongation that varies from
about 6 to 20 per cent of the length
being stretched. However, conduction
failure and the loss of axon and nerve
fibre continuity within fasciculi occur
well in advance of structural failure of
the nerve trunk;

iii. the rate of application as well as the
magnitude of the deforming force is
important. A greater increase in length
can be safely obtained when a nerve is
very slowly stretched;

iv. the gain in nerve length from stretching
depends on the length of the nerve free
to stretch. This explains why freeing the
nerve from surrounding scar tissue and

mobilising the nerve over a greater
distance adds to the length that can be
obtained by stretching;

v. the proximal segment of a severed nerve
and the denervated distal segment have
equivalent tensile strength and elasticity;

vi. nerve fibres and fine vessels begin to
rupture inside the fasciculi before the
elastic limit is exceeded. This damage
may extend irregularly over considerable
lengths of the nerve and may terminate
in extensive intrafascicular fibrosis.

4. When a limb is finally extended the suture
line should be under no more than the slightest
tension imposed by the normal elasticity of the
nerve; and the limb should always be extended
very slowly indeed. In general:

a. *excessive* traction to bring the nerve ends
together and *excessive* tension on the suture
line when they are united prejudice the
outcome of nerve repair by:

i. threatening the functional and structural
integrity of nerve fibres;

ii. compromising the intraneural
microcirculation at the suture site
(Miyamoto et al 1979, 1981);

iii. aggravating the formation of scar tissue
during suture line healing which creates
a formidable barrier to regenerating
axons.

b. *slight* tension at the suture line is not
necessarily incompatible with good recovery.
It could even have a beneficial effect on the
alignment of the collagen fibres that are
deposited in the interface tissue between the
nerve ends. Moreover, providing proper care
is taken to preserve regional nutrient vessels
and the longitudinal nutrient channels on the
surface of the nerve during mobilisation, the
blood supply to nerve fibres will not be
threatened.

Rodkey et al (1980), in a comparative
study of the relative merits of epineurial
suture under moderate tension and nerve
grafting, concluded that, because the results
were similar, the former should be preferred
on the grounds of its 'greater technical ease'.

5. Three points regarding the critical gap distance require re-emphasising.

a. It should be measured with the limb fully extended because this is the extreme that the repaired nerve will be obliged to cope with after joint mobilisation and postoperative stretching.

b. It should permit tension-free coaptation of the nerve ends after the judicious use of acceptable methods available for closing the gap.

c. It is pointless to embark unnecessarily on complicated auxiliary procedures to effect end-to-end union when this is neither possible nor desirable.

Experimental data

Generally speaking, animal experiments undertaken to determine the relative merits of nerve suture under tension and nerve grafting have been inconclusive other than to confirm a connection between excessive suture line tension and suture line scarring, and damage to the intraneural circulation at a suture line.

In a series of experiments by Terzis et al (1975), tension at the suture site was expressed as mild, moderate and severe according to the length of the nerve segments removed to create the gap to be closed: the lengths were 2, 4 and 6 mm, respectively. The effects of closing a gap of 6 mm were reported as being decidedly harmful. However, such conclusions become irrelevant when it is remembered that gaps of this dimension are regularly and readily closed clinically by end-to-end union without any untoward effect.

The best and most comprehensive experimental study is one by Orf (1978) in which he investigated the critical resection length and critical gap distance in peripheral nerves. Using an unusual technique to stretch sciatic nerves in rabbits, he concluded that autografting becomes necessary if a gap distance exceeds 5–8% of the total available nerve length. In some situations the critical limit could be as low as 4%. He further concluded that mobilisation and transposition are only justifiable if they are not too extensive and do not involve flexing neighbouring joints.

In their studies Millesi, Berger & Meissl (1972), Samii & Wallenborn (1972), Millesi and Meissl (1981) and Millesi (1988), have emphasised the importance of the harmful suture line scarring associated with suture line tension. They prefer to graft gaps exceeding 1.5–2 cm (Millesi 1981).

Clinical considerations

1. It should be noted that it is not possible to effect absolute tension-free end-to-end union, because the normal elasticity of nerves will always introduce some tension at the suture line when it is later recruited during a full range of normal limb movements.

What needs to be determined is the greatest gap distance that can be safely and consistently closed by end-to-end union without prejudicing the outcome and with results that are superior to those obtainable by grafting under identical conditions. This is a problem that will only be satisfactorily solved at the clinical level.

2. Various procedures are at the surgeon's disposal to assist him in closing the gap in a nerve. These include gentle stretching, mobilisation, transposition and slight joint flexion. Where feasible, advantage should be taken of any coexisting fracture, e.g. humerus or femur, to shorten the bone and therefore the distance between the nerve ends. However, shortening an intact bone solely to achieve end-to-end nerve union is now obsolete. This and extensive mobilisation, transposition and acute flexion are a dangerous coalition and should be avoided. This is particularly so now that the introduction of the operating microscope and group fascicular grafting are producing greatly improved results.

If after using all acceptable measures to close the gap, the nerve ends cannot be *easily* approximated, then there is no alternative to grafting.

3. Clearly, the postulated harmful effects of suture under tension are going to be difficult to evaluate because, with so many factors contributing to the end result, it is impossible to decide to what extent a residual disability is directly attributable to the tension. All that can be said is that good recoveries are often recorded when the length of nerve resected, and the various manipulative procedures required to close the gap

were such that some stretching of the nerve must have occurred when the limb was extended.

4. In the past, widely different views have been expressed in the literature on the greatest gap distances that can be closed by end-to-end union with the aid of mobilisation, transposition and joint flexion (Souttar & Twining 1918, Forrester-Brown 1921, Naffziger 1921, Babcock 1927, Forrester 1940, Highet & Holmes 1943, Fahlund 1946, Grantham et al 1948, De Angelis 1947, Schnitker 1949, Sunderland 1949, 1978, Zachary 1954, Clawson & Seddon 1960, Pulvertaft & Reid 1963, Seddon 1963, Collins 1967, Brown 1972). The spread of critical gap distances amongst these authors is so great that it is difficult to summarise the data other than to say that, in reports published prior to 1965, critical gap distances of 10, 12, 15 and 17 cm were common for all nerves. It should be noted, however, that these values were established over a period when the results of nerve grafting were, for many reasons, extremely discouraging. While gaps of this order have been closed by end-to-end suture with acceptable results, the outcome was always uncertain and the overall incidence of failures disturbingly high. The only realistic figures at that time were those of Sunderland (1949, 1978), which are given in Table 40.2.

By the late 1960s critical gap distances were now of the order of 4–8 cm. Since then they have been still further reduced, which reflects the greatly improved results of nerve grafting that have followed the control of infection, the introduction of improved microsurgical techniques and instrumentation, and the pioneering work of Millesi and others on group fascicular nerve grafting (Chapter 43, p. 479).

According to Millesi (1981) the views on this subject expressed at a Hand Meeting in Vienna in 1977 were as follows:

G. A. Urbaniak, Durham, North Carolina	5–7 cm
J. St. Gaul, Charlotte, North Carolina	4–6 cm
E. P. S. Wilgis, Baltimore, Maryland	4 cm
J. E. Kutz, Louisville, Kentucky	3–4 cm
M. Samii, Mainz, West Germany	1.5–2 cm
H. Millesi, Vienna, Austria	1.5–2 cm
G. Brunelli, Brescia, Italy	1.5 cm
D Buck-Gramcko, Hamburg, West Germany	1 cm

Hasse et al (1980) put the critical gap distance at 2.5 cm for the median and ulnar nerves. To Braun (1980) the closure of gaps of 4 cm in the median nerve in the lower forearm and at the wrist presents no problems and did not adversely affect the results. Orf (1978) gives a critical gap distance of 5–8 per cent of the available length of the nerve which in some situations should be reduced to 4 per cent. He reported that for human sciatic nerves of 91 cm the critical gap distance would be 4.6–7.3 cm and for a nerve 108 cm in length, 5.4–8.6 cm. These values are in general agreement with Sunderland's data (1978, Chapters 12 and 18). These give elasticity failing at elongations as low as 6 per cent of the test length which means that nerve fibres would have suffered earlier, probably at extensions of about 4 per cent.

A rough estimate of the critical gap distance can be obtained in another way.

a. The elastic recoil of the nerve ends following a clean transection leaves a gap of 1–2 cm between them. This can be easily reduced by gentle traction wihout jeopardising nerve fibres.

b. Further elongation by gentle traction is possible because of the sliding movement of the nerve in its bed and the taking up of the slack provided by the undulations in the

Table 40.2 Critical gap distances in cm (Sunderland 1949, 1978)

Nerve	Upper arm	Elbow Upper forearm	Lower forearm Wrist
Median	5	3.5	2
Ulnar	7	4	3.5

nerve trunk and fasciculi. These together provide at least another centimetre. This stretching does not threaten nerve fibres, which up to this point continue to run an undulating course within the fasciculi.

c. It is only when the nerve commences to take load and resists further stretching that forcible traction on the nerve ends becomes threatening. On the basis that nerve fibres rupture inside fasciculi well before the latter lose their elasticity, further stretching should be restricted to 4 per cent of the available length of the nerve. This provides about another 1.0–2 cm. These calculations would give a critical gap distance of somewhere between 3 and 5 cm for the median and ulnar nerves, and the tibial and peroneal nerves in the thigh.

General conclusions

Though there is a considerable range of individual variation in the percentage elongations possible within the normal elastic limits of nerves, there is no way of evaluating this feature in any individual patient. It would, therefore, be wise to accept the lowest ranges and, as a conservative estimate, to regard anything in excess of 3–5 cm as decidedly risky. Determining factors are the particular conditions prevailing in any particular case such as the proximity of the suture line to a joint, the mobility of the nerve in its bed and the ease with which the nerve ends can be brought together, aided where indicated by transposition and an acceptable degree of mobilisation and limb positioning.

This is of course setting a somewhat arbitrary value within what may be regarded as a safe range. However, despite what has been written, figures can be misleading and surgical experience and judgement, a 'feel for tissues', and a knowledge and appreciation of the behaviour of nerves under tensile loading, remain the most reliable guides to when traction is approaching a danger level. This subjective method and a gap distance of somewhere between 3 and 5 cm will prove to be about the same.

Additional points to be noted are:

1. end-to-end union is contraindicated where it is impossible to define the limits of third degree damage which is so extensive that excision of the involved segment would create an unbridgeable gap. This occurs, for example, in severe traction injuries of the brachial plexus and sciatic nerve which call for special methods of repair.

2. joint flexion to get the nerve ends together is not contraindicated providing it is not excessive, adequate time is allowed for suture line healing to be completed, and the limb is only then very slowly and never abruptly extended.

3. the gap distance should be measured with the limb extended.

4. regarding the adverse effect of joint movement on a suture line, these effects increase in severity as the suture line approaches the level of a joint. Suture lines at joint level are particularly at risk.

5. traction on the distal stump is transmitted to delicate branches leaving the nerve just below the suture line-to-be and pursuing a short course before entering a muscle. Care should be taken to ensure that these do not suffer a traction injury or become avulsed from muscle.

6. in general, the quality of the recovery declines as the length of the gap increases.

7. finally, and importantly, though the closure of gaps of the order of 3–5 cm would be tolerated by nerve fibres, the effect of tension introduced in this way on suture line healing is another matter. Despite much speculation on this point, precisely when tension reaches a level that introduces a hazard to axon regeneration in the form of scarring is not known. Tension is not the only factor resulting in scarring at the suture line and the participation of so many unknowns in the equation of useful regeneration makes an evaluation of this particular factor extremely difficult. Clinical experience tells us that closing gaps of this order by end-to-end union is often, all other things being equal, followed by an acceptable recovery.

WHEN SHOULD NERVE GRAFTING BE ABANDONED IN FAVOUR OF SOME OTHER FORM OF REPAIR?

There are occasions when, following the destruction of a considerable length of a nerve, the question arises as to whether the gap should be bridged by autografting or whether the preferred procedure should be some other method for getting regenerating axons to the distal stump. For example, following total destruction of the median nerve in the forearm there are three possibilities:

a. the use of a conventional group fascicular graft (Millesi, personal communication);
b. the use of a free vascularised nerve graft (Taylor and Ham 1976);
c. adopting a cross-union procedure by using the dorsal cutaneous of the hand branch of the ulnar nerve to provide regenerating axons to the sensory fasciculi of the median nerve at the wrist, and particularly to those fasciculi innervating the thumb and index finger (Sunderland 1974).

In other words the question at issue is, at what point does the length of a graft exclude its use as a bridging tissue?

Large gaps inevitably introduce the problem of:

  i. obtaining sufficient donor nerves to bridge the gap in a major peripheral nerve;
 ii. injuries causing extensive destruction of a nerve are usually associated with considerable damage to neighbouring structures resulting in a scarred nerve bed;
iii. the rate and degree to which long grafts are revascularised is impaired, particularly when a nerve is left occupying a badly scarred bed. Delayed revascularisation is a common cause of necrosis and graft failure.

Despite the occasional dramatic success, the track record of grafts in excess of 10–12 cm is not good, and if some worthwhile alternative is available it should be used.

WHEN SHOULD THE REPAIR BE JUDGED A FAILURE?

The answer is when:

1. recovery has failed to appear after adequate time has been allowed for this to occur and the nerve remains silent to electrical stimulation.

   The onset of recovery after nerve repair is sometimes unduly delayed but 3–6 months will cover most repairs, depending on the nerve and the level and circumstances of the repair. In some high sciatic nerve repairs this may need to be extended to 9 months;
2. recovery slows and is arrested well short of a functionally worthwhile and acceptable result. Though this might be regarded as the best achievable under the circumstances, it should still be recorded as a failure;
3. the electrodiagnostic evidence confirms a failed repair.

WHEN SHOULD A REPAIRED NERVE IN WHICH THERE HAS BEEN NO RECOVERY BE RE-EXPLORED?

Re-exploration of a repaired nerve is indicated:

1. when acute and disabling tenderness and pain at the suture site are due to involvement of this region in scar tissue and adhesions;
2. immediately suture line failure is suspected or confirmed by the separation of radio-opaque markers. The question of awaiting signs of recovery does not then arise and immediate re-exploration is indicated;
3. when signs of recovery fail to appear within the expected time, and particularly when:

   a. the first repair was performed under such unfavourable conditions that little recovery could be expected. The need to resuture at a later date may have been reported at that time;
   b. no information is available relating to:

      i. the conditions under which the nerve was originally repaired, or

ii. the qualifications of the surgeon performing the repair. There is always the possibility of a poor technique or, for example, the nerve having been sutured in error to a tendon or vice versa.

Assuming that local conditions were considered by an experienced surgeon to be favourable at the time, and that the repair was carefully and skilfully executed, what is a permissible delay before re-exploration? Unless this question can be answered with some certainty, nerves that would have recovered satisfactorily after the first repair will be unnecessarily subjected to a second repair.

A second repair should never be lightly undertaken. In addition to a second operation, the onset of recovery will be further delayed, denervated tissues will deteriorate still further, and the necessary preparation of the nerve ends will add to the retrograde neuronal reaction and create another gap that can be closed only by further stretching the nerve or by grafting. And there is no guarantee that the patient will fare any better.

The risk of performing a second repair or tendon transfer prematurely is of more than theoretical interest.

The only justification for early re-exploration and resuture before adequate time has been allowed for signs of recovery to appear are: (1) confirmed suture line rupture and, (2) when the first suture was performed under such favourable conditions that little recovery could be expected.

Excluding these two groups, it would be wise to refrain from re-exploration or any other premature surgical procedure, for example tendon transfers, until adequate time has been allowed for signs of recovery to appear after the first repair.

These considerations raise two important questions.

What is an acceptable interval between the first repair and the onset of recovery? Calculating a permissible delay is based on the level of the injury, the quality of the repair and accepted rates of regeneration. Such calculations can, for reasons given elsewhere, give only approximate values for any given patient. With this proviso, acceptable delays are 5 months for repairs in the lower half of the limb and 5–7 months for the forearm and leg muscles after repairs above the elbow and knee.

What is the significance of the delay factor in prejudicing the outcome after a second repair? Here the delay now becomes the interval between the original injury and the second repair and not the time elapsing since the first repair.

Estimates of the times within which a satisfactory recovery after nerve repair is still possible are discussed elsewhere in this chapter. On this basis a second repair does not appear to be a hopeful procedure if 3 years have elapsed since the time of the injury, though it could be undertaken as a procedure in desperation.

However delays of 5 and 7 months awaiting the onset of recovery after the first repair should not unduly prejudice the outcome if a second repair is ultimately required. In general, however, the results of second repairs in no way match those possible after a successful first repair.

WHEN SHOULD A REPAIRED NERVE THAT HAS SHOWN SOME RECOVERY BE RE-EXPLORED AND A SECOND REPAIR PERFORMED IN AN ATTEMPT TO OBTAIN A BETTER RESULT?

Where recovery has slowed and become arrested, should one be satisfied with the end result or should one feel justified in advising a second operation in an attempt to obtain a better result? This is often a matter of fine judgement. Guiding principles on which to base a decision are:

1. No matter how favourable the conditions for nerve repair or how well the repair has been performed, functional recovery is rarely complete in every respect and only so in very young. The residual defect usually is greatest in the case of:

a. those digital movements upon which manual dexterity depends and,
b. tactile and proprioceptor sensibility upon which skilled digital movements, the discriminative aspects of sensibility, and the stereognostic sense depend.

To expect complete recovery is therefore a forlorn hope. The question at issue is whether further attempts to obtain a better result will be any more successful. To answer this question recovery could be classed simply as negligible or useful. Negligible would then be regarded as recovery which is of no functional value to the patient and useful as recovery in which at least:

a. the proximal and forearm or leg muscles are contracting to give some useful movement;
b. some individual voluntary movements of the digits are possible as the result of recovery in the intrinsic muscles of the hand, and,
c. there is good protective sensation and cutaneous sensation has been restored to a level where trophic disturbances are fully corrected and some discriminative sensibility is present.

2. If there is negligible recovery after a suitable interval nothing is to be lost by proceeding to a second repair. This policy is justified even where conditions at the original operation were judged wholly favourable for repair, the technique for repairing the nerve was faultless and any subsequent separation at the suture line can be excluded.

Re-exploration is even more urgent when the original repair was faulty with the possibility of a nerve to tendon union and disruption at the suture line.

3. Where, on the other hand, some useful recovery has occurred, what is to be done? In these cases there is no way of knowing whether a second repair would be any more successful than the first. There are even grounds for believing that a second repair could still further complicate regeneration and impair recovery by introducing another round of retrograde neuronal changes, by creating even less favourable conditions at the suture line and by increasing the gap to be closed. Closing a larger gap would inevitably: (a) introduce further nerve stretching and increased tension at the suture line or, (b) necessitate grafting with the introduction of two suture lines. It would seem that if useful recovery has occurred one should rest content. In view of the uncertainties associated with a second repair, and the absence of any guarantee of an improvement, the risks should be fully explained to the patient before deciding on any further action.

WHEN SHOULD POSTOPERATIVE TREATMENT BE DISCONTINUED?

This subject is discussed in Chapter 37. Both clinician and patient should understand that recovery after nerve repair is an exceedingly slow and frustrating process demanding considerable patience, effort and perseverance. Where recovery is such a long-term business patients are easily discouraged.

Supervised treatment should, desirably, be intensive until reinnervated muscles are responding to voluntary effort and at least protective sensation has been restored, by which time a re-educational training regime can be commenced. The most intensive treatment will be reserved for the restoration of function of the hand. This will occupy at least 6 months depending on the level of the repair and the attitude and circumstances of the patient. By this time the patient should have learnt sufficient to manage his own treatment.

Closely supervised postoperative treatment should not be continued any longer than is absolutely necessary.

The progress of recovery should be followed by regular clinical examinations that should be continued for 5 years, monthly in the 1st year, quarterly in the 2nd year and then biannually.

REFERENCES

Babcock W W 1927 A standard technique for operations on peripheral nerves with especial reference to the closure of large gaps. Surgery Gynecology Obstetrics 45: 364
Braun R M 1980 Epineurial nerve repair. In: Omer G E, Spinner M (eds) Management of peripheral nerve problems. Saunders, Philadelphia, p 366
Brown P W 1972 Factors influencing the success of the surgical repair of peripheral nerves. Surgical Clinics of North America 52: 1137
Clawson D K, Seddon H J 1960 The results of repair of the sciatic nerve. Journal of Bone and Joint Surgery 42B: 205
Collins H R 1967 Damage of peripheral nerve associated with orthopaedic injuries. Southern Medical Journal 60: 355

De Angelis A M 1947 Surgical approach to the tibial nerve below the popliteal fossa. American Journal of Surgery 73: 568

Fahlund G T 1946 Suture of posterior tibial nerve below the knee with a follow-up study of the clinical results. Journal of Neurosurgery 3: 223

Forrester C R G 1940 Peripheral nerve injuries with results of early and delayed suture. American Journal of Surgery 47(ns): 555

Forrester-Brown M 1921 The possibilities of suture after extensive nerve injury. Journal of Orthopaedic Surgery 19: 277

Grantham E G, Pollard C, Brabson J A 1948 Peripheral nerve surgery. Repair of nerve defects. Annals of Surgery 127: 696

Haase J, Bjerre P, Simesen K 1980 Median and ulnar nerve transections treated with microsurgical interfascicular cable grafting with autogenous sural nerve. Journal of Neurosurgery 53: 73

Highet W B, Holmes W 1943 Traction injuries to the lateral popliteal nerve and traction injuries to peripheral nerves after suture. British Journal of Surgery 30: 212

Koschitz-Kosic H 1960 Chirurgie und Regeneration durchtrennter peripherer Nerven, S 37 VEB Fold und Gesundheit, Berlin

McQuillan W M 1965 Origin of fibrosis after peripheral nerve division. Lancet 2: 1220

Millesi H 1973 Microsurgery of peripheral nerves. Hand 5: 157

Millesi H 1981 Reappraisal of nerve repair. Surgical Clinics of North America 61: 321

Millesi H 1988 Importance of tension and epineurial tissue in scar formation and its effecting the results of nerve repair. In: Brunelli G (ed) Textbook of microsurgery. Masson, Milan, p 607

Millesi H, Berger A, Meissl G 1972 Experimentelle Untersuchung zur Heilung durchtrennter peripherer Nerven. Chirurgica Plastica 1: 174

Millesi H, Meissl G 1981 Consequences of tension at the suture line. In: Gorio A, Millest H, Mingrino S (eds) Post-traumatic peripheral nerve regeneration: experimental basis and clinical implications. Raven Pres, New York, p 277

Miyamoto Y 1979 Experimental study of results of nerve suture under tension vs nerve grafting. Plastic and Reconstructive Surgery 64: 540

Miyamoto Y, Tsuge K 1981 Grafting versus end-to-end coaptation of nerves. In: Gorio A, Millest H, Mingrino S (eds) Post-traumatic peripheral nerve regeneration. Raven Press, New York, p 351

Miyamoto Y, Watari S, Tsuge K 1979 Experimental studies on the effects of tension in intraneural microcirculation in sutured peripheral nerves. Plastic and Reconstructive Surgery 63: 398

Naffziger H C 1921 Methods to secure end-to-end suture of peripheral nerves. Surgery Gynecology Obstetrics 32: 193

Orf G 1978 Critical resection length and gap distance in peripheral nerves. Acta Neurochirurgica Supplementum 26

Petrov M, Solarov T 1965 Quoted by Orf, p 74

Pulvertaft R G, Reid D A C 1963 Surgery of the hand in Great Britain. British Journal of Surgery 50: 673

Rodkey W G, Cabaud H E, McCarroll H R 1980 Neurorrhaphy after loss of a nerve segment: comparison of epineurial suture under tension versus multiple nerve grafts. Journal of Hand Surgery 5: 366

Samii M, Wallenborn R 1972 Tierexperimentelle Untersuchungen über den Einfluss der Spannung auf Regenerationserfolg nach Nervennaht. Acta Neurochirurgica 27: 87

Schnitker M T 1949 A technique for transplantation of the musculospiral nerve in open reduction of fractures of the mid-shaft of the humerus. Journal of Neurosurgery 6: 113

Seddon H J 1963 Nerve grafting. Journal of Bone and Joint Surgery 45B; 447

Souttar H S, Twining E W 1918 Injuries of the peripheral nerves from the surgical standpoint. British Journal of Surgery 6: 279

Spielmeyer W 1918 Enfolge der Nervennaht. München Medizinische Wochenschrift 65: 1039

Stevens W G, Hall J D, Young V L, Weeks P M 1985 When should gaps be grafted? An experimental study in rats. Plastic and Reconstructive Surgery 75: 707

Sunderland S 1949 Observations on the course of recovery and late end results in a series of cases of peripheral nerve suture. Australian and New Zealand Journal of Surgery 18: 264

Sunderland S 1974 The restoration of median nerve function after destructive lesions which preclude end-to-end repair. Brain 97: 1

Sunderland S 1978 Nerves and nerve injuries, 2nd edn. Churchill Livingstone, Edinburgh

Taylor G I, Ham F J 1976 The free vascularised nerve graft. A further experimental and clinical application of microvascular techniques. Plastic and Reconstructive Surgery 57: 413

Terzis J, Faibisoff B, Williams H B 1975 The nerve gap: suture under tension vs graft. Plastic and Reconstructive Surgery 56: 166

Trail I A 1985 Delayed repair of the ulnar nerve. Journal of Hand Surgery 10B: 345

Woodhall B, Nulsen F E, White J C, Davis L 1956 Neurosurgical implications. In: Woodhall B, Beebe G W (eds) Peripheral nerve regeneration: a follow-up study of 3656 World War II injuries. VA Medical Monograph. Government Printing Office, Washington DC, p 569

Zachary R B 1954 Results of nerve suture. In: Seddon H J (ed) Peripheral nerve injuries. Special Report Series Medical Research Council No 282, HM Stationery Office, p 354

41. Strategies for improving the results of nerve repair

Those whose experience of nerve repair spans the last 50 years will be left with the conviction that the results following nerve repair today are far superior to those of 50 years ago.

There are many reasons for this impressive improvement (Chapter 36) but if one were pressed to nominate the five most important contributions to this improvement one could hardly do better than select:

1. The prevention and treatment of wound infection.
2. The recognition that nerves have an internal structure of considerable complexity that plays a significant part in influencing the quality of the recovery after nerve repair.
3. The recognition that a distinction should be drawn between axon regeneration and functional recovery (Chapter 15).

   For most transected tissues and structures of the body, once continuity has been restored by some mechanical means, natural processes attend to the restoration of function. In the case of peripheral nerves the surgeon can expect no such reward for his services. Here the restoration of function depends on far more than the simple restoration of nerve trunk continuity, requiring as it does the growth of new axons to replace those lost by degeneration below the transection.

   However, axon regeneration does not per se guarantee good functional recovery because many of the regenerating axons may, for different reasons, ultimately fail to make appropriate connections with peripheral tissues or with functionally related end organs so that the restored pattern of innervation is both imperfect and incomplete in comparison with the original. This immediately introduces a distinction between axon regeneration and functional recovery, the latter requiring orderly regeneration directed to re-establishing functionally useful pathways and connections. This is an entirely different proposition in that it introduces a new set of parameters into nerve repair involving a wide variety of microstructural arrangements and physiological processes.

4. The changing objective of nerve repair from the simple restoration of nerve trunk continuity to one strategically planned to maximise the re-establishment of functionally useful connections with the periphery.
5. The introduction of ingenious microsurgical techniques to give effect to changed surgical practices and designed to maximise the restoration of functionally useful axon pathways to the periphery.

Despite the overall improvement in the results of nerve repair generated by all this new knowledge and the introduction of new techniques, and despite the best efforts of experienced and skilled surgeons, the results of nerve repair sometimes fall short of expectations even to the point of being surprisingly and frustratingly disappointing.

All this means that nerve repair must now be strategically planned to prevent, or at least minimise, the wasteful regeneration of axons, and to maximise the restoration of functionally useful connections with the periphery. Only in this way will good results be made even better, the residuum of disappointing results greatly reduced and a persistent uncertainty removed from nerve repair.

If strategies for improving the results of nerve repair are to have any prospect of success, they must be based on a knowledge and understanding of, firstly, the complex structural arrangements and physiological processes involved and, secondly, the various factors that adversely affect the quality of the recovery after nerve repair. The adverse factors and the strategies planned to overcome or at least minimise them operate: (1) centrally, (2) at the interface between the nerve ends, (3) in the nerve below the repair, and (4) in the peripheral tissues.

CENTRAL FACTORS

The severity of the retrograde neuronal reaction determines how many neurons survive and recover to spin a new axon to the periphery. This is determined by the severity and level of the injury, both of which are beyond human influence. Though there is no way of preventing this central reaction, at least steps can be taken to avoid making it worse.

Preparing the proximal nerve end for repair inevitably involves further trauma to the nerve and adds to the severity of the retrograde neuronal reaction and the loss of neurons. For this reason great care should be taken to avoid a rough technique when preparing the proximal nerve end, particularly the unnecessary and repeated trimming of the nerve end when seeking a level where the tissue is considered suitable for repair.

This raises the intriguing question of whether any advantage is to be gained by pharmacologically blocking the nerve well above the site of the repair before proceeding to prepare the nerve ends.

Measures to accelerate axon growth

An advantage of accelerating axon regeneration would be to shorten the time for which muscles and skin are denervated and so hasten the onset of motor and sensory recovery. This would have particular value in the case of high repairs in the limb. This concept has resulted in a search for potentially effective axon growth accelerators.

The use of chemical agents, nerve growth factors, and pulsed electromagnetic and direct current stimulation for this purpose is discussed in Chapter 15.

Though these are interesting and promising lines of research, there are continuing reservations about their clinical value:

1. They do not contribute to the restoration of functionally useful connections and, therefore, useful functional recovery.
2. The formidable problem remains of directing the accelerating agent to the appropriate site, in an appropriate manner and in the right dosage.
3. With so many variables contributing to the end result it is difficult to assign a value to these ancillary methods of promoting axon regeneration.

All in all, the results of these studies have to date been inconclusive and, as the situation currently stands, it has yet to be convincingly shown that the agents under trial for accelerating axon regeneration have a worthwhile role as adjuncts to nerve repair.

STRATEGY DIRECTED TO THE INTERFACE BETWEEN THE NERVE ENDS

The objective of nerve repair is two-fold: (1) to restore continuity and the tensile strength of the nerve trunk by promoting sound healing at the suture line, and (2) to create an environment favourable for the ready and unimpeded passage of regenerating axon tips across the suture line and into the distal stump. It is here that regenerating axons commence their long journey down the nerve to their peripheral destination.

Suture line healing

Healing at the suture line and the restoration of nerve trunk continuity are effected principally by the activity of epineurial fibroblasts and to a lesser extent by endoneurial fibroblasts, the collagen fibres elaborated by the former being much thicker than those produced by the latter. These collagen fibres form a framework for the other components of the granulation tissue developing between the nerve ends. These include fibroblasts, myofibroblasts, capillaries, Schwann and perineurial cells, macrophages and tissue fluid. The end product of this activity is a suture line scar, the mechanical strength of which determines the tensile strength of the repaired nerve at the suture line. This property depends almost entirely on collagen fibres. The suture line is as strong as the rest of the nerve 4–6 weeks after the repair, depending on the size of the nerve.

Suture line scarring

Though sound healing at the suture line to restore the tensile strength of the nerve trunk is an important objective of nerve repair, it should not be forgotten that an equally if not more important function of the junctional tissue is to provide an effective framework for the unhindered passage of regenerating axon tips across the suture line and into the distal stump. In this latter respect suture line scarring impairs axon regeneration by:

1. obstructing the advance of some regenerating axons and delaying the entry of others into the distal stump;
2. constricting regenerating axons that have traversed it, thereby slowing their further progress. The rate of axon advance is slower after nerve repair than after second degree damage;
3. impairing the blood supply to the region, and particularly to the minifascicles of axons that are forming there.

Collagen formation at the suture line is, therefore, a mixed blessing, the dilemma being to control it in such a way as to facilitate the nutrition and passage of regenerating axons without mechanically weakening the union. What is needed is an optimal balance between these two opposing objectives but how to go about achieving this in a planned and purposeful way requires a more detailed knowledge of the cellular and structural mechanisms operating at the interface between the nerve ends than we currently possess.

Strategies directed to improving conditions at the suture site concern the malalignment of collagen fibres and the amount of collagen formed

The malalignment of collagen fibres

One problem relating to collagen formation at the suture line concerns the alignment of the collagen fibres as they are formed. When they are arranged longitudinally in the axis of the nerve, the passage of axon tips across the suture line is facilitated. However, the more usual meshwork arrangement constitutes a barrier to the orderly advance of axon tips. This raises the question of whether there is any way of influencing the alignment of collagen fibres in the developing scar tissue. In this respect it is conceivable that slight tension at the suture line could be an advantage by assisting the favourable alignment of collagen fibres. However, the point at which the beneficial effects of such tension would cease and tension take on a more damaging role is not known.

The amount of collagen formed

The collagen fibres are greater in number, thicker, more densely packed and irregular in their arrangement when:

1. the nerve trunk is composed mostly of epineurial tissue;
2. there is undue tension at the suture line;
3. there is wound infection;
4. the blood supply to the suture line is inadequate;
5. foreign material has been used to repair the nerve.

The overproduction of collagen and harmful scar tissue

This can be reduced by adopting the following precautions during the repair:

1. wound infection should be prevented or effectively treated. This is the worst offender;
2. avoiding rough handling and further traumatising the nerve ends when preparing them for repair;

3. careful attention should be directed to preserving the blood supply to the nerve ends. Assuming that the blood supply to nerves is as important as the evidence suggests (Chapter 10), then the following precautions should be taken during the repair to ensure an adequate continuing nutrient supply to the suture area:

   a. when mobilising the nerve, particularly over great distances, care should be taken to avoid interrupting the extrinsic longitudinal arterial anastomotic system that conveys blood to the nerve ends. In order to do this the main feeding nutrients should be identified and dealt with before each branches to participate in maintaining the longitudinal anastomotic systems.

   b. the most favourable bed available should be found for the repair site even if this means rerouting the nerve.

   c. the practice of surrounding the repair site with protective wrappings should be avoided unless there are sound reasons to the contrary. Wrappings inhibit revascularisation of the suture area from the nerve bed.

   d. major vessels severed by the injury should be repaired.

   e. every effort should be made to limit fibrosis at the suture line which impairs the transport of nutrient materials from capillaries to regenerating axons. This takes us back to suture line healing and fibrosis.

   f. where autografting is indicated:

      i. vascularised grafts should be used where feasible and
      ii. grafts composed of large fasciculi should be avoided because of the risk of central necrosis.

4. the repair site should be 'free running' and to facilitate this steps should be taken to prevent the formation of adhesions fixing the suture line to the nerve bed. The use of inert protective wrappings to achieve this is theoretically sound but carries some reservations in practice. The danger with inert wrappings is two-fold:

   a. they impair the restoration of an adequate blood supply to the suture area from the nerve bed;

   b. they do nothing to exclude epineurial fibroblasts that are the principal offenders. These continue to form collagen inside the wrapping.

5. the suture line should be provided with the best available bed.

6. undue tension at the suture line should be prevented by carefully planned and co-ordinated preparation of the nerve ends, mobilisation, transposition and limb positioning.

7. care should be taken to avoid drying out and heating of the suture area from theatre lighting.

8. the materials and methods currently used for uniting the nerve ends and the tissue reaction that develops about them remain a threat to axon regeneration. Suture materials should be of the finest calibre, kept to a minimum and peripherally placed. Those requirements should be consistent with the need to maintain union of the nerve ends. There is room for further improvement here and the search for less offending materials and methods is being continued. In certain situations the plasma glue and laser methods have advantages.

Fibroblast and collagen inhibitors

The results of experimental investigations directed to finding agents that would effectively limit fibroblast activity and the production of collagen at the nerve suture interface have not so far been encouraging.

The active agents in these investigations have included:

1. *Pyrogenic bacterial polysaccharide complexes (pyrogens and piromen).* It has been claimed that the administration of these agents in sufficient dosage to elevate the peripheral temperature accelerates

the growth and maturation of new axons, possibly because of an inhibitory action on the formation of collagen and scar tissue (Hoffman 1952, 1954). These claims have been denied by others.

2. *Triamcinolone (a synthetic corticosteroid)*. Graham et al (1973) have reported favourably on the use of this agent to reduce the formation of scar tissue and improve regeneration but this appears to be an isolated observation.

3. *Cis-Hydroxyproline*. Opinions on the efficacy of this agent as a collagen inhibitor are divided. Bora and his associates have explored the collagen inhibiting property of this agent by incorporating it in a bioerodable vehicle, Alzamer, in which it is conveyed to the suture site where it is slowly released and then diffuses locally (Pleasure et al 1974, Bora et al 1983). They reported that collagen formation was significantly reduced and the myelin content of the reinnervated distal segment increased with the further observation that electrodiagnostic studies showed normal nerve function. These have been preliminary results. Subsequently Nachemson et al (1985) reported unfavourably on this agent. Access to the suture site remains a problem.

4. *Penicillamine (Bucko et al 1981), and progesterone–oestrogen combinations and methylprednisolone acetate (Nachemson et al 1985)*. When tested these agents were found to have no beneficial effects.

5. *Allantoin*. This white crystalline substance is a normal end product of purine metabolism. It is found in small amounts in human urine. Loots & Joubert (1977) have reported that the application of this substance to the suture area inhibited the production of scar tissue, reduced the formation of adhesions and resulted in more regenerating axons crossing the suture line.

To date, there is very little in these results to indicate that a reliable scar suppressing agent for clinical use is in the offing. Furthermore, even when an effective agent is found, two problems remain:

1. getting the agent to the repair site in an appropriate manner and in the appropriate concentration, and ensuring that its action is confined to that site.
2. ensuring that the inhibition of fibroblast

activity does not so mechanically weaken the suture line as to predispose to postoperative suture line failure.

STRATEGIES DIRECTED TO MAXIMISING THE ORDERLY ENTRY OF REGENERATING AXONS INTO THE DISTAL STUMP, THE FASCICULI AND FINALLY FUNCTIONALLY RELATED ENDONEURIAL TUBES

Having negotiated the junctional tissue joining the nerve end, the next phase in axon regeneration is the entry of axons into the distal stump.

Though there is evidence that the distal stump is the source of neurotropic influences that attract regenerating axons from the proximal stump some distance away, this has no relevance to end-to-end repair because regenerating axons are already at the distal stump when they emerge from the proximal. Once at the distal stump, there are no neurotropic influences to attract axon tips back into their old tubes or even into fasciculi (Chapter 16).

The entry of axons into the distal stump is determined by propinquity and the physical features of the terrain through which they are growing. This means that the surgeon is forced to rely solely on his own initiative and resources in his efforts to minimise the wasteful loss of axons that occurs during this phase of their regeneration.

With this in mind, the strategy is now directed to aiding the entry of axons firstly into the distal stump, then into the fasciculi and not into the interfascicular tissue where they become lost, and finally into functionally related endoneurial tubes in those fasciculi.

Measures to promote the entry of regenerating axons into the distal stump

Here strategy is directed to the immediate repair of the nerve, or with the least possible delay, in order to circumvent nerve trunk and fascicular atrophy. The latter is well in evidence by the end of the 1st month, reaches a peak somewhere between the 3rd and 4th months and then levels out. The variable effect of fascicular atrophy on the cross-sectional area of the nerve trunk is discussed on p 85. Nerve trunk and fascicular atrophy are responsible for large numbers of regenerating axons going astray and failing to establish useful connections.

Measures to promote the entry of regenerating axons into the fasciculi of the distal stump

Here strategy is directed to techniques that will maximise the entry of regenerating axons into the fasciculi of the distal stump.

Only after clean transections will the fascicular patterns at the nerve ends correspond in every respect. All that is required under these favourable conditions is the correct apposition of the nerve ends and a simple epineurial repair.

After the loss of a length of the nerve, the nerve ends then present dissimilarities in the number, size and arrangement of the fasciculi so that even with correct apposition of the nerve ends, at least some fasciculi at the proximal nerve end will be opposed to interfascicular epineurial tissue in the distal stump into which axons will regenerate. Importantly, this mismatching of fasciculi is accentuated by the fascicular atrophy previously described. However, the mismatching is offset where the fasciculi are closely packed with little interfascicular epineurial tissue.

The only way of overcoming this complication is by some form of fascicular grouping at the nerve ends with the object of maximising fascicular apposition when the nerve ends are brought together or joined by a graft. This is the basis of selective group fascicular repair which, because of technical difficulties, has a limited application in end-to-end nerve repair. The merits and criteria for selecting this method of repair are discussed in the next chapter.

Measures to promote the entry of regenerating axons into functionally related endoneurial tubes

Here strategy is directed to taking advantage of any branch fibre localisation at that level by bringing groups of fasciculi with corresponding branch fibre compositions into apposition.

To be successful this manoeuvre requires: (1) a knowledge of the behaviour of the different branch fibre systems as they are traced along the nerve, and (2) the correct axial alignment of the nerve ends as they are brought together. This is the decisive factor in nerve repair.

Obtaining correct axial alignment and matching related fascicular groups is usually easy following clean transection but becomes more difficult as increasing lengths of the nerve are destroyed and particularly when retraction of the nerve ends, local scarring and mobilisation combine to confuse axial relationships. There is also the further problem of the translocation of fasciculi or fascicular groups as they are traced along the nerve (p 37).

Methods for establishing correct axial alignment of the nerve ends are based on one or more of the following:

1. matching blood vessels on the surface of the nerve. The extrinsic longitudinal nutrient arterial systems usually maintain the same quadrantic relationship as they run on the surface of the nerve and it is often possible to establish correct alignment of the nerve ends by lining up this interrupted longitudinal system.
2. careful inspection of the nerve ends may reveal some distinctive fasciculi that have retained their identity at each nerve end.
3. the electrical stimulation of fasciculi at the nerve ends in order to identify motor and sensory fasciculi (Chapter 42, p 454). Unfortunately, this does not overcome the problem of mixed motor and sensory fasciculi where the percentage representation of each is unknown.
4. histochemical methods to distinguish motor from sensory fasciculi (Chapter 42, p. 454). Again there is the problem of mixed fasciculi.

Each method has its limitations and its potential for error. Clearly, what is still needed is a foolproof method for obtaining correct axial alignment of the nerve ends during repair.

Though selective group fascicular repair undertaken to maximise the restoration of useful connections is logically sound, the question to be answered is whether or not it is feasible in practice. This question is discussed in Chapter 42.

THE NERVE AND PERIPHERAL TISSUES BELOW THE REPAIR

The changes occurring in the denervated section of the nerve below the level of the injury are discussed in Chapter 14. Nothing can be done to arrest these changes other than to repair the nerve at the earliest available opportunity in order to reoccupy endoneurial tubes with regenerating axons as soon as possible.

Failure to do this means that with increasing delays endoneurial tube atrophy, fascicular shrinkage and intrafascicular fibrosis will steadily continue until a point is reached where, despite the late regeneration of axons, the quality of the recovery will suffer.

Regarding the denervated peripheral tissues, strategy is directed to preserving them in the best possible condition pending their reinnervation and then to accelerating the restoration of function. The final strategy in the saga of nerve repair is directed to exploiting the capacity of central mechanisms to compensate for residual motor and sensory deficits in peripheral reinnervation. Measures to achieve these several objectives are discussed elsewhere (Chapters 37 and 39).

REFERENCES

Bora F W, Unger A S, Osterman A L 1983 The local inhibition of nerve scar by the bioerodable vehicle, Alzamer, carrying cis-hydroxyproline. Thirty-eighth Annual Meeting of the American Society for Surgery of the Hand, Anaheim, California, March 8

Bucko C D, Joynt R L, Grabb W C 1981 Peripheral nerve regeneration in primates during D-penicillamine induced lathyrism. Plastic and Reconstructive Surgery 67: 23

Graham W, Pataky P, Calabretta A et al 1973 Enhancement of peripheral nerve regeneration with triamcinolone after neurorrhaphy. Surgical Forum 24: 457

Hoffman H 1952 Acceleration and retardation of the process of axon sprouting in partially denervated muscles. Australian Journal of Experimental Biology and Medical Science 30: 541

Hoffman H 1954 Effects of a fibrosis-inhibiting substance on the innervation of muscles by nerve implants. Journal of Comparative Neurology 100: 441

Loots S M, Joubert W S 1977 The use of allantoin in peripheral surgery. In: Fisch H (ed) Facial nerve surgery. Kugler Medical Publications, Amstelveen, p 66

Nachemson A, Lundborg G, Myrhage R, Rank F 1985 Nerve regeneration after pharmacological suppression of the scar reaction at the suture site. An experimental study on the effects of oestrogen-progesterone, methylprednisolone acetate and cis-hydroxproline in rat sciatic nerve. Scandinavian Journal of Plastic and Reconstructive Surgery 19: 255

Pleasure D, Bora F W, Lane J, Prockop D J 1974 Regeneration after nerve transection. Effect of inhibition of collagen synthesis. Experimental Neurology 45: 72

42. End-to-end nerve repair

INTRODUCTION

Factors influencing the quality of the recovery after nerve repair and strategies for circumventing those adversely affecting recovery are outlined in Chapters 39 and 41. Decision making in relation to nerve repair is discussed in Chapter 40. The information contained in those chapters is basic to a rational and meaningful approach to the repair of a severed nerve. This makes them essential reading before proceeding to consider the contents of this chapter.

1. TERMINOLOGY

Neurotization. The operation of implanting a nerve into a muscle.

Neurotomy. The cutting of a nerve.

Neurectomy. The excision of a nerve.

Nerve repair. Refers solely to the restoration of continuity of a nerve, by one of several available methods or techniques. It does not in any way relate to the restoration of axon continuity and the restoration of function but is designed with those ends in view.

Nerve repair by reuniting the nerve ends

Nerve suture. Nerve end-to-end union. Nerve anastomosis. Bringing the ends of a severed nerve together and uniting them by using fine threads or filaments of a variety of materials. Union is preferable to suture in that it leaves unspecified the method used to maintain co-aptation of the nerve ends.

Neurorrhaphy. The suturing of a severed nerve. The simpler term nerve union is preferable.

External sutures. Those confined to the superficial epineurium.

Internal sutures. Those passing through the nerve or placed within it.

Through-and-through sutures. These are sutures that transfix the nerve.

Anchoring or stay sutures. These are sutures placed a short distance from the opposed nerve ends. They are designed to attach the nerve to its bed with the object of preventing or reducing tension at the site of coaptation, thereby preventing separation of the nerve ends postoperatively. They should not transfix the nerve but should be confined to the superficial epineurium.

Epineurial suture. The nerve ends are held together by sutures passed through the superficial epineurium. The term is synonymous with perineural which, however, should not be used lest it be confused with the perineurium and perineurial.

Epineurial suture becomes synonymous with fascicular suture when the nerve is composed of a single fasciculus.

Perineurial suture. Union is effected by means of sutures passed through the perineurium. This increases the risk of exposing the contents of the fasciculus to a harmful reactionary inflammatory reaction and fibrosis.

Sutureless nerve union. Adhesive nerve union. Sutures are dispensed with, the opposed nerve ends being held together with either a biological or non-biological adhesive material. The repair should be tension free in order to prevent the nerve ends from pulling apart.

Sleeve union. The opposed nerve ends are simply enclosed in a sleeve composed of a biological or artificial material.

Sleeve suture. Sleeve adhesive union. The nerve ends are held in apposition within the sleeve by sutures, by an adhesive or by anchoring sutures placed some distance away.

Laser union. Nerve continuity restored by sealing the nerve ends together by laser.

Fascicular repair. The ends of a severed fasciculus are reunited by suture or by some sutureless method. This is rarely possible because the numbers of fasciculi at the nerve ends do not correspond except after clean transection when fascicular repair is contraindicated for other reasons.

Group fascicular repair. The fasciculi at the nerve ends are appropriately grouped and the groups oriented and joined in a manner calculated to maximise fascicular apposition and to take advantage of any branch fibre localisation obtaining at the level of the repair.

Nerve gap. The interval separating the ends of a severed nerve after preparing them for repair. It comprises the length of nerve destroyed, the retraction factor involving the nerve ends and the amount of tissue removed from the nerve ends during their preparation for repair.

Nerve defect. This refers specifically to the length of the nerve destroyed and not to the gap separating the nerve ends.

Spontaneous recovery. Recovery that occurs in the absence of any form of nerve repair.

2. OBJECTIVES OF NERVE REPAIR

The objectives of nerve repair are not only to restore continuity of the nerve trunk but to do so in a strategically planned manner directed to:

1. maximising functional recovery by maximising the entry of axons into the distal stump, into fasciculi and, where possible, into functionally related endoneurial tubes;
2. minimising the loss of regenerating axons into the interfascicular epineurial tissue of the distal stump and into functionally unrelated endoneurial tubes at the suture line;
3. restoring correct axial alignment of the nerve ends;
4. taking advantage of any fascicular branch

fibre localisation present at the level of the repair;
5. minimising the further retrograde loss of neurons consequent on further trauma to the proximal nerve stump during its preparation for repair.

3. MICROSURGERY AND NERVE REPAIR

At the outset it should be emphasised that:

1. The unaided eye has a limited place in nerve surgery today.
2. Microsurgery should be taken to mean surgery under magnification and not surgery under an operating microscope. For this reason microsurgery should include conventional surgical loupe magnification of 4–6×. This is all that is required for the simple epineurial repair of most nerves.

   The operating microscope has no place in simple epineurial repair. It is an instrument for the refinements of nerve repair in certain special and specified situations such as:

   a. cranial nerve repair, nerve repair in the very young and, where indicated, the repair of fine peripheral nerves;
   b. group fascicular nerve repair;
   c. nerve grafting;
   d. nerve crossing.

3. Experimental studies designed to compare the relative merits of the surgical loupe and operating microscope by using clean transections and a simple epineurial nerve repair as the model have confirmed that the operating microscope confers no special advantages on the repair (Wise et al 1969, Gould 1979, Braun 1980, McManamny 1983, Omer et al 1986).

From a recent carefully planned experimental study, Omer (1984) concluded that the surgical loupe does permit a more accurate epineurial repair and does contribute to a better result. Where the clinical situation justifies a simple epineurial repair the high magnification provided by the operating microscope becomes an unnecessary extravagance.

Microsurgical techniques have greatly improved the quality of nerve repair (Kurtze 1964, Michon & Masse 1964, Smith 1964, 1975, Millesi 1973, 1975, Michon 1975, Allieu & Alnot 1978, Sunderland 1978, Merle et al 1984, 1988).

1. They have made internal neurolysis an easier and safer procedure.
2. Loupe magnification has increased the accuracy of conventional epineurial repair by improving the correct alignment of nerve ends and fascicular apposition. In this way it has greatly improved the prospect of obtaining better results.
3. Magnification provides a sharper definition of tissues at the nerve ends during their preparation for repair. In this way, overtrimming on the one hand and inadequate preparation on the other are minimised during the removal of pathological tissue to expose normal nerve. This greatly assists in conserving nerve tissue, in minimising the gap separating the nerve ends and in exposing conditions at the suture line that are favourable to the passage of regenerating axons across the interface.
4. Magnification facilitates the use of ultrafine needles and suture materials.
5. Postoperative fibrosis and neuroma formation at the suture site are reduced.
6. They have made group fascicular repair a practicable proposition.

There are two principal objections to the use of the operating microscope in nerve repair.

1. It has at times encouraged much time-consuming and unnecessarily complicated surgery with results that are in no way superior to those obtainable from a well-executed straightforward epineurial repair.
2. In some forms of group fascicular repair the suture line is left bristling with buried sutures which, no matter how fine, provoke collagen formation and fibrosis. These and other controversial issues are discussed in later sections.

4. TWENTY TENETS OF NERVE REPAIR

If one were asked to nominate the 20 most significant pieces of information relating to nerve repair the selection would immediately and inevitably introduce elements of personal interpretation and preference and individual bias. Accepting this proviso, the following is a list of those regarded by the author as taking priority over others.

1. Today it is not a question of what can be done but of what should be done.
2. There will be times when the surgeon will have only the best of human judgement to guide him. It is then that experience becomes the critical factor in nerve repair.
3. While the limits of nerve repair will ultimately be set by the molecular biologist, in the meantime anatomy remains the fundamental basis of the healing art.
4. Strategies directed to improving the results of nerve repair, to be meaningful and productive, require a detailed knowledge and understanding of the many complex anatomical factors influencing the quality of the recovery after nerve repair.
5. Nerve repair should not be undertaken without the aid of at least loupe magnification. For more intricate repairs the operating microscope has special advantages.
6. Axon regeneration is the key issue in any consideration of nerve repair. In this context:

   a. the destination of a regenerating axon is as important as the process of regeneration itself;
   b. a careful distinction should be drawn between axon regeneration per se and useful axon regeneration on which functionally useful recovery depends;
   c. the objective of nerve repair has now shifted from the simple restoration of nerve trunk continuity to the restoration of functionally useful connections with the periphery. To achieve this the repair must be designed to maximise the restoration of functionally useful

pathways and to minimise the wasteful loss of regenerating axons.

7. There are no neurotropic influences to sort out and organise axon growth in such a way as to ensure that each regenerating axon is successful in re-establishing its original terminal relationships.

8. In the absence of any neurotropic influence to assist him, the surgeon is forced to rely solely on his own resources and initiative when devising methods to satisfy the four essential requirements of nerve repair which are:

  a. to obtain correct axial alignment of the nerve ends. This is of critical importance in nerve repair;
  b. to maximise the entry of regenerating axons into the fasciculi of the distal nerve end;
  c. to minimise the wasteful loss of regenerating axons occurring at the suture line from their entry into the interfascicular tissue of the distal nerve end;
  d. to take advantage of any branch fibre localisation at the level of the repair in order to assist at least some axons to enter functionally related endoneurial tubes in the distal stump.

9. Nerve tissue should be treated at all times with the greatest care, gentleness and respect. Trauma to the nerve ends, which is inevitable during mobilisation and their preparation for repair, should be minimised.

10. During surgical procedures on the nerve care should be taken to avoid compromising the blood supply to the nerve from local nutrient vessels on which the structural and functional integrity of nerve fibres depends.

11. A cleanly severed nerve should be repaired with the least possible delay. This is standard practice when a nerve has been inadvertently severed during surgery or when a tumour has been resected. There are no biological contraindications to this practice. Other more serious injuries and life-saving measures naturally take priority.

12. A nerve should not be approached directly through scar tissue. It should first be identified above and below the scarred area and then each part traced through this tissue.

13. Respect the continuity of an exposed nerve and never resect too hastily.

14. Epineurial and group fascicular nerve repair are not interchangeable methods. Care should be taken to distinguish the criteria to be satisfied in each case before deciding which to use.

15. The gap that can be safely closed by end-to-end nerve repair remains a matter of personal judgement and experience. Preferably, the union should be tension free. However, light tension is permissible because this will not contravene the normal, safe range of elasticity of the nerve.

16. The nerve ends should be securely but loosely united. With tight unions the ends of fasciculi are inevitably forced into interfascicular tissues.

17. The thickness and number of sutures of a foreign material used to maintain coaptation of the nerve ends should be kept to a minimum and be of the finest, consistent with the size of the nerve.

18. Most of the serious hazards to useful axon regeneration occur at the suture line. It is there that efforts to improve the results of nerve repair should be concentrated.

19. The cardinal rule when repairing the nerve is: minimal interference, minimal use of foreign material, minimal tension at the suture line.

20. Regarding end results:

  a. young patients do better than old patients;
  b. early repairs do better than late repairs;
  c. low repairs do better than high repairs;
  d. pure nerves do better than mixed nerves;
  e. one suture line repairs do better than two suture line repairs;
  f. short nerve grafts do better than long grafts.

5. FREEING AND MOBILISING THE NERVE AND NERVE ENDS

1. The nerve should never be approached directly through scar tissue. It should first be identified and isolated well above and below where it is embedded in scar through which it can then be safely traced from above and below.
2. Before proceeding to free and isolate the damaged segment of the nerve from scar tissue and adhesions:

   a. the functional status of that segment of the nerve passing through scar tissue should be defined by stimulating the nerve above where it becomes lost in scar tissue. The procedure is repeated after the nerve has been freed;
   b. before the exposed nerve has been disturbed, any visible landmarks on the surface, such as the arrangement of blood vessels, should be noted. This could assist in restoring correct axial alignment of the nerve ends when they are finally brought together. This is further aided by placing four identification sutures through the superficial epineurium at corresponding and nearly equidistant points on the circumference of the proximal and distal stumps. These are sited at a convenient distance above and below the nerve ends or segment to be resected, so that the nerve ends can be prepared without interfering with the markers. The use of white suture material for one half of the circumference and black for the other helps in maintaining correct axial alignment.

3. Freeing the nerve ends from surrounding scar tissue requires careful, skilled, patient and gentle dissection:

   i. to avoid further trauma to the nerve;
   ii. to avoid damage to intact branches in the vicinity, and
   iii. to preserve the blood supply to the nerve, because an efficient blood supply at the suture line is essential for a sound and functionally successful union.

Further mobilisation of the nerve beyond freeing the nerve ends is discussed in Chapter 38, page 386.

6. PREPARATION OF THE NERVE ENDS

Conditions that affect the security of the union, the fate of regenerating axons and the quality of recovery include:

a. the relationship of the opposed nerve ends to one another in terms of cross-sectional areas, fascicular patterns, and the relative amounts of fascicular and epineurial tissue;
b. the extent of fascicular and endoneurial tube shrinkage;
c. the degree of fibre localisation prevailing at the level of the repair and the extent to which correct axial alignment of the nerve ends can be preserved during nerve repair;
d. the condition of the nerve ends after preparing them for end-to-end union;
e. the distance separating the nerve ends. This determines the ease with which they can be brought together, the tension introduced to do this and the amount of stretching to which the nerve is subjected postoperatively;
f. the nature of the bed in which the suture line finally rests;
g. the surgical technique and the method employed to unite the nerve ends.

Precautions

When preparing the nerve ends for repair, special care should be taken:

1. To preserve the blood supply to the repair site. This is essential for sound union.
2. To conserve nerve tissue because:

   a. increasing the length of nerve destroyed still further disturbs fascicular relationships at the nerve ends;
   b. unnecessarily trimming the nerve ends may prejudice recovery by increasing the distance separating them so that end-to-end union would then result in harmful and unacceptable tension at the suture line.

Assessing the suitability of the nerve ends for repair

The accepted practice is to trim the nerve ends carefully until 'healthy bundles or satisfactory cross-sections are exposed'. The terms 'healthy' and 'satisfactory', however, remain undefined. The term 'healthy' is also somewhat misleading, since the faces of the nerve ends will not present precisely the same appearance because of the changes, secondary to Wallerian degeneration, that have affected the distal segment. Ideally the proximal face should present fasciculi with well-defined outlines that glisten and pout somewhat from the nerve end. They should be set in normal-looking epineurial connective tissue and the overall appearance should be one of a recently cut normal nerve. In this respect the condition of the nerve ends for repair should be judged on the appearance and state of the fasciculi rather than on the amount and density of the interfascicular connective tissue. It is not possible to assess these features with the unaided eye. Magnification is necessary to determine when the transition from pathological to normal looking tissue is reached.

Because the destruction of fasciculi sometimes extends irregularly along the nerve stumps, sectioning the nerve ends may expose some normal looking fasciculi before others. In these cases the trimming should be continued until conditions are equally favourable across the entire face of the nerve. The fasciculi may also take on a healthy appearance while still surrounded by dense connective tissue. While it is desirable to obtain a normal-looking connective tissue field for the fasciculi, resecting more tissue in an attempt to do this adds to the risks of unnecessarily increasing the length resected and therefore the gap to be closed. It is generally agreed that some fibrosis between healthy looking fasciculi in the proximal stump is no obstacle to good regeneration.

It is the quality of the fasciculi which bears on regeneration and, immediately a level is reached where they present a favourable appearance, the nerve end may be regarded as suitable for repair.

It is more difficult to judge conditions at the face of the distal stump in delayed repair because the distinction between fibrous and fascicular tissue becomes less clear with the atrophy of the latter. Precisely where the section passes from unfavourable to favourable tissue is then not always clearly defined even under magnification and, to be on the safe side, it is preferable to remove more of the distal stump in order to be certain of establishing the most favourable conditions for repair.

Though oedema and swelling of the epineurium occasionally force fasciculi apart and cause them to be more widely separated, this is part of an acute reaction that has usually cleared by the time the nerve is repaired. What is more important is the normal variation in the amount of the epineurial tissue and in the number and arrangement of the fasciculi (Chapters 7 & 9). It is not unusual for fasciculi to be widely separated by a large amount of interfascicular connective tissue, and this feature should be noted lest it be interpreted as pathological. Failure to appreciate this introduces the risk of unnecessarily resecting normal tissue in an attempt to reveal a larger number of fasciculi with less interfascicular tissue which is an arrangement not normally present at that level. When assessing conditions at the distal nerve end for repair it is the quality of the connective tissue and the appearance of the exposed face of each fasciculus that are important.

Resection of the nerve ends during their preparation should not be overgenerous, for unnecessary trimming prejudices recovery by increasing the length of nerve destroyed and the gap to be closed. At the same time their preparation must be adequate even if this necessitates repair by grafting.

The thesis is developed elsewhere that the most mischievous factors militating against recovery are those that foster the wasteful regeneration of axons into the interfascicular epineurial tissue, and that these are introduced when the fascicular patterns of the nerve ends fail to correspond (Chapter 39). The dissimilarity is usually increased as the segment of nerve destroyed or resected increases and, for this reason, every attempt should be made to conserve nerve tissue when preparing the nerve ends for repair. Though the co-existence of other variables affecting regeneration makes it difficult to assess the influence of the distance separating the nerve ends, it is generally agreed that the results after the closure of small gaps are superior to those that follow the closure of large ones.

The condition of the nerve ends as an aid to prognosis

The condition of the nerve ends is best assessed under magnification during their preparation and by the histological examination of biopsy tissue which provides a more reliable basis for forecasting the success or failure of the repair and the quality of the end result. The examination should be directed with particular reference to:

1. the nature of the tissue;
2. the cross-sectional areas of the proximal and distal stumps;
3. the relative cross-sectional areas devoted to fasciculi and epineurial tissue at the nerve ends, and
4. a comparison of the fascicular patterns at the nerve ends to test for fascicular mismatching that results in fasciculi being opposed to interfascicular connective tissue. Despite such mismatching reasonable end-to-end apposition of fasciculi may still be attainable during repair if the fasciculi occupy most of the cross-sectional area of the nerve. On the other hand, where the fasciculi are small and widely separated the chances of some fasciculi in the proximal stump being unavoidably opposed to the interfascicular tissues of the distal stump are greatly increased.

7. RESTORING CORRECT ALIGNMENT OF THE NERVE ENDS

In the absence of any neurotropic influences that will attract regenerating axons into their respective endoneurial tubes in the distal stump it is important, when the nerve ends are being opposed, to take advantage of any fascicular branch fibre localisation at that level that would assist in the restoration of functionally useful connections. This is done by maintaining correct axial alignment of the nerve ends so that the general relationship between corresponding quadrants of the nerve are retained when the nerve ends are brought together and united.

In clean transection injury this does not usually present a problem because with negligible loss of nerve tissue the fascicular patterns at the nerve ends will be identical, or almost so. Under these favourable conditions there is no difficulty in restoring correct fascicular relationships when the nerve ends are opposed.

However, after the loss of a segment of the nerve restoring correct axial alignment of the nerve ends may be more difficult than is generally recognised. This is particularly so when the nerve ends are widely separated and normal relations are distorted by their involvement in scar tissue. A further complication may also be introduced by the translocation of some fasciculi within the lost segment so that they now occupy different sectors at the nerve ends (p. 37). Attempts to correct for this would only throw other fasciculi out of alignment.

The disappointing results that are the outcome of some nerve repairs could well be due to the failure to restore correct axial alignment of the nerve ends during the repair.

Faced with such difficulties, the restoration of correct axial relationships may be facilitated by:

a. the use of identification markers prior to freeing the nerve or nerve ends from scar tissue;
b. matching blood vessels on the surface of the nerve. The major longitudinal anastomotic chains of the extrinsic nutrient vascular system usually retain their position on the surface of the nerve for considerable distances. This arrangement may assist in establishing the correct axial alignment of the nerve ends;
c. matching the fasciculi at the nerve ends. Despite the rapid changes in the cross-sectional fascicular patterns brought about by fascicular plexus formations, not all fasciculi or groups of fasciculi participate in plexus formations at any one level. Consequently, some fasciculi or groups of fasciculi retain their identity over greater distances than others so that a distinctive fasciculus or group of fasciculi may be present at both nerve ends. These can be used to establish correct alignment of the nerve ends;
d. by taking advantage of any surviving strand of epineurial tissue linking the nerve ends

that may provide a useful guide to the restoration of correct axial relationships;

e. the use of electrical and histochemical methods to identify fasciculi and groups of fasciculi. These methods are discussed later in this chapter (p. 454).

8. METHODS FOR BRINGING THE NERVE ENDS TOGETHER

Several methods are available for bringing the nerve ends together when an injury or resection leaves them separated. Obviously it will not be necessary to use all methods in every case. A judicious and well-planned combination, in successive steps, of simple stretching, mobilisation and slight limb flexion is usually sufficient to correct moderate gaps, supplemented where necessary by transposition to give the nerve a shorter course, and by taking advantage in special circumstances of any co-existing fracture to shorten a bone. The successful record of nerve autografting in recent years has eliminated the need for bulb suture and nerve union under considerable tension.

When the nerve is exposed and the nerve ends have been prepared for repair, the gap between them is measured with the limb extended. The decision is then taken as to whether the repair should be by end-to-end union or by autografting. The critical gap distance that determines the point at which end-to-end repair is abandoned in favour of some alternative method of repair is discussed in Chapter 40.

The tension that may be safely applied when approximating the nerve ends, the distance for which mobilisation of the nerve should be continued, the degree to which a joint should be flexed and maintained in that position, and the rate at which the sutured nerve should be stretched postoperatively are difficult questions to answer in any individual case for there are only general principles and not precise rules to guide the surgeon. Much must, therefore, be left to his judgement and experience, and those with a respect and 'feel' for tissues, and an appreciation of what they will tolerate when deformed, will achieve better results than those who lack these essential qualities.

In this context it should be noted that some are so impressed by the harmful effects caused by suture line tension that they prefer to graft even short gaps in a nerve of the order of 2 cm (Millesi et al 1972, Orf 1978, Millesi & Meissl 1981, Millesi 1988).

Gentle traction on the nerve ends

The problem of closing the gap by gentle traction on the nerve ends introduces the subject of stretching peripheral nerves. Information relating specifically to the critical gap distance that can be closed by stretching the nerve is contained in a section devoted to this subject in Chapter 40.

The slack course taken by the nerve in its bed together with the undulations of the fasciculi within the epineurium and of the nerve fibres inside the fasciculi, along with the normal elasticity of the nerve, permit it to be stretched within certain limits without threatening the integrity of the contained nerve fibres. However, the extra length gained in this way is only suitable for closing smaller gaps in a nerve. This is because the undulations are soon taken up and the normal elastic limit reached. If stretching continues the nerve fibres suffer. In this respect it should be remembered that during stretching conduction and physiological failure in nerve fibres occur in advance of structural failure (Chapter 18).

For stretching to be effective the nerve stumps must first be freed from scar tissue and adhesions that limit elongation. Manual traction on the nerve to bring the nerve ends together should then be applied gently until the normal slack and undulations are taken up, at which point the nerve becomes taut and tension then falls directly on the fasciculi. Further elongation should be within the elastic range but to be on the safe side should not exceed 4 per cent of the mobilised length of the nerve. Clearly only small defects can be successfully closed in this way.

If this simple procedure fails then extended mobilisation, transposition, and limb flexion follow in successive steps as they are required. (Chapter 38).

Traction damage during nerve repair is caused by: (a) forcible attempts to bring the nerve ends together; and (b) careless postoperative extension after immobilisation in flexion.

The characteristic complications of excessive stretch or traction caused in this way are:

    i. the intrafascicular rupture of nerve fibres and such extensive intrafascicular fibrosis that few regenerating axons find their way through this barrier;

    ii. the often irregular but extensive longitudinal distribution of the lesions as the elastic limit of the nerve is approached and exceeded;

    iii. the rupture of nutrient blood vessels. This leads to extensive haemorrhage, particularly inside the fasciculi, which aggravates post-traumatic scarring;

    iv. more lasting retrograde neuronal effects.

Flexion of joints

Where nerves cross the flexor aspect of joints they are stretched when the limb is extended but are slackened when it is flexed. This feature is utilised in closing gaps in some nerves. The hazards of immobilising joints for the period necessary to establish sound union at the nerve ends, and the tension created within the nerve when the limb is extended, should not be overlooked when employing this manoeuvre to close the gap (see Chapter 40, p. 420).

Transposition

This procedure is undertaken in order to: (1) gain the additional length required to close the gap in a nerve; (2) provide a more satisfactory bed for the suture line; and (3) relieve tension on the nerve during movement. This procedure is discussed in Chapter 38.

Bone shortening

Bone shortening as a method of facilitating the end-to-end repair of a severed nerve requires consideration only when there is a co-existing fracture or non-union of the humerus or femur and a reasonable degree of bone shortening would permit effective end-to-end repair.

In these cases shortening of the order of 5 cm appears to be the upper limit. Whether such a drastic procedure should be preferred to autografting cannot be answered until the relative merits of the two procedures are known. To date, references to the quality of the recovery following end-to-end union made possible by bone shortening, and that achieved by autografting do not permit any such comparison, though the greatly improved recoveries after grafting in recent years are in its favour.

Shortening an *intact* bone by the removal of a segment to obtain end-to-end apposition of a nerve is unacceptable in view of the satisfactory record of nerve autografting.

Bulb suture

Bulb suture involves stretching the nerve in two stages. The fibrous or bulbous ends of the nerve stump are securely joined by stout sutures after full advantage has been taken of mobilisation, stretching, limb flexion and transposition to approximate the nerve ends. The limb is then gradually extended postoperatively. The wound is later reopened, the bulbs excised, and the nerve ends suitably prepared and sutured with the limb again flexed. Following the definitive repair the limb is gradually extended again.

With this method there is always the danger that the postoperative stretching, no matter how carefully performed, may cause considerable intraneural damage that is subsequently followed by extensive scarring. The strong fibrous ends of the nerve stumps are stronger than nerve tissue so that with excessive stretching the latter fails before the bulb sutures rupture or pull out.

Because the results following nerve autografting are so much better than in the past, bulb suture no longer has a place in nerve repair and the procedure is now of historical interest only.

9. METHODS FOR RESTORING AND MAINTAINING CONTINUITY OF THE NERVE TRUNK

It is now well established that:

1. a suture line represents a formidable barrier to the passage of regenerating axons, some being permanently blocked and others misdirected as they grow. It is in this zone that the greatest loss of axons occurs during regeneration.
2. the method of preparing the nerve ends for end-to-end union influences the microstructure of the tissue forming the junctional interface at the 'suture' line.

This formation has stimulated considerable and continuing interest over the years in suture repair technology, investigations being directed to devising methods of improving the quality of the recovery after nerve repair.

The methods available include both end-to-end repair by nerve suture and those using sutureless tension-free techniques.

Regardless of the method used:

1. further trauma to the nerve ends during the repair should be minimised.
2. all foreign material and blood clot should be carefully removed from the nerve ends.
3. where stay sutures are used to fix a nerve to its bed in order to prevent suture line separation, they should be confined to the superficial epineurium some distance from the nerve ends. Through and through sutures for any purpose should be avoided because they increase the risk of direct injury to fasciculi and nerve fibres.
4. the technique employed should not threaten the blood supply to the site of the repair.
5. the repair completed, the repaired site should be located in a bed of soft healthy tissue where it is protected and assured of a good blood supply, and where the risk of its becoming involved in scar adhesions is greatly reduced. If left occupying an unfavourable bed, the nerve should, where possible, be transposed to a more favourable site.
6. enclosing the site of the repair with a wrapping in order to protect it from becoming invaded by fibroblasts from injured tissue outside the nerve, and to confine regenerating axons to the nerve as they cross the suture line, has not been shown to confer any advantage on the repair. On the contrary, the practice may even have the opposite effect of promoting damaging fibrosis at that site. The routine use of such wrappings is not advocated where the suture site already occupies a favourable bed, but should be reserved for those occasions where the nerve must be left in a scarred bed to which it would otherwise become attached by adhesions (p. 459).
7. the use of radio-opaque markers. These are attached to each stump just beyond the repair site and the distance between them is measured. Radiological examination at intervals postoperatively will reveal whether the repair is holding or has failed. Separation of the nerve ends before postoperative stretching is commenced may occur owing to haemorrhage and tissue necrosis at the suture line, or inadequate healing. The period of greatest danger, however, is during postoperative extension of a limb flexed to facilitate end-to-end union.

10. END-TO-END NERVE UNION

Where the nerve ends can be brought together with little tension there is no substitute for a well-executed conventional epineural suture for repairing major peripheral nerves. This method could, however, be challenged in the future by the de Medinaceli technique. Under certain specified conditions the nerve should be repaired by the group fascicular method. Where the nerve ends can only be approximated under considerable tension there is no substitute for autografting or the use of one of the corrective procedures discussed in Chapter 43.

1. Nerve suture should be performed under loupe magnification.
2. The suture material and technique employed to effect union should be such as to minimise scarring at the suture line while at

the same time encouraging strong union and the development of bridging tissue that favours the passage of regenerating axons to the distal stump.

3. The local reaction to the material should be minimal. In the early stages this reaction interferes with the orderly advance of regenerating axons. At a later date the resulting fibrosis obstructs some axons and constricts others.

4. In order to minimise needle trauma, the needle should be of the finest atraumatic type that is consistent with technical efficiency and the size of the nerve to be repaired. The needle and suture tracks should not be too disproportionate. 8/0 sutures are suitable for the larger nerves and 10/0 for the finer. The former require a needle leaving a track of about 130 μm and the latter one of 70–80 μm.

5. Sutures should be confined to the superficial epineurium so that they, and the reaction they excite, are not in the track of regenerating axons. They should avoid transfixing the perineurium of fasciculi which increases the risk of involving nerve fibres either directly or in the ensuing inflammatory reaction.

6. The reaction that all suture materials promote is influenced, inter alia, by the surface area of the material in contact with the nerve. This should be kept to a minimum by using fine, interrupted sutures and only the number required to maintain union.

   The function of sutures is to hold the nerves ends *lightly opposed* until healing is completed. Only the number of sutures required to do this should be used. Two to six sutures are adequate for most repairs, the number depending on the size of the nerve. All that is necessary is that the nerve ends should be held lightly together.

7. The apposition should be loose and never tight. Tight unions result in buckling of the fascicular ends and force the cut ends of fasciculi into interfascicular tissues of both distal and proximal stumps.

8. Biodegradable have an advantage over non-absorbable materials in that the reaction to them is of shorter duration. They should remain until union is secure. This occurs by about week 4–6 depending on the size of the nerve.

9. The material should be available in the finest calibre compatible with ease of handling, technical practicability, and with the tensile strength to maintain secure union of the nerve ends.

Of all the materials available and tested (Sunderland & Smith 1950) silk, monofilament nylon and polyglycolic acid (Dexon & Vicryl) sutures best fulfil these conditions. All three excite some inflammatory reaction which is minimal in the case of the absorbable variety. Silk has the disadvantage of pulling on the tissues with a tendency to unravel. In the case of nylon, no matter how fine the suture, the adverse effects of the reaction and persisting fibrosis should never be under-estimated. Comparisons of absorbable and monofilament nylon sutures (6/0 & 8/0), based on experimental studies, have shown that the former has only a marginal advantage over the latter (Hudson & Hunter 1976, Bratton et al 1981, Cham et al 1984).

Epineurial and group fascicular repair

Preliminary comment

Many experimental investigations undertaken in recent years to test the relative merits of each of these methods have been ill conceived because:

1. they have been based on the erroneous assumption that they are alternative and interchangeable methods of repair;
2. the experiments have been based on clean transections under conditions in which group fascicular repair would normally never be considered;
3. they failed to recognise that each method has definite and specific criteria that must be satisfied before the method should be used;
4. the two sets of criteria are fundamentally different;
5. the two methods are not alternatives nor are they ever interchangeable (Sunderland 1979).

Epineurial repair

The criteria for the restoration of nerve trunk continuity by conventional epineurial repair are:

1. when the nerve has been cleanly severed. The fascicular patterns at the nerve ends are then identical. Providing correct axial alignment of the nerve ends has been established, fascicular continuity will be achieved when the nerve ends are brought together;
2. at levels where the fasciculi, though mismatched, are closely packed and there is little interfascicular epineurial tissue into which regenerating axons can grow and no branch fibre localization to be exploited. These conditions favour the coaptation of fascicular tissue when the nerve ends are united, while correct axial alignment of the nerve ends during repair will, despite any branch fibre mixing, at least go some way to assisting the restoration of functionally useful pathways.

Conventional epineurial repair also:

1. is a less complicated and time-consuming procedure than group fascicular repair and can be performed under surgical loupe magnification and without the need for highly specialized equipment and facilities;
2. under the conditions specified it effects fascicular coaptation that is in no way inferior to that obtainable by group fascicular repair;
3. minimizes interference with the nerve ends when they are prepared for union;
4. requires fewer sutures, which should be located peripherally, thereby leaving the nerve end interface free of foreign material;
5. permits the nerve ends to be held together under slight tension which dispenses with the need for a short graft and two suture lines instead of one.

There is general agreement among those who have written on the subject that, unless there are exceptional circumstances, a simple conventional epineurial repair is the preferred method.

Group fascicular repair

Fascicular repair is a misleading term in that it creates an erroneous impression that the nerve is repaired fasciculus by fasciculus, on a one-to-one basis, so that fascicular continuity is restored in every respect.

While it is technically possible to suture one fasciculus to another, nerve repair in this way is impracticable for the following reasons:

1. except with clean severance, the fasciculi at the nerve ends will not be equal in number nor will they correspond in size, size differences being increased by any atrophy of the fasciculi in the distal stump. Attempts to restore fascicular continuity, on a one-to-one basis, would inevitably leave some fasciculi unaccounted for, while size differences would make it impossible to match all fasciculi on the basis of their cross-sectional areas.
2. human nerves are usually multi-fasciculated structures. For example, the number of fasciculi comprising the median and ulnar nerves at the wrist varies from 6 to 37 and 8 to 36, respectively. Even if fasciculus to fasciculus repair were possible, the numbers of fasciculi to be united would leave the suture line crowded with suture material. This would aggravate and increase the formation of troublesome scar tissue.
3. some fasciculi are so fine that attempts to reunite them would be self-defeating.

While there may be occasions when nerve repair, fasciculus to fasciculus, is feasible these will be rare. Henceforth the term fascicular repair should be understood to mean group fascicular repair.

Objectives of group fascicular repair

What fascicular repair really means then is group fascicular repair in which the fasciculi at the nerve ends are grouped in a manner calculated to:

1. obtain the best possible fascicular apposition during union with the object of confining regenerating axons to fasciculi and, therefore, endoneurial tubes;
2. reduce the chances of fasciculi becoming opposed to interfascicular tissue;

3. take advantage of any localisation of branch fibres obtaining at the level of the repair in order to assist the entry of regenerating axons into functionally related endoneurial tubes.

In order to meet these objectives the following guidelines should be observed when grouping the fasciculi.

1. As with all other methods of repair, correct axial alignment of the nerve ends is crucial to the success of the repair. Group fascicular repair does not remove the necessity for doing this because it is the first step towards grouping the fasciculi at the nerve ends in a manner designed to exploit whatever branch fibre localisation is present at that level.

2. Where naturally occurring fascicular groupings can be identified at the nerve ends, these should be preserved even when the patterns of corresponding groups differ, for they are evidence of a spatial relationship. Such arrangements are found immediately above the site of branching.

3. However, where there are no naturally occurring fascicular groupings, the fasciculi are then arranged arbitrarily into groups in order to achieve the objectives listed above. This may necessitate grouping a number of fine fasciculi in order to match the cross-sectional area of a larger one but always in whatever combinations are necessary to give the best coaptation of fascicular tissue. At the same time corresponding sector relationships should be preserved in order to take advantage of any prevailing branch fibre localisation. However, expectations that group fascicular repair will assist regenerating axons to re-establish functionally useful connections at the periphery will only be realised where there is a worthwhile localisation of branch fibre systems at the level of the repair.

Grouping fasciculi at the nerve ends often becomes an exercise in interpreting the likely fascicular fibre content and concentration of the different branch fibres at the level of the repair.

Criteria for using group fascicular repair

Expecting more of a procedure than it has to offer is counterproductive. Group fascicular repair is not a method for all occasions and its limitations and disadvantages should be recognised and the criteria for its use clearly defined. It is pointless to embark on a long, tedious, complicated and difficult fascicular repair when it is contraindicated and a conventional epineurial repair would be more appropriate and effective.

Group fascicular repair should be reserved for those occasions when it is clear that conventional epineurial repair would in one way or another result in a serious loss of regenerating axons at the suture line. Group fascicular repair becomes the preferred method:

1. in nerve grafting and nerve cross-anastomosis where there is no alternative;
2. where the fascicular arrangement at the nerve ends is one in which much of the fascicular tissue at the proximal nerve end would be opposed to the interfascicular tissue of the distal nerve end if the nerve ends were brought together in a conventional epineurial repair. Under these conditions the loss of regenerating axons in the interfascicular tissue would be greatly increased;
3. where some measure of fascicular branch fibre localisation is present, thereby maximising the chances of regenerating axons entering functionally related endoneurial tubes. For this to be effective it is necessary to identify and unite fascicular groups composed of functionally related fibre systems. Suturing motor fascicular groups to sensory and vice versa must be avoided at all costs. This raises for consideration the accurate identification and matching of fascicular groups at the nerve ends and this, in turn, requires a knowledge of the internal anatomy of nerve trunks.
4. where there is a definite risk of sensory becoming opposed to motor fasciculi. The significance of this point is illustrated by reference to the loss of a segment of a radial nerve above the elbow (Fig. 7.7). Though the radial is often regarded as essentially a motor nerve, it should be remembered that, just above the elbow, the cross-sectional area of the nerve devoted to superficial radial

branch fibres (cutaneous) occupy from a quarter to a third of the cross-sectional area of the nerve. Numerically then, they are not a minor component of the radial nerve.

At the level in question, the superficial radial fibres are contained in a fascicular group located anteriorly in the nerve, the posterior interosseous nerve fibres in a group located posteriorly and the radial extensor branch fibres in a group located laterally.

Malalignment of the nerve ends during repair could bring sensory fasciculi into apposition with motor fasciculi and vice versa, a complication favouring faulty regeneration. In order to avoid such a complication the three functionally unrelated fascicular groups should be identified, isolated and sutured separately by group fascicular repair.

5. Where a branch fibre fascicular group is present in the proximal nerve end but is absent in the distal stump owing to the loss of a branch. Under these conditions bringing the nerve ends together could bring functionally unrelated fascicular groups into juxtaposition.

In some regions the nerve fibres representing individual branches, or functionally related branch systems, are localised in separate fascicular groups that are surrounded by slight thickenings of the epineurium. The arrangement is one that permits fascicular groups to be accurately identified and safely isolated at the ends of a nerve severed in that region. Under these conditions it is possible to suture fascicular groups separately. This improves the chances of reducing the wasteful growth of axons into foreign endoneurial tubes as well as into the interfascicular tissue of the distal stump. This is best illustrated by reference to an ulnar nerve injury in the lower third of the forearm where a 25 mm segment of the nerve has been destroyed along with the origin of the dorsal cutaneous branch (Fig. 42.1).

At the wrist, the bundle groups representing the superficial (predominantly cutaneous) and deep (predominantly motor) divisions of the ulnar nerve can be identified and separated for a distance of about 5–7 cm above the level of the wrist joint.

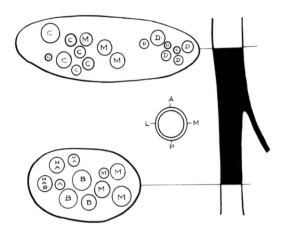

Fig. 42.1 Two sections from a serially sectioned specimen of an ulnar nerve. The sections are 25 mm apart and the dorsal cutaneous of the hand leaves the nerve from the intervening segment. If this segment of the nerve (blackened) were destroyed the proximal and distal stumps would present the fascicular patterns illustrated. The fasciculi for the dorsal cutaneous fibres would be present in the proximal stump but not in the distal and when the nerve was repaired these cutaneous bundles would be adjacent to those in the distal stump which are destined for the deep terminal (muscular) branch. *M*, Deep (muscular) division: *H*, Cutaneous fibres from the hypothenar eminence; *A*, Cutaneous fibres from the ulnar side of the little finger; *B*, Cutaneous fibres from the fourth interspace; *C*, Combined superficial (cutaneous) division fibres; *D*, Dorsal cutaneous fibres. *A*, *P*, *L*, and *M*, Anterior, Posterior, Lateral and Medial, respectively.

Under these conditions there are advantages in separately suturing the two different bundle systems in order to reduce the amount of wasteful fibre mixing that could occur during regeneration.

When an injury destroys a section of the ulnar nerve at the site of branching of the dorsal cutaneous branch, the fibres of the destroyed branch are represented by a bundle group in the proximal but not in the distal stump. This means that, when the axons of this branch regenerate, they are free to compete for endoneurial tubes in the distal stump that did not originally contain them.

In the proximal ulnar stump, the fasciculi are collected into three main groups that represent, from medial to lateral, the dorsal cutaneous fibres, the deep terminal division (predominantly motor), and the superficial terminal division (predominantly cutaneous). Only the two terminal divisions are represented at the distal nerve end.

Opposing the nerve ends in a conventional end-to-end epineurial repair under these conditions or even restoring continuity by autografting would result in: (1) the dorsal cutaneous bundle group at the proximal nerve end being opposed to the deep terminal motor division at the distal nerve end, and (2) the motor fascicular group becoming opposed to a group of sensory fasciculi. This would promote the entry of sensory axons into motor endoneurial tubes and motor axons into cutaneous sensory endoneurial tubes.

This complication should be prevented by excluding the dorsal cutaneous bundle group from the suture line or by bringing it into apposition with the cutaneous bundle group.

Group fascicular repair is, therefore, tailor made to meet special situations such as repairs of the median and ulnar nerves at the wrist and in the lower forearm and of the radial nerve above the elbow.

Expectations

When establishing a cause and effect relationship between group fascicular repair and the quality of the recovery it is important not to overlook the fact that:

1. the method should be used only when conditions meet the special criteria for selection. Assessments when the method is incorrectly used are worthless;
2. the method of repair is only one of many co-existing factors influencing and complicating regeneration and the quality of the recovery. Concentration on one factor to the exclusion of all others involves its abstraction from the total reality under investigation. Unless constant attention is given to what is being left out of immediate account, the results of evaluation studies are capable of serious misinterpretation. A worthwhile innovation may, for example, be inadvertently judged worthless and a worthless one incorrectly claimed to be of value.

Disadvantages of group fascicular repair

1. It calls for experience and skills in the use of microsurgical techniques and the related specialized equipment and facilities. These may not always be available.
2. It requires a detailed knowledge of the internal anatomy of nerve trunks.
3. It is a tedious and time-consuming procedure.
4. It preferably requires tension-free conditions at the suture line so that the group fascicular faces can be effectively maintained in contact.
5. It involves additional interference with the nerve ends during the preparation of the fasciculi. This increases the risk of trauma to fine nutrient vessels, fasciculi, and epineurial tissue, all of which are likely to intensify scarring at the suture line.
6. It may necessitate the use of internally located sutures that contribute to the formation of scar tissue at the suture line.

Grouping the fasciculi at the nerve ends for group fascicular repair

Anatomical, electrophysiological and histochemical methods are available for this purpose. Of the three the anatomical method remains the simplest.

Anatomical method

At the root of the limb the fibres of the different peripheral branches of a nerve are widely scattered throughout the fasciculi, each fasciculus containing fibres from most, if not all, of the branches in varying combinations and numbers. Only nerve fibres representing high branches are localised to a particular sector of the nerve but even these may be mixed with the fibres of more distal branches.

As the fibres of any given branch are followed distally they gradually become concentrated in fasciculi occupying a particular sector of the nerve where, however, they are still mixed .with other fibres. This partial localisation is worth exploiting when the fasciculi at the nerve ends are arranged into groups.

This sorting out process finally leaves some fasciculi composed solely of the fibres of a branch that is shortly to leave the nerve trunk. Thus the fibres of any particular branch are sharply localised and superficially located in a specific fasciculus or fascicular group for some distance only above the site of branching. For a short distance above the site of terminal branching the nerve fibres of each terminal branch are sharply localised and confined to separate fasciculi or groups of fasciculi. Charts are available that illustrate these features at the different levels along the major peripheral nerves (Sunderland 1978).

Electrophysiological method

This method involves stimulating individual fasciculi at the nerve ends as a means of differentiating between those that are sensory and those that are motor. Stimulation must be undertaken within 72 hours of severance because after that time severed nerve fibres no longer conduct (Hakstian 1968, Vandeput et al 1969, Nakatsuchi et al 1980, Gaul 1983, Jabaley 1984).

Exploration of the distal nerve ends. Failure to elicit a motor response is accepted as evidence that it is a sensory fasciculus. However, a motor response, although confirming the presence of motor fibres, does not exclude the presence of sensory fibres. Efforts to classify mixed fasciculi as predominantly motor or sensory on the response to stimulation have not solved the difficulty of interpretation.

Antidromic digital nerve stimulation to identify fasciculi containing sensory fibres at the distal nerve end has also been used.

Exploration of the proximal nerve end. This requires a conscious and co-operative patient because the detection of sensory fasciculi is based on the patient's reaction to stimulation. A negative response is regarded as evidence of a motor fasciculus. However, a positive response, although indicating the presence of sensory fibres, does not exclude the existence of motor fibres in the fasciculus.

The electrophysiological method loses its value at proximal levels where fasciculi usually contain a combination of motor and sensory fibres. Its strongest claim to consideration would be following transection of the median or ulnar nerve at the wrist, where fibre localisation in terms of separate

motor and sensory fasciculi is good. This, however, is a region where the motor and sensory fasciculi can usually be identified from a knowledge of fascicular anatomy. The electrical method, however, does have the advantage of facilitating the detection of motor fasciculi in the distal stump. In general, anatomical and electrophysiological methods of fascicular identification give similar results. The former is the simpler method.

Finally, the difficulty of electrical fascicular screening in children requires no elaboration.

Histochemical method of identification

In the early 1970s Gruber et al (1971) and Gruber and Zenker (1973) demonstrated that it is possible to differentiate between sensory and motor nerve fibres because of differing contents of acetylcholinesterase. This finding prompted Freilinger et al (1976) and Gruber et al (1976) to devise a histochemical method for distinguishing between sensory and motor fasciculi at the ends of a severed nerve. The method requires a preliminary biopsy on the nerve ends for histochemical examination within 72 hours of the transection.

The sections are treated for acetylcholinesterase which requires 25–30 hours incubation, by which time motor axons are stained while the sensory fibres are not. Only then can the information be used to match corresponding motor and sensory fasciculi at a later operation.

This method of identifying fasciculi has the following disadvantages:

1. It involves a delay of 25–30 hours in the repair.
2. It requires two operations.
3. Obtaining the biopsy specimens from the nerve ends increases the distance between them and adds to the mismatching of fascicular patterns.
4. It does not solve the problem of mixed motor and sensory fasciculi.
5. The test nerves were the median and ulnar at the wrist but the results only served to confirm the validity of anatomical methods of identification which offer a more practical guide to fascicular identification at that level.

Despite these objections, work to find a more reliable and practical histochemical method for the identification of fasciculi has continued.

Yun-Shao He and Shi-Zhen Zhong (1987, 1988) returned to the use of a staining technique for acetylcholinesterase and confirmed that motor and sensory fasciculi can be distinguished by their enzymatic activities. They confirmed the results obtained by Gruber but their modification of the method reduced the delay before a result could be obtained to 50 minutes. However, Shi-Zhen Zhong et al (1988) using the same method reported an incubation period of 24 hours.

Riley and Lang 1984 used a fixation technique that demonstrated acetazolamide-sensitive carbonic anhydrase activity in peripheral nerve axons and Engel et al (1980), Ganel et al (1981, 1982) and Ganel & Engel (1988) choline acetyltransferase to distinguish between motor and sensory fibres.

All that these methods achieved was to reduce the time delay to 50–80 minutes. The original objections to the method remain and the practicability and reliability of these new techniques in a clinical situation remains to be established.

11. SUTURELESS 'TENSION FREE' NERVE UNION

Concern over the reaction to suture materials and the hazards to nerve regeneration introduced by their use has resulted in the search for other methods of maintaining coaptation of the nerve ends. Some are concerned solely with securing the nerve ends in apposition until natural healing effects firm union. Others include tubular wrappings or sleeves to: (1) confine regenerating axons to the nerve by preventing them straying further afield, and (2) protect the repair site from invading fibroblasts and the formation of adhesions attaching the nerve to its bed.

The following methods have been used to effect sutureless nerve repair.

1. The de Medinaceli method.
2. Fibrin glue welding.
3. Laser welding.
4. Tubular or cuff union.
5. Various adhesives (fibrin adhesive, micropore

surgical tape, tissue adhesives) that have yet to establish an undisputed position in nerve repair. Their record to date has only served to confirm their unsuitability for the end-to-end repair of nerves.

Only the first four call for comment.
These methods all have the following limitations and disadvantages:

1. None prevents the erroneous cross-shunting of axons at the repair site.
2. All increase the technical difficulties of obtaining and maintaining correct apposition of the nerve ends and there is the continuing risk of their separation and malrotation postoperatively.
3. All demand tension-free conditions at the interface between the nerve ends, otherwise the latter will naturally pull apart. This, however, is not possible even with clean transection injuries because the normal elasticity of the nerve causes the nerve ends to retract and separate.

The practice of fixing the nerve to its bed by placing anchoring sutures some distance proximal and distal to the nerve end interface in order to eliminate tension at that site and nerve end separation is of questionable value, bearing in mind the need to avoid the formation of fixation adhesions.

Only the de Medinaceli method, by using an antitraction device to obtain tension free apposition of the nerve ends, overcomes this problem and by doing so offers the best prospects of success.

The De Medinaceli method of repair

In recent years de Medinaceli has returned to the challenging task of designing an improved method of nerve repair that would overcome the deficiencies of conventional methods. He and his associates have devised a 'reconnection' technique to minimise the physical and chemical damage to the nerve ends during their preparation and to ensure stress-free approximation of the nerve ends. Details of the technique and the results of their experimental studies have been detailed in a series of papers (1982, 1983, 1984, 1985, 1986, 1987, 1989)

In these papers the problem areas are correctly identified and their significance reconfirmed. They recognise the need to:

1. obtain the best possible face at each nerve end by minimising trauma during their preparation;
2. avoid the use of foreign materials at the suture line;
3. avoid all tension at the interface between the nerve ends;
4. maintain light apposition of the nerve ends throughout healing;

To achieve these objectives their reconnection method involves:

1. hardening the nerve ends by freezing in order to minimise physical damage when they are being trimmed;
2. using a vibration blade technique to trim the nerve ends which gives very smooth stump surfaces without further damaging the tissues;
3. irrigating the nerve ends during their preparation with a specially prepared fluid to minimise the damaging effects of freezing and thawing;
4. dispensing with the need to use suture materials to unite the nerve ends by replacing then with an antitraction device in which the nerve is attached, some distance from each nerve end, to a stretched rubber sheet which by its contraction neutralises the elastic recoil of the nerve ends and pulls them into light apposition. The rubber sheet was removed on the 20th postoperative day.

Theirs is a thoughtfully planned and carefully executed investigation. Using the walking gait of the rat to evaluate function and other tests to quantify axon regeneration, their findings pointed to decidedly improved results. According to Terzis & Smith (1986), who carried out a comparison of the de Medinaceli method and standard micro-suture methods, the former gave significantly superior results despite the fact that there was no statistical difference between the two groups in the number of regenerated axons in the distal stump. Wikholm et al (1988) have also reported favourab-

ly on the de Medinaceli technique but once again theirs was an experimental study using the rat.

Whether or not the de Medinaceli method brings any decisive advantage to the clinical repair of nerves remains to be established. Questionable aspects of the method are:

1. It is based on an experimental study using the sciatic nerve in rats which is an unsuitable experimental subject where the ultimate objective is the solution of a clinical problem.
2. In comparison with the major peripheral nerves in man, the sciatic nerve in the rat is very small with a much simpler fascicular structure.
3. Scarring during healing is less of a problem in the rat than in man.
4. The great problem in nerve repair is to create conditions at the suture line that will not only facilitate the passage of regenerating axons into the distal stump but will also, and more importantly, ensure the entry of axons into pathways that will lead them back to their original, or at least functionally related, end organs. The passage of regenerating axons across the nerve end interface and into the fasciculus or fasciculi of the distal stump is a far less complicated process in the rat than it is in man. Nor would the de Medinaceli reconnection method overcome the fascicular mismatching that is common with multifascicular human nerves and the consequent loss of regenerating axons into the interfascicular tissues and foreign endoneurial tubes of the distal stump. The de Medinaceli reconnection method does not address itself to this particular problem.
5. Freeze hardening and sectioning the larger nerve ends in human nerves presents problems not encountered in the rat. Edshage and Niebaurer's (1966) feasibility study of freezing the nerve ends to improve the quality of the cut surfaces indicated that this is not a satisfactory method for preparing nerve ends for repair.
6. Coaptation of the nerve ends and their correct alignment are more difficult to

maintain in large nerves by this method. The possibility of a widening of the nerve end interface and malalignment of the nerve ends remains a potential threat to useful regeneration.

7. The walking gait of the rat has been used to evaluate functional recovery. However, the problem is not with the function of the leg in the rat but with the function of the hand in man. Gait tracks are in no way comparable to the regeneration requirements to meet the delicate and co-ordinated movements involved in manual dexterity in man. The structure and function of nerves in the rat and man differ in such significant respects that extrapolation becomes unreliable.

8. A second operation appears to be necessary to remove the rubber sheet.

Despite these reservations the reconnection method of de Medinaceli has a sound theoretical basis and should be subjected to clinical trials which provide the only acceptable test on which to base the acceptance or rejection of the method. Until this is done, and knowing the many factors that influence the quality of the recovery after nerve repair that have not been taken into account in their studies, one remains to be convinced that the results will be consistently superior to those already obtainable by the meticulous use of the microsurgical procedures currently in clinical use. They will probably turn out to be no better and no worse.

Despite these critical comments, de Medinaceli is correct in emphasising the importance of obtaining optimal conditions at the nerve ends and he has demonstrated that the improved techniques advocated have achieved this — but in the rat.

Fibrin glue welding method

In this method fibrinogen coagulated blood plasma is used to glue and hold the nerve ends together. The method has been the subject of a protracted and searching study from the days when it was first proposed as a method of effecting end-to-end union by Young and Medawar and used clinically by Seddon and Medawar (Young & Medawar 1940, Seddon & Medawar 1942, Klemme et al 1943, Tarlov & Benjamin 1943, Tarlov et al 1943, 1948, Tarlov 1944, Hoen 1946, Lyons & Woodhall 1949, Indar & Fry 1958)

Despite improvements to the method and some early encouraging preliminary results the method soon lost favour, the chief objections to its acceptance being the difficulty of maintaining coaptation of the nerve ends, the need to have stress-free unions, the inflammatory response at the nerve interface resulting in obstructive fibrosis and a record of failed repairs.

To overcome the disadvantage of nerve end separation Bateman (1948) combined the plasma glue technique with a few silk sutures and reported good results but objections to the method persisted.

More recently Matras and his associates (1972, 1973, 1976) improved plasma glue welding and advocated its use in interfascicular grafting where obtaining tension free junctions is not a problem. They emphasised the necessity of preventing the spread of clotting substances between the fascicular nerve ends, a view shared by Millesi et al (1972). Unfortunately it is impossible to satisfy this proviso because the fasciculi at the nerve-graft junctions will not correspond in size, number or arrangement so that the spread of the glue between the ends of fasciculi is inevitable (Sunderland 1978).

Today improved techniques and the use of autologous fibrinogen coagulated blood plasma has given this method an established role in securing the nerve-graft junctions in interfascicular nerve grafting where the opposed nerve ends are slack and tension free (Kuderna et al 1979, Egloff & Narakas 1983, Gilbert 1988).

Even here one or two supplementary conventional sutures may be required to ensure a secure union. The method has proved particularly useful in complicated brachial plexus repairs involving multiple nerve grafts and nerve cross-anastomoses.

The lack of strength of the glue remains an unsolved problem and, as yet, the method has no place in end-to-end nerve repair (Cruz et al 1986). Moy et al (1988) in an experimental study (rabbit) reported that the fibrin seal did not provide a superior alternative method to 10/0 monofilament nylon sutures and was far less effective in maintaining nerve end approximation.

The transmission of hepatatis B and AIDS remains a threat and to overcome this problem the donor of the plasma glue preparation should be the patient.

Laser welding

Laser is an acronym for 'light amplification by the stimulated emission of radiation'. Laser light is produced by disturbing the resting state of a substance by exciting its atoms from a stable to an unstable condition. The effect of laser light on tissues is determined by its wave length. It has little effect on tissues that reflect or are transparent to it but is absorbed when its wave length matches the absorption spectrum of a tissue.

As blue green argon light passes through tissues it is almost completely reflected by or passes through white tissue but its specific wave length is absorbed by pigmented tissue such as the haemoglobin in red blood cells in vascular tissue. In this way the argon laser selectively coagulates blood.

Almquist and his associates (1984) have taken advantage of this feature of the argon laser to devise a method for the sutureless repair of severed nerves.

In their method, fasciculi were brought together and the junctional region coated with a film of autogenous blood which was then coagulated with a pulse of argon laser light. In this way the nerve ends were welded by the formation of a sleeve of coagulated blood around the repair site which adhered to the nerve. The sleeve was increased in thickness and strength by adding additional layers of blood to the sleeve and repeating the procedure. This bonding held the fasciculi and nerve ends together under light tension until healing was complete.

This method has the advantages of:

1. repairing the nerve at a fascicular or group fascicular level;
2. preventing the invasion of the junctional interface by scar tissue so that suture line scarring was non-existent;
3. confining regenerating axons within the sleeve;

4. permitting a more orderly growth of axons across the suture line.

Experimental trials in rats and lower primates confirmed the effectiveness of argon laser welding. The method has been used clinically to effect end-to-end repair and in group interfascicular nerve grafting with results that have been reported as encouraging.

Argon laser nerve repair appears to be a promising alternative to conventional nerve repair. However, its role in end-to-end repair remains limited because of the need to have an essentially tension-free union, while a fasciculus to fasciculus repair is only possible after clean transections without loss of nerve tissue.

The method is sound in principle and is worthy of extended clinical trials to establish the criteria for its use. In the final event only a wider clinical use of the method will determine whether it is entitled to an established place in nerve repair.

Almquist was well aware of all the difficulties involved when he wrote 'In all honesty, I cannot quantitate the nerve functions for several years with many cases. It is a big expense to set up a laser system and one must be quite certain if it is worthwhile before doing such' (Almquist, personal communication).

Tubular sleeve or cuff union

Here the nerve ends are maintained in apposition and the nerve end interface protected by an encircling wrapping, sleeve or cuff of some biological or non-biological material. What is written here about the use of tubular sleeves for repairing transacted nerves also applies to the treatment of the proximal and distal junctional regions of a nerve graft.

Nerve end approximation without tension brought about by anchoring sutures some distance from the nerve ends is now standard practice when this method is being used.

Biological sleeves

Arterial and venous sleeves

Arterial and venous sleeves have been investigated

for the sutureless repair of severed nerves and rejected because of their unsuitability.

Extended experimental trials have shown that the method does not have any advantage over conventional epineurial repair, which is easier technically and more reliable. Moreover, with the arterial sleeve technique the blood supply at the nerve end interface is threatened and there is the added risk of nerve constriction by the arterial coat. However, interest in the use of vessels as sleeves for nerve repair has recently been re-kindled, not as a means of effecting end-to-end repair, but as a bridging tube to convey regenerating axons across a gap in an injured nerve (see p. 486).

Collagen membrane and fabricated collagen tubes

These have been the subject of attention, not so much with the object of facilitating end-to-end union but in the form of tubes to guide regenerating axons across gaps in nerves (p. 486). Comment on Rosen et al's (1980) observations on tubulization repair using a hypoantigenic collagen membrane is deferred until protective wrappings are discussed in the next section. Reid et al (1978), reporting on biodegradable cuffs as an adjunct to nerve repair, remained undecided as to their value.

Epineurial cuff repair

To overcome these several difficulties Snyder et al (1974), Ploncard (1976) and Snyder (1981) have advocated creating a protective cuff of overlapping superficial epineurium about the suture site during the repair. However, this modified epineurial method does not address itself to the problem of epineurial fibroblasts contributing to suture line fibrosis.

Non-biological materials

The only non-biological material to survive exhaustive trials has been silastic (polymeric silicone), which many regard as the most suitable non-biological material for maintaining nerve end apposition and for protecting the repair site. The material is fashioned into microprosthetic

neurocuffs of different sizes that are applied around the suture site. Advantages claimed include strengthening the repair site, preventing adhesions and creating a favourable environment for regenerating axons. Again there is the risk of nerve compression, as has been reported by Birch (1979).

Temporary transfixion sutures appear to be needed to stabilise the nerve ends while the sleeve is being applied and secured, following which they are removed.

12. SUTURE LINE PROTECTION

What is written here about suture line protection applies equally to the use of protective wrappings at nerve-graft junctions. Enclosing the suture line with a protective shielding material has been advocated:

1. to protect this critical area from becoming involved in harmful scarring and adhesions;
2. to prevent regenerating axons straying outside the suture line;
3. to prevent the extension of extraneural scar tissue between the nerve ends where it would hinder the advance of growing axon tips;
4. to encourage the longitudinal alignment of the components of the junctional tissue, thereby facilitating the smooth passage of axons across the suture line;
5. to provide mechanical support for the suture line, thereby minimising torsion and displacement.

To date, the ideal wrapping has been regarded as one that is effectively ignored by the body and yet meets the conditions outlined above. However, by virtue of their inertness, such materials remain permanently as a potential mechanical irritant unless removed at a second operation. In this respect inertness can become a continuing liability. What is required is a biologically degradable membrane that would be absorbed once its primary function of ensuring sound, effective and uncomplicated union of the nerve ends has been fulfilled. In this way a second operation for its removal would be unnecessary. Whether protective shielding is effective in meeting these objectives is debatable.

Wrappings of the following materials have been given extended trials: blood vessels, cargile membrane, cellophane, fascia, fat, muscle flaps and segments, omentum and amnioplastin. They all endangered the blood supply to the suture line and were discarded. Tantalum cuffs were used extensively at one time but these were soon discontinued owing to fragmentation and the intense fibrosis associated with it.

The advantages claimed for millipore, a microporous cellulose acetate sheet were that:

  i. it was relatively inert in tissues;
  ii. its outer surface constituted a barrier against the invasion of the suture site by extraneural cells;
  iii. its inner surface favoured normal repair and the restoration of continuity at the suture line, and
  iv. the porosity of the membrane allowed the diffusion of fluids to meet the critical requirements of the junctional region.

Millipore was subsequently found to harden, become brittle and fragment. It was soon discarded in favour of silastic.

Silastic cuffing replaced millipore shielding for protecting the suture line with supporting claims reminiscent of those made earlier for millipore. The silastic tubing or cuff is likened to a synthetic perineurial tube and again there were reports of better longitudinal alignment of tissues at the suture line, superior axonal passage and less connective tissue proliferation and scarring.

As a further step towards improving the functional recovery after nerve repair, Campbell et al (1968) froze the nerve ends beneath the silastic cuff on the grounds that this minimised fascicular swelling and the accumulation of fibrin between the nerve ends. It was also postulated that the cryogenic destruction of all cells would leave an ideal collagen framework for the passage of regenerating axons unhindered by the proliferation of connective tissue. Nothing further has been heard of the method.

Kline and Hayes (1964) investigated the suitability of a collagen membrane as a protective wrapping for the suture site. They found that this material was associated with an increased cellular response which suggested the activation of an immune mechanism. Nevertheless, they felt that the potential of collagen membrane as a protective wrapping warranted further study. However, at a later date Millesi et al (1972) and Millesi (1975) reported that collagen membrane, millipore and silastic were all associated with an increased fibroblast reaction and functional results that were inferior to those obtained by simple end-to-end union. Rosen et al (1980) have since reported favourably on the use of a hypoantigenic collagen membrane for tubulization-nerve repair. However, it has suffered the fate of all such materials.

Many are opposed to enclosing the suture line with any foreign material (Barnes 1956, Madden & Peacock 1971, Brown 1972, Sunderland 1978). There is no substitute for a soft bed of viable healthy tissue and even inert foreign material is not problem free. There is already discussion of removing such protective sheaths once nerve union has consolidated and this means a second operation.

Further objections to the routine use of wrappings are:

1. With the condition of the nerve ends fluctuating during healing from oedema, cell proliferation and revascularisation the cuff could be too tight at one moment and too loose at another.
2. Their influence on the alignment of tissues at the junctional zone is questionable.
3. They carry the risk of impairing the blood supply to the suture area.
4. The inertness claimed for the material may in itself prove to be a disadvantage in that it persists as a foreign body and a source of mechanical irritation to produce harmful effects. Many advocating the use of protective sleeves concede that they should be removed at a second operation once nerve union has been consolidated.
5. The threat to the suture line in terms of scarring does not come from extraneural sources but from the proliferating fibroblasts of the epineurium and this is occurring *inside* the wrapping. The reason for this is clear when one considers the internal structure of nerve trunks (Fig. 42.2). In

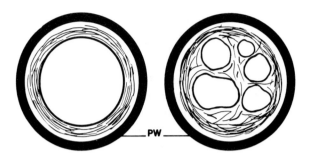

Fig. 42.2 Diagram to illustrate that the protective wrapping (*PW*) does not exclude epineurial tissue from the suture line. This tissue is the source of fibrosis which is more serious in the case of multifasciculated nerves.

human nerves, unlike in many animals used for experimental purposes, the monofascicular arrangement is uncommon, being confined to certain nerves in certain regions. The usual arrangement is of a multifascicular nerve trunk with varying, but large, amounts of epineurial tissue separating the fasciculi and enclosing the nerve trunk. This epineurial tissue is the source of the fibroblasts responsible for most of the harmful scarring involving the suture line. A protective wrapping does nothing to exclude this reaction and the fibrosis that follows.

The only advantage that can be claimed for isolating the suture in this way is to prevent the formation of troublesome adhesions that might attach the nerve to a scarred bed. It is important that the suture line should not become fixed in scar tissue or adherent to skin scar and tendons because this results in:

1. further scarring at the suture line itself;
2. deformation of the suture site during movements which causes pain and discomfort;
3. uneven distribution of forces along the nerve when it is stretched postoperatively during extension of the limb. The suture line may become so firmly adherent to adjacent tissues that forces are no longer evenly distributed along the entire nerve trunk but fall separately and unevenly on the proximal or distal segments; forces acting over shorter distances produce more serious effects.

13. POSTOPERATIVE NERVE STRETCHING

The use of radio-opaque markers to reveal whether the suture line is holding or has failed is referred to earlier. Suture line separation before postoperative stretching is commenced may occur owing to haemorrhage and tissue necrosis at the suture line, or inadequate healing. The period of greatest danger, however, is during extension of the limb. In this context it should be remembered that there is a limit to the size of the gap that can be closed effectively by a combination of mobilization, rerouting and limb positioning. If this limit is exceeded, either the nerve ends cannot be approximated or they are joined under such tension that postoperative stretching inevitably results in suture line failure or the disruption of nerve fibres elsewhere along the nerve.

Disruption at the suture line

If extension of the limb is commenced, or is accidentally or carelessly permitted, before union is consolidated, separation of the nerve ends may occur at the suture line. Regenerating axons are then faced with additional obstacles to their entry into the distal stump, while those that have already entered it are in an immature state and for this reason are probably more vulnerable to stretch. Premature postoperative stretching is a common cause of disruption at the suture line.

Tensile strength determinations of sutured nerves indicate that to be on the safe side, a delay of 4 weeks should be allowed for the ulnar and median nerves and one of 6–8 weeks for the sciatic before commencing to extend the limb.

The disruption of nerve fibres at levels other than the suture line

With sound healing the suture line scar becomes as strong as or even stronger than the remainder of the nerve. The denervated distal section of the nerve has the same tensile strength as the nerve above the repair. Providing the suture line holds, the tension developed during postoperative stretching is distributed along the entire nerve or, if the site of union has become adherent to adjacent structures, it will be concentrated either proximal or distal to the site of fixation depending on the position of the latter with reference to the joint.

Since there is a limit to which nerve fibres may be stretched, there is a grave risk during post-operative stretching of interfering with re-generation or even of rupturing nerve fibres and fine vessels within the fasciculi at levels elsewhere than at the suture line. In these cases, though con-tinuity is preserved, extensive intraneural damage and fibrosis seriously prejudice regeneration and there is little, if any, recovery.

14. SYMPATHECTOMY IN RELATION TO NERVE REPAIR

The value of sympathectomy as an aid to regen-eration requires further consideration and investigation. The benefits of sympathectomy could be:

1. to reduce the number of axons competing for endoneurial tubes in the distal nerve end;
2. generally to improve the blood supply to peripheral tissues when there is a co-existing injury to the main artery to the affected limb;
3. to prevent the early return of regenerating postganglionic sympathetic axons reimposing vasoconstrictor tone, particularly on digital vessels, that would further impair the circulation to denervated tissues.

15. COMMENT

Conditions at the suture line that affect the security of the union, the passage of regenerating axons and the quality of recovery are:

1. The relationship of the opposed faces of the nerve ends to one another in terms of cross-sectional areas, fascicular patterns, and the relative amounts of fascicular and epineurial tissue.
2. The state of the fasciculi and the endoneurial tubes.
3. The degree of fibre localisation prevailing at the suture line and the extent to which correct axial alignment of the nerve ends has been preserved during nerve suture.

4. The condition of the nerve ends after trimming in preparation for end-to-end union.
5. The length of the gap separating the nerve ends. This determines the ease with which they can be brought together, the degree of tension at the suture line and the amount of stretching to which the nerve is subjected postoperatively.
6. The nature of the bed in which the repair site finally rests.
7. Surgical technique. A standard technique in capable hands can still give inconsistent results because of the many factors adversely affecting recovery that are beyond the surgeon's control. Where so many variables operate to prevent, arrest, delay or accelerate recovery it might be argued that it is impossible to determine the influence of surgical techniques on the quality of the recovery. This is not so, for there is ample evidence confirming that much does depend on the knowledge, experience and skill of the surgeon.
8. With the foregoing considerations in mind it is possible to define conditions at the suture line that are either favourable or unfavourable for recovery after nerve suture.

Favourable conditions at the suture line

a. The segment of nerve trunk destroyed is no more than a few millimetres in length.
b. The nerve ends correspond in their cross-sectional areas and fascicular patterns.
c. Some fibre localisation is present and the fasciculi are tightly packed with a minimal amount of interfascicular connective tissue.
d. Correct axial alignment can be preserved during nerve repair.
e. Fascicular and endoneurial tube atrophy is minimal. This obtains only over the 1st month.
f. The amount of nerve tissue resected in order to expose tissue that is favourable for repair does not preclude satisfactory end-to-end union.
g. The nerve ends are easily united without tension.

h. A healthy bed is available for the nerve and there is no infection.

Unfavourable conditions at the suture line

a. The segment of nerve destroyed and later removed during the preparation of the nerve ends for suture leaves a gap that is too great to be closed except under unacceptable tension with no option other than to undertake a graft repair.

b. There is gross atrophy of the distal stump with inequalities in the dimensions of the nerve ends that complicate end-to-end union.

c. There is gross dissimilarity in the fascicular patterns at the nerve ends so that fasciculi in the proximal stump are opposed to the interfascicular connective tissue in the distal stump.

d. There is maximal atrophy of the fasciculi and endoneurial tubes which is reached about the end of the 3rd month.

e. There is no fibre localisation at the level of the repair and axial alignment has been irretrievably lost.

f. The nerve is left occupying a scarred bed and there is the further complication of postoperative wound infection.

g. Faulty technique such as rough handling of tissues, inadequate preparation of the nerve ends or unnecessary resection, the use of through and through sutures and suture materials that promote a reaction that terminates in considerable fibrosis, and faulty judgement in deciding to repair by end-to-end union when tension is such that postoperative stretching must inevitably lead to suture line failure.

REFERENCES

Allieu Y, Alnot J Y 1978 Résultats des sutures nerveuses sous microscope. Revue Chirurgie Orthopédique 64: 276

Almquist E E, Nachemson A, Auth D et al 1984 Evaluation of the use of the argon laser in repairing rat and primate nerves. Journal of Hand Surgery 9A: 792

Barnes R 1956 Peripheral nerve injuries. In: Platt H (ed) Modern trends in orthopaedics, 2nd Series. Butterworth, London

Bateman J E 1948 Plasma silk suture of nerves. Annals of Surgery 127: 456

Birch R 1979 Silicone rubber cuffs — a cause of nerve compression. The Hand 11: 211

Bratton B R, Kline D G, Hudson A R, Coleman W T 1981 Use of monofilament polyglycolic acid suture for experimental peripheral nerve repair. Journal of Surgical Research 31: 482

Braun R M 1980 Epineurial nerve repair. In: Omer G E, Spinner M (eds) Management of peripheral nerve problems. Saunders, Philadelphia, p 366

Brown P W 1972 Factors influencing the success of the surgical repair of peripheral nerves. Surgical Clinics of North America 52: 1137

Campbell J B, Pinner-Poole B, Tomasula J, De Crescito V 1968 Neurorrhaphy: improvement in neurolemmal alignment after application of cold at the time of surgery. Cryobiology 4: 272

Cham R B, Peimer C A, Howard C S et al 1984 Absorbable versus nonabsorbable suture for micro-neurorrhaphy. Journal of Hand Surgery 9A: 434

Cruz N I, Debs N, Fiol R E 1986 Evaluation of fibrin glue in rat sciatic nerve repairs. Plastic and Reconstructive Surgery 78: 369

de Medinaceli L 1987 How to correctly match 175,000 neurites; two postulates for a quick solution. BioSystems 20: 307

de Medinaceli L, Freed W J, Wyatt R J 1982 An index of the functional condition of rat sciatic nerve based on measurements made from walking tracks. Experimental Neurology 77: 634

de Medinaceli L, Freed W J 1983 Peripheral nerve reconnection: immediate histologic consequences of distributed mechanical support. Experimental Neurology 81: 459

de Medinaceli L, Wyatt R J, Freed W J 1983 Peripheral nerve reconnection: mechanical, thermal and ionic conditions that promote the return of function. Experimental Neurology 81: 469

de Medinaceli L, Freed W J, Wyatt R J 1983 Peripheral nerve reconnection: improvement of long term functional effects under simulated clinical conditions in the rat. Experimental Neurology 81: 488

de Medinaceli L, Church A C 1984 Peripheral nerve reconnection: inhibition of early degenerative processes through the use of a novel fluid medium. Experimental Neurology 84: 396

de Medinaceli L, Church A C, Wang Y N 1985 Posttraumatic autoimmune reaction in peripheral nerve: effects of two successive injuries at different sites. Experimental Neurology 88: 396

de Medinaceli L, Quach T, Duchemin A M, Wyatt R J 1986 Is vigor of regeneration a key factor in functional recovery from peripheral nerve injuries? Experimental Neurology 94: 788

de Medinaceli L, Rawlings R R 1987 Is it possible to predict the outcome of peripheral nerve injuries? A probability model based on prospects for regenerating neurites. BioSystems 20: 243

de Medinaceli L, Seaber A V 1989 Experimental nerve reconnection: importance of initial repair. Microsurgery (in press)

Edshage S, Niebauer J J 1966 Evaluation of freezing as a method to improve cut surfaces in peripheral nerves preparatory to suturing. Plastic and Reconstructive Surgery 37: 196

Egloff D V, Narakas A 1983 Nerve anastomoses with human fibrin. Preliminary clinical report. Annales Chirurgie Main 2: 101

Engel J, Ganel A, Melaned R et al 1980 Choline acetyltransferase for differentiation between human motor and sensory nerve fibers. Annals of Plastic Surgery 4: 376

Freilinger G, Gruber H, Holle J, Mandl H 1976 Differential funicular suture of peripheral nerves. Transactions of the Sixth International Congress of Plastic and Reconstructive Surgery, Paris, 1975. Masson, Paris, p 123

Ganel A, Engel J 1988 Nerve fascicle identification. In: Tubiana R (ed) The hand. Saunders, Philadelphia, Vol 3, p 430

Ganel A, Engel J, Luboshitz et al 1981 Choline acetyltransferase nerve identification method in early and late nerve repair. Annals of Plastic Surgery 6: 228

Ganel A, Farine I, Aharonson Z et al 1982 Intraoperative nerve fascicle identification using choline acetyltransferase — a preliminary report. Clinical Orthopaedics 165: 228

Gaul J S 1983 Electrical identification as an adjunct to nerve repair. Journal of Hand Surgery 8: 289

Gilbert A 1988 Nerve anastomosis and graft with fibrin glue. In: Tubiana R (ed) The hand. Saunders, Philadelphia, p 554

Gould J S 1979 Digital nerve repair with magnification technique. Quoted by Omer et al 1986

Gruber H, Zenker W, Hohenberg E 1971 Untersuchungen über die Spezifität der Cholinesterasen im peripheren Nervensystem der Ratte. Histochemistry 27: 78

Gruber H, Zenker W 1973 Acetylcholinesterase: histochemical differentiation between motor and sensory nerve fibres. Brain Research 51: 207

Gruber H, Freilinger G, Holle J, Mandl H 1976 Identification of motor and sensory funiculi in cut nerves and their selective reunion. British Journal of Plastic Surgery 29: 70

Hakstian R W 1968 Funicular orientation by direct stimulation: An aid to peripheral nerve repair. Journal of Bone and Joint Surgery 50A: 1178

Hoen T I 1946 The repair of peripheral nerve lesions. American Journal of Surgery 72: 489

Hudson A, Hunter D 1976 Polyglycolic acid suture in peripheral nerve. II Sutured sciatic nerve. Canadian Journal of Neurological Sciences 3: 69

Indar R, Fry R J M 1958 The experimental use of cortisone in peripheral nerve repair with plasma clot as a suture. Irish Journal of Medical Science 6: 136

Jabaley M E 1984 Electrical nerve stimulation in the awake patient. Bulletin of the Hospital for Joint Diseases Orthopaedic Institute 44: 248

Klemme R M, Woolsey R D, DeRezende N T 1943 Autopsy nerve grafts in peripheral nerve surgery. Journal of American Medical Association 123: 393

Kline D G, Hayes G J 1964 Use of resorbable wrapper for peripheral nerve repair. Journal of Neurosurgery 21: 737

Kuderna H, Redl H, Dinges H 1979 The repair of several peripheral nerves by means of a fibrin seal. Clinical experiences and results. European Surgical Research 11: 98

Kurtze T 1964 Microtechnique in neural surgery. Clinical Neurosurgery 11: 128

Lyons W R, Woodhall B 1949 Atlas of peripheral nerve injuries. Saunders, London

McManamny D S 1983 Comparison of microscope and loupe magnification: Assistance of the repair of median and ulnar nerves. British Journal of Plastic Surgery 36: 367

Madden J W, Peacock E E 1971 Some thoughts on repair of peripheral nerves. Southern Medical Journal 64: 17

Matras H, Dinges H P, Lassman H, Mamoli B 1972 Zur nahtlosen interfaszikulären Nerventransplantation im Tierexperiment. Wiener Medizinische Wochenschrift 122: 517

Matras H, Braun F, Lassman H et al 1973 Plasma clot welding of nerves (Experimental report). Journal of Maxillofacial Surgery 1: 236

Matras H, Kuderna H 1976 Glueing nerve anastomoses with clotting substances. I Experimental basis. Transactions of the Sixth International Congress of Plastic and Reconstructive Surgery, Paris, 1975. Masson, Paris, p 134

Merle M, Foucher G, Van Genechten F, Michon J 1984 The repair of peripheral nerve injuries in emergency. Bulletin of the Hospital for Joint Diseases Orthopaedic Institute 44: 338

Merle M, Amend P, Michon J 1988 Microsurgical repair in 150 patients with lesions of the median and ulnar nerves. In: Tubiana R (ed) The hand. Saunders, Philadelphia, Vol. 3, p 595

Michon J 1975 Nerve suture today. In: Michon J, Moberg E (eds) Traumatic nerve lesions of the upper limb. Churchill Livingstone, Edinburgh, p 69

Michon J, Masse P 1964 Le moment optimum de la suture nerveuse dans les plaies du membre supérieur. Revue de Chirurgie Orthopédique et Réparatrice de l'Appareil Moteur 50: 205

Millesi H 1973 Microsurgery of peripheral nerves. Hand 5: 157

Millesi H 1975 Treatment of nerve lesions by fascicular free nerve graft. In: Michon J, Moberg E (eds) Traumatic nerve lesions of the upper limb. Churchill Livingstone, Edinburgh, p 91

Millesi H 1988 Importance of tension and epineurial tissue in scar formation and its effecting the results of nerve repair. In: Brunelli G (ed) Textbook of microsurgery. Masson, Milan, p 607

Millesi H, Meissl G 1981 Consequences of tension at the suture line. In: Gorio A, Millesi H, Mingrino S (eds) Posttraumatic peripheral nerve regeneration: experimental basis and clinical implications. Raven Press, New York, p 277

Millesi H, Berger A, Meissl G 1972 Experimentelle Untersuchungen zur Heilung durchtrennter peripherer Nerven. Chirurgia Plastica 1: 174

Moy O J, Peimer C A, Koniuch M P et al 1988 Fibrin seal adhesive versus nonabsorbable microsuture in peripheral nerve repair. Journal of Hand Surgery 13A: 273

Nakatsuchi T, Matsui T, Handa Y 1980 Funicular orientation by electrical stimulation and internal neurolysis in peripheral nerve suture. Hand 12: 65

Omer G E 1984 Has the microsurgical technique improved the results of epineural repair? Limb Reconstruction Micro or Macrosurgery. Program for the Fifth American Orthopaedic Association International Symposium, Boca Raton, November 7–11. Copy kindly supplied by the author

Omer G E, O'Brien W J, Murray H M et al 1986 The technical factors influencing the results of the epineurial technique for peripheral nerve repair. Peripheral Nerve Repair and Regeneration. 3: 67

Orf G 1978 Critical resection length and gap distance in

peripheral nerves. Acta Neurochirurgica, Supplementum 26

Ploncard P 1976 Comparative study of circumferential nerve suture using the operating microscope. Acta Neurochirurgica 34: 175

Reid R L, Cutright D E, Garrison J S 1978 Biodegradable cuff as an adjunct to peripheral nerve repair. A study in dogs. The Hand 10: 259

Riley D A, Lang D H 1984 Carbonic anhydrase activity of human peripheral nerves: a possible histochemical aid to nerve repair. Journal of Hand Surgery 9A: 112

Rosen J M, Kaplan E N, Jewett D L 1980 Suture and sutureless methods of repairing experimental nerve injuries. In: Jewett D L, McCarroll H R (eds) Nerve repair and regeneration: its clinical and experimental basis. Mosby, St Louis, p 235

Seddon H J, Medawar P B 1942 Fibrin suture of human nerves. Lancet 2: 87

Shi-Zhen Zhong, Guo-Ying Wang, Yun-Shao He, Bo Sun 1988 The relationship between structural features of peripheral nerves and suture methods for nerve repair. Microsurgery 9: 181

Smith J W 1964 Microsurgery of peripheral nerves. Plastic and Reconstructive Surgery 33: 317

Smith J W 1975 Recent advances in the field of microsurgery. In: Michon J, Moberg E (eds) Traumatic nerve lesions of the upper limb. Churchill Livingstone, Edinburgh, p 79

Snyder C C 1981 Epineurial repair. In: Frykman G K (ed) The Orthopaedic clinics of North America 12: 267

Snyder C C, Browne E Z, Herzog B G 1974 Epineurial cuff neurorrhaphy. Journal of Bone and Joint Surgery 56A: 1092

Sunderland S 1978 Nerves and nerve injuries, 2nd edn. Churchill Livingstone, Edinburgh

Sunderland S 1979 The pros and cons of funicular nerve repair. Journal of Hand Surgery 4: 201

Sunderland S, Smith G K 1950 The relative merits of various suture materials for the repair of severed nerves. Australian and New Zealand Journal of Surgery 20: 85

Tarlov I M 1944 Plasma clot suture of nerves — illustrated technique. Surgery 15: 257

Tarlov I M, Benjamin B 1943 Plasma clot and silk suture of nerves: I An experimental study of comparative tissue reaction. Surgery Gynecology and Obstetrics 76: 366

Tarlov I M, Denslow C, Swarz S, Pineles D 1943 Plasma clot suture of nerves: experimental technic. Archives of Surgery, Chicago 47: 44

Tarlov I M, Boernstein W, Berman D 1948 Nerve regeneration: a comparative experimental study following suture by clot and thread. Journal of Neurosurgery 5: 62

Terzis J K, Smith K J 1986 'de Medinaceli' versus microsutures: a critical appraisal of nerve repair. Proceedings of the Annual Meeting of the American Society of Reconstructive Microsurgery 116: 51

Vandeput J, Tanner J C, Hypens L 1969 Electrophysiological orientation of the cut ends in primary peripheral nerve repair. Plastic and Reconstruction Surgery 44: 378

Wikholm R P, Swett J E, Torigoe Y, Blanks R H 1988 Repair of severed peripheral nerve: a superior anatomical and functional recovery with the reconnection technique. Journal of Otolaryngology — Head and Neck Surgery 99: 353

Wise A J, Topuzulu C, Davis P, Kaye I S 1969 A comparative analysis of macro- and microsurgical neurorrhaphy techniques. American Journal of Surgery 117: 566

Young J Z, Medawar P B 1940 Fibrin suture of peripheral nerves. Lancet 2: 126

Yun-Shao He, Shi-Zhen Zhong 1987 An exploration of the acetylcholinesterase histochemical method for intraoperative nerve fascicle identification. Chinese Journal of Clinical Anatomy 5: 13

Yun-Shao He, Shi-Zhen Zhong 1988 Acetylcholinesterase: a histochemical identification of motor and sensory fascicles in human peripheral nerve and its use during operation. Plastic and Reconstructive Surgery 82: 125. Discussion by Seckel B R, p 131

43. Nerve grafting and related methods of nerve repair

The subjects discussed in this chapter include: nerve grafting, tubal repair of nerves, muscle tissue interpositional grafting of nerves, nerve cross-union and direct neurotisation of muscles.

PART 1. NERVE GRAFTING

TERMINOLOGY

Nerve graft. This is provided by a length of a peripheral nerve.

Interpositional nerve graft. Any nerve graft interposed between the nerve ends.

Interpositional muscle graft. A length of muscle interposed between the nerve ends.

Heterograft. Xenograft. Heterologous graft. A nerve graft selected from an animal of a different species. The term used in this text is heterograft.

Homograft. Allograft. Allogenic graft. A nerve transferred from one individual, the donor, to another, the recipient, of the same species. The term used in this text is homograft.

Autograft. Autologous graft. Autogenous graft. A nerve graft obtained from another nerve in the same individual. The term used in this text is autograft.

Types of nerve autografts

Current terminology lists four main types of interpositional nerve autografts: full thickness, cable, group fascicular and free neurovascular grafts.

Full thickness nerve grafts. One composed of the full thickness of a donor nerve that matches the thickness of the recipient nerve.

Cable nerve graft. One composed of several parallel strands of a donor peripheral nerve suffi-

cient in number to match the thickness of the recipient nerve.

Fascicular nerve graft. Interfascicular nerve graft. Unqualified, these terms could be interpreted as meaning the grafting of individual fasciculi. This, however, is not possible because the numbers and arrangement of the fasciculi at both proximal and distal nerve-graft junctions will not correspond. The terms are, therefore, somewhat misleading and it would be better to discontinue using them.

Group fascicular nerve graft. Group interfascicular nerve graft. A nerve graft in which the fasciculi at the proximal and distal nerve ends of the injured nerve are appropriately grouped and the fasciculi of each cable of the graft so arranged in relation to them that fascicular apposition is maximised and quadrantic relationships maintained. In this way the chances are increased of regenerating axons entering fasciculi and advantage can be taken of any fascicular branch fibre localisation obtaining at the level of the repair.

In the past, the ends of each strand of the graft were applied in a random fashion to the free ends of the recipient nerve without any reference to fascicular structure or to fascicular apposition. In full thickness grafting the graft was attached by conventional epineurial suture. Both random cable and full thickness grafting disregard the importance of fascicular matching between the graft and nerve ends and should be discontinued in favour of group fascicular cable or group fascicular full thickness grafting. The greatly improved recoveries that can now be expected of autografting are the result of improvements in the method of junctional union and not to any change in the form of the graft.

The restoration of continuity by group interfascicular repair is discussed in Chapter 42 and what has been written there applies equally to autografting. Significant differences, however, are that end-to-end nerve union is replaced by two nerve to graft junctions while the destruction of a longer segment of the nerve means greater dissimilarities in the fascicular patterns and in the arrangement of the different branch fibre systems at the now well-separated nerve ends. This in turn reduces the chances of restoring useful functional connections during regeneration.

In practice, group interfascicular repair is more appropriate to grafting than to end-to-end nerve repair. Using the former, often to bridge quite small defects with a view to avoiding suture line tension, has given remarkably good results. The case for group interfascicular grafting has real merit, whereas end-to-end nerve repair by group fascicular suture remains controversial for reasons that are discussed in Chapter 42.

Free neurovascular nerve graft. One in which a selected length of the donor nerve, together with its main arteriovenous nutrient system, is mobilised, isolated, and then transferred en bloc to the recipient site, the circulation to the graft being restored by appropriate microvascular anastomoses in its new site.

Neurovascular pedicle nerve graft. Pedicle nerve graft. A full-thickness graft provided by an adjacent donor nerve in a two-stage procedure, designed to preserve the microcirculation of the graft. The donor nerve has been either irreparably damaged or is to be sacrificed depending on the circumstances. In the first stage, the proximal stumps of the donor and recipient nerves are attached to form a loop. In the second stage an appropriate length of the proximal segment of the donor nerve is freed and transferred to complete the closure of the gap in the recipient nerve.

Tubal nerve repair. This involves the use of a vein, artery, mesothelial tube or a tube of some biodegradable material as a conduit to facilitate the passage of regenerating axons across a nerve gap.

Nerve cross union. The procedure designed to provide regenerating axons from an adjacent donor nerve to the distal stump of the severed nerve. Anastomosis refers to vessels. Its use for nerves is not appropriate, though convenient.

Direct cross union. In this procedure, a normal donor nerve is sacrificed by transecting it and uniting its proximal end to the distal stump of the irreparably damaged nerve, which is then reinnervated from a new source. In complete cross-union the full thickness of the donor nerve is used. In partial cross-union only part of the donor nerve is used for the transfer.

Indirect cross-union. This method is required when the distance between the donor and recipient nerves is too great to be closed by direct cross-union. An intermediate nerve graft is then required to complete closure of the gap between donor and recipient nerves.

Neurovascular island graft. A graft in which an island of skin, with its neurovascular source of supply preserved, is transferred to an adjacent site.

Free neurovascular island graft. A graft in which an island of skin along with its neurovascular supply are isolated, transferred en bloc to a new site where, inter alia, the nerve and vessels are attached by appropriate microneural and microvascular repairs.

Neurotization. The operation of implanting a nerve directly into a denervated muscle.

Neurovascular muscle graft. A graft in which a muscle with its neurovascular supply left undisturbed is transferred to an adjacent site.

Free neurovascular muscle graft. A graft in which a muscle along with its neurovascular supply is isolated, transferred en bloc to a new site where, inter alia, the nerve and vessels are attached by appropriate microneural and microvascular repairs.

INTRODUCTION

Prior to the mid 1940s the results of nerve grafting were decidedly bad. There were many reasons for this disastrous record, the principal being the increased incidence of extensive open wounding in battle casualties, wound infection and the absence of fundamental data on the basics of nerve injury and repair. Wound trauma and infection produced their damaging effects by leaving a scarred poorly vascularised nerve bed, and by introducing long delays before repair could be undertaken.

Infection also involved the nerve ends in a spreading neuritis. This later necessitated sacrificing more nerve tissue when preparing the nerve ends for repair, thereby increasing the length of the graft required to bridge the gap.

Today the picture is very different, the scene having changed dramatically with: (1) the introduction of antibiotic therapy and the prevention and control of wound infection, and (2) the provision of much needed fundamental information relating to nerve injury, repair and regeneration.

The 'new look' for nerve grafting is largely the outcome of Hanno Millesi's enterprising and pioneering work on group interfascicular nerve grafting which has transformed nerve grafting from a procedure in desperation to one now seriously regarded by many as an alternative to suturing a nerve under any tension.

There are times when, after exhausting all possible benefits to be gained by mobilisation, transposition, posturing the limb and gentle stretching, all efforts to join the ends of a severed nerve by direct union fail. In the past these cases have represented a discouraging chapter in the saga of peripheral nerve repair but today the prospects for restoring functionally effective continuity by means of a graft have greatly improved.

However, the difficulties of nerve repair are greatly increased when a nerve graft is required. This is because:

1. a considerable length of the nerve has been destroyed;
2. the trauma responsible has been considerable so that retrograde neuronal and trans-synaptic effects are severe;
3. another nerve must be sacrificed to provide the graft;
4. two suture lines are involved instead of one;
5. injuries that necessitate nerve grafting usually cause extensive destruction of the neighbouring tissues and considerable scarring as healing occurs. The nerve ends, and subsequently the graft, are consequently left in an unfavourable bed and it is not always possible to find an alternative one of healthy tissue. Furthermore, in some cases the blood supply to the graft is still further embarrassed by a co-existing arterial injury.

On the other hand, the capacity of the surviving

axons of the proximal stump to sprout remains undiminished, and regenerating axons have a remarkable capacity to cross, unaided, considerable gaps in nerves. However, in the absence of any attempt at nerve repair, the growth of axons is disorganised, haphazard and incomplete and the results, from a functional point of view, usually negligible.

The success or failure of a graft can be judged only on the quality of the recovery and this is largely determined by the extent to which the original pattern of innervation is restored by axon regeneration.

The objective of restoring continuity between the nerve ends by a bridging graft is to take advantage of the remarkable capacity of axons to regenerate by providing them with a scaffolding that will not only guide them to the distal stump but will also do this in a manner that goes closest to restoring the original pattern of innervation.

The use of non-biological materials, non-neural tissue grafts and nerve heterografts has nothing to offer in terms of bridging materials. They do not warrant further consideration. Whether or not the use of skeletal muscle tissue to bridge the gap between nerve ends will come up with convincingly and consistently better results and justify a revision of this policy remains to be seen.

NERVE HOMOGRAFTING

If homografting were conclusively proved to be a successful alternative to autografting, this would represent a welcome advance in nerve repair. (1) It would allow banks of suitable nerves to be readily available on demand, and (2) it would dispense with the need to sacrifice a cutaneous nerve as an autograft.

Homografting was fully reviewed in the 1978 edition of *Nerves and Nerve Injuries* and it is not intended to retrace the ground covered in that account other than to list the general conclusions reached on that occasion.

1. While some regenerating axons reached and reinnervated the distal stump in some experiments, this regeneration was neither dependable nor predictable, its functional

value was unknown and it was impossible to evaluate the role played by the graft.

It was probably little better than that achievable by leaving a gap separating the nerve ends. This applies to all varieties of homografts: fresh, freeze dried and freeze-dried irradiated.

Clinically, homografts have to date been failures.

2. Predegenerating the graft has no place in the clinical situation.

3. Immunosuppression therapy involved:

   a. the use of immunosuppressive drugs available at that time. This was opposed on the grounds that nerve grafting is not a life-saving measure. The attendant risks of using immunosuppressive drugs and their failure to confer any decided advantages on homografting excluded their use.

   b. Histocompatibility testing (Singh et al 1977 a, b) to minimise antigenicity in the selection of a donor nerve was in the early experimental stages.

4. Ducker and Hayes (1970) concluded that the maximum length of a homograft was 4 cm and this has since been confirmed by Singh (1983) and Comtet (1988a). These are gaps, of course, that can be readily closed by end-to-end union.

5. There was nothing in these earlier studies to justify discontinuing autografting in favour of homografting.

With improved histocompatibility testing in relation to the graft-host reaction and with improvements in immunosuppressive therapy, and in particular the introduction of Cyclosporin A, there has been a resurgence of interest in nerve homografting (Singh et al 1977a,b, Levinthal et al 1978a,b, Aguayo & Bray 1980, Zalewski & Silvers 1980, Parekh 1981, Mackinnon et al 1982, 1984a,b, 1985a,b, 1987, Stearns 1982, Zalewski & Gulati 1982, 1984a,b, Singh 1983, Hirasawa et al 1984, Alnot et al 1988, Bain et al 1988, Gulati 1988). Gulati (1989) has reported that, in the cyclosporine-treated rat, an arterial allograft used to bridge a 10 mm gap in a nerve can serve as an effective conduit for regenerating axons.

Histocompatibility testing has been demonstrated to be of value in improving the selection and survival of nerve homografts and their usefulness as conduits (Singh et al 1977a,b, Singh 1983). Additionally, Cyclosporin A appears to be a more acceptable and effective immunosuppressive agent and, superficially, the results appear to be more encouraging. However, the old problems remain and the experimental approach is subject to the same objections.

1. Unbridged gaps of equivalent dimensions were not always included among the controls.

2. Gaps that have been allegedly successfully crossed by means of the graft are well within the range that regenerating axons will normally cross unaided.

3. The gaps did not exceed 3 cm and in many experiments were much less. Clinically, such gaps can be readily closed by end-to-end union. Comtet (1988a) has observed 'regeneration occurs only over short distances of less than 40 mm and is always of an inferior quality to that of an autograft.'

4. The structure of the nerves used in the experiments were less complicated than those in man and the results were based on less complex functions.

5. It is assumed that immunosuppressive therapy needs to be only temporary while axons are using the graft as scaffolding and that, when this contribution is complete, immunosuppression is no longer necessary and can be terminated. This overlooks the delayed antigenic reaction and rejection which is followed by fibrosis that could threaten the structural and functional integrity of the axons in the graft.

Clinically, recoveries attributed to the use of homografts are not necessarily the result of regeneration through the graft but could be explained in other ways, the misinterpretation of neurological findings being the most common. Nevertheless there are occasions when, after excluding those factors that could possibly confuse the issue, the homograft remains the only explanation to account for an unexpectedly favourable result. Here the relevant observation is not the consistently poor record of homografting but the fact that some recovery ever occurs at all. This justifies continuing the search to ascertain why so few homografts succeed. With a better understanding of the cellular and molecular basis of rejection, and with new and more dependable immunosuppressive measures it may be possible to introduce more effective methods of immuno-regulation that will make nerve homografting an acceptable proposition.

For homografts to replace autografts it will be necessary for the former to give results that are dependably and consistently better than, or at least as good as, those obtainable by autografting. This has yet to be convincingly demonstrated.

NERVE AUTOGRAFTS

A nerve autograft behaves in much the same way as does the distal segment of a severed nerve. Wallerian degeneration occurs somewhat more slowly in the former than in the latter, probably because of an impaired blood supply and the removal of debris.

The graft unites with the nerve ends and regeneration through it occurs in much the same way as after end-to-end repair. Regenerating axons are a little slower entering the graft than they are in crossing a suture line after end-to-end repair while their rate of growth through the graft is only slightly slower than in the peripheral segment. The new axons in the graft myelinate at about the same rate as in the distal segment, though not to the same degree as the parent axons in the proximal stump.

For reasons discussed elsewhere, studies of returning function are only of significance when the observations are made on man, for what the clinician is seeking is useful functional recovery. It is extremely difficult to relate the technical and biological features of autografting on the one hand to the quality of functional recovery on the other. Clinical records too frequently omit important details relating to the nature of the nerve injury, the graft selected, its length and method of implantation, the nature of the nerve bed and the presence or absence of infection, while references to recovery are often in the most vague and general terms.

The greatest advance in nerve grafting has come in recent years from a better understanding of the internal anatomy of nerve trunks, a better appreciation of the factors influencing the quality of the recovery after grafting and, significantly, the development of microsurgery. All of this has made possible group fascicular grafting and the introduction of this new method has resulted in greatly improved recoveries and has even led some to prefer this method for the closure of quite small gaps in severed nerves (Millesi et al 1967, 1972, 1976, Millesi 1968, 1969, 1973, 1975, 1980a,b, 1981a–c, 1984, 1988, Samii & Willebrand 1970, Buck-Gramcko 1971, Samii & Kahl 1972, Samii & Wallenberg 1972, Samii et al 1972, Samii 1973, Berger & Millesi 1978, Moneim 1982).

Features of nerve autografting and related matters that call for special comment are:

1. What gives a nerve autograft superiority as the bridge to close the gap in a nerve?
2. Group fascicular cable grafting of small gaps as opposed to nerve suture under slight tension.
3. When should end-to-end repair be abandoned in favour of nerve grafting?
4. When should nerve grafting be rejected as a method of repair?
5. Relevant structural features of a graft.
6. The relative merits of cable and full-thickness autografts.
7. The selection of a cutaneous nerve for cable autografting.
8. The blood supply to and survival of the graft.
9. Group fascicular repair in nerve grafting.
10. The graft bed.
11. The use of protective sleeves to enclose nerve-graft junctions.
12. The relative merits of fresh and predegenerated grafts.
13. The case for reversing the graft.
14. Timing the distal nerve-graft repair.
15. Factors influencing the quality of the recovery after nerve autografting.
16. The nerve-graft union.
17. Free neurovascular grafting.
18. Nerve pedicle grafting.

WHAT GIVES A NERVE AUTOGRAFT SUPERIORITY AS A BRIDGE TO CLOSE THE GAP IN A NERVE

Reference has been made elsewhere to the remarkable capacity of severed axons to regenerate, and the capacity of regenerating axons to cross unaided, considerable gaps in nerves. Quite clearly a graft is not necessary for this to occur. However, regenerating axons crossing the gap in an unaided way do so in a disorganised manner with the loss of large numbers en route. The function of a graft, as a definitive column of structured tissue, is to provide a more suitable terrain and environment for axon growth in which:

1. disorderly growth is converted into an orderly process with improved prospects of restoring functionally useful pathways and peripheral connections;
2. the loss of axons is reduced by providing them with a structured framework that facilitates their passage across the gap and into the distal nerve stump;
3. the nutritional needs of growing axon tips and newly formed axons are better met, particularly when the graft is rapidly revascularised.

However, something more than a structured bridge of tissue is required, otherwise a homograft, freeze dried and irradiated to reduce its antigenicity, would be just as effective as a fresh autograft and we know that this is not so.

What then are the elements in the nerve autograft that make it uniquely acceptable as a bridge for the passage of regenerating axons across a gap in the nerve?

Tissue compatibility and the rapid revascularisation are clearly important. In respect of the latter the cable variety has a distinct advantage over the full-thickness graft. However, there must be other elements in the autograft itself. This poses the question of whether or not neurotropic agents are liberated within the graft that confine regenerating axons to the graft once they have entered it.

There are three possible sources of such neurotropic agents: (1) the Schwann cells of the graft; (2) the products of axon-myelin breakdown; and (3) the activity of specialised cells of meso-

dermal origin: epineurial, endoneurial and perineurial.

Schwann cells

These are the most likely source because axons regenerating down endoneurial tubes fare far better than those that do not. However, what is the outcome should unduly delayed and severely impaired vascularisation of the graft lead to the loss of Schwann cells? This could be one explanation to account for the poorer results when the blood supply to the graft is severely impaired.

The products of axon-myelin breakdown

It is well established that the passage of regenerating axons down endoneurial tubes after a second degree injury is unimpaired by the presence of debris from the breakdown of axons and myelin. Moreover, the rate of advance is faster than after nerve repair when the endoneurial tubes are empty of all but Schwann cells. Admittedly, other factors are contributing to the slower rate after nerve repair. The question at issue is whether or not the faster rate in the presence of the breakdown products of Wallerian degeneration could be due to the liberation of neurotropic agents in the process. If this were the case, then fresh grafts would have an advantage over the predegenerated variety.

The activity of specialised mesodermal cells

Tello (Chapter 16) always maintained that neurotropic influences emanating from the distal stump were based on the mesodermal elements of the nerve end.

Reference has been made elsewhere to the observation that regenerating axons will enter epineurial tissue just as readily as fascicular tissue (Chapter 16). Though many of these end blindly in the epineurial tissue, others continue to advance and, providing the graft is not too long, may ultimately reach the distal stump and, hopefully, fasciculi. However, those axons that enter endoneurial tubes fare much better than those that find their way into epineurial tissue.

Conclusion

There is no doubt that nerve autografts confer special advantages on graft repair, even if we are at a loss to explain why this should be so.

GROUP FASCICULAR GRAFTING OF SMALL GAPS AS OPPOSED TO NERVE SUTURE UNDER SLIGHT TENSION

An as yet unanswered question is whether very short group fascicular grafting is preferable to end-to-end union under slight tension (Chapter 40). To date it has not been proven that the former provides consistently better recoveries than the latter which is, of course, the only reason for justifying its acceptance. Such superiority would be necessary to offset the following disadvantages of a graft procedure.

1. A somewhat longer and technically more difficult operation.
2. Regenerating axons have two suture line obstacles to overcome instead of one, while the chances of axons being misdirected into interfascicular epineurial tissue are doubled.
3. The loss of a donor nerve, usually the sural. While the cutaneous sensory defect is usually temporary and is, with time, corrected by sensory overlap and ingrowth, the formation of a troublesome neuroma at the end of the proximal stump is not unknown.

A final answer must await careful and reliable assessments of the recoveries that follow conventional epineurial repair and grafting under comparable conditions.

WHEN SHOULD END-TO-END REPAIR BE ABANDONED IN FAVOUR OF NERVE GRAFTING

This subject is discussed in Chapter 40.

WHEN SHOULD NERVE GRAFTING BE REJECTED AS A METHOD OF REPAIR

Deciding when to reject nerve grafting in favour of some other form of treatment depends on several factors and remains very much a matter of personal judgement.

Clearly, it is questionable to subject the patient to a long and tedious procedure if the prospects of obtaining any worthwhile improvement are indeed remote and alternative methods are available. In this context the following points are relevant:

1. The prospects of obtaining a useful recovery from nerve grafting decline as the length of the defect increases and the state of the nerve bed deteriorates.
2. As with nerve suture the results of grafting are better in the very young.
3. Are alternative forms of treatment available that would give a better result, e.g. tendon transfers in irreparable injuries of the radial nerve?
4. How incapacitating is the patient's disability? When the long-term effects of irreparable nerve injuries are carefully studied it is surprising how well and how often the intelligent patient learns to accept, adjust to, and compensate for his disability, given the benefits to be obtained from re-educational training and reconstructive surgery. This is certainly so for irreparable lesions of the radial, ulnar and lateral popliteal nerves. Sometimes the only persisting complaint is of a painful tender neuroma on the proximal stump.

5. In the doubtful situation, the particular nerve affected has some bearing on the final decision of whether to graft or not.

Permanent median nerve loss is a serious handicap and every reasonable attempt should be made to repair defects in that nerve by grafting. Extensive and complicated grafting of the brachial plexus is justified as an alternative to amputating the arm. As regards the radial, ulnar and lateral popliteal nerves, there is no point in attempting a graft repair except under the most favourable conditions. The results of grafting the sciatic and tibial nerves continue to be disappointing.

6. Each case should be carefully assessed with the object of deciding if grafting will benefit the patient. Clearly, for some nerves and

under some conditions not all large defects are worth repairing.

RELEVANT STRUCTURAL FEATURES OF A GRAFT

Three are worthy of special mention: (1) the cross-sectional area of the graft devoted to fasciculi; (2) the fascicular structure of the graft; and (3) the diameter of the nerve fibres constituting the graft.

The cross sectional area of the graft devoted to fasciculi

Fasciculi contain endoneurial tubes that provide the most effective channels for the growth of axons through the graft. Axons that miss fasciculi become lost in interfascicular tissue. Their entry into the fasciculi of the graft and subsequently into the fasciculi of the distal stump depends, inter alia, on: (1) the effectiveness of the union at the nerve-graft junctions, and (2) the degree to which fascicular apposition is attainable at the opposed ends of the graft and host nerve.

Since grafting is undertaken only when end-to-end repair is impossible, a considerable length of the nerve will have been lost, which means that the opposing nerve ends will present dissimilar fascicular patterns. Despite these dissimilarities the chances of axons entering fasciculi of the graft and distal stump will be facilitated when the fasciculi are closely packed for there is then less interfascicular tissue into which they may be misdirected.

In the case of the distal graft-nerve trunk junction, a further complication is introduced by atrophy of the distal stump which results in differences in the size of the opposed ends of the graft and distal stump.

The fascicular structure of the graft

The function of the graft is not only to guide regenerating axons to the endoneurial tubes of the distal stump but also to go as far as possible in assisting them to reach and enter functionally related endoneurial tubes. Three features are significant in this respect: (1) the branch fibre localisation obtaining in the damaged nerve at the site of the repair, (2) the fascicular structure of the graft, and (3) the number of nerve fibres representing individual branches.

Except when a short length of nerve is destroyed, the fibre localisation at the central stump will not be identical with that at the distal owing to the fascicular redistribution of fibres that has occurred in the lost segment. Correspondence, however, may be sufficiently close to warrant selecting a graft with a fascicular arrangement that goes closest to restoring axon-tubal relationships. One of parallel fasciculi would best meet requirements but this is an uncommon arrangement. However, the fewer the fascicular plexuses in the graft, the greater the chance of restoring useful connections. Finally, the greater the number of branch fibres representing a particular branch the greater the chances of restoring at least some useful pathways.

Group fascicular grafting aimed at restoring the original pattern of innervation is discussed in a separate section.

The diameter of nerve fibres constituting the graft

The restoration of the diameter of regenerated nerve fibres is important in view of the relationship between functional efficiency and nerve fibre diameter. Several factors are involved in this process, though only one relates to the autograft, namely the size of the endoneurial tubes that are to receive and convey the regenerating axons to the distal nerve end.

This raises the question of whether or not large myelinated fibres will be restricted in their development if the nerve graft contains fibres whose diameters are appreciably smaller than those of the host nerve.

Clinically, a study of the late results following regeneration along greatly shrunken endoneurial tubes can only be interpreted in one of two ways. Either large axons have the capacity to inflate small endoneurial tubes into which they regenerate, or normal function is not dependent on the restoration of the original diameter of the nerve fibres.

To be on the safe side, it would be wise to take advantage of the largest available endoneurial tubes by selecting for use as autografts those nerves that have the greatest number of large fibres.

THE RELATIVE MERITS OF CABLE AND FULL THICKNESS AUTOGRAFTS

The choice of a nerve autograft is, with few exceptions, restricted to cutaneous nerves and, since the diameter of the graft should equal or slightly exceed that of the host nerve, the cable variety is necessary to bridge a gap in a large nerve.

Under special conditions, however, full thickness autografting becomes possible and it is, therefore, of importance to examine the merits and disadvantages of each variety.

1. The cable graft required to bridge a long gap in a large peripheral nerve presents a problem, not only for technical reasons, but also because it may necessitate sacrificing more cutaneous nerves than can be justified.
2. Full-thickness grafts have the advantage of being easier to secure and retain in place in comparison with cable grafts.
3. One difficulty with a full-thickness graft is that, in order to match the calibre of a major peripheral nerve, it must come from another of corresponding dimensions and this is only possible when more than one major nerve has been irreparably damaged and one can be used to provide a length for bridging the gap in the other.
4. Revascularisation and graft survival. Central necrosis is more common following the use of full-thickness grafts, from which it is inferred that cable grafts fare better because the thin strands of which they are composed are revascularised more rapidly and effectively. While this is generally true it is not the complete story. Even cable grafts are sometimes in jeopardy. As is noted in the next section, an important factor determining the viability of the graft is the size of its constituent fasciculi and the relative amounts of epineurial and fascicular tissue composing the graft.
5. The fascicular structure of the graft. In full-thickness grafts fascicular

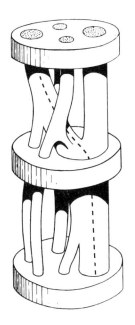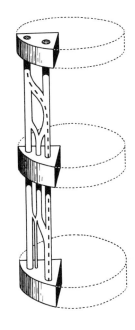

Fig. 43.1

communications may produce a considerable shift of fibres from one sector of the graft to another (Fig. 43.1). On the other hand, in the cable variety such a shift is confined to one strand only and therefore to only a limited sector of the graft. Thus axons growing down one strand of a cable cannot become widely dispersed as they regenerate, in contradistinction to those entering a fasciculus in a full-thickness graft where they may become so scattered. This bestows an advantage on the cable variety that increases as the number of strands increases.

However, though the overall effect of increasing the number of cable strands is to minimise the scattering of branch fibres brought about by fascicular plexuses in the full-thickness graft, a stage is ultimately reached when this advantage is offset by a greatly increased amount of non-fascicular tissue into which regenerating axons may be misdirected.

THE SELECTION OF A CUTANEOUS NERVE FOR CABLE AUTOGRAFTING

The choice of a nerve for cable autografting is limited to the cutaneous nerves of the limbs and their suitability for this purpose is based on the following criteria (Sunderland 1978).

1. Since the graft should be composed of strands of equal length and each should be a little longer than the distance between the nerve ends, a sufficient length of the nerve should be available to provide for a graft of adequate length and thickness.

2. Sometimes the gap is so great that autografting is impracticable. Here the only satisfactory alternative is some other method of conveying axons to the distal stump.

3. Each strand of the cable should be free from branches. Frequent branching reduces the thickness of the nerve and, if complicated, shortens its available length. A segment carrying a branch should only be used providing the branch extends the full length of the graft without itself branching, and can be secured against the parent stem. If branches are shorter than the full length of the graft, fasciculi will end abruptly and the axons descending along them will end in the supporting tissues, though some may continue on to enter the distal nerve end (Fig. 43.2). Reversing the graft when it is placed does not overcome this problem.

In general, cutaneous nerves give few branches while beneath the deep fascia and

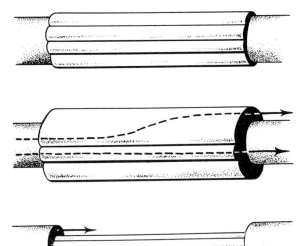

Fig. 43.3

only divide freely on entering the subcutaneous tissue. The most useful nerves are, therefore, those that run long courses beneath the deep fascia and are constant in structure and mode of branching.

4. The cable graft should just exceed, or at least equal, the diameter of the host nerve. Some overlap is required to compensate for any shrinkage in the graft, though its rapid occupation by axons would presumably arrest this shrinkage. The overlap, however, should not be too great lest descending axons are carried by interfascicular communications to bundles that, distally, lie external to the margin of the distal nerve end (Fig. 43.3).

5. The fasciculi should be large and tightly packed in order to reduce the interfascicular spaces that are responsible for the wasteful dispersal of regenerating axons. However, the size of fasciculi should be consistent with the effective revascularisation of the graft.

6. Each strand should, preferably, be composed of parallel fasciculi or, failing this, its fascicular pattern should be subjected to only minor modifications as the result of plexus formations.

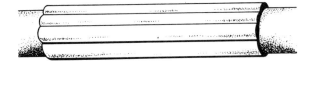

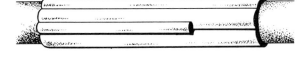

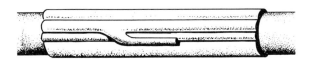

Fig. 43.2

7. The nerve should contain large numbers of large nerve fibres.

8. In a cable of suitable diameter, the greater the number of strands the greater will be the waste space between the fasciculi into which axons may be misdirected. Thus the cutaneous nerve selected should be as thick as possible in order to reduce the number of strands required but increased thickness is only of value when it is due to fascicular tissue and not interfascicular epineurial tissue, and the fasciculi are of a thickness consistent with rapid revascularisation.

9. The nerve should be readily accessible and constant in position so that it may be exposed rapidly and with confidence. A nerve subject to frequent variations will prove troublesome.

10. Unless there are good reasons to the contrary there are advantages in selecting an adjacent cutaneous nerve.

11. A cutaneous nerve should never be used when it innervates the skin adjacent to the area denervated by the nerve injury. For example, the superficial radial should not be used for repairing a gap in the median nerve. Such a nerve is responsible for some of the shrinkage occurring in the denervated area with the passage of time. If it is removed not only is this advantage lost but the area of skin originally rendered insensitive is greatly increased.

12. The resulting sensory defect should be minimal in quality and extent, and should affect an area where cutaneous innervation is not of great importance and its loss is not disturbing to the patient. If there is any doubt, the patient can experience, by first blocking the nerve, the sensory deficit that will follow loss of the cutaneous nerve.

13. The resulting scar should not involve a pressure-bearing area.

14. These features should be taken into consideration when evaluating the results of nerve grafting.

Comment

Since no cutaneous nerve possesses all the essential qualities required of a graft it is necessary to select, where possible, those in which the undesirable features are reduced to a minimum. On this basis the two outstanding are the superficial radial and sural nerves. Next in order of suitability are, in turn, the medial cutaneous nerve of the forearm, the lateral cutaneous nerve of the forearm and the lateral femoral cutaneous nerve, though these have only slender claims to selection. The medial cutaneous nerve of the arm and the posterior cutaneous nerve of the thigh should not be used if others are available. Where it is found necessary to use cutaneous nerves that do not conform to the standards required, then a reduction in the extent and quality of possible recovery must be expected.

As regards the undoubted claims of the superficial radial nerve for cable autografting, and the negligible sensory defect that follows its removal, this nerve should never be sacrificed for the repair of gaps in the median nerve because it is an important source for the compensatory sensory overlap and ingrowth into neighbouring denervated cutaneous areas, particularly the important radial side of the hand.

THE BLOOD SUPPLY TO AND SURVIVAL OF THE GRAFT

When a graft-to-be is removed from the donor nerve and transferred to its new site it is temporarily left without a blood supply and should, therefore, be adequately revascularised as rapidly as possible. If a blood supply is restored by the 3rd day the graft survives but after this period its viability steadily declines to the point of failure at the 5th day.

Inadequate and delayed revascularisation threaten graft survival by encouraging fibrosis, and particularly collagenisation of the endoneurium and ischaemic fascicular necrosis.

A nerve graft is revascularised by vessels entering, not only from across the proximal and distal junctions, but also by vessels that enter from the tissues of the bed in which the nerve is resting.

Blood vessels enter the graft from the proximal and distal stumps 3–4 days after implantation, and are prominent by the 5th day, by which time an occasional vessel has entered the epineurium from the tissues of the nerve bed. Vascularisation from the latter is well advanced 6–8 days after implanting the graft, following which the vessels from the tissues of the nerve bed become the main source for the blood supply to the graft. In approximately 3 weeks a free anastomosis develops between the longitudinal and regional arterial systems.

For this reason the graft should be located, wherever possible, in healthy well-vascularised tissue. The risk of ischaemia should not be increased by allowing the graft to remain in a badly scarred bed or by enclosing it in a sleeve of foreign material.

The manner in which the graft acquires a new blood supply indicates that the following factors influence its revascularisation and survival: (1) the length of the graft, (2) the thickness of the graft, and (3) the size of the constituent fasciculi and the amount of epineurial tissue composing the graft.

The length of the graft

Short grafts are rapidly revascularised from the nerve stumps and at a rate that maintains their viability. In long grafts the viability of the central portion will be entirely dependent in the early stages on revascularisation from the tissues of the nerve bed. Should effective penetration of the graft and the revascularisation of fasciculi be unduly delayed ischaemic necrosis will follow.

The thickness of the graft

Thin grafts fare better than thicker grafts. The latter are prone to central necrosis because of the delay in restoring an adequate circulation to the central part of the graft.

From this it is inferred that the thin strands of the former are revascularised more rapidly and effectively than the latter. While this is essentially correct, the important factor that determines the viability of the graft is not so much its total thickness as the size of its constituent fasciculi and the amount of epineurial tissue.

The size of the fasciculi and the amount of epineurial tissue

Revascularisation is greatly facilitated when the graft is composed of small fasciculi with a small

amount of epineurial tissue into which new vessels must first pass in order re-establish collateral circulations with the vessels there, from which the nerve fibres and endoneurium receive their blood supply.

Large amounts of epineurial tissue delay the effective revascularisation of fasciculi because of the additional time taken by new vessels to re-establish the collateral circulations in the epineurium from which the capillaries inside the fasciculi will be supplied.

Though full thickness grafts may survive, there is no doubt that central necrosis is more common in this variety. Clearly, there must be a critical graft and fascicular diameter beyond which it is not safe to go. The chances of full thickness grafts surviving is greatly improved if the constituent fasciculi are small enough and those at the centre are not separated from the surface by too great an amount of epineurial tissue. On the other hand, they run the risk of ischaemic damage if the nerve fibres are concentrated in one or a few large fasciculi. Thus it is the size of the fasciculi rather than the size of the nerve trunk itself that determines whether or not ischaemic necrosis is likely after free full-thickness grafting (Fig. 43.4).

Central necrosis has been reported after using a section of an irreparably damaged lateral popliteal

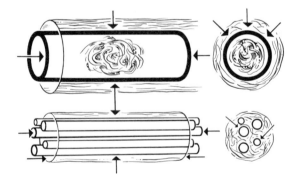

Fig. 43.4 Diagram to illustrate the effect of the fascicular structure of the graft on revascularisation. Revascularisation of the central portion of the graft is delayed when the nerve fibres are contained in one or two large fasciculi, each of which, because of its size, is encircled by a thicker perineurial sheath. Under these unfavourable conditions central necrosis of the graft is likely. The chances of satisfactory revascularization are greatly improved when the fasciculi are smaller. The arrows indicate the source of the new blood supply to the graft from the nerve bed and from the nerve at the nerve-graft junctions.

nerve as a free full thickness graft to repair a gap in a co-existing medial popliteal nerve injury. The central necrosis has been attributed to the use of a full-thickness graft. However, the lateral popliteal nerve is often composed of a single large fasciculus or a small number of large fasciculi in the distal half of the thigh. These are the conditions in which early revascularisation of the fasciculi is seriously impaired. This is a more likely explanation for the ischaemic fascicular necrosis than the fact that a full-thickness free graft has been used.

The strands of a cable graft and their contained fasciculi should be of such a calibre that they can be revascularised before central necrosis can occur. The critical size of fasciculi is not known but those provided by cutaneous nerves are rarely so large as to inhibit the rapid and effective vascularisation of the graft.

GROUP FASCICULAR REPAIR IN NERVE GRAFTING

There is no alternative to this method for maximising the entry of axons into fasciculi. At the same time, whether or not it will be effective in restoring useful connections will depend on the extent to which structural arrangements at the nerve ends and in the graft favour or restrict the erroneous cross-shunting of axons during regeneration.

The relative merits of cable and full-thickness nerve grafts are discussed in an earlier section in which it was shown that the cable graft is superior in many respects to a full-thickness graft.

Since each strand of a cable graft covers only a portion of the end of the host nerve, it can transmit only those axons emerging from that sector to which the strand is opposed. In this way the parallel strands of a graft would impose a measure of orderliness in the growth of axons through the graft.

Figure 43.5 illustrates the consequences of a number of possible branch fibre arrangements at widely separated nerve ends.

In general, the fascicular and branch fibre pattern in corresponding sectors at the proximal and distal nerve ends conform to one of four types:

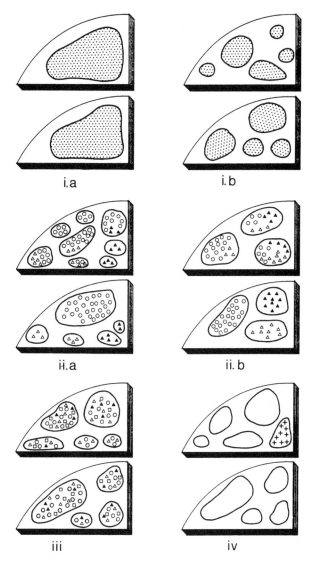

Fig. 43.5

1. The host sector, above and below, contains one or more fasciculi, presenting the same or dissimilar patterns but composed of fibres for the same branch. Though there is some rearrangement of axons as they enter and grow through a strand of the graft, this is of little functional consequence since it involves only fibres for the same branch (Fig. 43.5i, *a* and *b*).

2. The sector at the proximal nerve end contains fasciculi, some of which are

composed of fibres for the same branch while others are composed of a combination of fibres destined for different destinations. However, in the corresponding sector at the distal nerve end, each branch fibre system represented in the proximal sector is now confined to its own fasciculus or group of fasciculi. Despite the difference at the two levels some branch fibre localisation is retained and there is, consequently, a reasonable chance during regeneration of restoring at least some useful terminal connections. Another variant of this arrangement that gives the same result is shown in Fig. 43.5ii, *a* and *b*.

3. Each of the fasciculi in the opposing sectors contains fibres from several branches and all traces of localisation are lost (Fig. 43.5iii). Under these conditions one should not expect too much of the graft.

4. The sector at the proximal nerve end contains fibres not represented in the distal sector. Here there is no way of redirecting these axons into their old paths in the distal segment of the nerve (Fig 43.5 iv).

Discrepancies in fibre localisation at the nerve ends increase with the length of the graft, that is, the distance between the nerve ends. The fascicular arrangements described in (1), (2) and (3) above are more common at distal levels and are replaced, respectively, by (2), (3) and (4) at proximal levels.

The ideal graft would be one in which the fascicular arrangement was identical with that of the destroyed segment so that, after traversing the graft, the axons would be automatically directed to the appropriate endoneurial tubes in the distal segment. This would go a long way towards restoring the original fibre pattern. Though this ideal can never be realised, it is clear that the best cable graft would be one that has the simplest fascicular structure, preferably of parallel fasciculi. Such an arrangement would minimise the movement of regenerating axons between the fasciculi which tends to distort the pattern.

THE GRAFT BED

Injuries that call for nerve grafting usually cause extensive destruction of the neighbouring tissues and considerable scarring as healing occurs. The nerve ends, and subsequently the graft, are consequently left occupying an unfavourable bed and it is not always possible to find an alternative site amid healthy tissue.

There is no doubt that the critical factor determining the survival of a graft as a useful vehicle for the passage of axons to the distal stump is its blood supply. An inadequate blood supply imperils the graft by:

1. promoting fibrosis which is generalised but most harmful when the integrity of the endoneurium is destroyed by excessive collagenisation, and

2. resulting in necrosis which is most likely to involve the long full-thickness graft for reasons given elsewhere. The shorter and thinner the graft the better the result. Revascularisation of the graft is described in an earlier section, where attention is directed to the importance of vessels derived from the tissues in which the graft is resting. A nerve bed of well-vascularised healthy tissue favours the early and rapid revascularisation of the graft, whereas the contribution from this source is considerably impaired when the nerve occupies a scarred and poorly nourished bed.

In some cases the blood supply to the graft is still further embarrassed by a co-existing arterial injury such as occurs when a segment of a digital nerve and artery are destroyed.

THE USE OF PROTECTIVE SLEEVES TO ENCLOSE THE NERVE-GRAFT JUNCTIONS

The advantages and disadvantages of enclosing the nerve-graft junctions in protective sleeves are identical with those that have been outlined for end-to-end repair in Chapter 42.

In general, the use of protective sleeves is justified only when a favourable bed cannot be found for the repaired nerve, the intention being to prevent the formation of adhesions that would fix it to the nerve bed. The use of 'sleeves' is contra-indicated when a good, healthy bed can be found for the graft, largely on the grounds that they are then more likely to impair the restoration of a blood supply to regions of high metabolic activity. Usually, enclosing a long graft in an insulating material dooms it to failure.

THE RELATIVE MERITS OF FRESH AND PREDEGENERATED NERVE GRAFTS

Predegenerating a graft by nerve section in situ 8–15 days before its removal has been claimed to improve its qualities as a medium for conducting regenerating axons across the gap to the distal segment of the severed nerve. There is, a priori, no reason why this should be so and there is much evidence to show that the rates of axon advance through predegenerated and fresh grafts are not significantly different. If the predegenerated graft has any advantage over the fresh graft it is not based on a more rapid growth of axons into and through the graft.

The advantages claimed for grafts prepared in this way are:

1. They are firmer, which makes them easier to handle, thereby permitting a more effective union between the nerve ends.

2. It has been claimed that axon and myelin debris in degenerating nerve fibres in the graft obstruct the advance of axons and that, if sufficient time is allowed for the endoneurial tubes to be cleared of this debris, regenerating axons will then advance along them more easily and rapidly. A histological and clinical study of the pattern of recovery following a second degree nerve injury demonstrates that there is no foundation for this claim (pp. 94 and 420).

3. It seems reasonable to assume that the increased metabolic activity associated with Wallerian degeneration and the removal of axon-myelin debris would demand an increased blood supply. This is readily available when the graft is sectioned but left undisturbed in situ. When the graft is transferred to its new site, 8–15 days later, there is the further assumption that, by that time, the endoneurial tubes will have been cleared of axon-myelin debris, all of which means that the graft is then more likely to withstand the initial and temporary reduction or loss of a blood supply

pending its revascularisation. The difficulty of accepting this as an advantage is its reliance on assumptions. The products of Wallerian degeneration in the freshly transplanted graft are also removed, if somewhat more slowly, because revascularisation of the graft takes effect by about the 5th day. In any event the presence of such debris offers no obstacle to the advance of regenerating axons. On balance, the predegenerated graft has no decided advantage over the fresh graft. Moreover, the former has the disadvantage of necessitating a two-stage operation.

Clinically, the results from the use of fresh and predegenerated grafts have proved inconclusive in terms of deciding the relative merits of each.

Should anatomical considerations favour using the degenerated distal segment of an extensively damaged nerve there is no objection to doing so, providing that it has not been denervated for too long as this would reduce its usefulness for the transmission of regenerating axons.

THE CASE FOR REVERSING THE GRAFT BEFORE INSERTING IT

The rationale of this procedure is to prevent the loss of those regenerating axons that enter the endoneurial tubes of a branch that leaves the graft well short of the distal stump.

Whether or not such a manoeuvre enjoys any worthwhile advantages over the conventional method is debatable, particularly in view of the warning that cutaneous nerves that branch frequently over the selected length should be avoided. However, should conditions dictate otherwise, the branches should then extend to the distal end of the graft and should be closely applied to it. In their study of the effect of nerve graft polarity on nerve regeneration Stromberg et al (1979) concluded that nerve graft function was independent of polarity.

TIMING THE DISTAL NERVE GRAFT REPAIR

Normally the graft is attached proximally and distally at the same operation. However, there is always the risk that, by the time regenerating axons reach the distal suture line, scarring at that site will present an impenetrable barrier to their further advance. On this premise there is a case for treating the distal nerve-graft junction separately in one of two ways.

1. If it has been repaired at the original operation, the junctional zone is later excised, the graft and nerve ends are 'freshened' and then resutured. This is done just in advance of the calculated arrival of regenerating axons which are then confronted with a relatively fresh suture line which should favour their passage to the distal nerve end.
2. The distal graft and nerve ends are not united at the original operation but are tagged and left in juxtaposition. With the arrival of regenerating axons at the distal end of the graft a neuroma forms at that site. At this time the graft and nerve ends are freshened and sutured.

Comment

Calculations based on the graft length and regeneration rates can at best be only approximate, so that timing the arrival of regenerating axon tips at the distal level presents difficulties. If the nerve contains sensory fibres, tracking Hoffmann–Tinel's sign down the graft is a useful guide, while the formation of a neuroma at the distal end of the graft is evidence of active regeneration and the arrival of axons at that site.

If a delayed distal repair is performed prematurely then there is still time for damaging fibrosis to develop before axons arrive. If, on the other hand, axons have already crossed the suture site then what might have been satisfactory regeneration would have been lost by the second operation. This second possibility is avoided by not repairing the distal graft-nerve ends at the original operation.

Finally, there is always the risk when freshening the graft and nerve ends at the second operation of creating (1) a gap that now requires tension to close it, and (2) conditions that while allowing the passage of axons, will be followed later by a constrictive fibrosis little different from that originally assumed to be present.

Short grafts are not a problem and the repair should be completed in one operation. It is the long grafts that could present difficulties. Even under the most favourable conditions some fibrosis is inevitable at the distal anastomosis that could block axons.

Taking all factors into consideration, the preferable course of action is to complete the entire grafting procedure at the one operation. If sensory regeneration in involved, useful information can usually be obtained by carefully tracking the descent of Hoffmann–Tinel's sign, though there are now reliable electrophysiological techniques for detecting the presence of regenerating axons and of following their growth distally. If these methods confirm the speedy passage of axons across the distal suture line then no further action is required. It is only when axon growth is arrested at this site that the distal suture line should be resected and resutured.

FACTORS INFLUENCING THE QUALITY OF THE RECOVERY AFTER NERVE AUTOGRAFTING

The factors influencing the quality of the recovery after nerve autografting are essentially the same as those described for end-to-end nerve repair in Chapter 42 which should be consulted for this information.

THE NERVE-GRAFT UNION

Features of note:

1. The nerve-graft unions must be completely tension free. In order to ensure this:

a. the limb should be extended and not flexed when placing the graft;
b. the graft should be 10–20 per cent longer than the gap to be bridged. This is because elasticity causes an initial shortening of the graft when it is removed from the donor nerve and this shortening increases as the connective tissue of the graft contracts. After implantation the graft should be slack in its bed without tension at the nerve-graft junctions;

c. the limb should be immobilised until healing has given secure junctional zones. This takes about 4–6 weeks.

In their experimental study (cat sciatic nerve) of the biomechanical properties of the nerve-graft suture lines, Osterman et al (1986) found that the tensile strength of the distal suture line was decreased in comparison with the proximal over a period that was graft length dependent. There was much speculation on the reason for this without any clear explanation emerging.

2. There appears to be no bar, within reason, to the length of the graft, always remembering that its blood supply comes initially from the proximal and distal stumps and somewhat more slowly from the tissues of the nerve bed. Should the graft be unduly long, parts of the central portion may suffer ischaemic necrosis.

3. The graft should exceed the thickness of the nerve trunk being repaired in order to allow for the shrinkage that follows Wallerian degeneration. The rapid reinnervation of a fresh graft prevents or reverses this atrophy, while the use of a predegenerated graft would provide for this.

4. In preparing the graft and nerve ends for group fascicular repair:

a. avoid further unnecessary trauma to the nerve and graft ends;
b. preserve vasa nervorum;
c. restore fascicular continuity so far as this is possible within the limits imposed by discrepancies in the fascicular patterns at the opposed nerve and graft ends.

Epineurium is carefully removed from the nerve end under magnification, so that the fasciculi are freed, the large fasciculi individually and the smaller fasciculi in groups. In this way fasciculi are left protruding only slightly at the nerve end.

The manner in which fasciculi are grouped is determined by their number, size, position and arrangement. So far as fascicular apposition at the nerve-graft interface is concerned, the suture of individual fasciculi is rarely practicable. Each union will more commonly involve a group of fasciculi.

With short defects it is possible that a major fasciculus, or a group of small fasciculi, will correspond at the nerve ends and these should be connected by a cable of the graft. With long defects, however, there will be no corresponding groups at the nerve ends and the best that can be achieved under these circumstances is to arrange the fasciculi in a way that goes closest to restoring fascicular apposition when the graft is in place.

6. The methods of uniting large fasciculi and groups of small fasciculi are the same in nerve grafting as they are in end-to-end nerve repair. Suture materials should be of the finest calibre and used sparingly. So far as is possible, they should be placed facing the surface of the nerve, be confined to the perifascicular epineurium and should certainly go no deeper than the perineurium.

Plasma glue welding has advantages for consolidating the union of fasciculi though the need to avoid tension with such delicate unions is self-evident.

FREE NEUROVASCULAR GRAFTING

The greatest threat to the survival of a nerve graft relates to its blood supply. This is particularly so in the case of the long graft occupying an unfavourable bed. In order to counter this threat, and to ensure the best possible continuing blood supply to a long graft, a technique has been devised, tested experimentally and applied clinically, in which a donor nerve, together with the main arteriovenous system vascularising it, are transferred in toto to the graft site (Taylor & Ham 1976). The circulation is then restored by microvascular anastomoses and nerve trunk continuity by group fascicular suture at the nerve-graft junctions.

The method was also believed to carry an additional bonus in that an improved blood supply would promote the more rapid removal of axon and myelin debris that would otherwise obstruct and slow the advance of regenerating axons (Townsend & Taylor 1984). This concept is based on an earlier report by Seddon (1963) but is without foundation (pp. 94 and 420).

The test case was one of Volkmann's ischaemia involving total destruction of the median nerve, the superficial radial nerve and the radial vessels between the elbow and the wrist on the right side.

Using microsurgical techniques, the essential steps in closing the defect in the median nerve were:

1. a neurovascular bundle, comprising the superficial radial nerve, with its associated radial artery and venae comitantes, was isolated and removed from the sound forearm;
2. the neurovascular graft was transferred to the recipient forearm where its circulation was immediately restored by proximal and distal microvascular anastomoses. Large vessel continuity was re-established between the brachial artery and the radial artery by incorporating a 10 cm vein graft proximally;
3. the superficial radial nerve was inserted between the ends of the median nerve, suitable adjustments made at the nerve-graft junctions to establish the best possible fascicular apposition, and fascicular unions effected by suture.

Comment

Angiography postoperatively confirmed a good blood supply to the graft. The sensory recovery in the median field in this patient has been surprisingly good. Moreover, the rate of advance of regenerating sensory axons down the graft appeared to be faster than that recorded for a conventional nerve graft, though the comparison is based on inadequate data. However, the course of regeneration and the quality of the sensory recovery have endorsed the importance of an adequate blood supply to a nerve graft.

The technique of free vascularised nerve grafting was developed to ensure graft survival in situations where central or segmental necrosis of a conventional free nerve graft seemed likely.

In this respect the method is a special procedure reserved for special occasions.

Taylor and Ham's paper directed attention not only to the importance of the blood supply of grafts but also to a method of preserving that supply under particularly adverse conditions. Their paper stimulated considerable interest, and since that time at least 20 papers have appeared on the subject. In general the investigations reported have had two objectives:

1. To test the validity of the claims in favour of free neurovascular grafting.
2. To find additional neurovascular arrangements that would lend themselves to free neurovascular grafting. In the process the sural, saphenous and ulnar nerves were added to the superficial radial. The method has now been used for graft repairs to the brachial plexus following injuries in which a vascularised ulnar nerve has been available as the donor nerve (Bonney et al 1984, Alnot 1988, Birch et al 1988).

Experimental and clinical studies relating to the relative merits of vascularised and conventional nerve grafts have produced conflicting results. According to most reports the vascularised variety confers an advantage on the graft (Taylor & Ham 1976, Taylor 1978, 1979, Koshima & Harii 1981, 1985, Koshima et al 1981, Hunt 1983, Breidenbach & Terzis 1984, Townsend & Taylor 1984, Gu Yu-dong et al 1985, Restrepo et al 1985, Rose & Kowalski 1985, Lux et al 1988, Shibata et al 1986, Wood & Lind 1986, Boorman & Sykes 1987, Birch et al 1988). Others, however, find no significant difference between the two (McCullough et al 1984, Pho et al 1985, Seckel et al 1986, Comtet 1988b) and a third group found the conventional method to be superior (Settergen & Wood 1984, Daly & Wood 1985). Hunt (1983), in his experimental study, compared the effectiveness of short vascularised and nonvascularised grafts. Not surprisingly, he found little difference between them, with the former in some experiments having only a marginal advantage. Wood's (1988) discussion paper on Lux et al's 1988 paper is recommended reading.

Clearly, in these investigations much depends on the length of the graft and the nature of the graft bed. There is little point in devising and conducting experiments using short grafts in a favourable environment in order to compare the relative merits of the two methods for these are not the conditions in which free neurovascular grafting should be used. The latter should be reserved for those special occasions where a long graft is required to cross a considerable gap and the only available bed is composed of extensively scarred and poorly vascularised tissue.

Finally, in evaluating the method much will depend on whether or not the quality of the recovery consistently comes up to expectations, confirms the claimed advantages and proves to be superior to any other method for getting regenerating axons to the distal nerve end.

In the meantime free neurovascular grafting remains an innovatory procedure of considerable promise but only when the conditions justify its use.

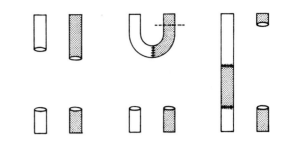

Fig. 43.6

NERVE PEDICLE GRAFTING

In general, a gap in a major nerve is best closed by a cable autograft. However, there are those exceptional injuries when alternative methods become necessary to repair a nerve. These involve sacrificing one nerve to repair another by using a nerve pedicle grafting technique in which the blood supply to the graft is preserved (Sunderland 1978).

Single nerve pedicle grafting

Here two adjacent major nerves have both been so extensively damaged that nerve repair by cable grafting each is impracticable. The gap in the more important nerve is then bridged by using a length from the less important nerve. The ulnar nerve is always sacrificed in favour of the median and the lateral in favour of the medial popliteal (Strange 1947, 1950).

Alpar and Brooks (1978) have recently used this method to good effect in nine patients with Volkmann's ischaemic lesions of the median and ulnar nerves where the ulnar has been used to repair the median.

The graft may be taken from either the proximal or the distal segment of the donor nerve depending on anatomical considerations, the length of the distal segment and the time for which it has been denervated. In general, it is preferable to use the proximal stump because it has not suffered changes that might prejudice regeneration.

The gap is bridged in two stages. In the first stage both proximal nerve ends are suitably prepared and then sutured in the form of an anastomotic loop (Fig. 43.6). The donor nerve is then divided above the anastomosis at a point that provides the length ultimately required to bridge the gap in the recipient nerve. This procedure leaves the contribution from the donor nerve trunk undisturbed in its own bed and with its blood supply from this source intact. In about 4 weeks' time the sutured proximal nerve ends have become securely united while the segment of the donor nerve has undergone Wallerian degeneration and been occupied by regenerating axons that have grown into it across the suture line of the loop from the proximal end of the recipient nerve. The second stage involves swinging the length of the donor nerve across the gap and suturing it to the distal nerve end of the recipient. This technique preserves the blood supply to the length of nerve which is to become the autograft. This is maintained in the first instance from the bed of the parent nerve and later from vessels that reach it from the proximal end of the recipient nerve across the suture line.

A variant of this method is illustrated in Fig. 43.7. The proximal segment of the donor nerve is divided superiorly and the upper end of the isolated section sutured to the proximal end of

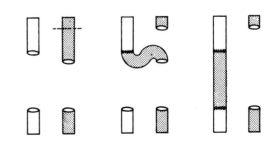

Fig. 43.7

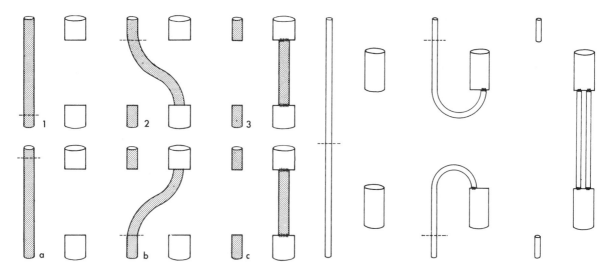

Fig. 43.8   **Fig. 43.9**

the recipient nerve. Subsequently, the lower end of the pedicle is swung down and sutured to the distal stump of the recipient nerve. The method is not without risk in that the graft pedicle must be temporarily deprived of a blood supply until it is revascularised across the suture line from above and from its new bed.

Using the same technique, a less important nerve in continuity is sacrificed to repair the gap in a more important nerve. For example, the medial cutaneous nerve of the forearm may be used to repair the median nerve in the upper arm. In this case a two-stage repair is performed by one of the two techniques illustrated in Fig. 43.8; both preserve the blood supply of what is to become the grafted section of the nerve and both ensure that the reinnervation of the median field will be by median nerve fibres. There is little to choose between them, though the second takes advantage of the earlier reinnervation and revascularisation of the proximal stump of the graft.

DOUBLE NERVE PEDICLE GRAFTING

Here a less important nerve is sacrificed to repair the gap in a more important neighbouring nerve. The technique is designed to interpose a double length of the cutaneous donor between the nerve ends. The selected length of, say, the medial

cutaneous nerve of the forearm is twice the length of the gap to be closed. At the first stage this length is divided in the middle, the upper and lower divisions being sutured to the proximal and distal stumps, respectively, of the median nerve. At a later second stage, the medial cutaneous nerve is divided superiorly and inferiorly and the freed sections then swung across the gap as illustrated in Fig. 43.9. The only advantage of this method over a conventional cable graft is that the blood supply is preserved, initially from the vasa nervorum of the donor nerve and later from across each suture line.

PART 2. THE TUBAL REPAIR OF NERVES

The use of sleeves to effect sutureless end-to-end nerve union is not relevant to this discussion, which is concerned exclusively with bridging widely separated nerve ends.

The concept of bridging widely separated nerve ends with tubes of a foreign material in order to assist regenerating axons to cross the gap has a long history dating back to the turn of the century (Sunderland 1978). The results were an unbroken succession of failures and the method abandoned.

However, Weiss and Taylor (1944, 1946) restored interest in the method in the 1940s by using arteries as the bridging material and they were later joined by others who introduced a wide variety of non-biological and biological materials for this purpose (veins, Swann 1941; millipore and reinforced millipore, Campbell et al 1956, 1961, Campbell and Bassett 1957, Noback et al 1958; amnioplastin, Chao et al 1962). It soon became clear that the only gaps that could be satisfactorily bridged in this way were those that could be more appropriately closed by an end-to-end repair or by nerve autografting. Clinical trials using the tubal repair techniques were again failures and the method abandoned.

But history has a habit of repeating itself and more recently many others have returned to this topic with, however, more carefully planned and controlled investigations, and more clearly defined objectives that are not confined to finding a guiding structure for regenerating axons and a device for excluding scar tissue from the repair site. They have been extended and elaborated to provide a very useful tool for studying regeneration growth patterns and, by modifying the environment in the chamber between the nerve ends, the factors, and particularly neurotropic influences, that control them.

Improved biodegradable and biological materials used for bridging the gap in these experiments have included: arterial allografts (Gulati 1989); veins (Chiu et al 1982); collagen membranes (Rosen et al 1980); various synthetic biodegradable materials (Reid et al 1978, Molander et al 1982, 1983, Nyilas et al 1983, Uzman and Villegas 1983, Seckel et al 1984, da Silva et al 1985, Dellon & Mackinnon 1988). Silicone, pseudosynovial and fabricated mesothelial tubes (Lundborg & Hansson 1979, 1980, 1981, Lundborg et al 1981a, b, 1982a–e, Danielsen et al 1983, le Beau et al 1983, 1986, Uzman & Villegas 1983, Varon & Lundborg 1983, Williams et al 1983, 1984, Jenq & Coggeshall 1985, Scaravilli 1984, da Silva et al 1985, Mackinnon et al 1985, Madison et al 1985, Williams & Varon 1985, Müller et al 1987a,b, Williams 1987, Dahlin et al 1988).

The mesothelial 'chambers' introduced by Lundborg and his associates have decided advantages over other materials and are proving a valuable asset for studying the biochemical and molecular aspects of axon regeneration and all that pertains thereto.

Though the subject is one of intense and continuing activity, it should not be overlooked that the tubular chamber is not without its limitations.

1. The use of improved tubes as a method of nerve repair has yet to emerge from the experimental stage and to find a clinical application.
2. In confirming the presence of neurotropic influences emanating from the distal nerve end that attract regenerating axons, effort has only served to confirm Cajal's observations of almost a century ago.
3. Tubal repair does not solve the overriding problem of the erroneous cross-shunting of axons and the loss of other axons into epineurial tissues at the distal nerve end.
4. Collectively, the investigations reveal that the critical gap distance that can be crossed using the method varies from 6 to 15 mm, though there is a report of axons crossing a 3 cm gap (Mackinnon et al 1984, Dellon & Mackinnon 1988). This should be checked. In any event these are all gaps that would be more readily and appropriately treated by nerve cable autografting or closed by end-to-end union.
5. Axon regeneration in a chamber is being studied in an artificial environment where it is not subjected to many of the constraints to which it is normally exposed in a clinical situation.

At the same time the model does provide an excellent tool for studying many of the parameters controlling axon regeneration.

PART 3. MUSCLE TISSUE AS AN INTERPOSITIONAL GRAFT FOR NERVE REPAIR

On the basis that the basement membrane of skeletal muscle fibres has a tubular structure reminiscent of the endoneurial sheath and basement membrane of nerve fibres, prepared skeletal muscle tissue is being investigated as an interpositional graft to guide regenerating axons across a nerve gap (Ide 1984, Keynes et al 1984, Ji-Ming Kong et al 1986, Fawcett & Keynes 1986, Glasby et al 1986, Ji-Ming Kong 1987, Ji-Ming Kong & Shi-Zhen Zhong 1988).

The experimental evidence indicates that this tissue can provide a scaffolding for the passage of regenerating axons, and according to Fawcett and Keynes the results are as effective as nerve autografting.

Additional claims include:

1. the basal lamina grafts are rapidly revascularised;
2. the graft tissue appears to be well tolerated;
3. the donor defect is minimal;
4. normal axon numbers were demonstrated in the grafts and in the distal nerve, with normal function returning across the graft at 6 months (Glasby et al 1986).

These claims, examined in isolation, make this method a serious challenger to more conventional methods of nerve autografting. However, before it is adopted for clinical use it needs to be evaluated more critically than appears to have been the case to date.

Fundamentally, it suffers from the defects inherent in all experimental studies using animals.

1. The nerve gaps were small and usually of an order that are readily corrected clinically by end-to-end nerve union.
2. It has not had to contend with the more complex internal structure that is a feature of human nerves. Nor does it solve the overriding problem of the erroneous cross-shunting of axons and the loss of many others en route and into the epineurial tissue of the distal nerve stump.
3. The evaluation of function is based on inadequate data.
4. Functional recovery in man requires far more than the passage of axons through a graft.
5. Long-term effects of potential scarring in the graft is unclear. Clearly it is too early to pass final judgement on an interesting innovatory procedure other than to say that it has a questionable future for clinical use.

PART 4. NERVE CROSS-UNION

In this method a normal nerve is completely or partially sacrificed and used for reinnervating the

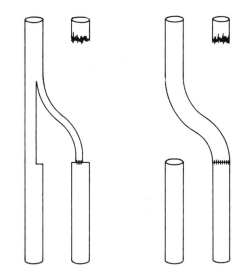

Fig. 43.10

distal segment of an irreparably injured nerve. Nerve crossing is complete when the donor nerve is completely divided and its proximal stump is sutured to the distal stump of the recipient; in partial crossing only part of the donor nerve is sutured to the distal stump (Fig. 43.10). The cross-union is completed by group fascicular repair designed to give the best possible fasicular apposition.

This method has three important limitations:

1. A suitable normal nerve that can be sacrificed is not always adjacent to the distal stump of the injured nerve to permit the cross-union.

2. The nerve fibre composition of the recipient and donor nerves should correspond, for nothing is to be gained by suturing a sensory nerve to one that is predominantly motor and vice versa. However, the two nerves are bound to differ as regards the numbers and relative proportions of motor and sensory fibres, branch fibre localisation and the function of the various structures innervated. Consequently the erroneous cross-shunting of axons into foreign and functionally unrelated tubes is more common and more disabling after cross-union.

3. Reinnervation is always incomplete and imperfect after nerve crossing because:

i. the donor nerve rarely matches the recipient nerve in size and fascicular structure, though a selected group fascicular repair may partly overcome discrepancies. This means that large numbers of axons are lost by erroneous cross-shunting into foreign functionally unrelated endoneurial tubes and by ending blindly in the epineurial tissues of the distal nerve end so that reinnervation of the periphery is both incomplete and imperfect and fails to provide adequately for either motor or sensory function.

ii. Even when motor axons reinnervate muscle fibres and cutaneous sensory 'axons' reinnervate the skin, the prospects of obtaining a useful functional result are not necessarily good. Movements that are regained by nerve crossing are difficult to control voluntarily, and though sensory recovery may be of some protective value to the patient, false reference remains a problem. Poor functional recovery is due to the disorganisation which affects the pattern of innervation when axons regenerate to structures that differ from those they originally supplied. Such reinnervation is only likely to be functionally useful if central adjustments can compensate for the altered patterns of innervation. The capacity to benefit from re-educational training depends on age and other factors and are clearly limited. This problem is accentuated after nerve-crossing when an injured nerve is reinnervated by a totally foreign nerve. Where the option is available it is preferable to have the distal stump innervated by the parent rather than a foreign nerve and for this reason group fascicular cable autografting is more likely to give a better result than nerve crossing.

Reference to three special injuries will illustrate the potential and special role of nerve cross-union in nerve repair.

THE FACIAL NERVE

The method has proved useful in correcting certain irreparable injuries of the facial nerve, the donor nerve being selected from the hypoglossal, descendens hypoglossi and spinal accessory nerves. Of these only the facio-hypoglossal cross-union has survived in clinical practice and this has been largely replaced by autografting.

THE BRACHIAL PLEXUS

Nerve cross-union, supplemented where necessary by interpositional grafts between the donor nerves and the plexus has been of particular value in the repair of traction rupture and avulsion injuries of the brachial plexus (see Chapter 46).

The donor nerves are provided by the 3, 4, 5 and 6 intercostal nerves and by the accessory nerve. The supplementary graft is usually from the sural but irreparably involved branches of the plexus, for example the ulnar nerve, may be salvaged and used.

The recipient part of the plexus may be the upper trunk, the lateral cord or the musculocutaneous nerve, though the procedure may be modified to meet the special requirements of individual injuries.

The long-term functional value of these complicated repairs has yet to be established, but to date they offer the only prospect of effecting any improvement and the results in well-selected cases are encouraging.

A word on the selection of the accessory nerve as the donor is not out of place here. One should caution against using this nerve for the following reasons. Sacrificing the accessory nerve paralyses the trapezius which is often the most important survivor, not only of the shoulder girdle elevators but also of the external rotators of the scapular.

1. With the loss of the elevators of the shoulder girdle, the latter sags and this puts tension on the repaired plexus which threatens repair sites.
2. Loss of the rotating action on the scapula removes the only remaining means of compensating for the loss of the true abductors at the shoulder joint.

THE MEDIAN NERVE

There are times when after examining the possible benefits to be gained by mobilisation, rerouteing, posturing the limb and stretching within physiological limits, it is clear that all attempts to bring the ends of the median nerve together would fail and a considerable gap would be left in the nerve. Such extensive destructive lesions in the upper arm and forearm do not lend themselves to surgical correction by autografting or nerve-crossing at the level of the injury.

If nerve-crossing is to have worthwhile prospects of a successful outcome then what is needed is the availability of a suitable sensory donor nerve and the cross-union to be performed at a level and in a manner that enhances the prospects of getting regenerating sensory 'axons' to, in particular, the thumb and index finger.

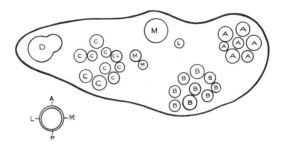

Fig. 43.11 Fascicular pattern and branch fibre composition of the median nerve at the wrist (not to scale). *M*. Thenar muscle fibres; *L*. lumbrical fibres; *A.B.C.* cutaneous fibres from the third, secound and first digital interspaces; *D*. Cutaneous fibres from the radial side of the thumb.

Nerve-crossing at the wrist using the dorsal cutaneous nerve of the hand (ulnar nerve) as the donor nerve

This method for restoring sensation to the median field in the hand involves a cross-union in which sensory axons of the fasciculi of the dorsal cutaneous branch of the ulnar nerve are used to reinnervate fasciculi in the median nerve and, in this way, the cutaneous area served by that nerve (Sunderland 1974). The method requires a knowledge of the internal anatomy of nerve trunks with particular reference to the fascicular structures and fascicular fibre composition of the median nerve at the wrist and the ulnar nerve in the lower forearm. (Fig. 43.11 & 43.12).

There are two essential pre-operative precautionary procedures.

1. The dorsal cutaneous nerve of the hand, which is to be the donor nerve, should be procaine blocked so that the extent and nature of the sensory deficit that will follow the sacrifice of this nerve can be experienced by the patient and assessed by the surgeon.
2. The median nerve should be procaine blocked at the wrist to discover if this alters sensation or motor function in the hand. This is necessary because aberrant median fibres may descend in the ulnar nerve as far as the forearm where they leave to join the median nerve by way of a communicating branch. The aberrant fibres then run in the

median nerve to the hand. These communicating branches are more common in the upper part of the forearm than in the lower forearm.

Since the cross-union involves transecting the median nerve at the wrist the presence of such aberrant motor fibres, though not necessarily excluding a modified cross-union, would nevertheless complicate it technically by making it obligatory at operation to identify the motor fasciculi in the median nerve by electrical stimulation. Having done this, the motor fasciculi should be isolated and preserved while the denervated sensory fasciculi making up the bulk of the nerve are prepared for the cross-union, the site of election for which is just above the wrist. The dorsal cutaneous nerve of the hand branch of the ulnar nerve is identified where it passes back beneath the tendon of the flexor carpi ulnaris muscle. It is cleanly divided at an appropriate level and mobilised over a suitable length by separation from the ulnar trunk to permit transposition of the proximal stump across to the median nerve.

The advantages of cross-union at the wrist

1. The repair is performed well away from the site of the injury so that the suture line is left in a clean field and occupies a favourable bed where post-operative scarring should be minimal.

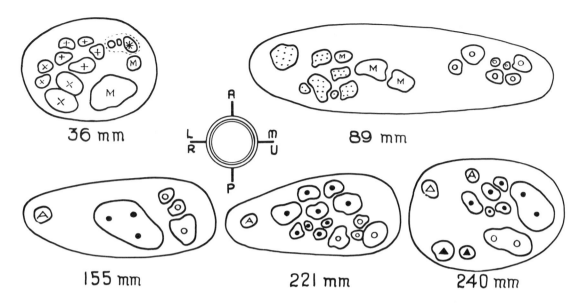

Fig. 43.12 Fascicular pattern and fascicular branch fibre composition of the ulnar nerve at the wrist and in the forearm. Branch fibre code. *M*, deep (muscular) division fibres; ⋆, cutaneous fibres from the hypothenar eminence; +, cutaneous fibres from the ulnar side of the little finger; X, cutaneous fibres from the fourth digital interspace; : : fine dots, combined terminal cutaneous fibres; ●●● heavy dots, combined terminal motor and cutaneous fibres; ○○, dorsal cutaneous fibres of the hand; △, flexor carpi ulnaris fibres; ▲, flexor digitorum profundus fibres; A, branch fibres to the ulnar artery.

2. Both the median nerve and the dorsal cutaneous of the hand from the ulnar nerve are cleanly severed, which gives the best possible conditions at the suture line.
3. The regenerating sensory processes have only one suture line to cross.
4. The regenerating sensory 'axons' have short distances to grow to reach cutaneous terminations.
5. The fibre localisation obtaining in the median nerve at the wrist permits a reasonable apposition to those sensory fasciculi whose constituent fibres serve the thumb and index finger.

Limitations and disadvantages of the method

1. The application of this method requires an intact uninjured ulnar nerve. All too often, unfortunately, the ulnar nerve suffers along with the median nerve in the extensive injuries of the type under consideration.
2. It involves the sacrifice of another cutaneous nerve which, though usually minimal in its

effects, does introduce another area of sensory deficit.
3. The emphasis is on sensory innervation in the hand and does not provide for the reinnervation of denervated muscles.

These disadvantages, however, are a small price to pay for restoring useful sensation to the thumb and index finger, useful in the sense that, though sensation remains imperfect, the affected parts are no longer insensitive but respond to a wide range and variety of stimuli, protective mechanisms are restored and the general condition of the reinnervated tissues improved. False reference remains a problem.

Nerve cross-union in the hand

Here the objective is to restore some sensation to the first three digital pads in irreparable injuries of the median nerve (Bedeschi et al 1984, Greene & Steichen 1985). In this procedure only selected terminal branches of the dorsal ulnar cutaneous and superficial radial nerves in the hand are used for reinnervating the appropriate terminal median branches. If the superficial radial fibres are used care is taken to avoid those branches innervating the dorsum of the thumb. Bedeschi et al reported surprisingly good results in their patients.

PART 5. DIRECT NEUROTISATION OF MUSCLE

Neurotisation is the direct implantation of the proximal stump of a transected nerve into a denervated muscle with the intention of reinnervating muscle fibres from that source. It is of limited value and should be regarded as a procedure of last resort. Fortunately, the occasions when it has claim for consideration will be few and far between.

The feasibility of reinnervating a muscle, in this way was investigated early in this century by Heineke (1914a,b) and Steindler (1915, 1916) but the results did not justify clinical acceptance and interest in the subject soon lapsed. In the 1970s and 80s neurotisation has been taken up again both experimentally (Sakurai & Campbell 1971, Brunelli et al 1976, Rubin & McCoy 1978, Brunelli 1982) and clinically (Brunelli & Monini 1985).

Just how effective the method is in reinnervating denervated muscle fibres to give a useful result remains a matter of conjecture. Denervated muscle fibres are certainly reinnervated, but the experimental evidence is essentially histological and the functional value of this reinnervation remains to be critically evaluated. To date, it appears to be without functional significance.

Brunelli and Monini have reported favourably on the clinical application of the method and in their paper list others with encouraging results. However, the documentation provided is incomplete and inadequate and the functional outcome of the procedure remains to be critically evaluated. There is also some doubt about the selection of cases, while the improvement attributed to the procedure could be accounted for in other ways such as reinnervation from the original source.

One situation where the method could, arguably, have some merit is in the treatment of some traction injuries of the upper brachial plexus in which long delayed spontaneous recovery of the biceps and brachialis muscles remains a possibility.

In such a situation, intercostal donors could be implanted directly into these muscles, thereby leaving the musculocutaneous nerve in continuity so that should delayed spontaneous recovery occur, regenerating axons will have an uninterrupted passage into these muscles. Theoretically, this would be preferable to suturing the intercostal donors into the musculocutaneous nerve because transecting the latter in order to complete the cross-union would forever exclude any spontaneously regenerating axons from ever reaching the muscle.

The method could also be used when the branch or branches have been avulsed from a muscle, though here the preferred procedure would be to reimplant the avulsed nerve back into the muscle either directly or indirectly by way of a nerve autograft. Another use is in the cross-over reinnervation of paralysed facial muscles.

PART 6. SOME CONCLUDING GENERALISATIONS

1. Grafting under magnification and using microsurgical techniques means a more carefully executed and therefore better repair, and a greatly improved result.
2. Reliability in the evaluation of end results is of critical importance if this is to be the basis for comparing the relative merits of different grafting procedures. Ignorance of anomalous innervations, sensory overlap and 'trick' movements, and the misinterpretation of neurological signs are all too often responsible for erroneously attributing improvement to the graft repair.
3. The co-existence of many variables influencing the quality of the recovery after grafting, and the nature of the inter-relationships existing between them, complicate the isolation of individual factors for separate evaluation.
4. Autografting remains the method of choice for bridging a gap in a nerve that cannot be safely closed by end-to-end union.
5. The advantages of homografting would be considerable could the method be shown to be a consistently reliable and worthwhile procedure.

6. Heterografting has no place in the repair of human nerves.

7. There are two basic types of nerve autografting — cable and full-thickness. Each has advantages and disadvantages. The choice of a donor autograft is limited to cutaneous nerves except under special circumstances. This means that autografts are more commonly of the cable variety.

8. Important factors determining the success of the graft are its blood supply and the restoration of fascicular continuity at the nerve-graft junctions.

9. The success or failure of the graft depends on it acquiring an adequate blood supply in the shortest possible time. To ensure this requires a careful microsurgical technique and a healthy well-vascularised bed. Ischaemic necrosis of the graft is related to the size of the constituent fasciculi rather than the thickness of the graft. Large fasciculi are more susceptible to central necrosis where there is delayed revascularisation of the graft.

10. Successful grafting demands more than the simple union of nerve and graft, the essential requirements being the restoration of fascicular continuity. This is necessary:
    a. because only those regenerating axons that enter fasciculi in the graft and in the distal stump reach the periphery;
    b. in order to take advantage of any branch fibre localisation that would favour regenerating axons ultimately entering functionally related endoneurial tubes in the distal stump because only these establish functionally useful connections at the periphery. This requires an appreciation of the internal anatomy of nerve trunks.

11. Suturing fascicular groups with the object of preventing the wasteful regeneration of axons into the interfascicular tissues has real merit. Combining and matching fasciculi in the expectation of restoring useful functional connections becomes guesswork when the repair is executed at levels where there is no fibre localisation.

12. With group fascicular cable grafting the union of *individual fasciculi* is rarely practicable. In most cases the procedure will involve joining matched *groups of fasciculi*.

13. Group fascicular cable grafting is a long and tedious procedure and should not be undertaken unless there are good prospects of significantly improving the patient's condition.

14. The choice between end-to-end union, autogenous grafting, some alternative method of conveying regenerating axons to the distal stump, reconstructive surgery or acceptance of the status quo may be difficult. The age of the patient, the length of the defect, the nature of the bed and the particular nerve affected are all significant factors.

15. As with nerve suture the results of grafting are better in the very young.

16. The prospects of obtaining useful recovery from nerve grafting decline as the length of the graft increases and the state of the nerve worsens.

17. Each case should be carefully assessed to determine its suitability for a graft repair. This requires an appreciation of what can and cannot be achieved by grafting under the prevailing conditions. It is pointless to expect more of a graft than it has to offer.

18. For some nerves, grafting long defects under unfavourable conditions is not worthwhile because the chances of obtaining any useful recovery are remote and alternative methods are available that offer better prospects of improving function. In these matters it is not a question of what can be done but of what should be done.

19. Some repair nerve gaps of more than 2 cm by grafting in order to avoid all tension across suture lines. Despite this view, slight tension at the suture line after end-to-end union has been shown to be acceptable.

20. Grafting has the great disadvantage of substituting two suture lines for one.

21. The interval between injury and grafting should be as short as possible, though grafting should not be performed as a primary procedure at the time of the injury,

except where excision of a segment of a nerve is necessary for reasons other than those due to trauma.

22. There appears to be no worthwhile advantage in predegenerating or reversing a graft.

23. Resecting and resuturing the distal suture line at the calculated time of arrival of regenerating axons in order to present them with a fresh suture line to negotiate is unnecessary, except on those occasions when there is clear evidence of obstruction at this site.

24. Neither the suture site nor the body of the graft should be routinely enclosed in protective sleeves.

25. The direct neurotisation of muscles has a limited clinical application.

26. Tubal techniques do not as yet have a role in the clinical repair of nerves, though they are a valuable experimental tool for studying environmental factors influencing and controlling axon regeneration.

27. Muscle tissue interpositional grafting is the most recent arrival on the nerve repair scene, but has a questionable future.

REFERENCES

Aguayo A J, Bray G M 1980 Experimental nerve grafts. In: Jewett D L, McCarroll H R (eds) Nerve repair and regeneration: its clinical and experimental basis. Mosby, St Louis, p 68

Alnot J Y 1988 The use of ulnar as a vascularized nerve graft in some peculiar conditions and particularly in total palsies of the brachial plexus with C7 C8 D1 avulsions. In: Brunelli G (ed) Textbook of microsurgery. Masson, Milano, p 637

Alnot J Y, Katz D, Henin D 1988 Frozen nerve allografts (experimental study in rats). In: Brunelli G (ed) Textbook of microsurgery. Masson, Milano, p 641

Alpar E K, Brooks D M 1978 Long term results of ulnar to median nerve pedicle grafts. The Hand 10: 61

Bain J R, Mackinnon S E, Hudson A R et al 1988 The peripheral nerve allograft. An assessment of regeneration across nerve allografts in rats immunosuppressed with cyclosporin A. Plastic and Reconstructive Surgery 82: 1052

Bedeschi P, Celli L, Balli A 1984 Transfer of sensory nerves in hand surgery. Journal of Hand Surgery 9B: 46

Berger A, Millesi H 1978 Nerve grafting. Clinical Orthopaedics 133: 49

Birch R, Dunkerton M, Bonney G, Jamieson A M 1988 Experience with the free vascularized ulnar nerve graft in repair of supraclavicular lesions of the brachial plexus. Clinical Orthopaedics and Related Research 237: 96

Boorman J G, Sykes P J 1987 Vascularized versus conventional nerve grafting: a case report. Journal of Hand Surgery 12B: 218

Bonney G, Birch R, Jamieson A M, Eames R A 1984 Experience with vascularized nerve grafts. Clinics in Plastic Surgery 11: 137

Breidenbach W, Terzis J K 1984 The anatomy of free vascularized nerve grafts. Clinics in Plastic Surgery 11: 65

Brunelli G, Brunelli M L, Antonucci A, Maraldi N 1976 Neurotizzazione in zona aneurale di miscoli denervati. Policlinico 83: 611

Brunelli G, 1982 Direct neurotization of severely damaged muscles. Journal of Hand Surgery 7A: 572

Brunelli G, Monini L 1985 Direct muscular neurotization. Journal of Hand Surgery 10A: 993

Buck-Gramcko D 1971 Wiederherstellung durchtrennter peripherer Nerven. Handchirurgie Praxis 15: 55

Campbell J B, Bassett C A L 1957 The surgical application of monomolecular filters (Millipore) to bridge gaps in peripheral nerves and to prevent neuroma formation. Surgical Forum 7: 570

Campbell J B, Bassett C A L, Girado J M et al 1956 Application of monomolecular filter tubes in bridging gaps in peripheral nerves and for prevention of neuroma formation: prelimary report. Journal of Neurosurgery 13: 635

Campbell J B, Bassett C A L, Husby J et al 1961 Microfilter sheaths in peripheral nerve surgery: a laboratory report and preliminary clinical study. Journal Trauma 1: 139

Chao Y C, Tsang Y C, Tsui C T 1962 Nerve regeneration through a gap. An experimental study. Chinese Medical Journal 81: 740

Chiu D T, Janecka I, Krizek T J et al 1982 Autogenous vein graft as a conduit for nerve regeneration. Surgery 91: 226

Comtet J-J 1988a Is there a future for nerve homograft? In: Brunelli G (ed) Textbook of microsurgery. Masson, Milano, p 629

Comtet J-J 1988b Vascularized nerve grafts. In: Tubiana R (ed) The Hand. Saunders, Philadelphia, Vol. 3, p 587

Dahlin L B, Danielsen N, Lundborg G, Ochi M 1988 Axonal growth in mesothelial chambers: effects of a proximal preconditioning lesion and/or predegeneration of the distal segment. Experimental Neurology 99: 655

Daly P J, Wood M B 1985 Endoneural and epineural blood flow evaluation with free vascularized and conventional nerve grafts in the canine. Journal of Reconstructive Microsurgery 2: 45

Danielsen N, Dahlin L B, Lee Y F, Lundborg G 1983 Axonal growth in mesothelial chambers. The role of the distal segment. Scandinavian Journal of Plastic and Reconstructive Surgery 17: 119

da Silva C, Madison R, Dikke S E et al 1985 An in vivo model to quantify motor and sensory regeneration using bioresorbable nerve guide tubes. Brain Research 342: 307

Dellon A L, Mackinnon S E 1988 An alternative to the classical nerve graft for the management of the short nerve gap. Plastic and Reconstructive Surgery 82: 849

Ducker T B, Hayes G J 1970 Peripheral nerve grafts. Experimental studies in the dog and chimpanzee to define homograft limitations. Journal of Neurosurgery 32: 236

Fawcett J W, Keynes R J 1986 Muscle basal lamina: a new graft material for peripheral nerve repair. Journal of Neurosurgery 65: 354

Glasby M A, Gschmeissner S E, Huang C L, De Souza B A 1986 Degenerated muscle grafts used for peripheral nerve repair in primates. Journal of Hand Surgery 11B: 347

Greene T L, Steichen J B 1985 Digital nerve grafting using the dorsal sensory branch of the ulnar nerve. Journal of Hand Surgery 10B: 37

Gulati A K 1988 Evaluation of acellular and cellular nerve grafts in repair of rat peripheral nerve. Journal of Neurosurgery 68: 117

Gulati A K 1989 Axon regeneration through blood vessel allografts after cyclosporine treatment. Journal of Neurosurgery 70: 115

Gu Yu-dong, Wu Min-ming, Xheng Yu-liu et al 1985 Vascularised free sural nerve grafting. Chinese Medical Journal 98: 875

Heineke H 1914a Die Einpflanzung des Nerven in den Muskel. Archiv für Klinische Chirurgie 105: 517

Heineke D 1914b Die directe Einpflanzung des Nerven in den Muskel. Zentralblat für Chirurgie 41: 465

Hirasawa Y, Tamai K, Katsumi Y, Sakaida 1984 Experimental study of nerve allografts: especially on the influence of histocompatibility in fresh nerve grafting. Transplantation Proceedings 16: 1694

Hunt D M 1983 A model for the study of free vascularised nerve grafts. Journal of Bone and Joint Surgery 65B: 659

Ide C 1984 Nerve regeneration through the basal lamina scaffold of the skeletal muscle. Neuroscience Research 1: 379

Jenq C B, Coggeshall R E 1985 Nerve regeneration through holey silicon tubes. Brain Research 361: 233

Ji-Ming Kong 1987 Preparation and application of an experimental model for guiding nerve regeneration with skeletal muscle. Chinese Journal of Clinical Anatomy 5: 17

Ji-Ming Kong, Shi-Zhen Zhong 1988 Long term observation of bridging nerve gap with skeletal muscle. Chinese Journal of Clinical Anatomy 6: 76

Ji-Ming Kong, Shi-Zhen Zhong, Bo Sun et al 1986 Experimental study of bridging the peripheral nerve gap with skeletal muscle. Microsurgery 7: 183

Keynes R J, Hopkins W G, Huang L H 1984 Regeneration of mouse peripheral nerves in degenerating skeletal muscle: guidance by residual muscle fibre basement membrane. Brain Research 295: 275

Koshima I, Harii K 1981 Experimental studies of vascularised nerve grafts in rats. Journal of Microsurgery 2: 225

Koshima I, Harii K 1985 Experimental study of vascularised nerve grafts. Multifactorial analyses of axon regeneration of nerves transplanted into an acute burn wound. Journal of Hand Surgery 10A: 64

Koshima I, Okabe K, Harii K 1981 Comparative study of free and vascularised nerve grafts transplanted into scar tissue in rats. Journal of Microsurgery 3: 126

le Beau J M, Longo F M, Ellisman M H 1983 Morphological assessment of myelination occurring in adult peripheral nerves regenerating through a silicone chamber. Neuroscience Abstracts 9: 49

le Beau J M, Schubert D, Powell H C, Ellisman M H 1986 Fluid conditioned by peripheral nerves regenerating in vivo stimulates Schwann cell migration and proliferation in vitro. Journal of Cell Biology 103: 2279

Levinthal R, Brown W J, Rand R W 1978a Fascicular nerve allograft evaluation. Part I: comparison with autografts by light microscopy. Journal of Neurosurgery 48: 423

Levinthal R, Brown W J, Rand R W 1978b Fascicular nerve allograft evaluation. Part II: comparison with whole nerve allograft by light microscopy. Journal of Neurosurgery 48: 428

Lundborg G, Hansson H A 1979 Regeneration of peripheral nerve through a preformed tissue space. Preliminary observations on the reorganisation of regenerating nerve fibres and perineurium. Brain Research 179: 573

Lundborg G, Hansson H A 1980 Nerve regeneration through preformed pseudosynovial tubes. A preliminary report on a new experimental model for studying the regeneration and reorganisation of peripheral nerve tissue. Journal of Hand Surgery 5: 35

Lundborg G, Hansson H A 1981a Nerve lesions with interruption of continuity. Studies on the growth pattern of regenerating axons in the gap between the proximal and distal nerve ends. In: Gorio A, Millesi H, Mingrino S (eds) Post-traumatic nerve regeneration. Raven Press, New York, p 229

Lundborg G, Dahlin L B, Danielsen N et al 1981b Reorganization and orientation of regenerating nerve fibres, perineurium and epineurium in preformed mesothelial tubes — an experimental study on the sciatic nerve of rats. Journal of Neuroscience Research 6: 265

Lundborg G, Longo F, Varon S 1982a Nerve regeneration model and neuronotrophic factors in vivo. Brain Research 232: 157

Lundborg G, Dahlin L B, Danielsen N et al 1982b Nerve regeneration across an extended gap: a neurobiological view of nerve repair and the possible involvement of neuronotrophic factors. Journal of Hand Surgery 7: 580

Lundborg G, Dahlin L B, Danielsen N et al 1982c Regeneration of nerve fibres in preformed mesothelial tubes — influence of distal nerve segment of a transected nerve on growth and direction. In: Lee A J C, Albrektsson T, Branemark P-I (eds) Clinical applications of biomaterials. Advances in Biomaterials, Vol. 4. Wiley, Chichester, p 323

Lundborg G, Gelberman R, Longo F et al 1982d In vivo regeneration of cut nerves encased in silicon chambers. Growth across a six-millimeter gap. Journal of Neuropathology and Experimental Neurology 41: 412

Lundborg G, Dahlin L B, Danielsen N et al 1982e Nerve regeneration in silicon model chambers: influence of gap length and of distal stump components. Experimental Neurology 76: 361

Lux P, Breidenbach W, Firrell J 1988 Determination of temporal changes in blood flow in vascularised and nonvascularised nerve grafts in the dog. Plastic and Reconstructive Surgery 82: 133

McCullough C J, Gagey O, Higginson B M et al 1984 Axon regeneration and vascularisation of nerve grafts. An experimental study. Journal of Hand Surgery 9B: 323

Mackinnon S E, Hudson A R, Falk R E et al 1982 Nerve allograft response: a quantitative immunological assessment. Neurosurgery 10: 61

Mackinnon S E, Hudson A R, Falk R E et al 1984 Peripheral nerve allograft: an immunological assessment of pretreatment methods. Neurosurgery 14: 167

Mackinnon S E, Hudson A R, Falk R E et al 1984 The peripheral nerve allograft: an assessment of regeneration across pretreated nerve allografts. Neurosurgery 15: 690

Mackinnon S E, Dellon A L, Hudson A R, Hunter D A

1985 Nerve regeneration through a pseudosynovial sheath in a primate model. Plastic and Reconstructive Surgery 75: 833

Mackinnon S E, Hudson A R, Falk R E, Hunter D A 1985 The nerve allograft response: an experimental model in the rat. Annals of Plastic Surgery 14: 334

Mackinnon S E, Hudson A R, Bain J R et al 1987 The peripheral nerve allograft: an assessment of regeneration in the immunosuppressed host. Plastic and Reconstructive Surgery 79: 436

Madison R, da Silva F, Dikkes P et al 1985 Increased rate of peripheral nerve regeneration using bioresorbable nerve guides and a laminin-containing gel. Experimental Neurology 88: 767

Millesi H 1968 Zum Problem der Uberbrückung von Defekten peripherer Nerven. Wiener Medizinische Wochenschrift 118: 182

Millesi H 1969 Wiederherstellung durchtrennter peripherer Nerven und Nerventransplantation. München Medizinische Wochenschrift 111: 2669

Millesi H 1973 Microsurgery of peripheral nerves. Hand 5: 157

Millesi H 1975 Treatment of nerve lesions by fascicular free nerve graft. In: Michon J, Moberg E (eds) Traumatic nerve lesions of the upper limb. Churchill Livingstone, London, p 91

Millesi H 1980a Interfascicular nerve repair and secondary repair with nerve grafts. In: Jewett D L, McCarroll H R (eds) Nerve regeneration and repair: its clinical and experimental basis. Mosby, St Louis, p 299

Millesi H 1980b Nerve grafts: indications, techniques and prognosis. In: Omer G E, Spinner M (eds) Management of peripheral nerve problems. Saunders, Philadelphia, p 410

Millesi H 1981a Different techniques of nerve grafting. In: Gorio A, Millesi H, Mingrino S (eds) Post-traumatic peripheral nerve regeneration: experimental basis and clinical implications. Raven Press, New York, p 325

Millesi H 1981b Interfascicular nerve grafting. Orthopedic Clinics of North America 12: 287

Millesi H 1981c Reappraisal of nerve repair. Surgical Clinics of North America 61: 321

Millesi H 1984 Nerve grafting. Clinics in Plastic Surgery 11: 105

Millesi H 1988 Technique of peripheral nerve repair. In: Tubiana R (ed) The hand. Saunders, Philadelphia, Vol. 3 p 557

Millesi H, Ganglberger J, Berger A 1967 Erfahrungen mit der Mikrochirurgie peripherer Nerven. Chirurgia Plastica et Reconstructiva 3: 47

Millesi H, Meissl G, Berger A 1972 The interfascicular nerve grafting of the median and ulnar nerves. Journal of Bone and Joint Surgery 54A: 77

Millesi H, Meissl G, Berger A 1976 Further experience with interfascicular grafting of the median, ulnar and radial nerves. Journal of Bone and Joint Surgery 58A: 209

Molander H, Olsson Y, Engkvist O et al 1982 Regeneration of peripheral nerve through a polyglactin tube. Muscle and Nerve 5: 54

Molander H, Engkvist O, Hagglund J et al 1983 Nerve repair using a polyglactin tube and nerve graft. An experimental study in the rabbit. Biomaterials 4: 276

Moneim M S 1982 Interfascicular nerve grafting. Clinical Orthopaedics and Related Research 163: 65

Müller H W, Shibib K, Friedrich H, Modrack M 1987a

Evoked muscle action potentials from regenerated rat tibial and peroneal nerves. Synthetic versus autologous interfascicular grafts. Experimental Neurology 95: 21

Müller H W, Williams L R, Varon S 1987b Nerve regeneration chamber: evaluation of exogenous agents applied by multiple injections. Brain Research 413: 320

Noback C R, Husby J, Girado J M et al 1958 Neuronal regeneration across long gaps in mammalian peripheral nerves: early morphological findings. Anatomical Record 131: 633

Nyilas E, Chiu T-H, Sidman R L et al 1983 Peripheral nerve repair with bioresorbable prosthesis. Transactions of the American Society for Artificial Internal Organs 24: 307

Osterman A L, Bednar J M, Bora F W et al 1986 Peripheral nerve grafts: the relationship of axonal growth cone and biomechanical properties. Journal of Hand Surgery 11A: 189

Parekh P K 1981 Homologous nerve transplantation and immunosuppression in rabbits. Research in Experimental Medicine (Berlin) 179: 121

Pho R W H, Lee Y S, Rujiwetpongstorn V, Pang M 1985 Histological studies of vascularised nerve graft and conventional nerve graft. Journal of Hand Surgery 10B: 45

Reid R L, Cutright D E, Garrison J S 1978 Biodegradable cuff, an adjunct to peripheral nerve repair. A study in dogs. The Hand 10: 259

Restrepo Y, Merle M, Michon J, Falligut B 1985 Free vascularised nerve grafts: An experimental study in the rabbit. Microsurgery 6: 78

Rose E H, Kowalski T A 1985 Restoration of sensibility to anaesthetic scarred digits with free vascularised nerve grafts from the dorsum of the foot. Journal of Hand Surgery 10A: 514

Rosen J M, Kaplan E N, Jewett D L 1980 Suture and sutureless methods of repairing experimental nerve injuries. In: Jewett D L, McCarroll H R (eds) Nerve repair and regeneration: its clinical and experimental basis. Mosby, St Louis, p 235

Rubin L R, McCoy W 1978 Neural neurotisation. Annals of Plastic Surgery 1: 562

Sakurai M, Campbell J B 1971 Reinnervation of the denervated muscle by direct nerve implantation in cats. Tohoku Journal of Experimental Medicine 105: 233

Samii M 1973 Interfaszikuläre autologe Nerventransplantation. Deutsch Arzteblatt 19: 1257

Samii M, Kahl R I 1972 Klinische Resultate der autologen Nerventransplantationen. Melsunger Medizinische Mitteilungen 46: 197

Samii M, Willebrand U 1970 Zur Indikation und Technik der interfaszikülaren autologen Nerventransplantation. Vortrag Jahrestag deutsche Gesellschaft für Neurochirurgie

Samii M, Wallenberg R 1972 Tierexperimentelle Untersuchungen über den Einfluss der Spannung auf den Regenerationserfolg nach Nervennaht. Acta Neurochirurgica 27: 87

Samii M, Wallenborn R, Scheinpflug W 1972 Experimentelle vergleichende Untersuchungen oder Nerventransplantation mit autologen u.lyophilisierten homologen Nerven. Symposium Kassel Wilhelmshöhe Feb 3–4

Scaravilli F 1984 The influence of distal environment on peripheral nerve regeneration across a gap. Journal of Neurocytology 13: 1027

Scaravilli F 1984 Regeneration of the perineurium across a

surgically induced gap in a nerve encased in a plastic tube. Journal of Anatomy 139: 411

Seckel B S, Chiu T H, Nyilas E, Sidman R L 1984 Nerve regeneration through synthetic biodegradable nerve guides: regulation by the target organ. Plastic and Reconstructive Surgery 74: 173

Seckel B R, Ryan S E, Simons J E et al 1986 Vascularised and nonvascularised nerve grafts: an experimental structural comparison. Plastic and Reconstructive Surgery 78: 211

Seddon H J 1963 Nerve grafting. Journal of Bone and Joint Surgery 45B: 447

Settergen C R, Wood M B 1984 A comparison of blood flow in free vascularised versus nonvascularised nerve grafts. Journal of Reconstructive Microsurgery 1: 95

Shibata M, Breidenbach W C, Tsai T M 1986 Comparison of functional results following vascularized and nonvascularized nerve grafting of the rabbit median nerve. Journal of Hand Surgery Proceedings 11A: 765

Singh R 1983 Histocompatibility matching and preserved nerve allografts in dogs. Doctoral Thesis, Erasmus University, Rotterdam

Singh R, Mechelse D, Stefanko S 1977a Role of tissue typing on preserved nerve allografts in dogs. Journal of Neurology, Neurosurgery and Psychiatry 40: 865

Singh R, Vriesendorp H M, Mechelse K, Stefanko S 1977b Nerve allografts and histocompatibility in dogs. Journal of Neurosurgery 47: 373

Stearns M P 1982 The effect of irradiation on nerve grafts. Clinical Otolaryngology 7: 161

Steindler A 1915 The method of direct neurotization of paralysed muscles. American Journal of Orthopaedic Surgery 13: 13

Steindler A 1916 Direct neurotisation of paralysed muscles. Further studies of the question of direct nerve implantation. American Journal of Orthopaedic Surgery 14: 707

Strange F G StC 1947 An operation for nerve pedicle grafting: preliminary communication. British Journal of Surgery 34: 423

Strange F C StC 1950 Case report on pedicled nerve-graft. British Journal of Surgery 37: 331

Stromberg B V, Vlaston C, Earle A C 1979 Effect of nerve graft polarity on nerve regeneration and function. Journal of Hand Surgery 4: 444

Sunderland S 1974 The restoration of median nerve function after destructive lesions which preclude end-to-end repair. Brain 97: 1

Sunderland S 1978 Nerves and nerve injuries, 2nd edn. Churchill Livingstone, Edinburgh

Swann J 1941 Discussion on injuries to the peripheral nerves. Proceedings of the Royal Society of Medicine 34: 521

Taylor G I 1978 Nerve grafting with simultaneous microvascular reconstruction. Clinical Orthopaedics and Related Research 133: 56

Taylor G I 1979 Vascularised nerve transfer in microsurgical composite tissue transplantation. In: Serafin D, Buncke H I (eds) Composite tissue transplantation. Mosby, St Louis, p 669

Taylor G I, Ham F J 1976 The free vascularized nerve graft. A further experimental and clinical application of microvascular techniques. Plastic and Reconstructive Surgery 57: 413

Townsend P, Taylor G I 1984 Vascularised nerve grafts using composite arterialised neurovenous systems. British Journal of Plastic Surgery 37: 1

Uzman B G, Villegas G M 1983 Mouse sciatic nerve regeneration through semipermeable tubes: a quantitative model. Journal of Neuroscience Research 9: 325

Varon S, Lundborg G 1983 In vivo models for peripheral nerve regeneration and the presence of neuronotrophic factors. In: Haber B, Perez-Polo J R, Hashim G A, Guffrida Stella A M (eds) Nervous system regeneration. Liss, New York, Vol. 19, p 221

Weiss P, Taylor A C 1944 Further experimental evidence against 'neurotropism' in nerve regeneration. Journal of Experimental Zoology 95: 233

Weiss P, Taylor A C 1946 Guides for nerve regeneration across gaps. Journal of Neurosurgery 3: 375

Williams L R 1987 Rat aorta isografts possess nerve regeneration-promoting properties in silicone Y-chambers. Experimental Neurology 97: 555

Williams L R, Varon S 1985 Modifications of fibrin matrix formation in situ enhances nerve regeneration in silicone chambers. Journal of Comparative Neurology 231: 209

Williams L R, Longo F, Powell H C et al 1983 Spatial-temporal progress of peripheral nerve regeneration within a silicon chamber. Parameters for a Bioassay. Journal of Comparative Neurology 218: 460

Williams L R, Powell H C, Lundborg G, Varon S 1984 Competence of nerve tissue as distal insert promoting nerve regeneration in a silicon chamber. Brain Research 293: 201

Wood M B 1988 Discussion on Lux et al's paper. Plastic and Reconstructive Surgery 82: 143

Wood M B, Lind R 1986 Comparison of the pattern of early revascularisation of conventional versus vascularised nerve grafts in the canine. Journal of Reconstructive Microsurgery 2: 229

Zalewski A A, Gulati A K 1982 Evaluation of histocompatibility as a factor in the repair of nerve with a frozen nerve allograft. Journal of Neurosurgery 56: 550

Zalewski A A, Gulati A K 1984a Failure of cyclosporin A to induce immunological unresponsiveness in nerve allografts. Experimental Neurology 83: 659

Zalewski A A, Gulati A K 1984b Survival of nerve allografts in sensitized rats treated with Cyclosporin A. Journal of Neurosurgery 60: 828

Zalewski A A, Silvers W K 1980 An evaluation of nerve repair with nerve allografts in normal and immunologically tolerant rats. Journal of Neurosurgery 52: 557

44. The course of recovery after nerve repair

In considering the course of motor and sensory recovery after nerve repair it is important not to confuse functional recovery with axon regeneration. The former involves complex processes at three levels.

1. The restoration of the axonal link between neurons and peripheral tissues.
2. Processes at the periphery involving the re-establishment of complex relationships between axon terminals and somatic tissues on which the further development and maturation of the new axons depend.
3. Central processes involving the restoration of complex patterns of activity on which the refinements of motor and sensory functions depend.

Recovery of motor function proceeds in six phases:

a. The regeneration of motor axons.
b. The reinnervation of muscle fibres which is revealed by alterations in the electrical activity of the muscle.
c. The maturation of motor nerve fibres. This only occurs when axons have established connections with functionally related end organs in the muscle.
d. The reappearance of contractions in response to voluntary effort and the return of voluntary movements.
e. The restoration of co-ordinated motor functions.
f. Complete recovery.

In the author's experience sweating of the digital pads was the slowest and last function to return.

Signs indicating the presence of regenerating sensory nerve fibres appear first in the nerve trunk and subsequently in the skin and deep tissues, the area of sensory loss being gradually but progressively reduced.

After nerve repair motor and sensory recovery proceed progressively through several stages, the ratings improving with the continuing arrival of more regenerating axons and the maturation of restored pathways. Since axons do not always commence to regenerate at the same time and grow at the same rate, the peripheral tissues are reinnervated in an irregular manner. This means that the various stages of recovery are not necessarily in step for different fibres, so that some overlap between the stages is to be expected.

STAGE 1 OF RECOVERY

This stage is taken up by the growth of axons down the nerve to reconstitute the pathway between the parent neuron and its terminal field in skin, muscle or other tissues. This process can be detected and followed by electrophysiological methods.

In the case of sensory 'axon' tips, their passage down the nerve can be followed by tracking the descent of the point at which Hoffmann–Tinel's Sign can be elicited. This sign is the tingling sensation referred to the cutaneous distribution of the nerve which is elicited by light percussion of the nerve trunk at the site of the regenerating axon tips. The sign is elicited by gently percussing the still denervated nerve trunk from below upwards until percussion first produces distal tingling. It is necessary when eliciting the sign to avoid simultaneously deforming nerve fibres at the site of damage. The sign is relevant only when it is clearly evident a short distance below the site of injury.

Though an advancing Hoffmann–Tinel sign indicates the progression of sensory 'axon' tips along the nerve trunk, it provides no clue as to whether or not they are in endoneurial tubes that will lead them to the skin, nor does it provide any evidence of the number of axons regenerating down the nerve. While, therefore, the sign is a useful indicator of regeneration it is not a reliable measure of *useful* regeneration, except in the case of pure sensory nerves.

Axon regeneration per se is completed when axons have reached and distributed their terminals in peripheral tissues. From this point onwards further improvement depends on the maturation of restored axonal pathways.

The first stage is completed within months or at most 2 years in the upper limb, or even 3 years in the lower limb, depending on the level of the injury or repair and favourable or unfavourable conditions at the suture line. Beyond this time there will be no significant addition of new axons to the system.

At this stage it is impossible to predict from the presence of regenerating axons what the outcome of this regeneration will be. This is because axon regeneration per se does not necessarily guarantee functional recovery. Of equal importance in the restoration of function is the final destination of those axons because, for axon regeneration to be functionally effective, each axon must reinnervate its old or at least a functionally related end organ. The important point is not to confuse axon regeneration with functional recovery. At this early stage there is no way of telling whether or not axons have established satisfactory terminal connections.

STAGE 2 OF RECOVERY

The second stage involves the re-establishment of those complex interrelationships between nerve terminals and the tissues innervated upon which the further development of restored axonal pathways depends. This only occurs when axon terminals re-establish connections with function-

ally related end organs. At this early stage all regenerating axons are non- or very finely myelinated.

The first signs of muscle reinnervation show up in records of the electrical activity of the muscle, reinnervated muscle fibres being detected before they are in sufficient numbers to produce a voluntary contraction.

During this stage muscles respond to stimulation of the nerve trunk but not to voluntary effort. Fibrillation potentials are being suppressed and reinnervation potentials can now be detected in muscles by electromyography and strength duration curve testing.

As increasing numbers of muscle fibres are reinnervated there is a further increase in the amplitude of the action potentials and their contour becomes smoother, the nerve conduction time is shortened and conduction velocity improves.

The completely denervated muscle is insensitive. The arrival of fine regenerating sensory terminals in muscles is revealed by tenderness when the muscle is firmly squeezed. Though this marks the presence of immature sensory fibres, these are usually accompanied by motor fibres, for voluntary contractions return soon after the appearance of muscle tenderness.

On arriving at the periphery regenerating sensory 'axons' track through the framework of the original nerve networks. Here, as immature non-myelinated and non-specific nerve fibre terminals, they first become exposed to superficial stimuli to which they are extremely sensitive. Their arrival is heralded by the reappearance of a crude form of sensation which presents certain distinctive characteristics. The previously insensitive area becomes acutely sensitive to pinprick and to extremes of temperature. Pinprick gives rise to an abnormal, extremely unpleasant, stinging sensation that radiates widely, defies localisation and lacks any qualitative features. The area is still insensitive to light touch; somewhat later, light stroking may elicit a diffuse tingling sensation.

STAGE 3 OF RECOVERY

This stage of recovery depends on the continuing maturation of regenerated axons. Axons slowly increase in calibre and degree of myelination. In man it is not known if the structural features of regenerated nerve fibres are ever fully restored after nerve repair; the evidence suggests that functional properties are not. The conduction velocity in restored pathways gradually improves but is never fully regained.

This stage sees the appearance of feeble palpable muscle contractions, and perhaps a flicker of movement, in response to voluntary effort.

The next stage in sensory recovery is the restoration of anatomical continuity with peripheral sensory endings. Some axons will be establishing functional connections with functionally related sensory endings, others will not. The new fibres, however, are still fine, inadequately myelinated and functionally immature. The findings of sensory testing are essentially the same as for the preceding stage but some subtle differences are beginning to make their appearance. A touch stimulus is recorded as a non-localised contact. While the response to pinprick and extremes of temperature is generally unpleasant, the response is less pronounced, hyperalgesia is not as consistent or uniform, and the application of the stimulus is sometimes recorded as a poorly localisable prick rather than as a diffuse widely radiating unpleasant sensation.

The extent to which radiation and false reference dominate the clinical picture at this stage largely depends on the nature of the nerve injury. It is marked and more lasting when considerable cross-shunting of axons occurs during regeneration and leads to errors in the restoration of spatial relationships between neurons and the periphery. It is less marked and of shorter duration when the axons have regenerated in an orderly way along the endoneurial tubes which they originally occupied and which return them to their original destination.

STAGE 4 OF RECOVERY

This phase of recovery is dependent on increasing numbers of 'axons' reaching muscles, joints and skin and their further development into mature nerve fibres.

Motor recovery is marked by a gradual increase in the range and power of individual movements. While individual muscles may be contracting quite strongly, their ability to participate in integrated movements, such as those on which manipulative skills depend, may be grossly defective owing to structural and physiological deficiencies in the restored pattern of innervation. Muscle wasting is gradually reduced.

The quality of sensation gradually improves as regenerating axon terminals re-establish functional relationships in increasing numbers with receptors and as restored neural pathways mature. This is reflected in the return of the proprioceptor sense and an appreciation of pinprick, light touch, warmth and cold. As the structural features of the regenerated fibres are gradually restored, the threshold to stimulation, the capacity to localise, and the remaining qualitative features associated with each of the sensory modalities all continue to improve.

STAGE 5 OF RECOVERY

This stage is dependent on the re-establishment of correct end-organ relationships and the completed maturation of fibres in sufficient numbers and combinations to improve the quality of the recovery. The latter is completed by the end of the 3rd year.

During this stage the range and power of individual movements are fully restored and individual muscles become integrated to permit the efficient performance of the more complex movements required to provide for a wide range of normal daily activities.

Finally, the recovery of sensory units in sufficient numbers and in appropriate combinations and patterns results in the restoration of those complex sensory mechanisms on which motor and sensory skills depend.

Sensory recovery during this phase is characterised by the reappearance and gradual improvement of the discriminative aspects of sensation such as the detection of marginal differences in joint movement, weight and pressure perception; the identification of degrees of sharpness; tactile, texture, and temperature discrimination and tactile localisation, all of which constitute the building blocks of the stereognostic sense and the return of refinements of sensory perception and acuity that are essential for object identification and the normal use of the hand in the efficient performance of daily tasks.

Because motor and sensory functions are interdependent it is important to remember that a residual motor disability may be due to a sensory defect rather than to muscle weakness. At the same time, objects must be handled as well as felt in order to give full scope to sensory discrimination and object identification.

After nerve repair the restored pattern of innervation is both incomplete and imperfect and beyond the capacity of central adjustments to correct. This is reflected in residual functional disabilities that, in the case of the hand, may limit its efficient use in the performance of normal daily tasks.

STAGE 6 OF RECOVERY

From this point onwards further improvement has nothing to do with nerve fibre regeneration. It now depends on the degree to which deranged central mechanisms, created by the nerve injury and by the incomplete and imperfect regeneration of axons, can be corrected by central adjustments.

It is a matter of common observation that, in everyday life, motor performance and sensory acuity can be improved by practice and experience. It should not, therefore, be surprising if, in well-motivated patients, a residual motor and sensory disability consequent on incomplete and imperfect axon regeneration can be reduced by intensive remedial training directed to increasing the patient's ability to use to greater advantage new and altered patterns of motor and sensory innervation. It is not due to a continuing regeneration of axons.

A possible explanation for the improvement brought about by remedial training could be the adaptive readjustment of flexible patterns of activity in the central nervous system that enable the patient to use incompletely reinnervated muscles more efficiently and to recognise and identify an altered profile of sensory signal patterns from the periphery and to relate the new sensations to a past experience.

These mechanisms differ in no significant respects from those operating when a normal individual is learning new skills where movements that are clumsily executed initially are, with time and practice, converted into well-regulated skilled movements. The only difference is that after nerve repair, central mechanisms have now to contend with a defective peripheral apparatus.

In this respect the very young are known to have a decided advantage over adults but there is no doubt that, with the passage of time, the motivated adult patient has a remarkable capacity for improving the quality of the recovery and for adjusting to a residual disability.

It is difficult to put a time limit on this last phase of recovery, depending as it does on a further set of factors such as the general attitude, intelligence, patience, perseverance and motivation of the patient. It is a slow process and certainly extends into the 5th year. In some patients it can extend well beyond this time.

CONCLUDING COMMENT

Though axon regeneration is an essential prerequisite for the functional recovery of reinnervated structures, such recovery requires far more than the restoration of axon pathways, depending as it does on the following additional events.

1. Further developments in regenerated nerve fibres resulting in an increase in calibre and degree of myelination. These changes depend on the destination of regenerating axons. If it is to their old, or functionally related end organs, development continues even if not to completion. If, on the other hand, the terminal relationship is with functionally unrelated endings then further development is arrested.

2. The quality of the recovery depends not only on the numbers of regenerating axons reinnervating muscles and skin, and the degree to which their structural features fall short of normal, but also on the restoration of those complex patterns of innervation involving motor and sensory fibres of diverse sizes and functions that constitute the neural basis of coordinated motor activity and the discriminative and stereognostic sense.

3. Providing structures and tissues survive denervation they have a remarkable capacity to recover and function efficiently on reinnervation after prolonged periods of denervation.

4. It is well established that recovery continues to improve steadily over many years and long after axon regeneration and the maturation of restored pathways have been completed. Contributing to this delayed improvement are:

a. the use hypertrophy of muscle fibres, that have been satisfactorily reinnervated and have fully recovered, to compensate for the loss of those muscle fibres that have failed to be reinnervated.

b. the continued efforts of the well-motivated patient to improve function by adhering to the principle that 'practice makes perfect'.

In the absence of factual information about the mechanisms involved one can only speculate that continued improvement of this nature is due to the existence of flexible central circuitry and mechanisms that can be readjusted and conditioned by repetitive effort to correct for persisting peripheral defects. In this way the motivated patient by consistent and persistent effort, improves motor performance and learns to correctly identify an altered profile of sensory signals from the periphery.

5. In the author's experience, the results in well-motivated patients are better at 5 years than at 3 years and even better at 10 years.

6. The end result evaluation of motor and sensory functions after nerve repair is discussed in Chapters 32, 33 and 45.

45. End result evaluation and its implications

Assessment of the end result is an essential element in the management of nerve injuries with implications relating to the determination of disability ratings, the monitoring of the effectiveness of surgical practices and procedures, the preservation of surgical standards, and to the evaluation of innovations introduced with a view to improving the often disappointing results of nerve repair.

An end result evaluation should include: (1) an evaluation of motor function (Chapter 32); (2) an evaluation of sensory function (Chapter 33); and (3) an evaluation of sympathetic function (Chapter 35). It should also take into consideration factors complicating the evaluation of motor and sensory function (Chapters 32 and 33).

ADDITIONAL FACTORS TO BE INCLUDED IN AN END RESULT EVALUATION

While attention is concentrated on the restoration of motor and sensory functions after nerve repair, it is important not to overlook the adverse effects that persistent pain and residual trophic changes can have on the final outcome.

Incomplete or failed sympathetic reinnervation

Sympathetic nerve fibre regeneration and reinnervation generally follow the same pattern as that recorded for somatic nerves. Sympathetic responses gradually improve, though secretion of sweat remains depressed in most patients.

Observations on patients with sympathectomised limbs indicate that the loss of sympathetic innervation does not adversely affect somatic motor or sensory function. However, troublesome trophic disturbances are more likely to develop and persist when sympathetic denervation is associated with a residual sensory defect. Furthermore, dry skin, consequent on the loss of sympathetic innervation, no longer offers the same resistance to the movement of objects over its surface and this adversely affects the performance of those manual daily tasks requiring a firm or strong grip.

Residual trophic changes

The trophic regulatory control that the nervous system exercises over the skin and subcutaneous tissues is served by sensory and sympathetic fibres which combine to control the complex nutritional requirements of these tissues.

Following denervation, the general appearance, colour and texture of the skin change, the terminal digital pads atrophy and the skin becomes dry and unduly susceptible to injury and ulceration from even minor trauma (Chapter 30). With reinnervation these trophic disturbances regress but in the absence of satisfactory reinnervation they persist and may severely restrict the usefulness of the part. The end result assessment should carry a reference to the adverse effects that any such trophic disturbances have on function.

Persistent pain and troublesome dysaesthesiae

Pain and discomfort often make an appearance during regeneration when a sensitive neuroma develops at the site of the repair, the previously insensitive cutaneous field becomes hyperalgesic and there are tenderness and aching in recovering muscles. These sensory disturbances normally regress with advancing recovery. However, the development of an exquisitely sensitive and painful neuroma at the suture line and/or the development and persistence of hyperalgesia and hyperpathia in the cutaneous field of the recovering nerve may severely restrict the usefulness of the hand or foot. Thus, the distressing hyperaesthesiae of the sole that often follows repair of the tibial nerve below the origin of the branches innervating the calf muscle may leave the patient worse off than before. The end result assessment should detail this information.

Causalgia is a special case. When it is present, spontaneous pain may be so severe and compelling that it incapacitates the patient regardless of the state of the motor and sensory function.

THE TIME FACTOR IN END RESULT EVALUATION

Recovery following nerve repair is a continuing process until an end point is reached beyond which no further improvement occurs. It is not possible to determine the end point in advance of the event because the time taken to reach it is influenced by many complex factors and so is subject to considerable individual variation.

Axon regeneration and the functional maturation of restored pathways are usually completed within 3 years after the repair. Further improvement then depends on the patient's ability to exploit the new but changed pattern of innervation prevailing after regeneration has ceased. This final phase of recovery, depending as it does on the general attitude, intelligence, patience, perseverance and motivation of the patient, is a slow process and continues steadily into the 5th year, and in some patients can extend well beyond this time. Therefore, although it is true that the effects of some 'methods on trial' may be apparent within a relatively short period of time, it may not be possible to assess others until many years after the repair. From this it is clear that many end result assessments have been, and continue to be, undertaken prematurely. With the foregoing proviso in mind, a 5-year end point may be regarded as a reasonable compromise for purposes of comparison. Alternatively, a condition that remains unchanged for 2 years is unlikely to show further improvement at a later date.

HOW MUCH OF THE RECOVERY IS DUE TO REINNERVATION FOLLOWING NERVE REPAIR AND HOW MUCH TO OTHER FACTORS

It is important to appreciate that the improvement following nerve repair is not due solely to axon regeneration and tissue reinnervation. Other factors are involved, the role and significance of which should be understood lest they confuse evaluation of the benefits conferred by the repair.

An all too common source of error in end result assessment studies is the failure to recognise the significance of anomalous motor and sensory innervations and the use of supplementary muscle actions to compensate for the continued paralysis or paresis of some muscles, for example, the capacity of the flexor pollicis longus to compensate for the loss of the adductor pollicis in ulnar nerve paralysis.

Non-neural factors in the form of loss of muscle substance, the division of tendons, the formation of restrictive scar tissue and adhesions, and joint and periarticular pathology should also be identified lest their contribution to a residual disability be attributed to a residual deficit in reinnervation.

Some of the improvement in motor performance following nerve repair could be due to the hypertrophy of reinnervated muscle fibres that compensate for those that are never reinnervated. The possible role of the sensory overlap from neighbouring intact cutaneous nerves, and the ingrowth of sensory terminals from the same source, in reducing the area of cutaneous sensory loss should also be constantly kept in mind.

That function can be further improved by remedial training after nerve regeneration has ceased has some interesting implications. It means, inter alia, that of two patients one may benefit still further from such training whereas the other will fail to do so despite the fact that reinnervation has progressed to the same degree in both. Expressed in another way it means that differences in the quality of the recovery do not necessarily reflect differences in reinnervation following regeneration.

Account should be taken of these factors when assigning a rating to a new method of repair on the basis of the quality of the recovery. In such studies some value, no matter how subjective, must be placed on one patient's capacity to benefit from remedial training as opposed to another's inability or unwillingness to do so.

THE EVALUATION OF INNOVATIVE PROCEDURES INTRODUCED TO IMPROVE THE RESULTS OF NERVE REPAIR

The results of nerve repair continue to be disturbingly uncertain and too often decidedly bad, the number of unsatisfactory recoveries increasing as more critical standards for testing and evaluating function are applied. This disappointing scenario explains the ceaseless search for new ways and means of removing the uncertainty from nerve repair and converting it into a more consistent and rewarding undertaking. In this search it is clear that any new method, procedure, technique or management policy directed to improving the results of such repairs should survive only if it can be conclusively shown that it, and it *alone*, is responsible for the improved results. In this respect accurate end result assessments of recovery provide the only acceptable yardstick by which to judge the effectiveness of any new method or procedure. In pursuing this theme, reference should be made to the difficulty of transferring experimental data to the clinical situation and to the limited role of animal experimentation in clinical problem solving (Chapter 3).

Turning to the clinical situation, experience reveals that assigning a value to a particular method or procedure on the basis of the end result is more difficult than it might at first appear. Another source of error is the common practice of concentrating exclusively on a particular feature of an injury or repair when investigating its influence on regeneration and the quality of the recovery and, in doing so, disregarding the influence of the many other co-existing variables that are known to combine in complex ways to influence the outcome after nerve repair (Chapter 39).

Concentration on one factor to the exclusion of others involves its abstraction from the total reality under investigation. Unless consideration is given to what is being left out of immediate account, the results of such studies are capable of grave misinterpretation. A worthwhile innovation may be inadvertently judged valueless and a worthless one incorrectly claimed to be of value.

This factor should be taken into consideration in any study or clinical trial undertaken to evaluate a new procedure. Disregarding it strikes at the credibility of the results.

END RESULT EVALUATION AND THE PRESERVATION OF SURGICAL STANDARDS

The outcome of any surgical procedure should always be subjected to a detailed and critical examination in order to determine in what respect the end result meets, exceeds or falls short of expectations. In the absence of this type of audit surgery degenerates into a thoughtless mechanical exercise devoid of any hope of improvement.

END RESULT EVALUATION AND THE COLLECTION OF CLINICAL DATA

In civilian practice it is unusual to find clinics specially created for the exclusive study and treatment of patients with peripheral nerve injuries. On the contrary, not only are such patients dispersed geographically but in any one area they are also treated in a variety of specialist surgical departments: orthopaedic, neurological, hand, plastic and so on. All this means that patients with nerve injuries are unlikely to accumulate in sufficient numbers in any one clinic or consulting room to satisfy the investigational instincts of a surgeon. Furthermore, where so many variables are interlocked in complex ways to influence the course of regeneration and the quality of the final recovery, it is difficult, when only a limited number of patients is available for study, to decide with certainty whether some selected variation in the repair is or is not responsible for an improved recovery.

One way of overcoming limitations imposed in this way would be to pool clinical data from several sources in order to create a series large enough to permit meaningful comparisons and correlations. An essential prerequisite for this sort of exercise, however, is the need for standardised, precise, accurate clinical documentation relating not only to the details of the injury and the repair but also to the quality of the final recovery.

CONCLUDING COMMENT

In the final analysis two questions are of critical importance: (1) Has the affected part protective sensation? (2) What is the patient's capacity to cope with a wide range of daily activities? Tests to evaluate this are limited only by the ingenuity of the clinician and the time at his disposal. How rapidly and efficiently can the patient pick up and handle dexterously a series of objects of varying sizes and shapes, both with and without visual assistance? How accurately can he recognise objects solely by feeling and handling them? Does the patient know whether or not he is holding an object when the act cannot be checked visually? Is he constantly dropping objects and injuring affected skin and joints? Does the hand become useless in the dark or when he is unable to see what he is attempting to do with it? Are movements clumsily performed because of a lack of sensory information and persisting muscle weakness and incoordination when carrying out such daily tasks as shaving, dressing and undressing, writing, sewing, cooking and handling cutlery,

tools and utensils? The list could easily be extended. Admittedly it is often difficult to put a value, other than one expressed in subjective terms, on these refinements of functional recovery, but unless end-result assessments include a reference to them, the evaluations will have limited value as a basis for comparing the relative merits of different procedures and techniques.

Finally, it is a matter of common observation in everyday life that motor performance and sensory acuity improve with training and practice. In evaluating the end-result it is, therefore, important not to overlook the fact that the residual motor and sensory disability consequent on incomplete and faulty axonal regeneration can be improved by increasing the patient's ability to use new and altered patterns of motor and sensory innervation to greater advantage. In this respect the very young are known to have a decided advantage. The younger teenager also enjoys some advantages in this respect and it is always well worth exploiting the regeneration that has occurred in the adult by intensive retraining.

In the author's experience, in well motivated patients the results at 5 years are better than at 3 and better at 10 years than at 5.

Generalising, it will be found that:

1. The very young patient does better than the old;
2. Early repairs do better than late repairs;
3. Low repairs do better than high repairs;
4. Pure nerves do better than mixed motor and sensory nerves;
5. End-to-end union repairs do better than nerve grafts;
6. Short grafts do better than long grafts.

46. Repair of the brachial plexus directed to restoring elbow flexion

From the recent literature on brachial plexus injury and repair, about which much more is being said and written than in the past, it is clear that there are few destructive lesions of the plexus that are now beyond the reach of the enterprising surgeon. The result has been a more active and adventurous approach to the surgical treatment of these lesions. In recent times the diagnosis, treatment and prognosis of brachial plexus injuries have been extensively discussed in numerous articles and reviews (Bonney, 1959, Seddon, 1963, Leffert & Seddon, 1965, Millesi, 1969, 1977, 1980, 1984, 1988a, b, Tsuyama et al., 1969, Kotani et al., 1971, 1972, Tsuyama & Hara, 1972, Tamura et al., 1974, Samii, 1975, Allieu, 1976, 1977, Alnot 1977, Alnot & Huten, 1977, Alnot et al., 1977a, b, Bonnel et al., 1979, Narakas, 1977a, c, 1978, 1980, 1981, 1982, 1984a, b, 1988a, b, Matsuda et al., 1978, Brunelli 1980, Tsuyama, 1980, Bonnel & Rabischong, 1981, Jesel et al., 1981, Sedel 1982, Kline & Judice, 1983, Solonen et al., 1984, Leffert, 1985, Kline et al., 1986, Allieu & Cenac, 1988, Birch et al., 1988, Kawai et al., 1988, Sedel, 1988 — and this list is far from complete). Today it is no longer a question of what can be done but of what should be done.

This chapter is included to illustrate some of the pitfalls that complicate the evaluation of the results after complex nerve cross-union repairs, supplemented where necessary by an intermediary nerve graft, of the brachial plexus undertaken to restore elbow flexion. It is devoted to an examination of two procedures employed to repair extensive rupture-avulsion injuries of the plexus with the intention of providing regenerating motor axons for, inter alia, the reinnervation of the paralysed biceps and brachialis muscles. Comment is, therefore, directed specifically and solely to the restoration of elbow flexion in these cases.

The first method involves the repair of the fifth and sixth cervical spinal nerves, or the upper trunk of the plexus, by some form of bridging graft. Even though the resulting reinnervation of the biceps and brachialis muscles is imperfect and incomplete, at least the regenerating axons that reinnervate these muscles reconnect them to their original motor centres.

The second procedure to provide regenerating motor axons for the reinnervation of the paralysed biceps and brachialis muscles involves cross-anastomosing a selection of the appropriate intercostal nerves to the lateral cord of the plexus or, preferably, to the musculocutaneous nerve. This is done either directly or, if this is not possible, by using an intermediary bridging graft to close the remaining gap.

Intercostal nerve cross-anastomosis to restore elbow flexion has a number of disadvantages which account for the limited success of the method.

1. Both the intercostal (donor) and musculocutaneous (recipient) are composed of motor and sensory nerve fibres in which the latter outnumber the former.
2. The nerve fibre composition of the donor and recipient nerves favours the erroneous cross-shunting of motor axons during regeneration and their failure to re-establish functionally useful connections with muscle.
3. The numbers of motor axons in the donor intercostal nerves fall short of those normally contained in the musculocutaneous nerve (Kotani et al, 1972, Bonnel et al, 1979).

While it is true that axon branching during regeneration would add to the number available for reinnervating the musculocutaneous, this would apply to both motor and sensory fibres. Nor should it be overlooked that such branching raises the question of overloading parent neurons and in this way reducing their regenerative capacity and functional efficiency.

4. Cross-anastomosis to the lateral cord means the entry of at least some regenerating motor axons into the lateral root of the median nerve. These play no part in the reinnervation of the biceps and brachialis muscles unless there is a feedback to these muscles by way of branches from the median nerve (see later). This explains why the cross-anastomosis is preferably to the musculocutaneous nerve itself. This may require the use of an intermediary graft which adds to the technical difficulties of the repair and necessitates two suture lines instead of one. This doubles the chances of axons going astray and becoming lost during regeneration. Even when the transfer is to the musculocutaneous nerve, some regenerating motor axons will be lost by entering the lateral cutaneous nerve of the forearm and the communications that the former frequently gives to the median nerve in the upper arm.

5. Regenerating motor axons that succeed in reinnervating the biceps and brachialis muscles now link them to foreign centres in the spinal cord. Under these circumstances the outlook is, from the functional point of view, distinctly less promising than that which can be expected when the repair is by way of a bridging graft between related nerve ends.

6. The recovery in the biceps and brachialis muscles takes the form of involuntary contractions that are synchronous with respiratory movements. Re-educational training may or may not be successful in converting these involuntary contractions into useful elbow flexion under voluntary control.

7. The all-in costs involved are considerable. In the final audit it could well be that, unless the prospects for upgrading the functional recovery and its value to the patient can be greatly improved, this method of repair could in the long term be discontinued.

Despite these comments it is obvious that, following *total* avulsion of *all* roots of the plexus, some form of nerve transfer would be required to provide a source of motor axons for the reinnervation of the biceps and brachialis muscles. As such, it offers the only chance of obtaining some elbow flexion after nerve root avulsion injuries that irreversibly destroy all motor pathways to those muscles.

Evaluating the effectiveness of extensive repairs for avulsion-rupture injuries of the upper roots and trunks of the plexus, which leave the remaining parts of the plexus in continuity but not necessarily undamaged, poses another problem. Here there is now the possibility that some or all of the postoperative recovery in elbow flexion could be due, not to the repair, but to delayed spontaneous recovery in unrecognised and unsuspected surviving nerve fibres. Such a possibility should be carefully considered and any contribution to the recovery originating in this way identified. Special care should also be taken to avoid misinterpreting neurological findings lest this, too, be responsible for erroneously attributing the recovery to the operation.

Any surgical procedure introduced with the object of restoring elbow flexion, lost as the result of a severe plexus injury, should be questioned unless it can be conclusively shown that it, and it alone, is responsible for the postoperative recovery. Possible sources of error to be avoided in reaching a correct judgement in this respect will now be examined.

TERMINOLOGY

Some of the terms used in discussion and reports on brachial plexus injuries are unsatisfactory in that they introduce an element of ambiguity that could be responsible for confusion and misunderstanding when analysing conflicting claims regarding management policy. The question of terminology is discussed in the section on Traction

Injuries of the Brachial Plexus (p. 151) and should be consulted.

ANATOMICAL CONSIDERATIONS

Standard textbooks and instructional manuals of anatomy provide standard accounts of structural arrangements without emphasising that these are but norms around which variations commonly occur. These variations often remain unrecognised, or their clinical significance unappreciated, until the introduction of a new surgical procedure directs attention to them. Such has been the case with the brachial plexus and the introduction of surgical methods of plexus repair planned and performed to restore elbow flexion. Points of particular interest in this context concern the form of the plexus, variations in the course taken by motor nerve fibres to reach their destination, and the segmental innervation of muscles. The following observations are based on the examination of more than 1000 dissections by the author during his 35 years' service as Professor of Anatomy, and subsequently as Professor of Experimental Neurology, in the University of Melbourne.

NERVE PATHWAYS

1. Anatomical dissection and histological fascicular studies do not distinguish between motor and sensory nerve fibres in the plexus. The inference is that those for a particular muscle are associated in their course through the plexus.

2. The manner in which the lower four cervical and first thoracic spinal nerves fuse to form trunks, the trunks divide to form divisions and the latter recombine to form cords is subject to considerable variation (Walsh 1877).

3. There is considerable variation as regards the length of the spinal nerve, trunk, divisions and cords of the plexus because they unite and divide at different levels in different individuals.

4. The effect of prefixation and postfixation of the plexus on its form and branch pattern is not fully understood. Prefixation is more common than postfixation.

5. The fasciculi of the spinal nerves, trunks, divisions and cords of the brachial plexus repeatedly divide and unite to form fascicular plexuses. This anatomical feature makes it impossible, by anatomical dissection, to follow the fibres of each spinal nerve outwards through the plexus. However, it is assumed, with some justification, that the fascicular plexuses, and the changing form of the brachial plexus itself, allow for the widespread redistribution, regrouping and re-arrangement of spinal nerve fibres within the plexus.

6. The features outlined above mean that the various trunks, divisions and cords of the plexus are subject to unpredictable variations with regard to their nerve root fibre composition.

7. The lateral cord may receive its contribution from the middle trunk (C7) low down in the axilla. In such a case this communication could escape damage in a high lesion of the upper plexus.

8. Communicating strands have been observed joining:

a. the seventh cervical spinal nerve-middle trunk of the plexus to: (i) the eighth cervical spinal nerve; (ii) the lower trunk of the plexus; (iii) the medial cord of the plexus (Fig. 46.1)

b. the lower trunk and lateral cord of the plexus.

Such communicating strands are a common feature of the brachial plexus.

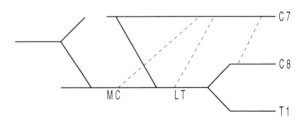

Fig. 46.1 Diagram of the lower plexus showing the aberrant communicating strands (Broken lines) by which nerve fibres from the seventh cervical nerve-middle trunk may pass to the lower trunk and medial cord of the plexus. *LT* = lower trunk; *MC* = medial cord.

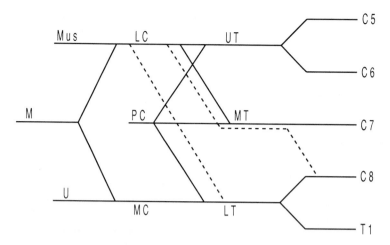

Fig. 46.2 Diagram of the brachial plexus showing the aberrant communicating strands (Broken lines) that have been found passing from (a) the eighth cervical nerve to the seventh cervical nerve-middle trunk, and (b) the lower trunk to the lateral cord of the plexus. Eighth cervical nerve fibres could reach the musculocutaneous nerve either directly by route (b) or indirectly by route (a), the fibres then travelling by way of the anterior division of the middle trunk to the lateral cord. *UT, MT* and *LT* = upper, middle and lower trunks respectively; *LC, PC* and *MC* = lateral, posterior and medial cords respectively; *MUS* = musculocutaneous nerve.

9. The lateral cord of the plexus may contain fibres from the eighth cervical nerve that reach it (Fig.46.2):

    i. over a communicating strand joining the eighth cervical nerve to the seventh cervical or middle trunk. The eighth cervical fibres could then enter the anterior division of this trunk in which they continue to the lateral cord;

    ii. by way of a direct communication from the lower trunk. This is consistent with Kerr's (1918) finding that this cord may receive fibres from nerves caudal to the seventh cervical and even as far caudally as the first thoracic.

10. The medial cord frequently receives fibres from the seventh cervical nerve, some of which innervate the pronator teres. Kerr (1918) reported that the medial cord may receive fibres from nerves cranial to the eighth cervical.

11. All roots of the plexus contribute nerve fibres to the posterior cord. Large numbers may come from the seventh and eighth cervical nerves but it is not known how many of these are involved in the innervation of the brachioradialis muscle.

12. The medial and lateral roots of the median nerve may be single or multiple.

13. The lateral root of the median nerve is composed of nerve fibres from the fifth, sixth and seventh cervical nerves but has been observed coming solely from the seventh. According to Herringham (1887) this root does not contain any fifth cervical nerve fibres.

14. The medial root of the median nerve may sometimes contain fibres from the seventh cervical in addition to its eighth cervical and first thoracic components.

15. The nerve fibres for the pronator teres muscle may come from the lateral root (usually) of the median nerve, the medial root or both. In the prefixed plexus the medial cord, now derived from the seventh and eighth cervical nerves, usually provides the nerve fibres for the pronator teres.

16. Kerr (1918), in his study, found that the musculocutaneous nerve contained fifth, sixth and seventh cervical fibres in 86 per cent of his specimens, eighth cervical fibres in 8.56 per cent and first thoracic fibres in 7.42 per cent.

17. Variations jointly involving the musculocutaneous and median nerves are common.

    i. Communications, of one sort or another,

between these two nerves are present in about 25 per cent of individuals;

ii. The musculocutaneous nerve may be thinner and the lateral root of the median much thicker than usual. In these cases the median nerve will be found to give:

a. a branch or branches lower in the arm to supply the biceps and brachialis muscles. The arrangement suggests that motor fibres to these muscles continue from the lateral cord to the median nerve via its lateral root. This may represent some or the entire motor supply to these muscles. In the latter event the musculocutaneous nerve, after sending a branch to the coracobrachialis, is composed solely of cutaneous fibres which continue as the lateral cutaneous nerve of the forearm;

b. a communication or communications back to the musculocutaneous nerve lower in the arm.

iii. As it courses between the biceps and brachialis muscles the musculocutaneous nerve may receive a communicating strand from the median nerve, which is composed of nerve fibres from its medial root. These fibres could be from the seventh cervical spinal nerve and conceivably the eighth.

18. The median nerve may send a branch or branches direct to the biceps and brachialis muscles. These branches could be composed of nerve fibres derived from the lateral cord of the plexus, from its medial cord, or from both.

Such arrangements as those just described mean that transection of the musculocutaneous nerve would be without effect on the biceps and brachialis muscles. Furthermore, any motor fibres reaching these flexor muscles by way of the medial root and trunk of the median nerve would not be disturbed during the preparation of the musculocutaneous nerve for a nerve cross-anastomosis repair.

19. The status of the branch which the radial nerve gives to the brachialis muscle is not clear, nor is the segmental origin of its fibres.

A study of these data on neural pathways reveals that the seventh and eighth cervical nerves could contribute to the innervation of the four elbow flexors (biceps, brachialis, brachioradialis and pronator teres). In the case of the biceps and brachialis muscles such motor fibres could, depending on the existence of the type of communicating strands previously referred to [(8) above] and certain variations in the form of the plexus, pass to these two elbow flexor muscles over the following pathways.

For seventh cervical spinal nerve fibres:

1. The middle trunk, its anterior division, the lateral cord and then to the muscles by way of: (a) the musculocutaneous nerve; (b) the lateral root of the median nerve, the median nerve and finally by those branches which the latter sometimes gives in the upper arm to the musculocutaneous nerve or direct to the muscles in question.

2. The communication to the lower trunk of the plexus, or to the latter by way of the communication to the eighth cervical nerve, the medial cord, the medial root of the median nerve, the median nerve and then by the branches of this nerve referred to in the previous section.

For eighth cervical spinal nerve fibres:

1. The lower trunk of the plexus, medial cord, medial root of the median and finally those branches which the median nerve sometimes gives in the upper arm to the musculocutaneous nerve or direct to the biceps and brachialis muscles.

2. The communicating strand which joins the eighth cervical nerve or lower trunk to the: (i) middle trunk and then by way of its anterior division to the lateral cord; (ii) the lateral cord.

Eighth cervical nerve fibres in the lateral cord may then proceed to the biceps and brachialis muscles by way of: (a) the musculocutaneous nerve; (b) the lateral root of the median nerve, the median nerve and finally by way of those branches from the median in the upper arm already referred to.

THE ELBOW FLEXORS AND THEIR INNERVATION

Flexion of the elbow is produced by the biceps, brachialis, pronator teres and brachioradialis muscles with the motor segmental innervation shown in Table 46.1.

The effect of prefixation and postfixation of the plexus on the segmental innervation of the elbow flexor muscles is not known. It could well be that, with prefixation, the seventh cervical nerve (now the fourth or second lowest root of the plexus) could be a major contributor to the innervation of the elbow flexors.

CLINICAL CONSIDERATIONS

While an injury that is sufficiently severe to avulse the fifth and sixth cervical nerve roots, or rupture the spinal nerves formed by them, might leave the neighbouring seventh cervical nerve in continuity, it is highly unlikely that its constituent fibres would escape without sustaining some damage. Such damage could be of first or second degree severity, from which the affected fibres would recover spontaneously after an interval which could be considerable depending on the time taken for the conduction block to be corrected or the affected muscles to be reinnervated.

Eighth cervical nerve fibres could also suffer in the same way following rupture — avulsion injuries of the fifth, sixth and seventh cervical nerves.

Important in these considerations is the fact that the preferred time for repairing the plexus in these

cases is well in advance of the time required by injured nerve fibres, which have survived in continuity, to regenerate spontaneously. Under these circumstances there is always the chance that the postoperative recovery could be erroneously attributed to the surgical repair when, in fact, it is the result of delayed spontaneous regeneration occurring in injured fibres.

It is for these reasons that the following procedure should be followed in order to provide the type of information that is required for determining whether the elbow flexion that returns postoperatively is, in fact, due to the surgical repair of the plexus or whether some other unrelated factor could be responsible.

1. In severe injuries involving the upper plexus it is important, both pre- and postoperatively, to ascertain, inter alia, the condition of all the elbow flexors. This can be done by simple clinical examination supplemented by electromyography.

2. When the plexus is explored, the exposure should be sufficient to enable any departures from the standard arrangement, as well as the nature and full extent of the damage, to be accurately defined and documented. This has been stressed by Narakas (1981), who also had in mind the identification of the two-level lesion.

3. Details of the grafting or intercostal nerve cross-anastomosis undertaken to restore, inter alia, the function of the biceps and brachialis muscles should be fully recorded.

4. Postoperatively, the ability of the patient to flex the forearm voluntarily against gravity should be critically examined in order to define the functional status of: (i) the pronator teres and brachioradialis muscles, and (ii) the biceps and brachialis muscles.

THE CONDITION OF THE PRONATOR TERES AND BRACHIORADIALIS MUSCLES

It is important at the outset to establish the status of these muscles lest their contribution to elbow flexion be overlooked. The nerve fibres to the pronator teres may have escaped injury in which case this muscle will continue to flex the forearm, contractions of the muscle being confirmed electrically or simply by palpation. If, on the other hand,

Table 46.1 Motor segmental innervation of muscles producing flexion of elbow

	Standard texts	Sunderland
Biceps	C 5, 6	C 5, 6, 7, (8)
Brachialis	C 5, 6	C 5, 6, 7, (8)
Pronator teres	C 6, 7	C 6, 7, 8
Brachioradialis	C 5, 6, (7)	C 5, 6, 7, (8)

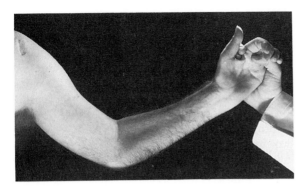

Fig. 46.3 Destructive lesion of the left musculocutaneous nerve with paralysis of the biceps and brachialis muscles. Powerful flexion of the forearm is performed by hypertrophied brachioradialis and pronator teres muscles.

the nerve fibres innervating this muscle have suffered first or second degree damage then the muscle will be temporarily paralysed (Fig. 46.3).

Second or greater degree damage is confirmed by electromyography approximately 3 weeks after the injury with the appearance of denervation fibrillation potentials.

Recovery in the paralysed muscle is delayed until either the conduction block is corrected or regenerating axons have reinnervated the muscle. In the event of the latter, reinnervation potentials and other electrophysiological evidence of advancing reinnervation and functional recovery would be present.

The same would apply to the brachioradialis.

If the pronator teres and/or brachioradialis are, in fact, responding to voluntary effort then this, rather than the repair, could account for the recovery of elbow flexion.

THE CONDITION OF THE BICEPS AND BRACHIALIS MUSCLES

Contractions in the biceps and/or brachialis muscles following the repair of destructive lesions of the upper plexus could be due to:

i. reinnervation by regenerating cervical axons using a bridging graft to reach their destination, and/or
ii. spontaneous recovery in damaged nerve fibres that have survived in continuity.

Nerve blocks to exclude or confirm the participation of these fibres would depend on a more detailed knowledge of aberrant pathways and innervation than is currently available.

The response to voluntary effort and the electromyographic evidence of reinnervation are the same in both cases so that there is no certain way of distinguishing between them. The onset of motor recovery well in advance of that to be expected from the repair would suggest spontaneous recovery in surviving pathways. However, it is not unknown for such spontaneous recovery to be delayed to a point where it would be indistinguishable from that due to the repair of interrupted pathways. It is then that extreme caution should be exercised in interpreting the neurological findings and any lingering doubt resolved before assigning a credit rating to the surgical repair.

iii. On the other hand, recovery which is based on muscle reinnervation by axons provided by an intercostal nerve cross-anastomosis shows a pattern with characteristic features which distinguish it from that described above. Now the biceps and brachialis muscles are innervated by foreign axons that are functionally unrelated to them. As a consequence, the recovery takes the form of involuntary contractions and electromyographic responses in these muscles that are synchronous with respiratory movements. Efforts directed to flexing the forearm are without effect unless the patient concentrates on respiratory movements of inspiration and expiration. Whether or not this can be corrected by re-educational training, and elbow flexion ultimately brought under direct voluntary control, is by no means clear.

If these distinguishing features of recovery are replaced by those characteristic of reinnervation by the cervical nerves then the cross-anastomosis should not be given credit for the postoperative improvement.

Obviously, the most suitable cases for testing the value of intercostal nerve cross-anastomosis are those of *total* avulsion of *all* roots of the brachial plexus. Under these extreme conditions any recovery in the biceps and brachialis muscles must then be due to the surgical repair.

Finally, any result short of elbow flexion against gravity should be regarded as a failure.

Nerve cross-anastomosis using part of, or the entire, accessory nerve to provide the regenerating axons for reinnervating the biceps and brachialis muscles has not been considered because of the contention that trapezius function should be preserved in view of its role in compensating for the loss of the normal abductors of the shoulder (deltoid and spinati). In the event, nerve cross-anastomosis, using the accessory nerve as the donor of regenerating axons, would be subject to the same reservations as those outlined for the intercostal nerves.

CONCLUSION

In this age of surgical innovation and advance, and at a time when adventurous approaches to the repair of extensive destructive lesions of the brachial plexus are increasing, it comes as no surprise that much of the reporting of new surgical methods has for its purpose the justification of operative procedures rather than the objective assessment of their value to the patient. In order to avoid this criticism and the uncritical acceptance of a method of repair that may be quite valueless, it is essential to subject every case to a searching review of the end result with a view to ensuring that the method is, in fact, responsible for the improvement claimed for it, that the result is worthwhile, that clinical findings are not being misinterpreted, and that other valid explanations for the improvement, quite unrelated to the repair, have not been overlooked.

The object of this chapter has been to direct attention to, and stress the clinical importance of, certain variations in the composition and structural features of the brachial plexus that provide several alternative routes for motor nerve fibres and regenerating axons to reach the elbow flexor muscles. The possibility that such aberrant pathways can exist should be taken into consideration when assessing the effectiveness and value of controversial methods of plexus repair for the restoration of elbow flexion.

Regarding those cases in which surgery ends in failure, these should also be carefully investigated before mistakenly accepting the method of repair as being at fault. The study of failures is often as revealing as the study of successes.

Finally, it is axiomatic that, in this field of surgery, it is no longer a question of what can be done but of establishing what should be done.

REFERENCES

Allieu Y 1976 Le traitement chirurgical dans les paralysies pour elongation du plexus brachial: Conceptions actuelles. Actualites en reeducation fonctionnelle et readaption. Masson, Paris, p 17

Allieu Y 1977 Exploration et traitement direct des lesions nerveuses dans les paralysies traumatiques par elongation du plexus brachial chez l'adulte. Revue de Chirurgie Orthopedique 63: 107

Allieu Y, Cenac P 1988 Neurotization via the spinal accessory nerve in complete paralysis due to multiple avulsion injuries of the brachial plexus. Clinical Orthopaedics and Related Research 237: 67

Alnot J Y 1977 Technique chirugicale dans les paralysies du plexus brachial. Revue de Chirurgie Orthopedique 63: 75

Alnot J Y 1988 Traumatic brachial plexus palsy in adults. In: Tubiana R (ed) The hand. Saunders, Philadelphia, p 607

Alnot J Y, Huten B 1977 La systemisation du plexus brachial. Revue de Chirurgie Orthopedique 63: 27

Alnot J Y, Allieu Y, Bonnel F et al 1977 a Symposium sur la paralysie traumatique du plexus brachial chez l'adulte. Revue de Chirurgie Orthopedique 63: 17

Alnot J Y, Augereau B, Frot B 1977b Traitement direct des lesions nerveuses dans les paralysies traumatiques par elongation du plexus brachial chez l'adulte. Chirurgie 103: 935

Birch R, Dunkerton M, Bonney G, Jamieson A M 1988 Experience with the free vascularized ulnar nerve graft in repair of supraclavicular lesions of the brachial plexus. Clinical Orthopaedics and Related Research 237: 96

Bonnel F, Rabischong P 1981 Anatomy and systematization of the brachial plexus in the adult. Anatomica Clinica 2: 289

Bonnel F, Allieu Y, Sugata Y, Rabischong P 1979 Anatomico-surgical bases of neurotization for root avulsion of the brachial plexus. Anatomica Clinica 1: 291

Bonney G 1959 Prognosis in traction lesions of the brachial plexus. Journal of Bone and Joint Surgery 41B: 4

Brunelli G 1980 Neurotization of avulsed roots of the brachial plexus by means of anterior nerves of the cervical plexus (preliminary report). International Journal of Microsurgery 2: 55

Herringham W P 1886 The minute anatomy of the brachial plexus. Proceedings of the Royal Society of London 41: 423

Jesel M, Merle M, Petry D et al 1981 Paralysies proximales du plexus brachial d'orgine traumatique. Resultats fonctionnels apres reparation par greffes fasciculaires dans les ruptures des racines C5, C6 et du tronc primaire superieur ou apres neurotisation du nerve musculocutane par le spinal. Personal communication

Kawai H, Kawabata H, Masada K et al 1988 Nerve repairs for traumatic brachial plexus palsy with root avulsion. Clinical Orthopaedics and Related Research 237: 75

Kerr A T 1918 The brachial plexus of nerves in man, the variations in its formation and branches. American Journal of Anatomy 23: 285

Kline D G, Judice D J 1983 Operative management of selected brachial plexus lesions. Journal Neurosurgery 58: 631

Kline D G, Hackett E R, Happel M H 1986 Surgery for lesions of the brachial plexus. Neurobiological Review 43: 170

Kotani P T, Matsuda H, Suzuki T 1972 Trial surgical procedures of nerve transfers to avulsion injuries of plexus brachialis. Proceedings of the 12th Congress of the International Society of Orthopaedic Surgery and Traumatology. Tel Aviv, p 348

Kotani T, Toyoshima H, Matsuda H et al 1971 Postoperative results of nerve transposition in brachial plexus injury. Orthopaedic Surgery (Tokyo) 22: 963

Leffert R D 1985 Brachial plexus injuries. Churchill Livingstone, Edinburgh

Leffert R D, Seddon H J 1965 Infraclavicular brachial plexus injuries. Journal of Bone and Joint Surgery 47B: 9

Matsuda H, Hirose T, Nishiue et al 1978 A new diagnostic method and operative treatment for brachial plexus palsy with root avulsion. Proceedings of the Twenty-First Annual Meeting. Japanese Society for Surgery of the Hand, p 43

Millesi H 1969 Verletzungen des Plexus brachialias. München Medizinische Wochenschrift 3: 26

Millesi H 1977 Surgical management of brachial plexus injuries. Journal of Hand Surgery 2: 367

Millesi H 1980 Trauma involving the brachial plexus. In: Omer G E, Spinner M (eds) Management of peripheral nerve problems. Saunders, Philadelphia, p 548

Millesi H 1984 Brachial plexus injuries: management and results. Clinics in Plastic Surgery 11: 115

Millesi H 1988a Brachial plexus injuries: Nerve grafting. Clinical Orthopaedics and Related Research 237: 36

Millesi H 1988b Brachial plexus lesions: classification and operative technique. In: Tubiana R (ed) The hand. Saunders, Philadelphia, Vol 3, p 645

Narakas A 1977a Paradoxes en chirurgie nerveuse peripherique au niveau du plexus brachial. Medicine et Hygiene 35: 833

Narakas A 1977b The surgical management of brachial plexus injuries. In: Daniel R K, Terzis J K (eds) Reconstructive Microsurgery. Little Brown, Boston, p 443

Narakas A 1977 Indications et resultats du traitement chirurgical direct dans les lesions par elongation du plexus brachial de l'adulte. Revue de Chirurgie Orthopedique 63: 88

Narakas A 1978 Surgical treatment of traction injuries of the brachial plexus. Clinical Orthopaedics 133: 71

Narakas A 1980 The surgical treatment of traumatic brachial plexus lesions. International Surgery 65: 521

Narakas A 1981 Brachial plexus surgery. Orthopaedic Clinics of North America 12: 303

Narakas A 1982 Les neurotisations ou transferts nerveux dans les lesions du plexus brachial. Annales de Chirurgie de la Main 1: 101

Narakas A O 1984a Operative treatment for radiation-induced and metastatic brachial plexopathy in 45 cases, 15 having an omentoplasty. In: Bulletin of the Hospital for Joint Diseases Orthopaedic Institute 44: 354

Narakas A 1984b. Traumatic brachial plexus lesions. In: Dyck P J, Thomas P J, Lambert E H, Bunge M B (eds) Peripheral neuropathy. Saunders, Philadelphia, p 1394

Narakas A O 1988a Neurotization or nerve transfer in traumatic, brachial plexus lesions. In: Tubiana R (ed) The hand. Saunders, Philadelphia, Vol 3, p 656

Narakas A O, Hentz V R 1988b Neurotization in brachial plexus injuries: indication and results. Clinical Orthopaedics and Related Research 237: 43

Samii M 1975 Modern aspects of peripheral and cranial nerve surgery. In: Krayenbühl H (ed) Advances and technical standard in neurosurgery. Springer, New York, Vol. 2; p 53

Seddon H J 1963 Nerve grafting. Journal of Bone and Joint Surgery 45B: 447

Sedel L 1982 The results of surgical repair of brachial plexus injuries. Journal of Bone and Joint Surgery 64B: 54

Sedel L 1988 Repair of severe traction lesions of the brachial plexus. Clinical Orthopaedics and Related Research. 237: 62

Solonen K A, Vastamäki M, Ström B 1984 Surgery of the brachial plexus. Acta Orthopaedica Scandinavica 55: 436

Tamura K, Inoue N, Matsumoto S et al 1974 Intercostal nerve transfer to restore the finger sensation and its anatomical basis in the treatment of irreversible plexus injuries. Proceedings of the Seventeenth Annual Meeting, Japanese Society for Surgery of the Hand, Tokyo, p 20

Tsuyama N 1980 Further studies on nerve crossing in irreparably damaged peripheral nerve. 1st Congress of the International Federation of Societies for Surgery of the Hand, Rotterdam

Tsuyama N, Hara T 1972 Intercostal nerve transfer in the treatment of brachial plexus injury of root avulsion type. Proceedings of the 12th Congress of the International Society of Orthopaedic Surgery and Traumatology. Tel Aviv, pp 351 and 504

Tsuyama N, Hara T, Maehiro S et al 1969 Intercostal nerve transfer for traumatic brachial nerve palsy. Orthopaedic Surgery (Japan) 20: 1527

Walsh J F 1877 The anatomy of the brachial plexus. American Journal of Medical Sciences 74: 387

47. The future

Who shoots at the midday sunne, though he be sure
he shall never hit the mark, yet as sure he is he shall
shoot higher than who aymes but at a bush.

Sir Philip Sydney

World War II provided an impetus to peripheral nerve research that greatly increased our knowledge of the neurobiological background of nerve injury and repair from which emerged many remarkable advances in the management and surgical treatment of these injuries. As a consequence, the results of nerve repair today are vastly superior to those obtainable prior to 1940.

It is essential that the momentum created in this way should be maintained because, despite all this new knowledge, the introduction of improved techniques and the best efforts of skilled and experienced surgeons, the results of nerve repair at times still fall short of expectations even to the point of being surprisingly disappointing or even decidedly bad. Again, following digital nerve repair under the most favourable conditions of a clean transection injury and primary end-to-end union, recovery is never complete in every respect, sensation being different even when it is not diminished. Furthermore, this is the case even where a nerve is composed solely of cutaneous sensory and sympathetic nerve fibres and at a peripheral level where it might reasonably be expected that the intraneural rearrangement and sorting out of fibres taking place along the limb would have been completed.

This prompts the question of whether complete recovery after nerve repair can ever be expected except, perhaps, in the very young where the capacity of the nervous system to compensate for the permanent loss of some axons appears to be unlimited.

Whether or not it will ever be possible to restore axonal continuity, axon by axon to its correct partner, is for the future to answer. At this time it is not even possible to restore fascicular continuity, fasciculus by fasciculus, because their numbers and arrangement at the opposing nerve ends will not correspond except after a clean transection injury. From this and other related observations, it would appear that for the time being, we must rest content in the belief that the restoration of all original connections is currently beyond the reach of human endeavour. Despite this pessimistic scenario, the curiosity of man, his inventiveness and the search for perfection will not allow the matter to rest there. At the same time it should be recognised that there will be those occasions when the nature, level and severity of the nerve injury, and the particular nerve involved, impose conditions that inevitably predicate a poor result.

This directs attention to the need to have a clear understanding of the distinction that should be drawn between complete recovery and an acceptable recovery, given the conditions imposed by the injury and presented as a fait accompli to the clinician. The challenge, then, is to devise measures that can offset the adverse effects of harmful factors introduced in this way.

The study of axon regeneration as a biological phenomenon will remain the star attraction for the neuroscientist. Others, however, concerned more specifically with the restoration of function will direct their efforts to devising ways to maximise the restoration of functionally useful pathways and to minimise the loss of axons that occurs during regeneration. The challenge is to ensure the best achievable result under the prevailing conditions.

Personal experience and the critical overview of nerve injuries and their repair undertaken in the preparation of this book have revealed several obstacles to further progress. No doubt there are others as yet unformulated. However, before proceeding to identify these obstacles, some over-riding generalisations should be noted.

GENERALISATIONS

1. There is no difficulty in getting axons to regenerate. The problem is preventing them from doing so, as those people involved in the treatment of painful neuromas will testify. The core of the problem is not promoting axon regeneration but in getting them back to where they belong.

2. When the influence of a particular factor is under investigation it is well to remember that it may have been abstracted from the totality of a situation in which a plurality of variables is combined and interlocked in complex ways to influence the outcome of nerve repair. The isolation of any particular factor for special study and evaluation then becomes an exceedingly difficult and risky exercise. Unless consideration is given to what has been left out of immediate account, the results can be very misleading. The omission of this precaution is a conspicuous feature of many experimental programmes and reports.

3. A continuing problem in improving the results of nerve repair on a broader front is the failure to appreciate and apply information that is already available. The future should see an expansion of training and continuing educational programmes specifically designed and directed to reducing the gap between what is known and what is practised. Today this concept has its most constructive fulfilment in the structured training programmes and educational courses organised and conducted in North America by such bodies as the American Society for Surgery of the Hand and the American Academy of Orthopaedic Surgeons.

4. Despite the restrictions inherent in the study of nerve injury in man, it is in the clinic and hospital wards where problems originate and where the answers should be sought. Despite the difficulties of a terrain where nature and not man dictates the terms of the experiment, patients with nerve injuries continue to offer a veritable treasure house for the investigator. However, the unique opportunities provided in this way are all too often neglected in favour of the search for an experimental model from which it is confidently hoped that important clues and answers will inevitably flow.

Admittedly, animal experimentation has a continuing and important role to play in the search for new knowledge. However, the limitations of this approach should be recognised (Chapter 3). Animal experiment rarely provides definitive answers to clinical problems though it may well provide important clues to their solution.

5. The experimentalist, seeking to satisfy only his biological curiosity, is all too often unaware of the pressing practical demands of the clinical situation. On the other hand, the clinician, preoccupied with the needs and realities of clinical practice, and burdened with patient care responsibilities, will advance at a much slower pace and often in a different direction. Faced with the risk of a widening gap between clinical and experimental studies, these two groups of investigators should be brought into a productive and harmonious coalition where meaningful dialogue can be encouraged and maintained between them so that each is kept aware of the interests and needs of the other, especially with reference to the contributions that the basic scientist can make to the solution of clinical problems. The future should see a continuing and expanding dialogue between the two groups.

6. Today much of the reporting of surgical cases appears to have for its purpose the justification of operative procedures rather than the objective assessment of their value. In this technological age there is always a risk of nerve repair becoming increasingly concerned with technical details to the point where technique triumphs over reason.

SOME UNRESOLVED PROBLEMS

1. The retrograde neuronal reaction to nerve injury

This reaction, as expressed in terms of cell death or a permanent residual defect, is a significant factor adversely affecting axon regeneration and recovery. It is known that the severity of this reaction is proportional to the nature, severity and level of the injury to the nerve. However, we are, as yet, no closer to an understanding of the nature and pathogenesis of this reaction though increasing knowledge of axon transport systems may lead us to some of the answers.

What we need to know is whether or not the retrograde reaction to the original injury is increased by further interference and trauma to the nerve during the repair. If so, what steps should be taken to minimise this effect and would there be any advantage in blocking the nerve preoperatively above the site of the repair?

2. Axon regeneration

a. What is meant by the vague statement 'improving axonal regeneration' which often appears in reports? Does it mean hastening the onset of regeneration, accelerating the advance of regenerating axons, increasing the numbers of regenerating axons or assisting them to find and enter functionally related endoneurial tubes? Reporting needs to be more specific on this point.

b. The advantage to be gained by being able to accelerate axon regeneration would be to reduce the time for which peripheral tissues are left denervated, particularly after high repairs. This would hasten the onset of recovery. To date, the agents and measures tested have either been failures or have given inconclusive results (Chapter 15). Despite this, the concept is sound and the search should be continued. However, even if an effective accelerating agent is found, it will not contribute to the overriding problem of aiding regenerating axons to grow back to where they belong.

c. What are the relative roles of axon transport systems and the local blood supply in providing the nutritional requirements of regenerating axons?

d. Regarding the axon branching that occurs during regeneration, more information is required on such features as:

i. The level at which it commences.
ii. Does it occur following second degree injuries or is it confined to nerve transection injuries?
iii. Sprouting certainly occurs where the axon is obstructed in its passage through the tissue between the nerve ends. Is this branching repeated at more distal levels? If so, what is the ultimate fate of the multiple daughter axons that now occupy the same endoneurial tube?
iv. When an endoneurial tube becomes occupied by several axon sprouts, what is the outcome when all are from the same regenerating axon and when the sprouts are from different axons?

e. What is the effect on a neuron when the peripheral field which it innervates is greatly increased as a result of axon sprouting?
f. Does axon sprouting impair or aid recovery?

3. Neurotropism

There are no known neurotropic influences acting to direct each regenerating axon back to its original pathway in the distal nerve stump, thereby ensuring the restoration of a pattern of innervation that would be identical with the original (Ch. 16).

All this means that, when repairing a nerve, the surgeon is forced to rely solely on his own resources and initiative in devising methods to minimise the loss of axons from fruitless regeneration. Here there is scope for further improvement.

4. The use of in vivo nerve guide chamber models for the study of axon regeneration

These devices, composed of silicone or structured mesothelial tissue tubes, are designed to provide a conduit for the passage of regenerating axons across the gap between the nerve ends. They have proved a valuable tool for continuing research into those elements that contribute to a complex biological process — in particular axons, Schwann cells, fibroblasts and blood vessels. The model allows the contents of the chamber, and therefore the microenvironment in which axons regenerate, to be modified at will and in a manner calculated to reveal factors and mechanisms influencing nerve regeneration, the ultimate objective being to improve the results of nerve repair. The model also facilitates the continuing search for effective growth promoting agents.

Whether such nerve guide tubes will ever prove suitable for clinical use is conjectural. In the case of the complex multifasciculated nerves of man they would certainly do nothing to prevent the loss of large numbers of regenerating axons occasioned by their entry into the interfascicular epineurial tissue of the distal stump as well as into functionally unrelated foreign endoneurial tubes.

Despite this reservation, they will remain a valuable tool for continuing neurobiological research.

5. Central mechanisms

Frequent references have been made in this book to the continued improvement in function that occurs long after nerve regeneration has been completed. What is the explanation for this? Clearly, the improvement must be due to some central neural mechanisms which can be exploited by patient motivation and retraining programmes. There is increasing need for more detailed information on the processes involved, how they compensate for imperfect and incomplete axon regeneration, and the ways and means of modifying them in order to improve function and provide new skills. If they are to be exploited to the full in an effort to maximise recovery, much more must be learnt about them. The search for answers will be the last great frontier to cross and will take investigators well into the 21st century.

6. Nerve repair

a. End-to-end union

The search will continue for more effective ways of repairing nerves — effective in the sense of still further reducing the loss of regenerating axons that occurs at the site of the repair and of maximising the restoration of functionally useful connections with the periphery.

The de Medinaceli Reconnection Technique is the most recent to have been devised for this purpose (Chapter 42, p. 455). This method of repair comes closest to satisfying the principles that should govern nerve repair. However, its reputation to date is based solely on experimental studies in the rat. It is now time for it to be applied clinically where useful axon regeneration and functional recovery are far more complicated and demanding than in the experimental animal.

In the clinical situation the method can be subjected to the type of detailed and critical examination which is not possible in an experimental situation. In any event it should be noted that, like all other methods of nerve repair, the de Medinaceli method does nothing to overcome the problem of fascicular mismatching at the nerve ends or to prevent the escape and loss of regenerating axons into the interfascicular tissue of the distal stump as well as into functionally unrelated endoneurial tubes.

b. Nerve grafting

Nerve autografting inevitably involves sacrificing one or more cutaneous nerves. This disadvantage alone justifies the continued search for an acceptable substitute.

The present difficulty is that nerve autografts do confer special advantages on graft repair even if we are at a loss to explain why this should be so. What are the elements in an autograft that make it uniquely acceptable as a bridge to conduct regenerating axons across a gap in a nerve? Until there is an answer to this question, attempts to find an acceptable substitute will be stalled. To state that it is the property of 'self' begs the question.

Much work is currently in progress on the use of homografts as a substitute. For these to replace autografts they must give results that are consistently superior to, or at least as good as, those obtainable by using autografts. This has yet to be convincingly demonstrated. However, improved histocompatibility testing and advances in immunosuppressive therapy have narrowed the gap between the two. Importantly, if clinical trials undertaken to test the merits of homografting are to have any validity, the gaps to be closed should be considerably larger than those that currently appear to be the subject of investigation. This is because of the remarkable capacity of regenerating axons to cross, quite unaided, large gaps in nerves.

c. *Suture line problems*

This is where the greatest loss of axons occurs during regeneration. The principal offender in this respect is a sequela of tissue healing, namely scar tissue (Chapter 41). Suture line healing has a dual function: (1) to restore nerve trunk continuity and to impart tensile strength to the suture line, and (2) to provide a framework for the passage of regenerating axons across the interface between the nerve ends. This second function is most favourable when the collagen content is minimal and collagen fibres are openly arranged in parallel. However, when collagen is excessive and the collagen fibres are densely and irregularly packed, the scar then forms a serious barrier to the free and orderly passage of regenerating axons through it.

There is as yet no clear or complete picture of the factors influencing the activity of fibroblasts in the healing tissue. Excessive tension is known to have a deleterious effect though there is also the chance that slight tension could have a beneficial effect by promoting a parallel alignment of collagen fibres. Other factors are also clearly involved such as the fibrosis resulting from an inadequate blood supply to the region. More detailed information is required on these matters.

A question of more immediate interest is whether it is possible to reduce the amount of harmful scarring at the repair site by artificially controlling fibroblast activity at that site. Corollaries of such a proposition are: (i) finding an effective fibroblast–collagen inhibitor; (ii) getting the agent to the repair site in the appropriate concentrations; (iii) eliminating the risk of weakening the suture line to a point where postoperative suture line failure would be inevitable.

These are three formidable conditions and, to date, attempts to control the activity of fibroblasts and the deposition of collagen by artificial means have not been encouraging. The problem remains of being able to reduce collagen formation without jeopardising the integrity of the suture line.

The beneficial effect on suture line healing claimed for pulsed electromagnetic field therapy is disputed. In this respect it is worth noting that, in wound healing in general, these field effects involve an increase in fibroblast activity.

d. *Suture line tension*

Expressed in another way, the problem relates to the greatest gap between the nerve ends that can be safely closed by end-to-end union without prejudicing the end result.

All are agreed that one suture line is preferable to two. The question at issue is the point at which end-to-end union should be abandoned in favour of some alternative method of repair.

There is abundant evidence that at times good and acceptable results have followed the closure of quite large gaps by end-to-end union when the suture line must have been left under considerable tension. It is the high failure rate in this group of cases that is disturbing. How is the discrepancy to be accounted for where some results are good even though outnumbered by poor results? Obviously, factors other than tension are participating and this must surely introduce an element of uncertainty when evaluating the harmful effects attributed to tension.

The bald statement that any tension at the suture line is harmful is not, as yet, good enough. What is needed is more precise information on the role of tension in impairing regeneration and the point at which the harmful effects associated with it become significant. This problem should be studied in a clinical context and not left to animal experiment, where the results are often difficult to interpret and can be misleading.

e. *Obtaining correct axial alignment of the nerve ends during repair*

This is a crucial step in the repair of a nerve because any malalignment of the nerve ends can lead to the apposition of unrelated fasciculi and fibre systems, and the consequences of such an error can be serious. This is particularly the case when the error involves opposing motor to sensory and sensory to motor systems.

The clean transection injury presents no problems but, as increasing lengths of a nerve are destroyed, the chances of error in aligning the nerve ends are correspondingly increased.

Procedures currently available to assist in securing correct axial alignment at the suture site are discussed in Chapter 42. Each procedure has its limitations and defects. What is urgently needed is a method that will consistently guarantee the accuracy of alignment with the minimum of fuss.

7. The painful nerve lesion

a. It has not yet been possible to settle the vexed question of why some nerve lesions, and neuromas in particular, are painful and others are not, even in the same individual.

   The pathogenesis of painful nerve lesions has yet to be clarified, particularly the role of central mechanisms in sustaining the painful state.

b. Regardless of the method selected from the many available for the treatment of painful neuromas, the best results appear to carry a residual failure rate of at least 20 per cent. What is needed is a method that will consistently give good results at all times.

c. There is general agreement that the sympathetic nervous system is involved in the genesis of causalgia and other painful states such as reflex sympathetic dystrophy. The nature of that involvement continues to elude us.

8. Miscellaneous

a. The survival of denervated muscle

Presuming that a denervated muscle has been maintained in the best possible state by appropriate therapy, it is still not possible to put a limit on the time for which it will survive, and later respond satisfactorily when reinnervated. Until this information is available, it will not be possible to decide with any certainty when nerve repair would no longer serve a useful purpose.

b. The value of electrotherapy in the treatment of denervated muscle

Opinions on the value of electrotherapy continue to be divided and will remain so until a conclusive study can be instigated (Chapter 28). The costs of providing such treatment demand confirmation of its value.

c. The brachial plexus

Complicated, time-consuming and costly nerve repairs undertaken to restore function lost as the result of rupture avulsion injuries of the brachial plexus are becoming more common, thanks to an active and more adventurous approach to the surgical treatment of these injuries pioneered in particular by Japanese surgeons and by Narakas in Europe (Chapter 46).

When evaluating the end result of these procedures it is essential that all potential sources of error in making a correct judgement should be excluded before attributing the recovery to the surgical repair. To do this requires detailed and accurate information on cutaneous dermatomes and the motor root innervation of individual muscles along with related variations. The information currently available is incomplete and probably misleading, largely because the final destination of root fibres is concealed by plexus formations.

A critical study of the motor and sensory disturbances following localised lesions of the plexus could provide much needed information.

d. Sensory testing

The tests currently in use for evaluating sensory function should be critically examined with a view to discarding those that are irrelevant and promoting those that bear a closer relationship to the needs and practicalities of daily living.

EPILOGUE

Sufficient has been said in this chapter and elsewhere in this book to show that, despite the many remarkable advances in recent years, much remains to be done in an investigational way to clean up a residue of unsolved problems.

All that has been done here is to identify and highlight some of the major areas most urgently in need of attention. They are but an expression of the author's personal thoughts and, as such, are subject to limits set by one's personal knowledge and experience.

It is hoped that the observations recorded in these pages will prompt the reader to further thought, study and investigation.

Index